Upper Gastrointestinal Surgery

2nd Edition

Take a look at the other great titles in the *Companion Series...*

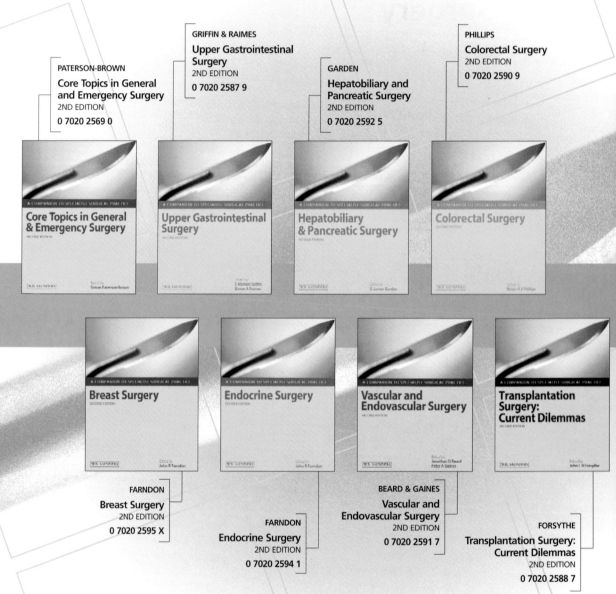

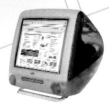
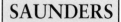

A Companion to Specialist Surgical Practice

Series editors

O. James Garden
Simon Paterson-Brown

Upper Gastrointestinal Surgery

2nd Edition

Edited by

S. Michael Griffin

Professor of Gastrointestinal Surgery and Consultant Surgeon
Northern Oesophago Gastric Unit
Royal Victoria Infirmary
Newcastle upon Tyne

Simon A. Raimes

Consultant Surgical Gastroenterologist
Department of General Surgery
Cumberland Infirmary
Carlisle

Saunders

London   Edinburgh   New York   Oxford   Philadelphia   St Louis   Sydney   Toronto 2001

SAUNDERS
An imprint of Harcourt Publishers Limited

First edition 1997
Reprinted 1999
Second edition 2001
Reprinted 2002
Reprinted 2003

ISBN 0 7020 2587 9

British Library Cataloguing in Publication Data
A catalogue record for this book is available from the British Library

Library of Congress Cataloging in Publication Data
A catalog record for this book is available from the Library of Congress

Note
Medical knowledge is constantly changing. As new information becomes available, changes in treatment, procedures, equipment and the use of drugs become necessary. The editors/authors/ contributors and the publishers have, as far as it is possible, taken care to ensure that the information given in this text is accurate and up to date. However, readers are strongly advised to confirm that the information, especially with regard to drug usage, complies with the latest legislation and standards of practice.

Existing UK nomenclature is changing to the system of Recommended International Non-proprietary Names (rINNs). Until the UK names are no longer in use, these more familiar names are used in this book in preference to rINNs, details of which may be obtained from the British National Formulary.

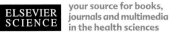 your source for books, journals and multimedia in the health sciences
www.elsevierhealth.com

Printed in China

Commissioning Editor: Miranda Bromage
Associate Editor: Paul Fam
Project Development Manager: Sheila Black
Project Manager: Joanne Scott
Design Direction: Jayne Jones

Contents

Contributors

Derek Alderson MD FRCS
Professor of Gastrointestinal Surgery
Division of Surgery
Bristol Royal Infirmary
Bristol, UK

William H. Allum BSc MD FRCS
Consultant Surgeon
Epsom General Hospital
Dorking Road
Epsom, Surrey, UK

John R. Anderson FRCS MB ChB
Consultant Surgeon
Dept General Surgery
Southern General Hospital NHS Trust
Glasgow, UK

C. Paul Barham MD FRCS (Gen.)
Consultant Surgeon
Department of Surgery
Bristol Royal Infirmary
Bristol, UK

Hugh Barr MD ChM FRCSE FRCS
Professor and Consultant Surgeon
Gloucestershire Royal Hospital
Gloucester, UK

John Baxter MD FRCS
Professor of Surgery
Morriston Hospital
Morriston
Swansea, UK

Mark Bennett FRC Path
Consultant Histopathologist
Department of Histopathology
The Newcastle upon Tyne Hospitals
NHS Trust
Newcastle upon Tyne, UK

Jane M. Blazeby BSc MD FRCS (Gen.)
MRC Clinial ScientistHonorary Consultant
Senior
Lecturer in Surgery
Division of Surgery
Bristol Royal Informary
Bristol, UK

Adrian Crellin FRCP FRCR
Consultant Clinical Oncologist
Leeds Cancer Centre
Cookridge Hospital
Leeds, UK

Petra Dildey MRCPath
Specialist Registrar in Histopathology
Department of Histopathology
The Newcastle upon Tyne Hospitals
NHS Trust
Newcastle upon Tyne, UK

Samuel M. Dresner FRCS
Northern Oesophago-Gastric
Cancer Unit
Royal Victoria Infirmary
Newcastle upon Tyne, UK

Jonathan I. Ferguson MA FRCS
Specialist Registrar Thoracic Surgery
Norfolk and Norwich Hospital
Norwich, UK

S. Michael Griffin MD FRCS FRCSE
Professor of Gastrointestinal Surgery and
Consultant Surgeon
Northern Oesophago Gastric Unit
Royal Victoria Infirmary
Newcastle upon Tyne, UK

Glyn G. Jamieson MS FRCS FACS FRACS
Dorothy Mortlock
Professor of Surgery
University of Adelaide
Department of Surgery
Royal Adelaide Hospital
Adelaide, South Australia

Simon Paterson-Brown MBBS MPhil MS FRCS(Ed)
FRCS(Engl) FRC(HK)
Consultant General and Upper Gastrointestinal Surgeon
Department of Clinical and Surgical Sciences (Surgery)
Royal Infirmary
Edinburgh, UK

Simon A. Raimes MD FRCS
Consultant Surgical Gastroenterologist
Department of General Surgery
Cumberland Infirmary
Carlisle, UK

Ian H. Shaw BSc PhD MB BChir FRCA
Consultant Anaesthetist
Department of Anaesthesia and Intensive Care
Newcastle General Hospital
Newcastle upon Tyne, UK

David Watson MD FRCS
Associate Professor of Surgery
Department of Surgery
University of Adelaide
Royal Adelaide Hospital
Adelaide, South Australia

John Wayman MD FRCS
Specialist Registrar in Surgery
Northern Oesophago Gastric Cancer Unit
Royal Victoria Infirmary
Newcastle upon Tyne, UK

Foreword

In their Preface to the first edition, the series editors expressed the hope that the series would meet the needs of the higher surgical trainee and busy practising surgeon, providing up-to-date information on recent developments and succinct coverage of key topics within each speciality area. The outstanding success of the first edition suggests that these ambitions have been fulfilled and that the product is indeed meeting demand and expectations. Throughout the initiative there has been great emphasis on rapid publication, with all of its attendant stresses and strains, so that the reader could be provided with the very latest information. The fact that the second edition is now emerging within three years of the first indicates that James Garden and Simon Paterson-Brown and their now established team of volume editors are determined to follow through and maintain the momentum of this excellent series.

Contributors have been hand-picked with great care. They are a widely respected and authoritative group of surgeons and supporting specialists who are at the very forefront of their respective fields. The second edition retains the attractive format of the first, is well illustrated and eminently readable. The needs of the general surgeon are balanced nicely with those of the true surgical sub-specialist, and there are significant additions to the range of topics covered. The series has been expanded from seven to eight volumes due to the separation of breast and endocrine surgery. There will be a widespread welcome for the emphasis on evidence-based practice and the highlighting of key references both within the text and the supporting bibliography. I am pleased to see that the authors have endeavoured to use references that are as up-to-date as possible, and readers will welcome their consistent emphasis on recent developments.

A Companion to Specialist Surgical Practice series has filled an important niche in surgical publishing and with the quality and industry of the team now established, it seems destined to continue to do so. I am proud to have been associated with the first edition of the series and feel privileged to have been asked to provide this introduction to its successor. I congratulate all those who have worked so hard to ensure the continued success of the series and wish it well over the years to come. I have no doubt that the second edition will be very well received and recommend it unreservedly.

Sir David Carter, MD, Hon DSc, Hon LLD, FRCS (Ed), FRCS (Eng), FRCS (Glas), Hon FRCS (Ire), Hon FACS, Hon FRACS, FAMedSci, FRSE
Vice Principal, University of Edinburgh, Formerly Chief Medical Officer in Scotland and Regius Professor of Clinical Surgery, Royal Infirmary, Edinburgh, UK

Preface

The Companion to Specialist Surgical Practice series has been designed to meet the needs of the higher surgeon in training and busy practising consultant surgeon who require access to up-to-date information on recent developments in relation to their sub-specialty surgical practice. Many major surgery texts cover the whole of 'general surgery' and may contain information which is not of specific interest to the specialist surgeon. Similarly specialist texts may be outwith the reach of the trainee's finances and, though comprehensive, may fall out-of-date during production or as a consequence of rapid new developments in practice. As for the successful 1st edition, this edition has also been written and produced in a very short time frame, so that the contents are as up-to-date as possible.

Each volume in the *Companion to Specialist Surgical Practice* series provides succinct summaries of all key topics within a specialty and concentrates on the most recent developments and current data. A specialist surgeon, whether in training or in practice, need only refer to the volume relevant to his or her chosen specialist field in addition to the *Core Topics in General and Emergency Surgery*.

We are grateful to our series editors for their perseverance and for their outstanding response to our repeated promptings over the last year. We would like to thank Rachel Stock and Linda Clark from WB Saunders, for their help in getting this project safely launched in the past and would give special thanks to Sue Hodgson, Sheila Black, Paul Fam and Miranda Bromage for piloting this series to its second edition. We appreciate very much the guidance and assistance of Sir David Carter as a series editor in the 1st series and for writing the foreword to this second series.

We hope that our aim − of providing affordable up-to-date specialist surgical texts − has been met and that all surgeons, in training or in practice, will find the 2nd edition of this series to be a valuable resource.

O. James Garden BSc, MD, FRCS(Glasg), FRCS(Ed)
Regius Professor of Clinical Surgery, Department of Clinical and Surgical Sciences (Surgery), Royal Infirmary, Edinburgh

Simon Paterson-Brown MBBS, MPhil, MS, FRCS(Ed), FRCS(Engl), FCS(HK)
Consultant General and Upper Gastrointestinal Surgeon, Department of Clinical and Surgical Sciences (Surgery), Royal Infirmary, Edinburgh

S. Michael Griffin MD, FRCS, FRCSE
Professor of Gastrointestinal Surgery and Consultant Surgeon, Northern Oesophago Gastric Unit, Royal Victoria Infirmary, Newcastle upon Tyne

Simon A. Raimes MD, FRCS
Consultant Surgical Gastroenterologist, Department of General Surgery, Cumberland Infirmary, Carlisle

Evidence-based Practice in Surgery

The second edition of the *Companion to Specialist Surgical Practice* series has attempted to incorporate, where appropriate, **evidence-based practice in surgery**, which has been highlighted in the text and relevant references. A detailed chapter on evidence based practice in surgery written by Jonathan Michaels and Kathryn Rigby has been included in the volume on *Core Topics in General and Emergency Surgery* to which the reader is referred for further information on assessing levels of evidence. We are grateful to them for providing this summary for each volume.

Critical appraisal for developing evidence-based practice can be obtained from a number of sources; the most reliable being randomised controlled clinical trials, systematic literature reviews, meta-analysis and observational studies. For practical purposes three grades of evidence can be used, analogous to the levels of 'proof' required in a court of law:

1) **Beyond reasonable doubt** – such evidence is likely to have arisen from high-quality randomised controlled trials, systematic reviews, or high-quality synthesised evidence such as decision analysis, cost effectiveness analysis or large observational data sets. The studies need to be directly applicable to the population of concern and have clear results. The grade is analogous to burden of proof within a criminal court and may be thought of as corresponding to the usual standard of 'proof' within the medical literature (i.e. $p < 0.05$).

2) **On the balance of probabilities** – in many cases a high-quality review of literature may fail to reach firm conclusions due to conflicting or inconclusive results, trials of poor methodological quality, or the lack of evidence in the population to which the guidelines apply. In such cases it may still be possible to make a statement as to the best treatment on the 'balance of probabilities'. This is analogous to the decision in a civil court where all the available evidence will be weighed up and the verdict will depend upon the balance of probabilities.

3) **Not proven** – insufficient evidence upon which to base a decision or contradictory evidence.

Depending on the information available three grades of recommendation can be used:

a) strong recommendation, which should be followed unless there are compelling reasons to act otherwise.

b) a recommendation based on evidence of effectiveness, but where there may be other factors to take into account in decision-making, for example the user of the guidelines may be expected to take into account patient preferences, local facilities, local audit results or available resources.

c) a recommendation made where there is no adequate evidence as to the most effective practice, although there may be reasons for making a recommendation in order to minimise cost or reduce the chance of error through a locally agreed protocol.

 Having highlighted the text and references which are considered to be associated with reasonable evidence in this volume with a 'scalpel code', the reader can then reach his or her own conclusion.

Dedication

I wish to thank my wife, Alison and children Kathleen, Jeannie and Robbie for enduring even more prolonged absences from my fatherly duties.

S. Michael Griffin

To Theresa and our children.

Simon A. Raimes

1 Pathology of benign, malignant and premalignant oesophageal and gastric tumours

Petra Dildey
Mark K. Bennett

INTRODUCTION

Malignant tumours of the upper gastrointestinal tract appear as irregular mucosal ulcers, polypoid masses or diffuse thickenings. Most arise from the endoderm and so are classified as carcinomas. Dysplasia is regarded as the tumour precursor and is defined in terms of cytological (individual cell) and as architectural (gland or mucosal) atypia. Other mucosal changes, which predispose to the development of dysplasia, may be present. Investigations of the genetic/molecular changes in the mucosa confirm the stepwise progression from normal to dysplasia and cancer.

Squamous carcinoma is the commonest tumour of the oesophagus, accounting for a death rate of 221 per million per annum in the UK. Although the incidence is falling, carcinoma of the oesophagus is the 5th and 7th most common cause of death in men and women respectively. Other tumours are thought to arise from basal cells or from the submucosal glands. Carcinoma *in situ* is full thickness atypia and is regarded as an irreversible change. Lesser degrees of dysplasia are more difficult to define and sometimes confused with regenerative changes. The metaplasia of squamous epithelium to a glandular mucosa (Barrett's oesophagus) occurs as a result of reflux of gastric and duodenal contents. The premalignant potential and the malignant transformation to adenocarcinoma are being actively investigated.

Gastric adenocarcinoma is the commonest tumour of the stomach and is derived from the lining mucosa. In the UK gastric carcinoma presents late in its natural history; it is the sixth most common cancer and causes 230 deaths per million per annum.[1] Throughout the Western world the incidence has been falling for several decades, which may in part be accounted for by a reduction in the intestinal type of tumour. Most tumours are sporadic, though there are some familial cases (associated with hereditary non-polyposis colorectal cancer or HNPCC). Environmental factors are more important than genetic influences (such as blood group A or a family history) in the development of carcinoma. No linkage studies have been possible, as large kindred have rarely been reported. There are significant difficulties in the interpretation of dysplasia and intramucosal cancer.[2] One of the most important changes is the recognition of early gastric cancer, with its better patient survival. In countries with a low incidence of gastric cancer such as the UK the proportion of early tumours still remains disappointingly low (10–20%).[3]

Epithelial tumours of the oesophagus

Squamous carcinoma

The aetiology of these tumours is unknown though there is a strong association between squamous cancer, alcohol intake and smoking in different parts of the world. Up to 80% of the male cases in USA, Latin America and Japan have a history of either one or the other factor while in Iran and China these are not considered to be major causative agents.[4] Potential carcinogens (N-nitrosamines), which may be of environmental origin, have been found in areas where there is a high incidence of tumours. Similarly diets lacking fresh fruit and vegetables and with an increased consumption of pickled foods are also found in these areas. This may reflect deficiencies in vitamins A, C and riboflavin and trace elements (zinc, molybdenum and selenium). There is evidence to suggest the human papilloma virus (HPV 16 and 18) may be important in some tumours.

Several predisposing factors have been reported (**Table 1.1**). Achalasia has a reported risk of cancer development of up to 33 times that of the normal population with an incidence of 88 per 100 000 population.[5] The progression from a benign fibrous stricture as a result of chemically induced damage (e.g. Lye ingestion),[6] to tumour has reported to occur in between 0.8 to 7.2% with a latent period of up to 40 years. Tylosis, a rare autosomal dominant condition of abnormal keratinisation affecting the palms and soles of the feet, has been associated with oesophageal cancer.[7] Post-cricoid dysphagia with hypochromatic (iron deficiency) anaemia associated with mucosal webs is known as Plummer Vinson or Patterson Brown Kelly syndromes. The webs consist of thin mucosal folds with some epithelial changes extending into the oral mucosa. This consists of epithelial atrophy or hyperkeratinisation and could account for the high incidence (up to 16%) of these patients having aerodigestive cancers.[8] The pharyngo-oesophageal (Zenker's) diverticulum found at the border of the cricopharyngeus and the inferior constrictor muscles has a reported incidence of cancer between 0.3 and 0.8%.[9] The tumours tend to be at the apex of the diverticulum and by the time of diagnosis are usually in an advanced stage with extension through the wall. Barrett's oesophagus can occasionally be associated

---

Achalasia

Chemical strictures

Tylosis

Plummer Vinson or Patterson Kelly syndrome

Oesophageal diverticulae

Barrett's oesophagus

Irradiation treatment

Table 1.1 *Predisposing factors for oesophageal carcinoma*

with a squamous carcinoma, though an adenocarcinoma is more usual.[10] There is a slightly increased incidence of squamous cancer in patients with coeliac disease though more frequently this condition has been complicated by small bowel lymphoma.[11] The least frequent possible aetiology is that of irradiation treatment, 13 cases have so far been reported.[12]

The tumours are found in the upper, middle and lower thirds in ratios of approximately 1:5:2 respectively. They appear as fungating, ulcerating or infiltrating masses though occasional verrucous (polypoid) or multifocal tumours are seen. Ulcerating lesions (**Fig. 1.1**) have raised rolled edges with necrotic centres while the stenosing variety show a diffuse full circumferential infiltrating mass, often with a grey-white fibrous cut surface. The endoscopic appearances of early tumours which may be better appreciated by use of the vital stains (toluidine blue or iodine) have been reported as showing a mosaic or hypervascular pattern or remain occult.[13] The pathological findings of these early tumours are similar to the advanced stages with erosions, plaques or polypoid masses within the lumen.[14] The macroscopic appearances change with chemoradiation as a result of tumour shrinkage and scarring.

Tumour infiltration and spread will depend on the site of the primary.[15] Approximately three-quarters of the tumours at presentation will extend through the submucosa and deep muscle layers into adventitial tissue. Lymph-node involvement increases with the depth of invasion; there is a 10-fold increase in lymph metastases in submucosal tumours in comparison with those that are intramucosal. Because of the complexity of the mucosal lymphatic system approximately 40% of the upper third tumours will spread to the abdominal nodes while similar numbers from the lower third will metastasise to the cervical lymph nodes. Metastatic tumour to visceral organs is a reflection of venous invasion,[16] most frequently to lung and liver and has been demonstrated in 40 to 75%. There is an increase in second tumours within the aero-digestive tract as

Figure 1.1
Oesophageal carcinoma with a central ulceration and an irregular margin. To one side there is a smaller nodule that represents intramucosal spread.

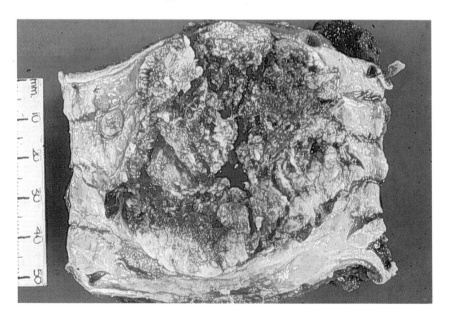

Figure 1.2
Squamous carcinoma of the oesophagus that is formed from lobulated islands of prickle cells

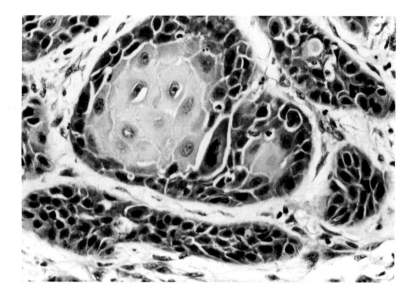

well as head and neck region and in some this may be related to a family history or to the use of tobacco and alcohol. Depending on the degree of keratinisation, keratin whorl formation and the cytological atypia present, the histological appearances can be described as well, moderate or poorly differentiated (**Fig. 1.2**). Two variants of the squamous carcinoma are seen:

1. *Verrucous carcinoma* is similar to that found at other sites such as the head and neck. It has a predominantly exophytic papillary appearance which forms an intraluminal fungating mass. Difficulties in histopathological interpretation of this tumour occur when superficial biopsies have been taken. The main differential diagnoses of this indolent malignant tumour are pseudo-epitheliomatous hyperplasia, which is a benign reactive change and the squamous papilloma which is very uncommon in humans.

2. *Carcinosarcoma* (also known as sarcomatoid carcinoma and spindle cell carcinoma),[17] which appears as an exophytic mass composed of a mixture of both squamous and spindle cells. The histogenesis of the spindle cells is unclear as electron microscopy and immunocytochemistry suggest an origin from either squamous or mesodermal cells. Although the microscopic features are worrying, the tumour behaves in a less aggressive manner than the pure squamous carcinoma.

Molecular aspects

The multistep progression from normal mucosa to cancer shows that in up to half the cases of squamous carcinoma, the p53 gene has been found to be abnormal. p53 is found on the short arm of chromosome 17 and normally acts as a brake on DNA replication and as a trigger for apoptosis (programmed cell death). As p53 expression is found in normal and dysplastic epithelium, it has been suggested that abnormalities occur early in the pathway leading to malignancy. Several defects are found, the most frequent being mutations of A:T base pairs, with a high prevalence of G to T transversions and or loss of heterozygosity. Similar mutations are found in adenocarcinoma of the oesophagus.[18] The mutations allow abnormal cell growth and are associated with further damage to the genome, especially to the important tumour suppressor genes. This includes deletions or loss of heterozygosity (LOH) of the retinoblastoma (Rb, 48%), mutations in colorectal carcinoma (MCC, 63%), adenomatous polyposis coli (APC, 67%) and deletions in colorectal cancer (DCC, 24%) genes. In nearly all cases one of these defective tumour suppressor genes is present, while nearly three-quarters of the squamous carcinomas have two abnormalities.

Continued cell growth will occur as a result of amplification and over expression of growth factors and oncogenes. One of the most important is the protein kinase, epidermal growth factor receptor (EGFr), which shows amplification in 40–70% of squamous carcinomas. The ligands for EGFr, EGF and TGFα act on the receptor in an autocrine manner, further increasing the cellular proliferation. In addition to this important effect, EGF has at least one other effect on the tumour by phosphorylation of beta-catenin.[19] This reduces the cellular adhesion and may account for more aggressive tumour behaviour. The ras oncogene family, unlike other gastrointestinal tract cancers, appears not to have an important role in the genesis of squamous carcinoma.

Precancerous conditions: dysplasia

Dysplasia and carcinoma *in situ* are regarded as precancerous conditions of the oesophagus and the atypia is similar to that found in other squamous epithelia such as the cervix or bronchial epithelium. There is irregular maturation of the keratinocytes with abnormally situated mitotic figures accompanied by nuclear enlargement and variation in size. If there is evidence that the squamous cells show some abnormality of maturation this is regarded as dysplasia, while a full thickness abnormality is classified as carcinoma *in situ*. The suggestion that these two conditions are premalignant has come from the finding of dysplasia in up to 8% of the population in high-risk areas and the abnormalities of DNA within the mucosa.[20]

The finding of dysplasia is sufficiently worrying for surveillance to be contemplated as the risk of developing carcinoma is increased.[21] In screened high-risk populations the finding of dysplasia predates the development of carcinoma by approximately 5 years.

Carcinoma *in situ* can also be found at a distance from the primary tumour in up to 14% of resections. This is associated with the development of the secondary oesophageal malignancy or other tumours in the aero-digestive tract. The precursor lesion for development of dysplasia is not well identified although in areas of high risk there is an increased incidence of moderate to severe chronic oesophagitis suggesting luminal damage may be in part responsible for this preneoplastic change.

Adenocarcinoma of the oesophagus

A significant rise in the incidence of adenocarcinoma of the oesophagus and gastric cardia has been reported. The tumours of the oesophago-gastric junction share common epidemiological features: having a significant male predominance they are more frequently associated with hiatus hernia, reflux and peptic strictures. Although smoking and alcohol are common factors they are less constant features than with squamous carcinoma. To improve the epidemiological and demographic understanding, the following classification of these tumours has been suggested.[22,23]

Type I	Adenocarcinoma of the distal oesophagus that usually arises from an area of specialised intestinal metaplasia of the oesophagus (Barrett's oesophagus) and which may infiltrate the oesophago-gastric junction from above.
Type II	True carcinoma of the cardia arising from the cardiac epithelium or short segments with intestinal metaplasia at the oesophago-gastric junction; this entity is also referred to as 'junctional carcinoma'.
Type III	Subcardial gastric carcinoma, which infiltrates the oesophago-gastric junction and distal oesophagus from below.

Adenocarcinoma in Barrett's oesophagus (Type I tumour)

First described in 1950[24] Barrett's oesophagus is defined as the replacement of the squamous epithelium by a columnar-lined mucosa in the lower oesophagus (**Fig. 1.3**). Initially this was restricted to a 3 cm length but with time there has been recognition that short segment (i.e. less than 3 cm) metaplastic change occurs. The metaplastic change develops as a consequence of chronic oesophago-gastric reflux with the replacement of the squamous epithelium by the characteristic intestinal type mucosa.[25] The differential diagnosis includes ciliated cell rests, tracheobronchial remnants and ectopic gastric mucosa. Further details of Barrett's oesophagus can be found in Chapter 11.

The incidence of malignancy in cases of Barrett's has been estimated to vary between 1 in 80 and 1 in 440 cases. From these figures it has been suggested that the risk of developing an adenocarcinoma is between 30 and 40 times that of the general population. This suggests that patients with Barrett's oesophagus may benefit from a screening programme, although the risk is questioned by others.[26,27] In particular, the area of involvement by the metaplasia and its duration appear

Figure 1.3
Barrett's oesophagus in which the squamous epithelium is displaced uniformly away from the oesophago-gastric junction and the mucosa takes on the macroscopic appearances of that of the gastric mucosa.

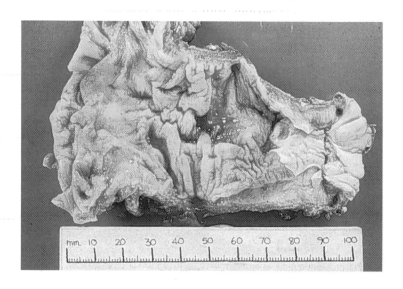

Figure 1.4
Barrett's oesophagus with an adenocarcinoma showing an irregular ulcerating tumour, which is encroaching upon the metaplastic mucosa. The residual squamous epithelium has been left as grey-white mucosal islands separated by the bands of metaplastic mucosa.

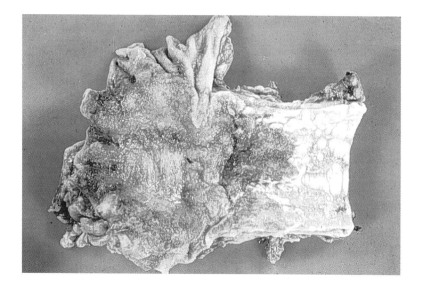

insufficient to identify those patients at risk of developing malignancy.[28] The majority of the tumours are found in the lower third, though up to one-fifth are found in the middle third. Most appear as exophytic masses, ulcers (**Fig. 1.4**) or endophytic irregular masses. At presentation most are found to be at a late stage with infiltration past the deep muscle layer in 70% of cases and lymphnode metastases in up to three-quarters. Histologically the majority of these tumours show features similar to the intestinal type of gastric carcinoma.

Adenocarcinoma of the oesophago-gastric junction (Type II tumour)

These tumours form a distinct group from the more common subcardial tumours, occurring in slightly younger patients with a male predominance. As with type I tumours, symptoms related to hiatus hernia and reflux are common as is a history of smoking and drinking alcohol. These tumours show an aggressive behaviour with a worse prognosis than cancers in the rest of the stomach. There are several factors which might explain this including large size (> 5 cm) at presentation, early submucosal invasion, extension into the oesophagus and, because of their large size, the more frequent involvement of the serosa and lymphnode metastases. Unlike the more distal tumours they are not associated with atrophic gastritis or intestinal metaplasia, suggesting that demographic and pathological features of these tumours are similar to the adenocarcinoma found in Barrett's oesophagus. The histological features of these tumours are similar to the other gastric adenocarcinomas. Multivariate analysis has shown that the staging of tumours is the most significant prognostic variable[26] together with lymphnode metastases. The majority of the nodal involvement is intra-abdominal though metastatic spread to thoracic nodes was found in 7% of cases. Up to 80% of the tumours are aneuploid and have a shortened survival when compared with diploid tumours (10.6 versus 20.4 months). A few studies have looked at the oncogenes and growth factors in adenocarcinoma; EGFR is amplified and there is over expression of TGFα, h-ras and erb-B2. These factors are expressed in greater amounts with progression from normality to malignancy.

Other oesophageal tumours

In addition to the squamous and adenocarcinoma of the oesophagus there are several other uncommon tumours to be considered in the differential diagnosis. Very uncommon tumours such as melanoma, choriocarcinoma, Paget's disease, squamous papilloma, cysts and also metastatic tumours to the oesophagus are not included in this discussion.

Granular cell tumours are found in the skin, mouth and throughout the gastrointestinal tract but most frequently in the oesophagus. They present with dysphagia or pain, the clinical symptoms possibly related to the size of the lesion (up to 4 cm in diameter). Nearly two-thirds of these tumours have been found in the lower third of the oesophagus and arise from the submucosa. The covering squamous epithelium is often thickened and the characteristic tumour cells fill the subjacent stroma. These are uniform plump cells with granular cytoplasm and stain with PAS and S-100 protein. These benign tumours are thought to be derived from Schwann cells.

Basaloid carcinoma (also known as adenoid cystic carcinoma and cylindroma) is an uncommon tumour usually found in males of over 60 years. Most have been reported in small series and are thought to represent between 0.75% and 5% of oesophageal cancers. They are thought to arise from the ducts or acini of submucosal glands and present as ulcerating, infiltrating or fungating masses in the distal oesophagus. Microscopically they are similar to those found in the salivary gland and composed of islands of basophilic cells with thickening of the basement membrane and microcystic structures. Most tumours show minor degrees of squamous differentiation and so are regarded as variants of squamous carcinoma. Similar neoplasms are reported in the trachea, breast, skin and cervix. They have a variable survival, though most of the patients with oesophageal tumours die within 2 years. In a recent report the prognosis is similar to the squamous carcinoma.[29]

Mucoepidermoid carcinoma is an uncommon aggressive tumour found in males in the 7th decade. As the name implies, the tumour is composed of a mixture of glandular tissue which forms cystic spaces and squamous elements.[30] They are most likely to have arisen from the submucosal glands (analogous to salivary gland tumours) and are found most frequently in the middle and lower third. There is extensive invasion with lymph-node metastases and a prognosis equivalent to the squamous carcinoma.[31]

Small cell carcinoma is a similarly infrequent tumour representing 0.05% to 7.6% of all oesophageal cancers; approximately half of reported cases have come from Japan.[32] They present in the lower and middle third and are more usually found in males in the 5th to 6th decade. As with the equivalent lung lesion, ectopic hormone secretion (ACTH, calcitonin, somatostatin or gastrin) has been reported. Macroscopically they appear as exophytic or ulcerative growths measuring on average 6 cm at presentation. Histologically these may appear as homogeneous tumours (**Fig. 1.5**) or as a mixture of squamous or mucoepidermoid elements. As a result of this heterogeneity it is unclear whether they arise from totipotential reserve cells at the base of the squamous epithelium or from oesophageal/tracheobronchial mucosa in the embryonic foregut. The possibility of metastatic or direct spread from the lung should also be considered. The prognosis is poor with fewer than 14% of patients surviving 2 years.

Figure 1.5
Oat cell carcinoma of the oesophagus that is composed of sheets of undifferentiated cells with little cytoplasm showing streaming of the cells within the tumour. The appearances are similar to the more common bronchial oat cell from which they must be differentiated.

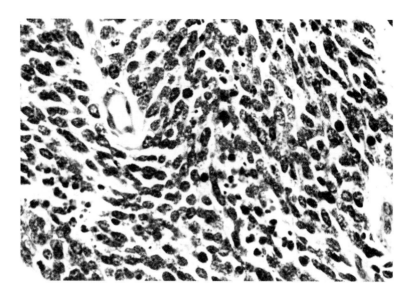

Epithelial tumours of the stomach

Precursors of gastric carcinoma

The pathogenesis of gastric carcinoma is complex and multifactorial with several potential precursor lesions (**Table 1.2**). Correa proposed a pathway from normal mucosa to cancer[33] and this is discussed in detail in Chapter 2.

Chronic atrophic gastritis and intestinal metaplasia

Chronic atrophic gastritis (**Fig. 1.6**) and intestinal metaplasia are a consequence of continuing inflammatory damage to the mucosa. They can result from a bacterial infection (*H. pylori*), chemical irritants or as a consequence of an auto-immune process (pernicious anaemia). *H. pylori* survive within gastric mucus (**Fig. 1.7**), inducing damage by several mechanisms, which include the production of urease and ammonia, acetaldehyde, a vacuolating toxin and mucolytic factors. *H. pylori* has a strong chemotactic effect for polymorphs and other

---

Chronic gastritis

Intestinal metaplasia of gastric mucosa

Gastric polyps

Gastric remnants (post-gastrectomy state)

Ménétrier's disease

Chronic peptic ulcer

Gastric epithelial dysplasia

Table 1.2 *Precursors of gastric carcinoma*

Figure 1.6
The pyloric mucosa showing a quiescent atrophic gastritis with complete intestinal metaplasia. This has an irregular surface with elongation of the pits in which there are goblet cells. The normal serous glands are not present while in the lamina propria there is a mild mononuclear cell inflammatory infiltrate.

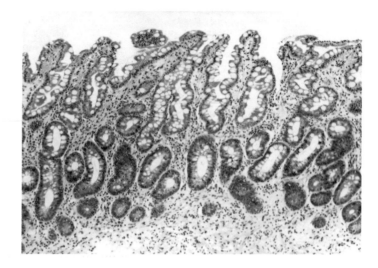

Figure 1.7
Helicobacter pylori. The bacteria are found at the surface and in the mucus of the pits; in this silver stain they appear as black rods often curved at the apex of the cell.

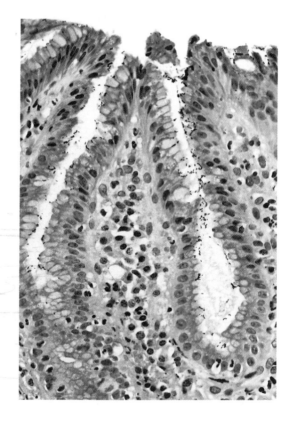

inflammatory cells, which can produce reactive oxygen metabolites. These cause cellular damage and result in an acute then chronic gastritis. Accumulation of lymphocytes results in lymphoid follicle formation and this, together with the continuing cellular damage, lead to an atrophic gastritis. Eradication of *H. pylori* reduces the inflammatory reaction and halts the development of intestinal metaplasia. Recently *H. pylori* has been linked with gastric carcinogenesis.[34,35,36,37]

There are several epidemiological studies showing a greater incidence of previous infection with *H. pylori* in gastric cancer patients than in controls. At present there is no direct evidence linking *H. pylori* to the later phases of carcinogenesis. In particular the bacterium avoids areas of intestinal metaplasia, which is a common associated feature of gastric cancer. In the past environmental factors such as a high dietary intake of salt, dried or pickled food were thought to enhance the development of the gastritis. The changes of an atrophic gastritis are a thinning of the mucosa, with loss of the specialised glands in the deeper portion and a compensatory increase in turnover of cells in the proliferative zone.[38] The incidence of atrophic gastritis increases with age, being present in up to 40% of patients older than 60 years and who are otherwise normal, indicating that further changes are required before malignant transformation can occur.

In addition to the inflammatory damage, the cells of the pits may undergo metaplasia towards intestinal epithelium.[39,40] This is seen as a change from the production of neutral to acid mucins, a change in function from a secretory to an absorptive cell type and the production of Paneth cells (which are usually found in the small bowel). The initial production of acid sialomucins is referred to as *complete intestinal metaplasia (type II)* and is found in association with Paneth cells and absorptive cells. With continuing damage, the pit cells change their morphology and produce an acid sulpha mucin. This is more characteristic of colonic mucosa, and is accompanied by the loss of the Paneth cells, this appearance being known as *incomplete intestinal metaplasia (type III)* (Fig. 1.8).

Figure 1.8
Intestinal metaplasia (type III). The superficial pits show both large solitary and multiple smaller secretory vacuoles within the apical portions of the cells. (Stained with alcian blue and PAS.)

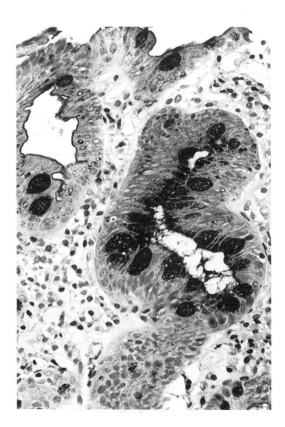

There is continuing controversy as to the value of identifying this colonic-type mucin and its predictive value in identifying patients at risk of developing cancer.[41]

There is a significant difference in the expression of the sulpha mucins between the intestinal and diffuse type of carcinomas (80% and 20% respectively), which has suggested differences in the underlying aetiology. It should be noted that intestinal metaplasia increases in prevalence and extent with age and is not infrequently associated with non-malignant disease, for example benign peptic ulceration. In these situations as well as those associated with the cancers, there are abnormalities of the mucin genes and cell kinetics.[42,43]

Although it is possible to reverse the inflammatory changes, atrophy and more especially the colonic-type intestinal metaplasia are regarded as irreversible. The mechanism by which damage to the nuclear DNA occurs is unclear, though several potential means are recognised. With the loss of the fundic glands, hypochlorhydria is found. In this changed environment there exists the possibility for nitrosating bacteria to proliferate.[44,45,46] These bacteria are able to convert nitrates to nitrites, as well as creating N-nitroso compounds by catalysing reactions between amines and amides and the nitrites. Ascorbic acid, the reduced form of vitamin C, appears to protect against neoplasia, possibly by scavenging both nitrites and reactive oxygen metabolites. H. pylori block the secretion of ascorbic acid and hence would allow any carcinogen to exert an effect on the mucosa. A further potential mutagenic pathway is the production of potent N-nitrosating agents from nitric oxide by H. pylori. Both of these have been shown to cause mutations in p53 with its secondary effects on uncontrolled cell proliferation. The hyperproliferative state found in atrophic gastritis would perpetuate any damage to the genome. This could result in genomic instability[47] and together would initiate the steps required to convert the atrophic to a dysplastic mucosa.

Gastric mucosal polyps

Gastric polyps are found with increasing incidence with age, in some series they are present in up to 7% of patients over 80 years. The classification is important as it indicates whether or not they are premalignant or are just incidental and sometimes associated with tumours.[48,49] Gastric mucosal polyps fall into three main groups; the hyperplastic polyps, fundic gland polyps and neoplastic polyps or adenomas.

Hyperplastic polyps are the most frequently found, usually with an equal sex distribution and occurring in later life usually in the 7th decade. They represent between 80 and 85% of all gastric polyps, are found more often in the antrum than in the corpus, are often multiple and usually less than 1 cm in diameter. Histologically they are composed of disorganised and hyperplastic glandular elements which are lined by regular epithelium and have an adjacent chronic gastritis. The risk of malignant transformation overall is approximately 0.5% and with rare exceptions this occurred in those polyps greater than 2 cm in diameter.[50] The risk of detecting coexistent cancer in prospective studies varied from 4.5–13.5%.

Fundic gland polyps are present in up to 3% of endoscopies and form multiple sessile lesions confined to the body of the stomach. Originally described in association with familial adenomatous polyposis.[51] they are now found sporadically more frequently. They show alteration in mucin synthesis, increase in proliferation and expression of the sialyl-Tn epitope. There is no evidence that there is an increased risk of gastric cancer and they are regarded as hyperproliferative hamartomatous lesions.

Neoplastic polyps are also referred to as adenomas and histologically have a tubular configuration. They occur predominantly in the antrum, with no sex preference and more frequently in the elderly. They have been found in up to 0.23% of endoscopic studies, most are smaller than 2 cm. They are often associated with atrophic gastritis and intestinal metaplasia. Histologically the polypoid epithelium shows dysplastic features with hyperchromasia, irregularity of maturation and abnormally situated mitoses, there is no evidence to suggest infiltration through the basement membrane. The risk of malignant transformation has been reported to occur in up to 40% of those adenomas greater than 2 cm. Although often found in isolation, coexistent cancers have been found in 3–25% though the malignant change is generally reported in the range 5–10%.[52]

Gastroduodenal polyps are found with familial adenomatous polyposis (FAP), and are mainly fundic gland or hyperplastic types. These are often multiple and occur at an earlier age than the sporadic cases. Adenomas have been reported (between 35–100% of cases), they are less frequent in the stomach than duodenum and occur at a younger age (mean 37 years) than the sporadic adenoma. The lesions are usually small and multiple; with time they increase in number and exhibit frequent malignant transformation.[53] Except in Japan the risk of gastric carcinoma is not increased in patients when compared with controls though the relative risk of duodenal and periampullary carcinoma is markedly increased.

Flat adenomas similar to those found in the colon are another form of tubular adenoma with variable degrees of dysplasia.[54] Macroscopically, they appear as irregular impressions being mistaken for a healing ulcer or depressed type of early gastric cancer. They occur in the distal two-thirds of the stomach, having similar demographic features to the more common polypoid adenomas. A larger percentage of the adenomas are described as having high-grade dysplasia though the prevalence is unknown. In the Japanese literature, these lesions may represent up to 10% of all neoplastic polyps.

Gastric remnant

Following distal gastrectomy with gastroenteric anastomosis there has been a high incidence of carcinoma reported (2%) in the gastric remnant. There has been a wide variation in the reported incidence most likely related to the time factor. Those who are at most risk have been identified as patients who have undergone surgery before the age of 40 and who have had a post-surgery interval of between 15 and 20 years.[55] The type of gastrectomy and the nature of the preoperative disease are not factors. The risk of cancer is increased in countries with a high intrinsic rate of gastric cancer and is approximately twice that of the control population. There are a variety of benign histological changes associated with gastric remnants; these include a chronic gastritis and atrophy, fundic gland polyps, xanthomas, hyperplasia of the surface/foveolar epithelium and hyperplastic polyps with gastritis cystica profunda.

Cancers are termed 'stump cancers' and the majority are found at or close to the stoma site, rarely extend into the intestinal side of the anastomosis and show equal proportions of intestinal and diffuse histological type. Nearly 40% of cases have been restricted to the submucosa, in other words an early gastric cancer. It has been suggested that selective surveillance should be considered for those patients who are symptomatic, who underwent surgery at a young age, those who are 20 years or more after surgery and for those who have high-grade dysplasia on endoscopy. In addition, cases of lymphoma of the stomach are now being described in the gastric stump.[56] A variety of non-gastric malignancies have been identified in follow-up series, and these have been predominantly lung, pancreatic ductal and colorectal cancers.

Ménétrier's disease (hypertrophic gastropathy)

This is a rare cause of rugal hypertrophy characterised by hyperplasia of the surface cells, hypochlorhydria and a protein-losing enteropathy. A review of the cases shows that approximately 10% are associated with cancer, diagnosed either simultaneously or within 12 months. However follow-up in a total of 16 cases shows the risk of malignancy to be low or negligible.[57] A few cases however have been associated with gastric dysplasia.

Chronic peptic ulcer disease

Chronic gastric ulcers were previously considered to be precancerous, but this is no longer supported by evidence as less than 1% of ulcers undergo malignant transformation.[58] The epidemiological evidence would suggest that ulcers do not have a significant role in gastric carcinogenesis. The natural history of early gastric carcinoma may explain why there was an initial over-reporting of the malignant change, since these tumours undergo episodes of mucosal ulceration followed by repair, some of which may be related to active medical therapy. It is essential, therefore, to ensure that any mucosal ulcer is adequately sampled before making a diagnosis of a benign ulcer.

Gastric epithelial dysplasia

Dysplasia may occur in an epithelium, which shows intestinal metaplasia and may be flat, depressed or polypoid.[59] It has been previously classified in three grades, mild, moderate or severe.

There are several problems associated with histological interpretation that include inter-observational variation, distinguishing regenerative atypia from true dysplasia, the ability to differentiate high-grade dysplasia from intramucosal carcinoma and a lack of experience due to the rarity of dysplasia (especially in low incidence areas). This may be overcome with the recently published Padova classification of gastric dysplasia; see Table 1.3.[60]

The natural history of dysplasia is not relentless progression to cancer, as regression to normal mucosa occurs in mild and moderate dysplasia in 60 and 70% of cases respectively. Severe dysplasia can also regress but this is less common; the majority of the patients progress to carcinoma (50–80%).[61] From retrospective studies high-grade dysplasia is closely associated with gastric carcinoma in the adjacent mucosa.

1. Negative for dysplasia (reactive)
    1.0 Normal
    1.1 Reactive foveolar hyperplasia
    1.2 Intestinal metaplasia (IM)
        1.2.1 IM complete type
        1.2.2 IM incomplete type

2. Indefinite for dysplasia
    2.1 Foveolar hyperproliferation
    2.2 Hyperproliferation IM

3. Non-invasive neoplasia (flat or elevated [synonym adenoma])
    3.1 Low-grade
    3.2 High-grade
        3.2.1 Including suspicious for carcinoma without invasion (intraglandular)
        3.2.2 Including carcinoma without invasion (intraglandular)

3. Suspicious for invasive carcinoma

4. Invasive adenocarcinoma

Table 1.3 *Padova classification of gastric dysplasia*

Between 40 and 100% of early gastric cancers and 5 and 80% of advanced tumours show dysplasia. In comparison only 1 to 3% of gastric ulcers with an atrophic gastritis are associated with dysplasia. A diagnosis of severe dysplasia is a frequent marker of coexistent cancer when a gross endoscopic lesion such as an erosion, ulcer or polyp accompanies it. In this situation 50% of the tumours were diagnosed within 3–24 months of the initial finding of dysplasia on biopsy.

Early gastric cancer

This is defined as a malignant tumour limited to the mucosa or submucosa and is independent of any lymph-node metastasis. The penetration of the muscularis mucosae allows subdivision of the tumours into those that are intramucosal or submucosal types.

 The Japanese Endoscopic Society introduced a macroscopic classification of these tumours (**Fig. 1.9**). This divided the lesions into predominantly protuberant (type I); a superficial type where there is minimal mucosal thickening (type II); or where there is a significant ulcerating lesion (type III).[62]

Type I protruding polypoid tumours appear as sessile smooth hemispherical nodules with a broad stalk, less than 3 cm in diameter and are often paler than the adjacent mucosa. Type II tumours are subdivided into three subsets: the slightly elevated (IIa, in which the mucosal thickness is no greater than twice that of the adjacent mucosa), the flat (IIb, where no mucosal elevation or depression is seen) and the depressed group (IIc, in which there is mucosal erosion but no deep ulceration). More than one appearance can be found, especially if the tumours cover a large area. In this situation they are classified by the predominant type followed by the subsidiary type(s) e.g. IIa + IIc (**Fig. 1.10**). The appearances of these early gastric cancers was further studied by Inokuchi and Kodama who showed that the small tumours which penetrated the submucosa

Figure 1.9
Schematic representation of the different types of early gastric carcinoma.

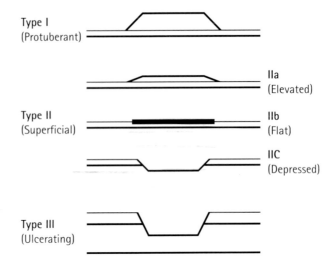

Type I
(Protuberant)

Type II
(Superficial)

IIa
(Elevated)

IIb
(Flat)

IIC
(Depressed)

Type III
(Ulcerating)

Figure 1.10
An early gastric carcinoma of the antrum showing areas of both an elevated and superficially depressed tumour (type II a+c).

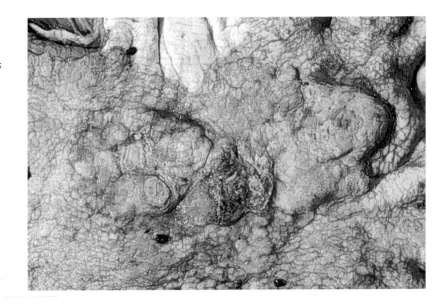

with an expanding margin (Pen A) tended to have more lymphatic and blood-borne metastases than the infiltrative type of tumour (Pen B).[63] The latter tumour had greater peritoneal recurrences.

Early gastric cancers are found predominantly within the lower two-thirds of the stomach and vary in size from 3–5 mm to more than 8 cm, although most are between 2–5 cm. Those lesions that are less than 5 mm in diameter are referred to as minute carcinomas. Mori *et al.*[64] have reported a small series of 21 patients with early carcinoma of the cardia. The ulcerating tumours (types III and IIc) are the most frequent, accounting for 64% of the neoplasms, followed by the exophytic lesions. The entirely flat IIb lesion is the least common and represents 14% of the tumours. Histologically the exophytic tumours tend to have a better differentiated intestinal type while the ulcerating tumours are more frequently

Figure 1.11
The macroscopic appearances of advanced gastric cancer a) Polypoid (Borrman type I) and b) ulcerating (Borrman type III).

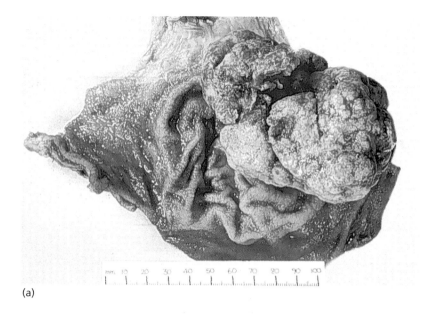

(a)

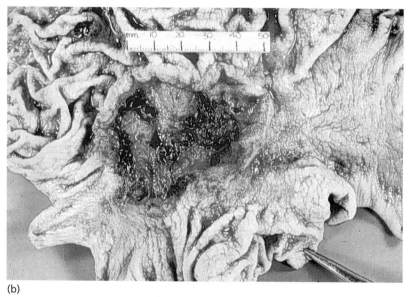

(b)

associated with the signet ring or poorly differentiated histology. The flat lesions have a mixed histological pattern.

The prognosis for EGC is excellent with a reported 5-year survival of 92%.[65] Long-term studies have shown that tumours confined to the mucosa have a 15-year survival of 87% and slightly less when there is infiltration into the submucosa (75%).[66] Despite this, reports from Japan indicate a recurrence rate of up to 2%, which is thought to be due either to residual tumour in the gastric remnant or haematogenous metastatic disease.[67,68] The features that are associated with haematogenous metastases are intestinal-type tumours, submucosal invasion

Figure 1.12
A linitis plastica (Borrman type IV) in which there is diffuse infiltration of the wall of the stomach by tumour and apparent thickening of the rugal folds.

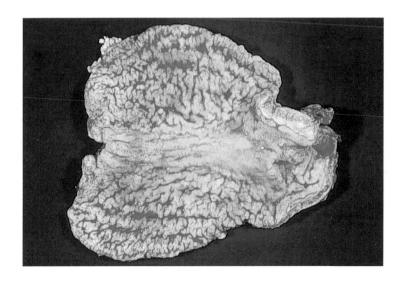

and involvement of the epigastric lymph nodes. Intramucosal EGC rarely have perigastric nodal metastasis (less than 5%) due to the paucity of intramucosal lymphatics. Invasion of the submucosa is however associated with 10–20% nodal metastases,[69,70] although reports from the UK have suggested even higher rates.[45] Interestingly DNA analysis shows that aneuploid changes are more frequent in types I and IIa tumours though the ploidy status and nodal metastasis have not been shown to be consistently correlated.[71]

Advanced gastric cancer

Approximately 90% of all malignant tumours of the stomach are adenocarcinomas. The majority of the remaining tumours are either malignant lymphoma or smooth muscle tumours. There are in addition a wide variety of other primary tumours arising from the stomach, which reflects the tissue present within the mucosa and deeper structures. These include squamous and oat cell carcinomas, carcinoid tumours, benign and malignant mesodermally derived tumours (i.e. those coming from blood vessels, fat cells and neural elements) and an assortment of rare tumours more often associated with extra-gastrointestinal sites such as the malignant fibrous histiocytoma, glomus tumours, teratoma and choriocarcinoma.

Advanced gastric cancer has shown significant changes over recent decades with an overall decline in incidence, increase in tumours of the cardia and oesophagogastric junction over the distal stomach and finally an increase in the diffuse type (see below) which now represents up to 30% of all gastric neoplasms.[72]

Macroscopic features

The macroscopic appearances of an advanced gastric cancer have been divided into four types by Bormann[73] (Table 1.4, Figs 1.11 and 1.12); although this classification is commonly used in Germany and Japan it has never gained general acceptance throughout the English-speaking world. Approximately 50% of the tumours are confined to the antrum while a third are at the oesophago-gastric

Type 1 or fungating. A polypoid protrusion with a broad base, often soft, red in colour and may be slightly ulcerated.

Type 2 An excavated carcinoma, which is dominated by the crater with slightly, elevated margins. There is no definite infiltration of the adjacent mucosa.

Type 3 This also is ulcerative with mildly elevated margins and infiltrated.

Type 4 A diffusely thickened (scirrhous type) and is also known as linitis plastica. The macroscopic appearances allow an assessment of similar types of tumour and whether it is diffusely infiltrated and possibly may be able to aid in the understanding of the natural history of the tumour.

Table 1.4 *Macroscopic appearances of advanced gastric carcinoma (Borrman).*

junction. The tumours are large: more than a half are 6 cm in diameter with 1 in 7 reaching 10 cm or more.

Histological features

The complexity of the histological features of gastric tumours is a reflection of the multiple cell types present. These include mucous and goblet cells, immature absorptive cells, pyloric gland cells, Paneth, parietal and endocrine cells.

This has led to a variety of classifications, the most widely accepted being that proposed by Lauren.[74] The tumours were divided into two main types: those which formed glandular structures are known as *intestinal* (53%) while those with no structure that secrete mucin are referred to as *diffuse* carcinomas (33%: see **Table 1.5**).

Features	Intestinal	Diffuse
Sex ratio M:F	2:1	Approximately 1:1
Mean age of detection in years	55	48
Decreasing incidence in Western countries	Yes	No
5-year survival rate (all cases)	20%	Less than 10%
Major gross appearances	Intraluminal growth, fungating	Ulcerative infiltrating
Microscopic features differentiation	Well differentiated, glandular, papillary, solid	Poorly differentiated signet ring cells
Growth pattern	Expansile	Non-cohesive diffuse
Mucin production	Confined to gland lumen	Extensive often prominent in stroma around glands
Associated intestinal metaplasia	Almost 100%	Less frequent
Aetiological factors	Diet, environmental, *H. pylori*	Unknown,? genetic factors associated with blood group A, *H. pylori*

Table 1.5 *Comparative histological features of advanced gastric carcinoma*

Figure 1.13
A diffuse (signet ring) adenocarcinoma in which the tumour cells are widely dispersed and separated by a variable amount of stroma. Occasional cells show that their nuclei are displaced by the intracytoplasmic secretory vacuoles.

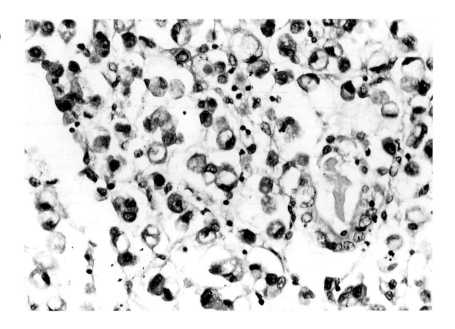

Figure 1.14
An intestinal adenocarcinoma is composed of irregular glands, which are lined by attenuated cuboidal epithelium showing in a well-differentiated case minimal nuclear pleomorphism or pseudostratification of the cells. There is invasion of the muscle layer and a mixed inflammatory infiltrate between the tumourous glands.

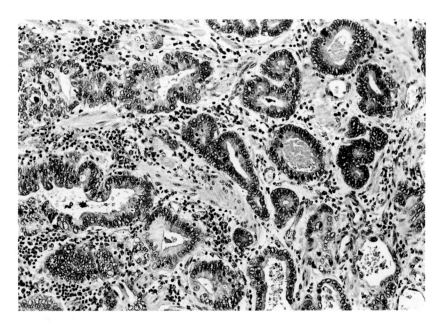

The remaining 14% had a mixed appearance with elements from both types and were regarded as unclassified. The intestinal type of adenocarcinoma is associated with an increased incidence of chronic atrophic gastritis and gastric atrophy, while the diffuse cancers do not have this association. The macroscopic appearance of these tumours depends on the relative proportions of stromal collagen and mucus produced. There are several other classification schemes proposed including those of Ming, in which the tumours are split into expanding and infiltrating types,[75] and that of the World Health Organisation where the tumours are organised into several different histological types (papillary, tubular, mucinous, signet ring cell adenocarcinomas).[76] Unfortunately these have not been conclusively shown to be independent factors in the prognosis of gastric cancer. In addition Goseki *et al.* classified gastric carcinoma into four groups based on the degree of glandular differentiation and amount of intracytoplasmic mucin produced.[77] In the initial studies they were able to show that liver metastases were more frequent in group 1 tumours (well-differentiated tubules with little mucin) while direct infiltration of peritoneum and lymph-node metastases were seen in group IV tumours (little attempt at tubule formation with mucin rich cells). A group of poorly differentiated tumours with a prominent lymphoid infiltrate, the lymphoepithelioma-like carcinoma, have been described.[78] In more than 80% of these tumours EBV has been demonstrated, while it is found in only 9% of other adenocarcinomas.

Prognostic pathological features

Careful assessment of gastrectomy specimens has shown several prognostic features in advanced gastric cancer, the most important being the depth of tumour invasion (TNM stage).[79]

Involvement of the resection margin by tumour, the presence of lymph node metastasis[80] and recently the Goseki classification has been shown to provide further prognostic information.[81] Survival of patients with cancers of the cardia and upper third of the stomach are worse than those of the body and antrum (5-year survival of 15, 25 and 30% respectively). Serosal involvement is an ominous feature with a 5-year survival of just 7% while tumour infiltration restricted to the subserosa is about 29%. Transcoelomic dissemination and direct infiltration of adjacent structures may occur as a result of serosal involvement. Several authors have investigated the area of serosal involvement. Most have taken less than 2 cm in diameter as the limit that indicated a better prognosis. Abe *et al.*[82] showed that serosal involvement of less than 3 cm had a 5-year survival of 59.6% compared with 11.5% with tumours more than 3 cm. They have also suggested that if both the serosa and lymph nodes were involved then the diameter of serosal involvement is the more important factor in predicting the ultimate survival. A significant under-estimation of serosal involvement at surgery has been reported.[83] This tended to occur with large undifferentiated tumours and showed nearly 10% of cases had positive microscopic serosal involvement when the macroscopic appearances were thought to be tumour free.

The rate of lymph-node metastases in early gastric cancer is related to the size, growth pattern and the presence of ulceration. Survival is dependent upon the number of nodes involved,[84] the extension of metastasis through the capsule of nodes and involvement of the adjacent fibrovascular and fatty tissue and whether or not the metastasis were judged to be present microscopically.[85]

Involvement of the duodenum in tumours of the distal stomach has been reported from 9–69% of the resections.[86,87] When present, it is regarded as a poor prognostic sign with a significant reduction in the 5-year survival rate to 8%, in comparison with those tumours restricted to the stomach. These tumours also show an increased involvement of the serosa, with evidence of lymphatic and vascular invasion. The suggestion that relaparotomy should be undertaken to achieve a tumour-free resection line is controversial.

Other independent factors to show positive predictive value have included blood and lymphatic invasion,[88] intratumoural vessel count, patient age over 70, tumours with a diffuse infiltrating pattern and tumours involving the entire stomach or that measure more than 10 cm in diameter.[87] The only histological tumour type showing a worse prognosis is the adenosquamous carcinoma – this is an uncommon tumour, which is composed of both glandular and squamous elements. Those tumours which macroscopically appear as early gastric carcinoma, but histologically are advanced cancers, have a prognosis that is intermediate between the two groups.

Molecular aspects

It has been suggested, as with most other tumours, that a stepwise development of gastric cancer occurs. This is shown in Fig. 1.15 and indicates that the underlying mechanisms may be different for the diffuse and intestinal types of tumour.[89] The development of gastric cancer requires that there is disruption of the genome and participation of many cancer-associated oncogenes, regulatory genes and proteins to perpetuate the uncontrolled cell growth.[90] The consequence of these changes is the alteration and aberrant expressions of mucins, enzymes and hormones by the tumour epithelium.

Cytogenetic studies have failed to identify consistent chromosomal abnormalities, suggesting that many of the changes are non-specific or are secondary to the malignant transformation. Aneuploid tumours are common (60–70%) being more frequent in intestinal type tumours. The most common abnormalities, apart from those mentioned below, are on chromosome 3 (rearrangement), chromosome 6 (deletions distal to 6q21), chromosome 8 (trisomy), chromosome

Figure 1.15
Genetic pathway for development of gastric carcinoma.

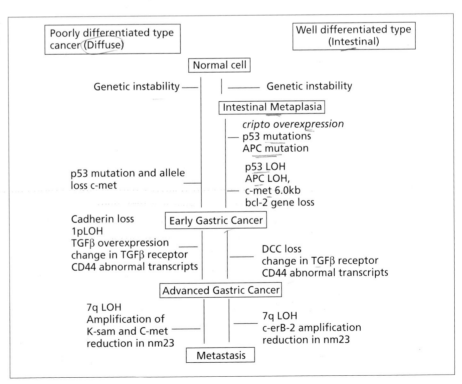

11 (aberration (11p13–11p15)), and on chromosome 13 (monosomy and translocations). The most consistent abnormality has been p53 in gastric cancer. Allelic loss and/or mutations of the p53 gene are found in intestinal metaplasia, adenomas and adenocarcinoma (14%, 33% and over 60% respectively). Other tumour suppressor genes show LOH on chromosome 5p near the APC gene. Between 30–40% of tumours show this defect and this suggests a possible further suppressor gene at this site. There is significant allelic loss noted at the DCC gene locus on 18q (more than 60%).

Microsatellite instability has been found in a proportion of sporadic tumours from which there is the potential to establish multiple gene abnormalities. These changes are more frequently found in intestinal than diffuse-type tumours and in particular in subcardial intestinal tumours. There is a negative association with p53 suggesting this is a different pathway of accumulating genetic abnormalities. The target for the instability has been reported to be the transforming growth factor beta (TGFβ) type II receptor. Oncogene expression appears early in tumour formation and may be the cause for increased cell division, though the significance of the genes and gene products is unclear at present. Two oncogenes c-myc and cripto show amplification and over-expression in intestinal metaplasia, some cases of dysplasia and advanced gastric cancer. C-met is amplified and present in 30% of intestinal cancers especially the scirrhous tumours. The gene encodes a tyrosine kinase receptor for the hepatocyte growth factor but it interacts with EGF, TGFα, interleukin-1-α, amphiregulin, K-sam and others.[91] A member of the fibroblastic growth factor receptor family, K-sam is amplified in both diffuse and scirrhous carcinomas but not other types of tumours.[92] The fibrosis seen in these tumours suggests interaction between receptors and oncogenes of the stromal and tumour cells.

Genetic abnormalities of e-cadherin gene and reduced expression of the protein have been found in up to 90% of carcinomas, especially the diffuse type. E-cadherin is a transmembrane calcium-dependent cell-adhesive molecule that is important in epithelial cell interactions. Loss of its binding properties could result in tumour infiltration and dissemination. Other molecules that have an anchoring function such as CD44 are also found to be defective.[93]

Finally it is being recognised that patients with hereditary non-polyposis colorectal cancer (HNPCC) are at risk not only of the colorectal tumours but also of tumours in the stomach, endometrium, small bowel, ovary and ureter and to a lesser extent kidney and hepatobiliary system. The criteria for the diagnosis of HNPCC are:

1. At least three affected relatives with verified colorectal cancer;
2. At least one of the above is a first-degree relative of the other two;
3. Familial adenomatous polyposis has been excluded;
4. At least two successive generations are affected;
5. One of the patients is younger than 50 years of age.

This is an autosomal dominant inherited genetic disease due to a germ-line mutation in one of the four DNA mismatch repair genes.[94] The tumours develop as a result of the loss of large relative segments of chromosomes, which are thought to include tumour suppressor genes. As a consequence the tissue becomes more liable to mutations and this accelerates carcinogenesis; the relative risk of developing gastric cancer is reported as 4.1 and the median age is 54 years.

Mesenchymal tumours of oesophagus and stomach

The stomach is the most frequent site within the gastrointestinal tract for these tumours and the largest series has recently been published.[95] In the stomach they range in size from under 1 cm, where they are clinically asymptomatic, to bulky 20 cm masses. Multivariate analysis showed that the tumour location, size and mitotic index were all independent prognostic factors. Approximately three-quarters in the stomach and even more in the oesophagus are benign. It is important to recognise that these tumours may be part of other clinical syndromes such as Carney's triad. This affects young women and consists of extra-adrenal paraganglioma together with pulmonary chondroma and stromal tumours of the stomach. The triad may be diagnosed if two of the three features are present. The stromal tumours and paragangliomas are often multiple.

Initially the tumours were thought to be leiomyomas or leiomyosarcomas as they were composed of spindle cells with close resemblance to the muscle layers (**Fig. 1.16**), with a variable amount of extracellular collagen. Electron microscopy shows heterogeneous features suggesting smooth muscle or neural differentiation, both or no differentiation. This has led to problems of classification, which is now being addressed by the use of immunocytochemisty. Variable expression of the markers of muscle (desmin and smooth muscle actin), nerve (S100, NSE and PGP 9.5) and interstitial cells of Cajal (CD 34 and CD 117; also known as c-kit protein) has allowed classification into three major groups. Leiomyomas and leiomyosarcomas are positive for desmin and actin and negative for CD 34, neurofibroma and other neural tumours will be positive for S100 but negative for the other markers. The largest group of these tumours are positive for CD 34 and CD 117 and negative for the others and are referred to as gastrointestinal stromal tumours (GIST).

Carney's triad

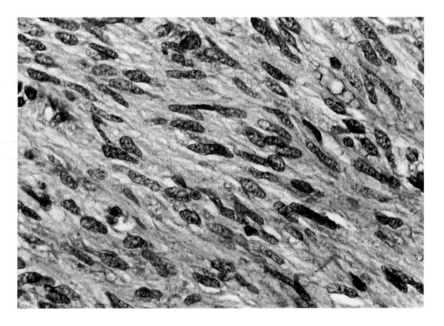

Figure 1.16
Gastrointestinal stromal tumours (GIST) the spindle cells have irregular nuclei with rounded ends and form loosely associated bundles separated by a collagenous matrix.

Apart from the histiogenesis of the tumours, predicting clinical behaviour is problematical. Because of the bland cytological features clinical information such as the presence of metastases or local invasion are important in indicating malignancy. Although size is important, with 60% of the tumours more than 10 cm in diameter showing metastatic spread within 5 years, benign tumours of a similar size have been described. The most important histological feature after multivariate analysis has been the mitotic index; malignant behaviour being most likely when there are more than 5 mitotic figures per 10 high-power fields. Recent developments have shown that mutations of the c-kit gene in stromal tumours have a worse prognosis.[96]

The inflammatory fibroid polyp is a benign lesion reported throughout the gastrointestinal tract with a predilection to the distal stomach and ileum. The gastric lesions typically present in the 6th decade, with slightly more males than females affected. The larger tumours cause outlet obstruction although most measure less than 3 cm in diameter. They present as polyps or expansile lesions in the submucosa, at or just proximal to the pyloric sphincter muscle. Plump spindle cells, numerous small blood vessels and a mixed inflammatory infiltrate, which includes eosinophils, are the cellular components of the tumour. The adjacent mucosa often shows features of atrophic gastritis. The underlying cause for the lesion is unknown. Ultrastructural features of the spindle cells shows them to be fibroblasts or myofibroblasts, suggesting that the tumours are reactive in nature; possibly an exuberant granulation tissue response.

In addition, small numbers of vascular tumours, glomus tumours, angiomas and Kaposi's sarcoma – the latter associated with AIDS – have been reported.

Gastric mucosa associated lymphoid tissue (MALT) lymphoma

The stomach is the commonest site for gastrointestinal lymphomas, representing 3–6% of all gastric malignancies. The majority of the tumours are B-cell non-Hodgkin's lymphomas with occasional T-cell lymphoma and Hodgkin's disease. These tumours arise from lymphoid tissue acquired as the result of *H. pylori* infection.[35] The majority occur in patients over the age of 50 years with equal sex distribution who present clinically with symptoms suggesting a diagnosis of gastritis or peptic ulcer disease.[97] The tumours appear macroscopically as an ill-defined thickening of the mucosa with erosions, sometimes ulcerated (**Fig. 1.17**) and frequently multifocal. The gastric MALT lymphoma remains localised to the stomach and rarely spreads to lymph nodes or bone marrow though the frequency of this spread may have been underestimated.[98] The lymphoma cells resemble follicle centre cells and are termed centrocyte-like, with other cells showing plasma cell differentiation and occasional blast cells. The characteristic lymphoepithelial lesion (**Fig. 1.18**) is composed of small to medium-sized tumour cells with irregular nuclei which infiltrate the pit epithelium. This lesion is not pathognomonic of a lymphoma as it can also be demonstrated in an *H. pylori*-associated gastritis, Sjögren's syndrome and Hashimoto's thyroiditis. It is thought that the development of lymphoma is a multistage process, which results from the interaction of the *H. pylori*, neutrophils, B- and T-cells. Continuing B-cell proliferation, which is T-cell dependent, results from the antigen (*H. pylori*) stimulation. It has been postulated that in the presence

Figure 1.17
Non-Hodgkin's lymphoma that shows superficial ulceration of the antrum with fibrous scarring of the adjacent mucosa.

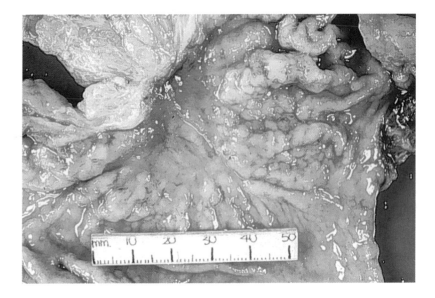

Figure 1.18
Lymphoepithelial lesion – an intense mononuclear cell infiltrate is present within the mucosa which extends into the pits. There is partial destruction of these (arrowhead).

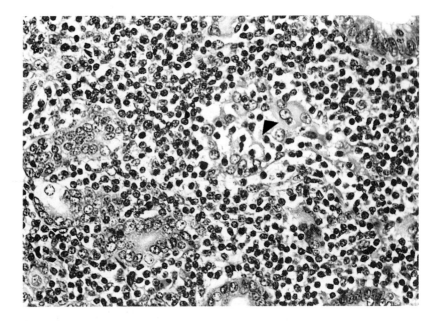

of a mutator phenotype (from defective mismatch repair machinery) nuclear damage is caused by neutrophils generating oxygen radicals, and resulting in genetic instability. The early chromosomal abnormalities include trisomy 3 (in up to 60% of cases), translocations t(11;18), p53 mutations or loss of heterozygosity and c-myc mutation. This results in an abnormal clone which undergoes clonal expansion and gives rise to a low-grade MALT lymphoma, the early phase of which is responsive to *H. pylori* eradication.[99] Most low-grade MALT lymphomas are associated with localised disease confined to the gastric mucosa with slow dissemination. The favourable clinical behaviour may reflect the partial dependence on the *H. pylori* antigenic drive. In a minority of cases accumulation of further genetic abnormalities (such as inactivation of p53 and p16) can be identified, however in the majority the changes have not been recognised. The progression to the more common high-grade MALT lymphoma is thought to require the development of T-cell and *H. pylori* independence of the B-cell clone together with further genetic abnormalities.[100] Generally there are excellent survival rates with reported 5- and 10-year survival rates of 91% and 75%, though at present the best treatment has not yet been defined. Some of the high-grade lymphomas have been reported as having a more favourable prognosis than their equivalent nodal disease though this is not as good as the low-grade tumours (75% at 5 years).

Gastric carcinoids

The gastric mucosa contains several endocrine cells and these give rise to carcinoid (neuroendocrine) tumours. The endocrine cells have a characteristic distribution, staining pattern and electron microscopic appearance[101] and most of the tumours are derived from enterochromaffin-like cells. Multistep progression from simple hyperplasia through nodule formation to dysplasia and tumour is thought to occur. The separation of benign from malignant tumour depends on the histological grade, size, depth of invasion and mitotic activity.[102] Recently it has been found that there is an increased incidence of gastric carcinoids although at present this still represents only 0.54% of all malignant tumours.[103]

At least four groups of patients with carcinoid tumours can be identified:

1. Multiple well-differentiated tumours affecting predominantly middle-aged females are associated with pernicious anaemia and hypergastrinaemia.[104] Where the tumours are invasive they tend to be limited to the submucosa and metastases are usually confined to the local lymph nodes (7–12%). No reported deaths are associated with these tumours. The possibility of reversibility, by antrectomy (to reduce the hypergastrinaemia) or with octreotide, has demonstrated a reduction in the endocrine cell numbers at 1 month although there tends to be a rebound phenomenon at 3 months after stopping treatment.

2. Carcinoid tumours associated with the Zollinger–Ellison syndrome or those patients with MEN type I have hypergastrinaemia and are predominantly middle-aged females. The tumours tend to be multicentric with a minimal gastritis but both hyperplasia and endocrine-cell dysplasia are present. These tumours often extend into deep muscle, have lymph-node metastases and have occasionally caused death. The loss of the MEN-1 gene locus is seen in the majority of these tumours, a defect also found in those tumours of the gut, pancreas and parathyroid associated with MEN-1.[105]

3. Solitary lesions that occur in middle-aged men and tend to be larger (2 cm) and have a more aggressive behaviour. The adjacent mucosa shows a minimal non-specific gastritis and only focal neuroendocrine hyperplasia and no dysplasia. Serosal infiltration with lymphatic and vascular invasion is more common. Liver metastasis with an accompanying carcinoid syndrome has been reported. Metastases are present in 52% of cases and approximately one-third of the patients will have died in a median of 51 months.

4. The fourth type of tumour showing neuroendocrine differentiation is the poorly differentiated carcinoid. These also tend to be solitary and affect the corpus mucosa with an accompanying chronic active gastritis. At presentation these patients tend to be slightly older than the other groups (median 65 years) and again males predominate. This is sometimes associated with a hypergastrinaemia or G-cell hyperplasia. The lesions tend to be large, deeply invasive and as a consequence the median survival is short (6.5 months), death frequently being tumour related.

References

1. Anonymous. Mortality statistics 1998. Office for National Statistics. Series DH2 no. 25.

2. Schlemper RJ, Itabashi M, Kato Y *et al.* Differences in diagnostic criteria for gastric carcinoma between Japanese and Western pathologists. Lancet 1997; 349 (9067):1725–9.

3. Everett SM, Axon AT. Early gastric cancer in Europe. Gut 1997; 41 (2):142–50.

4. Munoz NC, Grass M, Wang Guo A *et al.* Precursor lesions of oesophageal cancer in high-risk populations in Iran and China. Lancet 1982; 1:876–9.

5. Streitz J Jr., Ellis F Jr, Gibb SP *et al.* Achalasia and squamous cell carcinoma of the esophagus: analysis of 241 patients. Ann Thor Surg 1995; 59 (6):1604–9.

6. Applequist P, Salmo M. Lye corrosion carcinoma of the esophagus. A review of 63 cases. Cancer 1980; 45:2655–8.

7. O'Mahony ME, Hellier JP, Mann M *et al.* Familial tylosis and carcinoma of the oesophagus. J R Soc Med 1984; 77:514–17.

8. Chisholm M. The association between webs iron and post-cricoid carcinoma. Postgrad Med J 1974; 50:215.

9. Huang BS, Unni KK, Payne WS. Long term survival following diverticulectomy for cancer in pharyngooesophageal (Zenker's) diverticulum. Ann Thorac Surg 1984; 38:207–10.

10. Tamura HS. Barrett-type esophagus associated with squamous carcinoma. Chest 1971; 59:330–3.

11. Swinson CM, Slavin G, Coles EC *et al.* Coeliac disease and malignancy. Lancet 1983; 1:111–15.

12. Sherrill DG, Galal BA, Zajtchuk FS *et al.* Radiation induced associated malignancies of the oesophagus. Cancer 1984; 54:726–8.

13. Contini SC, Di Lecee GF, Chiapasco F *et al.* Vital staining of oesophagus in patients with head and neck cancer: still a worthwhile procedure. Ital J Gastroenterol 1991; 23:5–8.

14. Bogomoletz WT, Gayet G, Molas G *et al.* Superficial squamous cell carcinoma of the esophagus. A report of 76 cases and review of the literature. Am J Surg Pathol 1989; 13:535–46.

15. Jaskiemdcz KB, Mafungo L, Knobel V *et al.* Oesophageal mucosa in a population at risk of oesophageal cancer: postmortem 72 studies. Int J Cancer 1992; 50:32–5.

16. Sarbia M, Porschen R, Borchard F *et al.* Incidence and prognostic significance of vascular and neural invasion in squamous cell carcinomas of the esophagus. Int J Cancer 1995; 61 (3):333–6.

17. Balercia G, Bhan AK, Dickersin GR. Sarcomatoid carcinoma: an ultrastructural study with light microscopic and immunohistochemical correlation of 10 cases from various anatomic sites. Ultrastruct Pathol 1995; 19 (4):249–63.

18. Montesano R, Hainaut P. Molecular precursor lesions in oesophageal cancer. Cancer Surv 1998; 32:53–68.

19. Shiozaki H, Kadowaki T, Doki Y *et al.* Effect of epidermal growth factor on cadherin-mediated adhesion in a human oesophageal cancer cell line. Br J Cancer 1995; 71 (2):250–8.

20. Matsuura HKH, Morita M *et al.* Predicting recurrence time of esophageal carcinoma through assessment of histologic factors and DNA ploidy. Cancer 1991; 67:1406–11.

21. Muir CS, McKinney PA. Cancer of the oesophagus: a global overview. Eur J Cancer Prev 1992; 1 (3):259–64.

22. Ruol A, Merigliano S, Baldan N *et al.* Prevalence, management and outcome of early adenocarcinoma (pT1) of the esophago-gastric junction. Comparison between early cancer in Barrett's esophagus (type I) and early cancer of the cardia (type II). Dis Esoph 1997; 10 (3):190–5.

23. Siewert JR, Stein HJ. Classification of adenocarcinoma of the oesophagogastric junction. Br J Surg 1998; 85:1457–9.

24. Barrett N. Chronic peptic ulcer of the oesophagus and 'oesophagitis'. Br J Surg 1950; 38:175–82.

25. Womack C, Harvey L. Columnar epithelial lined oesophagus (CELO) or Barrett's oesophagus: mucin histochemistry, dysplasia, and invasive adenocarcinoma. J Clin Pathol 1985; 38 (4):477–8.

26. Thomas P, Doddoli C, Lienne P et al. Changing patterns and surgical results in adenocarcinoma of the oesophagus. B J Surg 1997; 84 (1):119–25.

27. Van der Burgh A DJ, Hop WCJ, van Blankenstein M. Oesophageal cancer is an uncommon cause of death in patients with Barrett's oesophagus. Gut 1996; 39:5–8.

28. Iftikhar SY, James PD, Steele RJ et al. Length of Barrett's oesophagus: an important factor in the development of dysplasia and adenocarcinoma. Gut 1992; 33 (9):1155–8.

29. Sarbia M, Verreet P, Bittinger F et al. Basaloid squamous cell carcinoma of the esophagus: diagnosis and prognosis. Cancer 1997; 79 (10):1871–8.

30. Matsuki A, Nishimaki T, Suzuki T et al. Esophageal mucoepidermoid carcinoma containing signet-ring cells: three case reports and a literature review. J Surg Oncol 1999; 71 (1):54–7.

31. Mafune K, Takubo K, Tanaka Y et al. Sclerosing mucoepidermoid carcinoma of the esophagus with intraepithelial carcinoma or dysplastic epithelium. J Surg Oncol 1995; 58 (3):184–90.

32. Takubo K, Nakamura K, Sawabe M et al. Primary undifferentiated small cell carcinoma of the esophagus. Hum Pathol 1999; 30 (2):216–21.

33. Correa P, Chen VW. Gastric cancer. Cancer Surv 1994; 20:55–76.

34. Correa P, Shiao YH. Phenotypic and genotypic events in gastric carcinogenesis. Cancer Res 1994; 54 (7 Suppl):1941s–3s.

35. Eidt S, Stolte M. The significance of *Helicobacter pylori* in relation to gastric cancer and lymphoma. Eur J Gastroenterol Hepatol 1995; 7 (4):318–21.

36. Genta RM, Graham DY. *Helicobacter pylori*: the new bug on the (paraffin) block. Virchows Archiv 1994; 425 (4):339–47.

37. Parsonnet J, Friedman VD, Vandersteen DP et al. *Helicobacter* infection and the risk of gastric carcinoma. N Engl J Med 1991; 325:1127–31.

38. Wyatt JI. Gastritis and its relation to gastric carcinogenesis. Sem Diag Pathol 1991; 8 (3):137–48.

39. Silva S, Filipe M. Intestinal metaplasia and its variants in the gastric mucosa of Portuguese subjects. A comparative analysis of biopsy and gastrectomy material. Hum Pathol 1986; 17:955–88.

40. Sipponen P, Kimura K. Intestinal metaplasia, atrophic gastritis and stomach cancer: trends over time. Eur J Gastroenterol Hepat 1994; 6 (1):S79–83.

41. Stemmermann GN. Intestinal metaplasia of the stomach. A status report. Cancer 1994; 74 (2):556–64.

42. Ho SB, Shekels LL, Toribara NW et al. Mucin gene expression in normal, preneoplastic, and neoplastic human gastric epithelium. Cancer Res 1995; 55 (12):2681–90.

43. Saegusa M, Takano Y, Okayasu I. Bcl-2 expression and its association with cell kinetics in human gastric carcinomas and intestinal metaplasia. J Cancer Res Clin Oncol 1995; 121 (6):357–63.

44. Sipponen P, Hyvarinen H. Role of *Helicobacter pylori* in the pathogenesis of gastritis, peptic ulcer and gastric cancer. Scandinavian Journal of Gastroenterology (Suppl) 1993; 196:3–6.

45. Antonioli DA. Precursors of gastric carcinoma: a critical review with a brief description of early (curable) gastric cancer. Hum Pathol 1994; 25 (10):994–1005.

46. Hill MJ. Bacterial N-nitrosation and gastric carcinogenesis in humans. Ital J Gastroenterol 1991; 23 (1):17–23.

47. Correa P, Fox J, Fontham E et al. *Helicobacter pylori* and gastric carcinoma: Serum antibody prevalence in populations with contrasting cancer risks. Cancer 1990; 66:2569–74.

48. Ming S-C. Malignant potential of epithelial polyps of the stomach. In: Ming S-C (ed.): Precursors of gastric cancer. New York: Praeger, 1984; pp. 219–31.

49. Nakamura T, Nakano G. Histopathological classification, and malignant change in gastric polyps. J Clin Pathol 1985; 38:754–64.

50. Hattori T. Morphological range of hyperplastic polyps and carcinomas arising in hyperplastic polyps of the stomach. J Clin Pathol 1985; 38:662–30.

51. Iada M, Yao T, Watanabe H et al. Fundic gland polyposis in patients without familial adenomatosis coli: Its incidence and clinical features. Gastroenterol 1984; 86:1437–42.

52. Kolodziejczyk P, Yao T, Oya M et al. Long-term follow-up study of patients with gastric adenomas with malignant transformation. An immunohistochemical and histochemical analysis. Cancer 1994; 74 (11):2896–907.

53. Sarre RG, Frost AG, Jagelman DG et al. Gastric and duodenal polyps in familial adenomatous polyposis. A prospective study of the nature and prevalence of upper gastrointestinal polyps. Gut 1987; 28:306–14.

54. Xaun Z, Ambe K, Enjoji M. Depressed adenoma of the stomach revisited: Histologic, histochemical and immunohistochemical profiles. Cancer 1991; 67:2382–89.

55. Fujiwara T, Hirose S, Hamazaki K et al. Clinico-pathological features of gastric cancer in the remnant stomach. Hepato Gastroenterol 1996; 43 (8):416–19.

56. Sebagh M, Flejou JF, Potet F. Lymphoma of the gastric stump. Report of two cases and review of the literature. J Clin Gastroenterol 1995; 20 (2):147–50.

57. Johnson MI, Spark JI, Ambrose NS et al. Early gastric cancer in a patient with Menetrier's disease, lymphocytic gastritis and *Helicobacter pylori*. Eur J Gastroenterol Hepatol 1995; 7 (2):187–90.

58. Lee S, Iada M, Yao T et al. Long-term follow-up of 2529 patients reveals gastric ulcers rarely become malignant. Dig Dis Sci 1990; 35:763–8.

59. Morson BS, Grundmann LH, Johansen E et al. Precancerous conditions and epithelial dysplasia in the stomach. J Clin Pathol 1980; 33:711–21.

60. Rugge MC, Dixon P, Hattori MF et al. Gastric dysplasia; The Padova International Classification. Am J Surg Pathol 1999; 24 (2):167–76.

61. You WC, Zhao L, Chang YS et al. Progression of precancerous gastric lesions. Lancet 1995; 345:866.

62. Murakami T. Pathomorphological diagnosis. Definition and gross classification of early gastric cancer. Gann Monogr 1971; 11:53–5.

63. Kodama Y, Inokuchi K, Soejima K et al. Growth patterns and prognosis in early gastric carcinoma. Superficial spreading and penetrating growth types. Cancer 1983; 51:320–6.

64. Mori M, Sakaguchi H, Akazawa K et al. Correlation between metastatic site, histological type, and serum tumor markers of gastric carcinoma. Hum Pathol 1995; 26 (5):504–8.

65. Saragoni L, Gaudio M, Vio A et al. Early gastric cancer in the province of Forli: follow-up of 337 patients in a high risk region for gastric cancer. Oncol Reports 1998; 5 (4):945–8.

66. Tsuchiya A, Kikuchi Y, Ando Y et al. Lymph node metastases in gastric cancer invading the submucosal layer. Eur J Surg Oncol 1995; 21 (3):248–50.

67. Kitamura K, Yamaguchi T, Okamoto K et al. Total gastrectomy for early gastric cancer. J Surg Oncol 1995; 60 (2):83–8.

68. Sano T, Sasako M, Kinoshita T et al. Recurrence of early gastric cancer. Follow-up of 1475 patients and review of the Japanese literature. Cancer 1993; 72 (11):3174–8.

69. Kim JP, Hur YS, Yang HK. Lymph node metastasis as a significant prognostic factor in early gastric cancer: analysis of 1136 early gastric cancers. Ann Surg Oncol 1995; 2 (4):308–13.

70. Hayes NK, Scott D, Raimes D et al. Radical lymphadenectomy for early gastric carcinoma. Br J Surg. 1996; 83:1421–3.

71. Brito M, Filipem I, Williams GT et al. DNA ploidy in early gastric carcinoma (T1). A flow cytometric study of 100 European cases. Gut 1993; 34:230–4.

72. Ikeda YM, Kamakura M, Haraguchi T et al. Improvements in diagnosis have changed the incidence of histological types in advanced gastric cancer. Br J Cancer 1995; 72 (2):424.

73. Borrmann R. Makroskopische Formen des vorgeschritteten Magenkrebses. In: Henke F, Lubarach O (eds.) Handbuch der speziellen pathologischen Anatomie und Histologie, vol 4/1. Berlin: Springer, 1926.

74. Lauren P. The two histological main types of gastric carcinoma: diffuse and so called intestinal-type carcinoma. Acta Path Microbiol Scand 1965; 64:31–49.

75. Ming S-C. Gastric carcinoma. A pathobiological classification. Cancer 1977; 39:2475–85.

76. Watanabe HJJ, Sobin LH. Histological typing of gastric and oesophageal tumours. WHO International Histological Classification of Tumours, 2nd edn. Berlin: Springer-Verlag, 1990; pp. 20–6.

77. Goseki N, Maruyama M, Takizawa T et al. Morphological changes in gastric carcinoma with progression. J Gastroenterol 1995; 30 (3):287–94.

78. Matsunou H, Konishi F, Hori H et al. Characteristics of Epstein–Barr virus-associated gastric carcinoma with lymphoid stroma in Japan. Cancer 1996; 77 (10):1998–2004.

79. Kinugasa S, Abe S, Tachibana M et al. Surgically curable and incurable scirrhous carcinomas of the stomach. J Surg Oncol 1997; 65 (3):194–200.

80. Boku T, Nakane Y, Minoura T et al. Prognostic significance of serosal invasion and free intraperitoneal cancer cells in gastric cancer. Br J Surg 1990; 77 (4):436–9.

81. Songun I, van de Velde CJ, Arends JW et al. Classification of gastric carcinoma using the Goseki system provides prognostic information additional to TNM staging. Cancer 1999; 85 (10):2114–18.

82. Abe S, Shiraishi M, Nagaoka S et al. Serosal invasion as the single prognostic indicator in stage IIIA (T3N1M0) gastric cancer. Surgery 1991; 109 (5):582–8.

83. Ichiyoshi Y, Maehara Y, Tomisaki S et al. Macroscopic intraoperative diagnosis of serosal invasion and clinical outcome of gastric cancer: risk of underestimation. J Surg Oncol 1995; 59 (4):255–60.

84. Noda N, Sasako M, Yamaguchi N et al. Ignoring small lymph nodes can be a major cause of staging error in gastric cancer. Br J Surg 1998; 85 (6):831–4.

85. Di Giorgio A, Botti C, Sammartino P et al. Extracapsular lymphnode metastases in the staging and prognosis of gastric cancer. Int Surg 1991; 76 (4):218–21.

86. Kakeji Y, Korenaga D, Baba H et al. Surgical treatment of patients with gastric carcinoma and duodenal invasion. J Surg Oncol 1995; 59 (4):215–19.

87. Nakamura K, Ueyama T, Yao T *et al*. Pathology and prognosis of gastric carcinoma. Findings in 10 000 patients who underwent primary gastrectomy. Cancer 1992; 70 (5):1030–7.

88. Setala LK, Marin V-M, Lipponen S *et al*. Prognostic factors in gastric cancer: the value of vascular invasion, mitotic rate and lymphoplasmacytic infiltration. Br J Cancer 1996; 74:766–72.

89. Correa P. Human gastric carcinogenesis: a multistep and multifactorial process–First American Cancer Society Award Lecture on Cancer Epidemiology and Prevention. Cancer Res 1992; 52 (24):6735–40.

90. Tahara E, Yokozaci H, Yasui W. Stomach – Genetic and epigenetic alterations of preneoplasia and neoplastic lesions. Molecular pathology of early cancer. Srivastava S, Henson DE, Gasdar A (eds.). Amsterdam: IOS Press, 1999, pp. 341–61.

91. Tahara EY. Genetic alterations in human gastrointestinal cancers. The application to molecular diagnosis. Cancer 1995; 75 (6 Suppl):1410–7.

92. Stemmermann G, Heffelfinger SC, Noffsinger A *et al*. The molecular biology of esophageal and gastric cancer and their precursors: oncogenes, tumor suppressor genes, and growth factors. Hum Pathol 1994; 25 (10):968–81.

93. Harn HJ, Ho LI, Chang JY *et al*. Differential expression of the human metastasis adhesion molecule CD44V in normal and carcinomatous stomach mucosa of Chinese subjects. Cancer 1995; 75 (5): 1065–71.

94. Aarnio M, Salovaara R, Aaltonen LA *et al*. Features of gastric cancer in hereditary non-polyposis colorectal cancer syndrome. Int J Cancer 1997; 74 (5):551–5.

95. Emory TS, Sobin LH, Lukes L *et al*. Prognosis of gastrointestinal smooth-muscle (stromal) tumors: dependence on anatomic site. Am J Surg Pathol 1999; 23 (1):82–7.

96. Taniguchi M, Nishida T, Hirota S *et al*. Effect of c-kit mutation on prognosis of gastrointestinal stromal tumours. Cancer Res 1999; 59 (17):4297–300.

97. Montalban C, Castrillo JM, Abraira V *et al*. Gastric B-cell mucosa-associated lymphoid tissue (MALT) lymphoma. Clinicopathological study and evaluation of the prognostic factors in 143 patients. Ann Oncol 1995; 6 (4):355–62.

98. Du MQ, Isaacson PG. Recent advances in our understanding of the biology and pathogenesis of gastric mucosa associated lymphoid tissue (MALT) lymphoma. Forum 1998; 8.2:162–73.

99. Wotherspoon A, Doglioni C, Diss TC *et al*. Regression of primary low-grade B-cell gastric lymphoma of mucosa associated lymphoid tissue type after eradication of *Helicobacter pylori*. Lancet 1993; 342:575–7.

100. Zucca E, Bertoni F, Roggero E *et al*. Molecular analysis of the progression from *Helicobacter pylori*-associated chronic gastritis to mucosa-associated lymphoid-tissue lymphoma of the stomach. New Engl J Med 1998; 338 (12):804–10.

101. Solcia E, Fiocca R, Villani L *et al*. Hyperplastic, dysplastic, and neoplastic enterochromaffin-like-cell proliferations of the gastric mucosa. Classification and histogenesis. Am J Surg Pathol 1995; 19 (1):S1–7.

102. Rindi G, Azzoni C, La Rosa S *et al*. ECL cell tumor and poorly differentiated endocrine carcinoma of the stomach: prognostic evaluation by pathological analysis. Gastroenterology 1999; 116 (3):532–42.

103. Modlin IM, Sandor A, Tang LH *et al*. A 40-year analysis of 265 gastric carcinoids. Am J Gastroenterology 1997; 92 (4):633–8.

104. Sculco D, Bilgrami S. Pernicious anemia and gastric carcinoid tumor: case report and review. Am J Gastroenterology 1997; 92 (8):1378–80.

105. Debelenko LV, Emmert-Buck MR, Zhuang Z *et al*. The multiple endocrine neoplasia type I gene locus is involved in the pathogenesis of type II gastric carcinoids. Gastroenterology 1997; 113 (3):773–81.

2 Epidemiology and screening for oesophageal and gastric cancer

William H. Allum

INTRODUCTION

The last century saw remarkable changes in cancer of the oesophagus and stomach. Both are major health problems worldwide and much effort has been directed at improving our understanding of the aetiology and to detecting disease at an early and treatable stage. Oesophageal cancer is considerably less common than gastric cancer, although it is highly prevalent in parts of the world with high population density, such as China. Incidence in more developed countries has shown increases in the latter part of the last century. The tumour type has shown corresponding changes with increased numbers of adenocarcinoma compared with squamous cell cancers particularly affecting the lower third of the oesophagus.

Gastric cancer has shown an overall worldwide decrease in incidence, but has only recently been overtaken by lung cancer as the commonest worldwide malignancy. Latterly, developing countries have tended to predominate in incidence although 50 years ago gastric cancer was very common in more socially advanced populations. Dietary and hygiene changes are likely to have been responsible. Nevertheless in more developed countries gastric cancer remains a significant health problem largely because of the plateau in age-standardised incidence reflecting the increase in the ageing population. The incidence of proximal tumours has markedly increased. Indeed the downward migration of oesophageal cancer and a proximal shift in gastric tumours suggests a common aetiology. Furthermore, this has resulted in tumours of the gastric cardia being considered as separate entities.

The overall poor results of treatment have reflected the advanced stage of most cases at presentation. Those parts of the world with high incidence have developed and pursued active mass screening programmes. These have certainly identified precursor lesions and premalignant conditions. Indeed, application of these programmes has produced a significant improvement in survival rates for gastric cancer, particularly in Japan. The knowledge of these changes and underlying conditions has enabled areas of lower incidence to pursue examination of those at estimated high risk. Not only has this begun to increase the number of earlier stage cancers but has also suggested ways in which primary and secondary prevention can begin to reduce overall disease incidence.

Oesophageal cancer

Incidence

In 1985, carcinoma of the oesophagus (ICD Code 150) was the ninth common-est form of malignancy worldwide comprising 4.0% of all cancers.[1] This report from the International Agency for Research in Cancer evaluated cancer incidence by type of country. In developed countries 61 000 cases were registered contrast-ing with developing countries where 243 000 cases were recorded, representing the fourth most common cancer in these countries. Males predominated with a male to female ratio of approximately 2:1. The highest rates were recorded in China; 47% of all new cases occurred there. Incidence was not uniform. In western Europe (France, the former West Germany and the Benelux countries: population 155.0 million) there were approximately 9000 new cases, contrasting with northern Europe (the UK and Scandinavia: population 83.2 million) where 6100 new cases were registered. The sex incidence was significantly different with a male to female ratio in western Europe of 4.3:1 compared with 1.3:1 in north-ern Europe. Subsequent studies have shown a steady increase in European inci-dence. Cheng and Day[2] have reported a 60% increase in age-standardised mortality for men in England and Wales between 1956–60 and 1986–90 with a corresponding increase of 35% for women. (Although mortality rates do not pre-cisely correspond to incidence rates the overall poor survival justifies this method of estimation.)

Similarly in a 25-year review of oesophageal cancer in the West Midlands, UK, Matthews *et al.*[3] reported a rising incidence. The crude incidence over the whole period of study (1957–81) was 5.01 per 100 000 with an age-standardised rate of 3.31. Increasing incidence is apparent for the figures documented for 1957–61 (crude rate 3.63; age-standardised 2.74) compared to those for 1977–81 (crude rate 6.65; age-standardised 4.11). The increases occurred in both sexes with a trend towards a greater increase in women. Factors influencing this increase were partly improvements in registration efficiency but also the effect of the increasing age of the population and an overall increase in the incidence of the disease itself.

Changes in incidence and the actual burden of new cases over time are the result of changes in the size and composition of population and in the actual risk for a specific cancer. The influence of age has already been identified. In the Birmingham study the population was divided into groups (cohorts) according to their year of birth. There is a tendency in both sexes for those born more recently to have high incidence rates. This implies that the risk in younger people is greater at each age than it was for their elders when they were at the same age. This trend together with the greater longevity of the population has significant implications for both clinical workload as well as the needs for general, social and health care with a predicted increased number of cases of oesophageal cancer.

The increase in incidence in the UK of oesophageal cancer has occurred in both histological subtypes. However, the rate of increase has been greatest for adenocarcinoma (**Fig. 2.1**).[4] Within the oesophagus there have been corres-ponding increases in each of the principal subsites. However, the greatest increase by approximately a factor of 5 has occurred in the lower third. When analysed by gender these changes are generally equally distributed although the rate of rise in the lower third has been greater in men.[3]

Figure 2.1
Incidence changes for squamous cell carcinoma and adenocarcinoma of the oesophagus, 1962–1986.

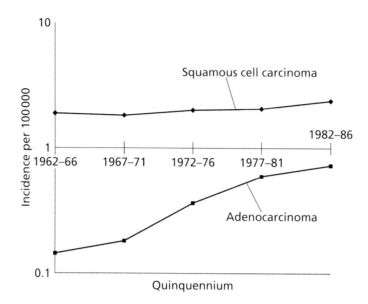

Demography of oesophageal cancer

Oesophageal cancer shows a remarkable preponderance for variation in prevalence and incidence. Differences between countries have already been described. However, enormous variations are seen between provinces or even districts within certain countries: In the West, for instance, the incidence in France is three times greater than in Spain. Within France the national average of 10 per 100 000 rises to 30 per 100 000 in Burgundy and Normandy. These rates are dwarfed by the rates in Iran and China. In Linxian county of northern China the age-adjusted incidence for men is 151 per 100 000 and 115 per 100 000 for women. In parts of Iran the highest world incidence rates have been recorded of 195 cases per 100 000 for females and 165 per 100 000 for males. These rates have tended to be stable throughout the twentieth century. However, in South Africa there have been significant increases in the last 40 years. This has particularly occurred in black people where incidence rates of 28.4 per 100 000 men and 17.8 per 100 000 women have been recorded. Furthermore, Yang and Davis[5] reported an increase in incidence in black men and women in the USA. This was most marked for squamous cell carcinoma which was 4–5-fold more common, yet the incidence of adenocarcinoma in the black population was 30% that of the white population. The incidence of squamous cell carcinoma in the black population increased by 30% between 1973 and 1982 with a parallel increase for adenocarcinoma in white men. Recent data from the USA show that adenocarcinoma incidence in white men has now surpassed that of squamous cell carcinoma affecting 3.2/100 000. Between 1974 and 1994 there has been a 350% rise in incidence of adenocarcinoma.[6]

Although traditionally oesophageal cancer has occurred in the 7th and 8th decades, in those parts of the world where the disease is becoming more prevalent, the age at diagnosis is decreasing. McGlashan[7] reviewed death certification in South Africa and found very few cases of oesophageal cancer under 40 years of age for 1980–82. However, during 1986–88 8.8% of oesophageal cancer deaths occurred in the 3rd and 4th decades.

These striking variations in incidence and the age of onset which occur in geographically related parts of the world have led to extensive studies searching for common aetiological factors which have resulted in the identification of several premalignant conditions (see Chapter 1).

Aetiology

Squamous cell carcinoma

Worldwide squamous cell carcinoma is the commonest histological subtype. It is found predominantly in the areas of highest incidence. These areas are in those countries of low socioeconomic level where poverty and malnutrition predominate. Aetiological studies in Iran and China have evaluated the identification of oesophagitis as a premalignant lesion. It is a different type of oesophagitis from that found in the West and is often complicated by atrophy and dysplasia (see Chapter 1). It is not usually associated with gastro-oesophageal reflux and is often asymptomatic.

In an attempt to identify the underlying cause of these histological changes Chang-Claude et al.[8] investigated a population of 15–26 year olds in a high-risk area. Using a multivariate case–control analysis they compared a series of factors in those with mild and moderate oesophagitis with those with very mild oesophagitis and normal subjects. Significant changes were associated with ingestion of very hot beverages, a family history of oesophageal cancer, prevalence of oesophagitis among siblings and a low intake of fresh fruits and wheat flour products. Cigarette smoking and the use of cottonseed oil for cooking were usually observed in those with oesophagitis but there was no striking difference according to level of risk.

Other similar studies have identified riboflavin deficiency and vitamin A and C deficiency[9] as risk factors that are particularly important at a young age. Conversely vitamin C intake confers a protective benefit; Hu et al.[10] in a case–control study found that 100 mg vitamin C per day decreased risk by 39%. Overall, those with a nutritionally deficient diet have a higher incidence of oesophageal cancer in the high-risk areas.[11]

Dietary habits and customs are additionally important to nutritional content. Hot drinks and coarse foods have been implicated. In both Iran and China wheat contains silica fibres and millet bran contains silica plates. Furthermore, nitrosamine precursors associated with mouldy or pickled foods are commonly ingested in areas of high risk. Not only do nitrosamines come from foodstuffs but also some other ingested substances. In France apple brandy, in Northern Italy heavy tar-coated cigarettes and in Iran opium smoke are potent sources. The significance of nitrosamines is supported by work in animal models in which ingestion of nitrosamine induces similar lesions to those found in patients in Iran and China.

It has thus been postulated that chronic oesophagitis is the common pathway towards oesophageal cancer. This may be induced directly by mechanical irritation, thermal injury or vitamin deficiencies. Alternatively the inflammatory injury producing oesophagitis increases the sensitivity of the oesophageal mucosa to carcinogens and hence malignant transformation.

Squamous cell carcinoma is also associated with a variety of uncommon conditions that can equally be explained by this hypothesis, relating to some form of inflammatory injury. Oesophageal strictures developing after ingestion of corrosive agents particularly in childhood are associated with a 1000-fold increase in the risk of carcinoma. There is a time delay of 20–40 years after ingestion of the corrosive and as a result tumours are seen at a younger age than normal.

Achalasia is associated but the magnitude of the risk is unclear. Again the risk appears to relate to retention oesophagitis secondary to stasis and exposure to possible carcinogens in fermenting food residue. There is a lead time of approximately 15–20 years and these cases probably warrant long-term surveillance. Treatment of the achalasia does not seem to reduce the risk.

The Plummer Vinson syndrome of dysplasia, iron-deficiency anaemia, koilonychia and oropharyngeal mucosal atrophy is associated with an increased risk of cervical oesophageal cancer. There are associated vitamin deficiencies including riboflavin that predispose to the carcinogenic tendencies already described.

Finally there is a familial tendency suggesting a genetic predisposition. Tylosis palmarum is a rare inherited autosomal dominant condition in which there is a very high incidence of squamous cell cancer. Perhaps of greater significance is the finding of the increased risk in low-risk areas for offspring of parents with oesophageal cancer.[12] There are numerical and structural chromosomal aberrations in patients with a family history not seen in those without a family history.

Adenocarcinoma of the oesophagus

The different populations affected by adenocarcinoma of the oesophagus and the changes in disease pattern over recent years suggest a different aetiology to squamous carcinoma. Although there are ectopic islands of gastric mucosa that in theory can undergo malignant change, the most commonly associated histological change is the development of metaplastic columnar lined epithelium (Barrett's metaplasia) (see Chapter 1). Gastro-oesophageal reflux is now the commonest symptomatic presentation of all conditions affecting the upper gastrointestinal tract. Estimates suggest that 4–9% of all adults experience daily heartburn and up to 20% experience symptoms on a weekly basis. Many are self-treated and do not attend for further investigation so it is difficult to determine the true incidence of Barrett's metaplasia. Endoscopy studies suggest that 3–5% of patients with symptomatic reflux have metaplasia. The overall incidence may be slightly greater as some patients presenting with oesophageal adenocarcinoma have associated columnar epithelium yet have never experienced symptomatic reflux. Results from endoscopy series of all-comers suggest that Barrett's may be seen in 1% of all those undergoing symptomatic examination. Furthermore studies from autopsies of the general population indicate a prevalence of approximately 370/100 000, which is equivalent to 17 times higher than the clinically diagnosed prevalence.[13]

The implication of Barrett's in the aetiology of oesophageal adenocarcinoma arises from a difference in prevalence between the sexes. Barrett's is twice as common in men and men have an 8-fold greater incidence of cancer than women. The median age for developing Barrett's is 40 years and the peak prevalence occurs at just over 60 years. Since oesophageal cancer has a peak incidence at 60 years of age or older, it is likely that Barrett's change will have been present for at least 20 years before cancer diagnosis. Evidence from the Mayo clinic[13] suggests that the mean length of the involved segment of oesophagus was similar at all ages implying that the full extent of the change occurs quickly and then remains stable over many years.

The relationship of GORD and oesophageal adenocarcinoma has been evaluated in case–control studies. Chow *et al.*[14] found a relationship between oesophageal and cardia cancer associated with a past history of oesophageal reflux, hiatus hernia, oesophagitis or dysphagia, with an odds ratio of between 2 and 5. The individual cancer risk is small because of the high frequency of GORD. Barrett's probably represents an intermediate change between GORD and cancer. It is a common finding near to areas of carcinoma occurring in up to 86% of cases.[15]

Despite the association of Barrett's with adenocarcinoma, the outcome for the patient with Barrett's remains an enigma. Survival data for patients with Barrett's metaplasia have shown little difference from the general population. Most patients die from causes other than oesophageal cancer largely reflecting the age and concurrent medical conditions of the patient at diagnosis. From a review of the literature Tytgat[16] estimates that in affected patients the median incidence of cancer was 1 per 100 patient years of follow-up. This may be an overestimate as follow-up in the reviewed series was short. In longer follow-up the rate falls to 1 per 180 patient years. Such data will be considered further in the discussion of screening (see below).

Predisposing factors to malignant transformation include male gender, race (more common in white people), tobacco smoking, alcohol abuse, obesity, length of the columnar lined segment and previous gastric surgery with associated alkaline reflux. Alkaline reflux appears to discriminate between those at risk of progressing from metaplasia and those not progressing.[17] Furthermore antireflux surgery may actually arrest the progression of Barrett's metaplasia and in principle this should reduce the risk of progression to cancer (see Chapter 11).

Gastric cancer

Incidence

Gastric cancer (ICD Code No 151) has shown a dramatic decrease in incidence over the past 100 years. In 1980 the IARC survey documented it as the commonest form of malignancy world-wide accounting for 10.5% of all registered cancers, a total of almost 670 000 cases per year worldwide. The follow-up survey from 1985 showed it to have fallen to second place behind lung cancer yet it still accounts for 755 000 new cases of cancer worldwide each year.[1] Comparison with incidence data shows a decrease from 36 per 100 000 to 20 per 100 000 for men and from 31 to 11 per 100 000 for women between 1920 and 1985[18] in England and Wales. These rates of decline have been similarly documented in other Western series.[19] However, the incidence according to type of country relative to socioeconomic status shows little difference. In 1980 for developed countries, gastric cancer was fourth commonest and for developing countries

for storage and transportation and by the 1950s and 1960s for domestic use. Indeed, the reduction in mortality observed in Japan shows an inverse relationship with the increase in ownership of domestic refrigerators (**Fig. 2.4**).[29] The effect of refrigerators is likely to be 2-fold, increasing the intake of fresh and frozen produce and altering the consumption of salted and pickled foods.

Helicobacter pylori

The Correa hypothesis implicates other factors that may induce gastric mucosa change. The identification and characterisation of the effect of *Helicobacter pylori* on gastric mucosa has raised the potential for a role in gastric carcinogenesis. The initial effect is acute inflammation. Since the infection does not resolve spontaneously, an effect is likely to persist for a long time and may proceed to chronic gastritis and associated mucosal atrophy and intestinal cell metaplasia. Furthermore *H. pylori* induces tissue monocytes to produce reactive oxygen intermediates which are potent carcinogens. In addition infection is associated with a significant reduction in gastric juice ascorbic acid further implicating antioxidant activity.[30]

Evidence for a relationship with gastric cancer comes from epidemiological studies identifying previous *H. pylori* infection by the detection of IgG antibodies to *H. pylori* in sera. In South America in areas with a high incidence of gastric cancer, *H. pylori* infection is endemic particularly in the young.[31] In rural China there is a significant correlation between gastric cancer mortality and *H. pylori* infection.[32] Communities throughout the world selected for their gastric cancer rates have been randomly examined for *H. pylori* infections. A significant correlation was found between *H. pylori* seropositivity and both incidence and mortality of gastric cancer.[33] These authors concluded that there was an approximately 6-fold increased risk of gastric cancer in populations with 100% *H. pylori* infection compared with populations that have no infection. Furthermore, the presence of *H. pylori* in poor communities reflects the established associations between low socioeconomic groups and gastric cancer. As a result of all of these and other

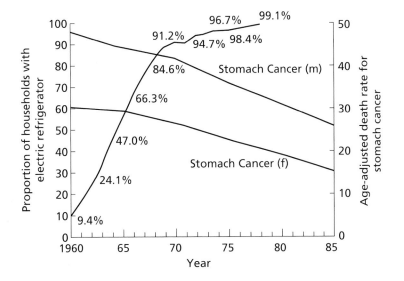

Figure 2.4
Annual trends for proportion of households with electric refrigeration and age-adjusted death rates for stomach cancer in Japan, 1966–1985.[29]

findings, the International Agency for Research on Cancer has classified *H. pylori* as a group I carcinogen and a definite cause of gastric cancer in humans.

Although the relationship between *H. pylori* and gastric cancer has been established[34] there remains some conflicting evidence. Firstly several at-risk populations do not have high *H. pylori* infection rates. Secondly, there is a significant difference in disease pattern from duodenal ulceration that is strongly associated with *H. pylori*.[35] Finally, there is an inverse relationship between the rate of *H. pylori* infection and the increasing severity of precancerous lesions; chronic gastritis (72% *H. pylori* positive), intestinal metaplasia (63%), dysplasia (44%) and carcinoma (35%).[36]

Nevertheless, there is sufficiently strong evidence to propose a role for *H. pylori* in gastric cancer development. Simple eradication of the infection may have a major impact on gastric cancer incidence. However, this has major methodological implications as *H. pylori* seropositivity is very common and many of those infected are unlikely to progress. Targeting of high-risk populations for eradication programmes may be of importance and a number of studies are currently investigating such an approach. As with other factors it is likely that *H. pylori* is an initiator for gastric carcinogenesis and acts in combination with other agents.

Oesophago-gastric and cardia cancers

The incidence data have shown that oesophago-gastric cancers are slowly merging to occur principally at the cardia. These are adenocarcinomas and many authorities are beginning to consider them as separate tumours from more proximal oesophageal cancers and more distal gastric cancers. Siewert and Stein[37] have proposed a classification of these tumours, describing them in three groups. Type I is adenocarcinoma of the distal oesophagus which usually arises from an area of Barrett's metaplasia and which may infiltrate the oesophago-gastric junction from above. Type II is true carcinoma of the cardia arising from the cardiac epithelium or short segments with intestinal metaplasia at the oesophago-gastric junction, often referred to as 'junctional carcinoma'. Type III is subcardial gastric carcinoma that infiltrates the oesophago-gastric junction and distal oesophagus from below.

Although there are a number of common features shared by these tumour types, there are some important differences. Type I cancers are more common in men and are associated with hiatus hernia, a long history of GORD and the presence of Barrett's metaplasia. There are also differences in growth pattern and direction of lymphatic spread, which have important consequences on treatment (see Chapters 5 and 6).

Mass surveys have demonstrated that cardia adenocarcinoma has a high incidence in areas where oesophageal cancer is common.[38] The natural history of the two sites appears to be similar. Guanrei *et al.*[39] reported on a group of patients with early oesophageal squamous carcinoma and early adenocarcinoma of the cardia who refused any treatment. Progression to advanced disease was similar at 4–5 years. Survival from diagnosis was also similar with a median of 74 months. Aetiologically there may also be a difference in *Helicobacter* infection which is less likely in cardia tumours. Lifestyle may be equally relevant. Powell and McConkey[4] demonstrated that the increase of adenocarcinoma of the lower third of the oesophagus and the cardia was mainly in social classes I and II, i.e. professional and managerial occupations.

Such evidence suggests that the tumours are similar. This has a significant implication for management, as each site should be considered in a similar manner. Furthermore, with the projected increases in incidence there are significant effects on workload and health-care planning. The separation of management and treatment of oesophageal and gastric cancer should no longer occur, particularly if improvement in overall outcome is to be achieved. These cancers therefore need to be assessed by the same multidisciplinary team.

Screening for oesophageal and gastric cancer

Screening programmes for any disease are dependent on a number of criteria. First, the disease must be common in the target population. A reliable and accurate test that is as sensitive and specific as possible is required. The test should be acceptable to the screened population. There should be an effective treatment for the screened abnormality with minimum morbidity and mortality. Finally, not only does the treatment need to show an improvement in results but implementation of the screening programme should also result in an overall benefit for the screened population.

The worldwide differences in incidence of oesophageal and gastric cancer allow the implementation of screening programmes for asymptomatic populations only in those areas where the incidence is high. However, lessons from these programmes have increased knowledge of natural history and have allowed high-risk groups to be targeted in low-risk areas in order to detect disease at an earlier stage.

Oesophageal cancer screening

Asymptomatic screening

Evaluation of asymptomatic screening for carcinomas of the oesophagus has centred on those parts of China with highest incidence. The screening test involves swallowing a small deflated balloon which is then inflated at the lower end of the oesophagus. The balloon surface is covered with a fine mesh; on withdrawal from the oesophagus, this scrapes the mucosa to collect cells. A cytological smear is then made from the scrapings for microscopic examination. Those individuals found to have abnormalities are then subjected to endoscopy and appropriate biopsy. Radiology has very little place. In 132 subjects with early oesophageal cancer detected in this way 26% had normal radiological appearances.[40]

The efficiency of this technique has had varying reports. Reviewing data based on 500 000 examinations, Shu[41] suggested an accuracy for the differentiation of benign from malignant of 90%. Mass surveys have shown that 73.8% of detected cancers were either *in situ* or minimally invasive. In a provincial review, Huang[42] reported on 17 000 examinations screened during a one-year period. Abnormalities were found in 68% of the population, with low-grade dysplasia in

37%, high-grade in 26% and *in situ* cancer 2%. A group with high-grade dysplasia were followed for up to eight years. Regression to normal or low-grade change was observed in 40%, 20% remained as high grade, 20% fluctuated between high and low grade and 20% developed cancer. In the absence of dysplasia, 0.12% developed cancer. Progression from dysplasia to *in situ* cancer occurred over 3–12 years and from *in situ* to invasive cancer over 3–7 years. Tumour risk was consistent with a known distribution of middle third chronic oesophagitis in 76%. It would seem that the duration of severe dysplasia is the greatest risk for malignant transformation. Follow-up by endoscopy is, therefore, important and in order to ensure biopsy of the same site vital stains have been used. Huang[43] reported that staining with toluidine blue was effective for identifying neoplastic epithelium; 84% of cancers were identified in positively staining areas.

The problem associated with this approach is the management of dysplasia. Oesophageal dysplasia is a dynamic process with both spontaneous regression and progression. Furthermore, even if *in situ* cancer develops, progress to advanced disease is often prolonged and may be associated with prolonged survival. In one series of 23 untreated patients, 11 developed late-stage disease at a mean of 55 months. In the remainder there was no change for over 6 years and the 5-year survival of the group was 78%.[44] Five-year survival needs to be considered with caution as detection of asymptomatic slowly progressive disease introduces lead-time bias and this can falsely give the impression that treatment results for screen-detected cases are better.

As a result a UICC recommendation has been to limit oesophageal cancer screening to areas of high risk.[45] The aim is to identify the natural history of dysplasia more completely. Common standards are required for the classification of dysplasia to identify those changes with greatest risk. Once the assessment is more reliable, control studies should be developed to determine whether screening intervention could reduce mortality for oesophageal cancer.

Symptomatic screening

Symptomatic endoscopic screening is useful for those individuals whose symptom profile suggests a high risk for oesophageal cancer. Thus for tylosis, achalasia and corrosive stricture, regular endoscopies are recommended. This should start 10 years after diagnosis for achalasia and ingestion of the corrosive agent.

Barrett's metaplasia is usually combined with dysplasia prior to development of invasive malignancy. Surveillance programmes have, therefore, been instituted that attempt to diagnose malignant transformation at an early, preinvasive stage. Current emphasis is on repeated biopsy although there is much interest in gene alterations, which may occur before cancer develops. There appears to be a time scale of progressive change from low- to high-grade dysplasia over a median of 29 months and from high-grade dysplasia to cancer over 14 months.

The interval between endoscopies is contentious. A consensus from the International Society of Diseases of the Esophagus[46] suggests that all patients with Barrett's should be considered for surveillance irrespective of the length of the abnormal segment. Biopsies should be taken at 2 cm intervals from all quadrants of the circumference of the oesophagus.[47] In the absence of dysplasia endoscopy and biopsy should be repeated every 2 years. In those with low-grade dysplasia annual endoscopy and biopsy should be undertaken. High-grade dysplasia warrants a review of the endoscopy, repeat biopsy and if confirmed then careful consideration should be given to resection. In such patients re-evaluation will demonstrate malignant change in up to 60%. Patients managed in this way have an overall survival that is superior to those with cancer in a segment of Barrett's oesophagus not detected by surveillance.[48]

Although such a policy provides appropriate guidance, there are areas that warrant careful consideration. Low-grade dysplasia can be confused with inflammatory atypia. This is likely to reverse after treatment with acid suppression. Thus patients diagnosed with low-grade dysplasia at their first endoscopy should receive full acid suppression for 3 months prior to re-examination. Regression of dysplasia may occur and the frequency of surveillance may be adjusted accordingly. In those with high-grade dysplasia the decision to recommend resection should be considered in the context of likely surgical outcome. Such patients should be fully appraised of the risks of the procedure in terms of both morbidity and mortality together with the risks of not undergoing resection. Most would therefore recommend that surveillance should only be undertaken in those fit for radical surgery and the majority of surveillance programmes start at age 50.

In practice surveillance programmes have had varying success. For example, Wright *et al.*[49] found an incidence of one cancer per 59 male and 167 female patient-years follow-up. They subsequently reported a definite financial advantage by screening at-risk males compared with diagnosis made on symptomatic presentation. Macdonald *et al.*[50] were less convinced as from their experience of following 144 patients with Barrett's metaplasia alone over a 10-year period they only detected one case of cancer. Ferraris *et al.*[51] reported similarly, yet achieved equivalent figures to Wright *et al.* when only those with dysplasia were included.

Endoscopic appearance of Barrett's oesophagus

The ability to recognise Barrett's oesophagus is fundamental to diagnosis, surveillance and proposed approaches to treatment. This ability does require experience, as appearances at the oesophago-gastric junction can be confusing.

Most endoscopists will agree with identification of the proximal limit of the gastric rugae and the junction with pale oesophageal mucosa. Oesophageal columnar metaplasia is recognised by a salmon pink colour that is less glossy and paler than gastric mucosa. There may be residual patches of squamous pale mucosa to mark the original squamo-columnar junction. There are often varying degrees of inflammation depending on the degree of reflux damage. This includes patches of erythema and superficial ulceration, which will resolve after appropriate acid suppression thus leaving only the metaplastic change. Hiatus hernia can confuse as the lower end of the hernia may be mistaken for the oesophago-gastric junction. Partial deflation may aid identification of gastric folds in the hernia and hence the junction.

The extent of the metaplastic change is variable. Short or ultra short (<2 cm) segment change presents with islands of pinkish mucosa extending into the squamous layer. In longer segments the pink mucosal appearances extend for a variable distance even up to the upper oesophageal sphincter. Metaplasia may also only affect one side of the oesophagus. Assessment of the extent can be difficult particularly with short segment change and may vary from one examination to the next. The specific identification of columnar change can be enhanced with vital dyes such as methylene blue that may also help detection of dysplasia, which can otherwise be very difficult. Early malignant change has been classified similarly to early gastric cancer. Type I is elevated or protruding and can be high (>3 mm) or low (<3 mm). Type II is superficial or flat and Type III is depressed or excavated.

Gastric cancer screening

Asymptomatic

The size of gastric cancer as a public health problem in Japan led to the development during the 1960s of a mass screening programme for all men over the age of 40 years. The programme has been based on double-contrast radiology with endoscopy assessment of any abnormalities.[52] Members of the public are invited to undergo radiology in mobile units at which seven films are taken after the ingestion of an effervescent contrast agent. Screening is undertaken annually or biannually depending on the area of Japan and the associated risk of disease. Government recommendations set a target of 30% for the annual examination rate. In 1985 over 5 million were examined representing 13% of the at-risk population. Therein lies one of the problems with any screening programme, namely the cooperation of the public. Despite recognition of gastric cancer as a public health problem, attendance for screening is low.

Screening in this way detects disease at an early stage. Approximately half the cases diagnosed are limited to the mucosa or submucosa (early gastric cancer). Interestingly half of those detected are symptomatic and an alternative approach could be envisaged. In keeping with the criteria for a screening programme there has been a highly significant decrease in mortality since mass screening was introduced. However, as already discussed there may be other reasons for the decline in mortality.

Oshima et al.[53] compared screened and unscreened populations to determine whether screening was important over and above the other influences on the decrease in mortality. In a case–controlled study they found that the risk of dying from gastric cancer among screened cases was at least 50% less than that for non-screened cases. Other Japanese groups have reported similar results.

However, the actual effect on mortality remains to be proven as none of the studies have been randomised or controlled. Again, as with oesophageal screening there is the risk of lead-time bias. Nevertheless, as Hisamichi observes, the Japanese could not wait to see if their incidence would follow the trends of decreasing incidence observed in the West as they wished to speed up the decline in mortality.

As a result the UICC recommended that studies should be continued in Japan to resolve the problem, but screening in this way should not be adopted as public health programmes in other parts of the world.[45] Despite this recommendation other countries have developed similar programmes to cope with their high incidence. In Chile, for example, where incidence is 75% that of Japan, there has been an increase in early detection after the introduction of mass screening.[54] Furthermore, the Chileans have found that mass contrast radiology is efficient despite its critics. They recommend its use as an inexpensive assessment particularly in poor countries with high risk.

Symptomatic screening

In areas of low risk, asymptomatic screening is not justifiable. There is a small group who should be considered for regular assessment by virtue of their concurrent conditions. Pernicious anaemia imposes a 3- to 4-fold risk over the normal population. However, screening of such individuals may be limited, as in one survey of gastric cancer 1.3% had pernicious anaemia. Patients who have undergone gastric resection for benign disease have been considered to have a greatest risk possibly because of increased alkaline reflux. However, again this group provides only a small portion of gastric cancers detected in a screening programme.[55]

Since half of those that were detected in Japan through screening had symptoms, efforts have been made to further evaluate symptoms in low-risk populations. In the UK increased availability of endoscopy has been assessed as an influence on gastric cancer diagnosis.[56] However, large numbers of endoscopies in the population with dyspepsia have been performed without significant findings. Many of the diagnoses have been of functional disorders. Subsequently groups have assessed symptomatic scoring symptoms to form a profile of the at-risk patient.[57,58] Unfortunately these profiles have tended to identify only those with advanced disease or have proven too cumbersome for routine use.

Since EGC in the UK tends to peak in incidence approximately 10 years younger than advanced disease[59] and since dyspepsia as a new symptom is associated with early disease or dysplasia[60] those over 40 with dyspepsia can be considered as a high-risk group. A recent study evaluated endoscopic examination of such a group of patients before any treatment had been started. During a 4-year period 2600 patients were examined from a 100 000 population. Gastric cancer was diagnosed in 57 (2%) with 12 (22%) being limited to the mucosa and submucosa. In a further 49 (19%) precursor lesions were identified in whom six were subsequently found to have early gastric cancer on follow-up endoscopy.[61] Those with gastric cancer proceeded to resection and comparison of this group with those diagnosed in the five years prior to the study shows an overall 20% survival advantage for the 'screened' population[62] (**Fig. 2.5**). This survival benefit suggests application of similar schemes to other areas of low incidence.

The problem with the approach in this study remains the large number of examinations for limited clinical benefit to the patient. Certainly a diagnosis can be achieved and management pursued appropriately. Indeed, this has significant health economic implications particularly for prescribing practice. However, there are limitations as regards early diagnosis of cancer. It remains to be seen if improving the accessibility of symptomatic patients to diagnostic services as currently proposed in the UK will actually affect outcome by increasing the numbers with early disease. There may be a hidden benefit of increasing awareness of doctors and patients alike to pursue significant symptoms which hitherto have been ignored. Christie *et al.*[63] have reviewed the symptom profile of a series of young patients in an attempt to improve detection rates and reduce the number of examinations. In 25 patients under 55 years of age with gastric cancer,

Figure 2.5
Survival after early detection of gastric cancer (study population) compared with historical control population (pre-study population).

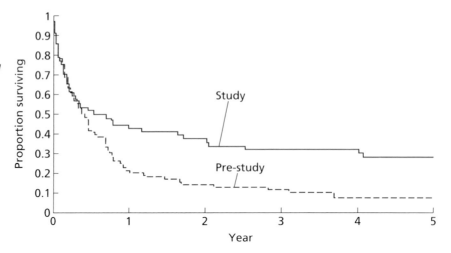

24 had dyspeptic symptoms that were complicated by alarm symptoms such as weight loss, dysphagia, anaemia or an abdominal mass. As only one of their patients with gastric cancer had uncomplicated dyspepsia, they argue that early endoscopic assessment should be restricted to those under 55 with complicated dyspepsia. A concern with this approach, however, is the potential for missing an early oesophageal cancer presenting with reflux-type symptoms.

A variety of markers have been assessed to aid prediction of significant gastric mucosal change and so enable more specific use of endoscopy. Tumour markers such as the oncofetal antigens have been extensively assessed. However, none have the required sensitivity or specificity for either early or advanced disease.

Serum levels of gastric hormones have been investigated as changes in pepsinogen and gastrin levels appear to relate to mucosal change. Two types of pepsinogen have been identified as having a potential role: pepsinogen I arising from cells of the gastric body and pepsinogen II from cells of the body and antrum. Stemmerman et al.[64] found low pepsinogen I levels to be specific for extensive intestinal metaplasia. Furthermore, low serum pepsinogen I and raised gastrin levels were found in pernicious anaemia complicated by gastric atrophy.[65] Kekki et al.[66] have suggested that low serum pepsinogen I is useful for screening as it is markedly reduced in atrophy of gastric body mucosa.

In gastric cancer low pepsinogen I is found with a moderate elevation in pepsinogen II. A ratio of the two has been proposed as a screening test.[67,68] Farinati et al.[69] found similarly for pepsinogen levels but also found reduced gastrin concentrations. This equally has been assessed as a ratio with reasonable sensitivity and specificity. However, although there appears to be a relationship with prediction for precursor changes or malignancy, when these parameters have been assessed in an early detection programme, limitations were observed because of false positive values.[70] Recently Kitahara et al.[71] have reported a sensitivity and specificity of pepsinogen screening for gastric cancer of 84.6% and 73.5% respectively. They also found limitations such that cancers in combination with mild gastric atrophy were overlooked, as were small cancers in the gastric fundus.

The role of *H. pylori* as a marker for endoscopy is receiving considerable attention. Both serological estimation and breath tests depending on exhalation of urea have been investigated. Serology has been assessed for concordance with the underlying histological presence of *H. pylori*. Farinati *et al.*[36] found 82% agreement between a measurable antibody response and histological evidence of *H. pylori* infection. Urea breath tests are in routine use in *Helicobacter* eradication programmes for duodenal ulceration. Again the problem is one of specificity and sensitivity.

H. pylori seropositivity does not necessarily imply active infection. Equally seropositivity is a common finding and may not be specific for the at-risk population. It increases with age and to a certain extent parallels gastric atrophy, which is equally an age-related phenomenon and in the majority does not progress to cancer. However, evidence of infection at an early age does identify a group at risk and therefore worthy of consideration for endoscopic follow-up. Whiting *et al.*[72] reported a retrospective analysis of *H. pylori* seropositivity in cancer patients compared with a group of undiagnosed dyspeptics. Although the cancer patients were significantly more likely to be seropositive, this was very much site related. Cardia cancers were not usually seropositive. Thus any screening programme based on *H. pylori* serology would miss the proximal tumours, which are currently the more common cancers. Further investigation is required and longitudinal studies may resolve the issue of whether patients with *H. pylori* seropositivity warrant close endoscopic follow-up.

Endoscopic appearance of early gastric cancer

The experience of the endoscopist is critical. In the early phase a low threshold for biopsy of any abnormality is appropriate. Improvements in resolution with video endoscopy have aided diagnosis of small lesions, as has the descriptive morphology from Japanese studies.

As well as producing a significant influence on the way in which the disease is managed in Japan, the Japanese screening approach has enabled greater understanding of the endoscopic appearances of early gastric cancer and precursor lesions. Macroscopically EGC has been described as protruding (type I), superficial (type II) and excavated (type III).[73] Type II is further divided into elevated (IIa), flat (IIb) and depressed (IIc) (**Fig. 2.6**). A further subclassification of the type I/IIa (protruding lesion) has been designed – sessile (I), semi-spherical (II), spherical (III) and pedunculated (IV). Pedunculated lesions less than 20 mm are usually benign, but sessile and semi-spherical are usually malignant. Spherical lesions greater than 10 mm and all lesions greater than 20 mm are likely to be malignant.

Knowledge of the morphological appearances is useful in areas of high incidence where screening is active. However, for areas of low incidence where more often than not type IIc or III lesions are seen, more practical advice has been given by Sano *et al.*[74] An elevated lesion is likely to be limited to the mucosa if the surface is regular and not ulcerated. Small depressed lesions that are shallow with either slight or no gastric fold convergence are likely to be mucosal. However, more depressed lesions with a stiff base and irregular nodularity and fold convergence will penetrate at least to the submucosa. Finally, irregular ulcerating lesions are most likely to show full thickness wall penetration.

Screening assessment can be supplemented by endoluminal ultrasound (EUS). Experienced endoscopists with EUS can identify the four layers of the gastric

Figure 2.6
Classification of macroscopic subtypes of early gastric cancer.

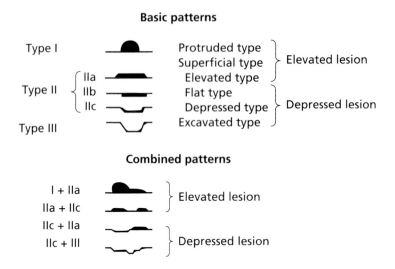

wall.[75] Shallow lesions are usually straightforward to assess. However, limitations are inherent as fibrosis secondary to ulceration can be difficult to differentiate from penetration by tumour.

The identification and review of precursor lesions has equally been advanced by experience from screening. Areas of gastric atrophy, intestinal metaplasia and dysplasia need to be actively surveyed. Again, as with the oesophagus the changes are in a dynamic equilibrium and spontaneous regression can occur. However, once severe dysplasia has been identified on more than one biopsy on two separate occasions, surgery should be recommended, as progression to cancer is inevitable.[76]

In order to ensure the same site is assessed, vital dye sprays have been used during endoscopy. Intestinal metaplasia shows highly reproducible rates of positive staining after spraying with methylene blue.[77] The frequency of repeat endoscopy is contentious. However, the increased risk of intestinal metaplasia type III (colonic type) and dysplasia merits repeat endoscopy every 12 months.[78]

Summary and future

Oesophageal cancer incidence is increasing with a particular change in adenocarcinoma. Although gastric cancer is decreasing, the workload is staying constant. Management principles of the two diseases particularly in the developed world are converging. Thus distinction between the two diseases is becoming blurred and this has important implications for health planning.

In developing countries the results of primary and secondary prevention programmes are eagerly awaited to determine specifically if *H. pylori* eradication and improvements in diet can reduce incidence. In developed countries the role of *H. pylori* remains to be evaluated particularly as an indicator of early diagnosis. The concentration of disease at the oesophageal hiatus strongly implicates reflux as an important factor. However which patients are at high risk, requiring careful assessment and review, remains to be established. It may be that with appropriate intervention those with complications of reflux may be spared the development of invasive malignancy.

The poor end results of the past remain as potent influences on the philosophy towards treatment of gastro-oesophageal cancer. Greater appreciation of the curability of early disease by both medical and public education must become a priority.

References

1. Parkin DM, Pisani P, Ferlay J. Estimates of the worldwide incidence of eighteen major cancers in 1985. Int J Cancer 1993; 54:594–606.

2. Cheng KK, Day NE. Oesophageal cancer in Britain. Br Med J 1992; 304:711.

3. Matthews HR, Waterhouse JAH, Powell J et al. Cancer of the oesophagus. Clinical Cancer Monographs vol. 1. London: Macmillan, 1987.

4. Powell J, McConkey CC. The rising trend in oesophageal adenocarcinoma and gastric cardia. Eur J Cancer Prevent 1992; 1:265–9.

5. Yang PC, Davis S. Incidence of cancer of the oesophagus in the US by histologic type. Cancer 1988; 61:612–7.

6. Devesa SS, Blot WJ, Fraumeni JF. Changing patterns in the incidence of esophageal and gastric carcinoma in the United States. Cancer 1998; 83:2049–53.

7. McGlashan WD. Oesophageal cancer in the black peoples of South Africa 1980–82. South African Journal of Science 1988; 84:92–9.

8. Chang-Claude JC, Wahrendorf J, Liang QS et al. An epidemiological study of precursor lesions of oesophageal cancer among young persons in a high risk population in Huixian, China. Cancer Res 1990; 50:2268–74.

9. Iran – IARC Study Group. Oesophageal cancer studies in the Caspian Littoral of Iran: results of population studies. A prodrome. J Natl Cancer Inst 1979; 59:1127–38.

10. Hu J, Nyren O, Wolk A et al. Risk factors for oesophageal cancer in northeast China. Int J Cancer 1994; 57:38–46.

11. Yang CS. Research on oesophageal cancer in China: a review. Cancer Res 1980; 40:2633–44.

12. Li JY, Ershaw AG, Chen ZJ et al. A case-control study of cancer of the oesophagus and gastric cardia in Linxian. Int J Cancer 1989; 43:755–61.

13. Cameron AJ. Epidemiology of columnar-lined of oesophagus and adenocarcinoma. Gastroenterol Clin North America 1997; 26:487–94.

14. Chow WH, Finkle WD, McLaughlin JK et al. The relation of gastro-oesophageal reflux disease and its treatment to adenocarcinomas of the oesophagus and gastric cardia. JAMA 1995; 274:474–7.

15. Haggitt RC, Tryzelaar J, Ellis FH. Adenocarcinoma complicating columnar epithelium-lined (Barrett's) oesophagus. Am J Clin Path 1978; 70:1–5.

16. Tytgat GNJ. Does endoscopic surveillance in oesophageal columnar metaplasia (Barrett's Oesophagus) have any real value? Endoscopy 1995; 27:19–26.

17. Attwood SEA, Ball CS, Barlow AP et al. Role of intragastric and intraoesophageal alkalinisation in the genesis of complications in Barrett's columnar lined lower oesophagus. Gut 1993; 34:11–15.

18. Davis DL, Hoel D, Fox J et al. International trends in cancer mortality in France, West Germany, Italy, Japan, England and Wales and the USA. Lancet 1990; 336:474–81.

19. Howson CP, Hiyama T, Wynder EL. The decline in gastric cancer: epidemiology of an unplanned triumph. Epidemiol Reviews 1986; 8:1–27.

20. Parkin DM, Laara E, Muir CS. Estimates of the worldwide frequency of sixteen major cancers in 1980. Int J Cancer 1988; 41:184–97.

21. Fielding JWL, Powell J, Allum WH et al. Cancer of the stomach. Clinical Cancer Monographs vol. 3. London: Macmillan, 1989.

22. Allum WH, Powell DJ, McConkey CC et al. Gastric cancer: a 25-year review. Br J Surgery 1989; 76:535–40.

23. Antonioli DA, Goldman H. Changes in the location and type of gastric adenocarcinoma. Cancer 1982; 50:775–81.

24. Paterson IM, Easton DF, Corbishley CM, Gazet J-C. Changing distribution of adenocarcinoma of the stomach. Br J Surg 1987; 74:481–2.

25. Sedgwick DM, Akoh JA, Macintyre IMC. Gastric cancer in Scotland: changing epidemiology, unchanging workload. BMJ 1991; 302:1305–7.

26. Correa P, Sasano N, Stemmerman N et al. Pathology of gastric carcinoma in Japanese populations: comparisons between Miyagi prefecture, Japan and Hawaii. J Natl Cancer Inst 1973; 51:1449–59.

27. Correa P. A human model of gastric carcinogenesis. Cancer Res 1988; 48:3554–60.

28. Munoz N, Vivas J, Buiatti E *et al.* Chemoprevention trial of precancerous lesions of the stomach in Venezuela. Eur J Cancer Prevention 1993; 2 (Suppl 1): 5.

29. Hirayama T. Actions suggested by gastric cancer epidemiological studies in Japan. In: Gastric Carcinogenesis. P.I. Reed and M.J. Hill (eds.) Amsterdam: Excerpta Medica, 1988; pp. 209–28.

30. Sobala GM, Schorah CJ, Shires S. Gastric ascorbic acid concentration and acute *Helicobacter pylori* infection. Rev Esp Enf Digest 1990; 78 (Suppl 1): 63.

31. Correa P, Fox J, Fontham E *et al. Helicobacter pylori* and gastric carcinoma. Serum antibody prevalence in populations with contrasting cancer risks. Cancer 1990; 66:2569–74.

32. Forman D, Sitas F, Newell DG *et al.* Geographic association of *Helicobacter pylori* antibody prevalence and gastric cancer mortality in rural China. Int J Cancer 1990; 46:608–11.

33. Eurogast Study Group. An international association between *Helicobacter pylori* infection and gastric cancer. Lancet 1993; 341:1359–62.

 34. Forman D, Newell DG, Fullerton F *et al.* Association between infection with *Helicobacter pylori* and risk of gastric cancer: evidence from a prospective investigation. Br Med J 1991; 302:1302–5.

35. Forman D. *Helicobacter pylori* infection: a novel risk factor in the aetiology of gastric cancer. Journal of the National Cancer Institute 1991; 83:1702–3.

36. Farinati F, Valiante F, Germania B, Della Libera G, Baffa E, Rugge M *et al.* Prevalence of *Helicobacter pylori* infection in patients with precancerous changes and gastric cancer. Eur J Cancer Prevention 1993; 2:321–6.

 37. Siewert JR, Stein HJ. Classification of adenocarcinoma of the oesophago-gastric junction. Br J Surg 1998; 85:1457–9.

38. Guanrei Y, Sunglian Q. Incidence rate of adenocarcinoma of the gastric cardia and endoscopic classification of early cardial carcinoma in Henan province, the People's Republic of China. Endoscopy 1987; 19:7–10.

39. Guanrei Y, Songliang Q, He H *et al.* Natural history of early oesophageal squamous carcinoma and early adenocarcinoma of the gastric cardia in the People's Republic of China. Endoscopy 1988; 20:95–8.

40. Wang G-Q. Endoscopic diagnosis of early oesophageal carcinoma. JR Soc Med 1981; 74:502–3.

41. Shu Y-J. Cytopathology of the oesophagus. Acta Cytol 1983; 27:7–16.

42. Huang G-J. Recognition and treatment of the early lesion. In: International Trends: General Thoracic Surgery 4. Oesophageal cancer. NC Delarae, EW Wilkins, Wong J (eds.). St Louis: Mosby, 1988; pp. 149–52.

43. Huang GJ. Early detection and surgical treatment of oesophageal carcinoma. Jpn J Surg 1981; 11:399–405.

44. Yanjun M, Li G, Xianzhil G *et al.* Detection and natural progression of early oesophageal carcinoma – preliminary communication. JR Soc Med 1981; 74:884–6.

45. Chamberlain J, Day NE, Hakama M, Miller AB, Prorok PC. UICC workshop of the project on evaluation of screening programmes for gastrointestinal cancer. Int J Cancer 1986; 37:329–34.

46. Stein HJ *et al.* Oesophageal cancer: screening and surveillance. Dis Esoph 1996; 9 (Suppl 1): 3–19.

47. Reid BJ, Weinstein WM, Lewin KJ *et al.* Endoscopic biopsy can detect high-grade dysplasia or early adenocarcinoma in Barrett's oesophagus without grossly recognisable neoplastic lesions. Gastroenterology 1988; 94:81–90.

48. Peters JH, Clark GWB, Ireland AP *et al.* Outcome of adenocarcinoma arising in Barrett's oesophagus in endoscopically surveyed and non-surveyed patients. J Thorac Cardiovasc Surg 1994; 108:813–22.

49. Wright TA, Gray MR, Morris AI *et al.* Cost effectiveness of detecting Barrett's cancer. Gut 1996; 39:574–9.

50. Macdonald CE, Wicks AC, Playford RJ. Ten years experience of screening patients with Barrett's oesophagus in a university teaching hospital. Gut 1998; 41:303–7.

51. Ferraris R, Bonelli L, Conio M *et al.* Incidence of Barrett's adenocarcinoma in an Italian population: an endoscopic surveillance programme. European J Gastro Hepatol 1997; 9:881–5.

 52. Hisamichi S. Screening for gastric cancer. World J Surgery 1989; 13:31–7.

53. Oshima A, Hirata N, Ubakata T *et al.* Evaluation of a mass screening programme for stomach cancer with a case-control study design. Int J Cancer 1986; 38:829–34.

54. Llorens P. Gastric cancer mass survey in Chile. Sem Surg Oncol 1991; 7: 339–43.

55. Oshima A, Sakagami F, Hawai A *et al.* Evaluation of a mass screening programme for gastric cancer. In: Epidemiology of Stomach Cancer (WHO-CC Monograph) Hirayama T (ed.). Tokyo: WHO, 1977; pp. 35–45.

56. Gear MWL, Barnes RJ. Endoscopic studies of dyspepsia in a general practice. BMJ 1980; 280:1136–7.

57. Mann J, Holdstock G, Herman M, Machin D, Loehry CA. Scoring system to improve cost-

effectiveness of open access endoscopy. BMJ 1983; 287:937–40.

58. Davenport PM, Morgan AG, Darkborough A, De Dombal FT. Can preliminary screening of dyspeptic patients allow more effective use of investigational techniques? BMJ 1985; 290:217–20.

59. Fielding JWL, Ellis DJ, Jones BG et al. Natural history of 'early' gastric cancer: results of a 10-year regional survey. Br Med J 1980; 281:965–7.

60. De Dombal FT, Price AB, Thompson H et al. The British Society of Gastroenterology early gastric cancer/dysplasia survey: an interim report. Gut 1990; 31:115–20.

 61. Hallissey MT, Allum WH, Jewkes AJ et al. Early detection of gastric cancer. Br Med J 1990; 301:513–5.

62. Hallissey MT, Jewkes AJ, Allum WH et al. The impact of the dyspepsia study on deaths from gastric cancer. In: Nishi M, Sugano H, Takahashi T (eds). International Gastric Cancer Congress, Bologna. 1995; vol. 1.

63. Christie J, Shepherd NA, Codling BW et al. Gastric cancer below the age of 55: implications for screening patients with uncomplicated dyspepsia. Gut 1997; 41:513–7.

64. Stemmerman GM, Ishidata T, Samloff IM et al. Intestinal metaplasia of the stomach in Hawaii and Japan. Am J Dig Dis 1978; 23:815–20.

65. Varis K, Samloff IM, Ihamaki T et al. An appraisal of tests for severe atrophic gastritis in relatives of patients with pernicious anaemia. Dig Dis Sci 1979; 24:187–91.

66. Kekki M, Samloff IM, Varis K, Ihamaki T. Serum pepsinogen I and serum gastrin in the screening of severe atrophic corpus gastritis. Scand J Gastroenterol 1991; 26 (Suppl 186): 109–16.

67. Nomura AMY, Stemmerman GM, Samloff IM. Serum pepsinogen I as a predictor of stomach cancer. Ann Int Med 1980; 93:537–40.

68. Huang SC, Miki K, Furihata C et al. Enzyme linked immunosorbent assays for serum pepsinogens I & II using monoclonal antibodies – with data on peptic ulcer and gastric cancer. Clin Chim Acta 1988; 175:37–50.

69. Farinati F, Di Mario F, Plebani M et al. Pepsinogen A/pepsinogen C or pepsinogen A multiplied by gastrin in the diagnosis of gastric cancer? It J Gastroenterol 1991; 23:194–6.

70. Hallissey MT, Allum WH, Fielding JWL. Serum screening tests for gastric cancer and high risk groups. Euro J Surg Oncol 1986; 12:398.

71. Kitahara F, Kobayashi K, Sato T et al. Accuracy of screening for gastric cancer using serum pepsinogen concentrations. Gut 1999; 44:693–7.

72. Whiting JL, Hallissey MT, Fielding JWL et al. Screening for gastric cancer by *Helicobacter pylori* serology: a retrospective study. Br J Surg 1998; 85:408–11.

73. Murakami T. Pathomorphological diagnosis. Definition and gross classification of early gastric cancer. In: Early Gastric Cancer, Gann Monograph on Cancer Research 11. T. Murakami (ed.). Tokyo: University of Tokyo Press, 1971, pp. 53–66.

74. Sano T, Okuyama Y, Kobori O et al. Early gastric cancer: endoscopic diagnosis of depth of invasion. Dig Dis Science 1990; 35:1340–4.

75. Tio TL, Schowink MH, Cikot RJML et al. Preoperative TNM classification of gastric carcinoma by endosonography in comparison with the pathological TNM system: a prospective study of 72 cases. Hepatogastroenterol 1989; 36:51–6.

76. Landsdown M, Quirke P, Dixon MF et al. High grade dysplasia of the gastric mucosa: a marker for gastric carcinoma. Gut 1990; 31:977–83.

77. Suzuki S, Suzuki H, Endo M et al. Endoscopic dyeing method for diagnosis of early cancer and intestinal metaplasia of the stomach. Endoscopy 1973; 5:124–9.

78. Rokkas T, Filipe MI, Sladen GE. Detection of an increased incidence of early gastric cancer in patients with intestinal metaplasia type III who are closely followed up. Gut 1991; 32:1110–3.

3 Staging of oesophageal and gastric cancer

Jonathan I. Ferguson
Simon Paterson-Brown

INTRODUCTION

Accurate preoperative staging of patients with oesophageal and gastric cancer is essential in order to identify which patients should undergo surgery, and if so which procedure is the most appropriate. With the recent introduction of alternative potentially curative treatments for early tumours, which include endoscopic techniques, laparoscopic surgery, photodynamic therapy and various regimens of chemotherapy and radiotherapy, very accurate preoperative staging is required in order to identify suitable patients and assess results. Although there remains controversy as to the role of neo-adjuvant therapy (see Chapter 7), accurate preoperative staging is essential in order to enter appropriate patients into relevant trials.

In the past, surgical resection where possible has always been considered to provide the best palliation, and in some patients, such as those with gastric outflow obstruction and/or bleeding, this remains true. However one cannot underestimate the morbidity of oesophago-gastric resection without hope of cure and in particular in those who undergo an 'open and close' operation. Recent data confirm this view and only those patients who remain recurrence free after oesophagectomy appear to reach preoperative quality of life levels.[1] With the introduction of better staging investigations alongside improved methods of non-surgical palliation, no patient should now be subjected to an 'exploratory operation' without very careful preoperative assessment.

Following resection, accurate histological staging should be obtained in order to provide a prognosis for each patient, in addition to identifying those who might benefit from adjuvant therapy. This chapter will explore the various options open to the clinician for preoperative staging of patients with oesophageal and gastric cancer and compare them to final histological staging from resected specimens.

Staging classifications

In order to understand and compare the results of various preoperative staging investigations it is important to first describe the various classifications that are used for staging both oesophageal and gastric cancer. The final staging of a cancer relies on a combination of the results of preoperative investigations, the intraoperative macroscopic findings and the pathological microscopic analysis of the resected specimen. The staging systems for gastric and oesophageal cancer are different and there are several systems presently in use for each.

Gastric cancer

There are three main staging systems presently used in different countries, although since 1986 there has been an attempt to use an agreed unified TNM system. It is, however, important to be aware of the various systems.

The Japanese Research Society for Gastric Cancer: the PHNS system

This is the most systematised and detailed system for staging gastric cancer. There are rules for both the macroscopic intraoperative findings and the histological findings. The PHNS system is derived from the TNM system, but takes into account four factors.[2]

P factor – Grade of peritoneal dissemination (**Table 3.1**).
H factor – Presence of liver metastases (**Table 3.1**).
N factor – Extent of lymph node involvement (**Table 3.2**).
S factor – Extent of invasion of serosal surface of the stomach (**Table 3.2**).

P factor
P_0 no evidence of peritoneal spread
P_1 peritoneal spread limited to supracolic area including greater omentum but not the diaphragm
P_2 small number of nodules on diaphragm and/or below mesocolon
P_3 numerous nodules on diaphragm or below mesocolon

H factor
H_0 no liver metastases
H_1 metastases in one lobe
H_2 small number of metastases in both lobes
H_3 multiple metastases in both lobes

Table 3.1 *Clinical staging of gastric cancer – PHNS system*

N factor
N_0 no lymph node involvement
N_1 group 1 nodes involved
N_2 group 2 nodes involved
N_3 group 3 nodes involved
N_4 nodes involved extending beyond group 3

S factor
S_0 no serosal invasion
S_1 suspected serosal invasion
S_2 definite serosal invasion
S_3 serosal invasion and invasion of contiguous structures

Table 3.2 *Clinical staging of gastric cancer – PHNS system*

Anatomical description

The stomach is subdivided into three sections – upper (C), middle (M) and lower (A) (**Fig. 3.1**). When the carcinomatous infiltration is completely limited to one of the three sections this is expressed by indicating the appropriate letter. If the lesion extends across the dividing line the section primarily involved is listed first followed by the less involved section or sections. For example MCA indicates a tumour arising in the middle portion but extending into the upper third and to a lesser extent the lower third. In describing the site of the primary lesion the stomach is also separated into four parts looking at the cross-section of the stomach.

Pathological description

It is with regard to the N factor that the Japanese have carried out considerable research and revision over that in the original TNM classification. Essentially the lymph-node drainage is divided into three tiers around each part of the stomach. Each lymph-node group has been numbered and named (**Fig. 3.2**). **Table 3.3** lists the N1, N2 and N3 node groups in relation to the site of the primary tumour. Any nodal metastases outside these groups are classed as N4. Nodal involvement can be assessed intraoperatively, but only very detailed histological studies can accurately determine the N factor, after which it is designated as pN.

Although serosal involvement and peritoneal dissemination can be assessed at operation, histology is still needed to confirm this aspect of staging. Serosal involvement is described on the basis of both the macroscopic findings (**Table 3.2**)

Figure 3.1
Location of primary gastric cancer.

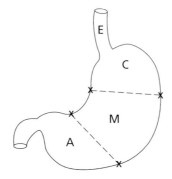

	Location of tumour			
Lymph node group	**AMC, MAC, MCA, CMA**	**A, AM**	**M, MA, MC**	**C, CM**
N1	1,2,3,4,5,6	3,4,5,6	1,3,4,5,6(2MC)	1,2,3,4s
N2	7,8,9,10,11	1,7,8,9	2,7,8,9,10,11	4d,5,6, 7,8,9,10,11
N3	12,13,14,110,111	2,10,11,12,13,14	12,13,14	12,13,14,110,111

Table 3.3 *Lymph node groups in relation to site of gastric cancer*

Figure 3.2
(a) Perigastric lymph nodes; (b) extra-gastric lymph nodes.

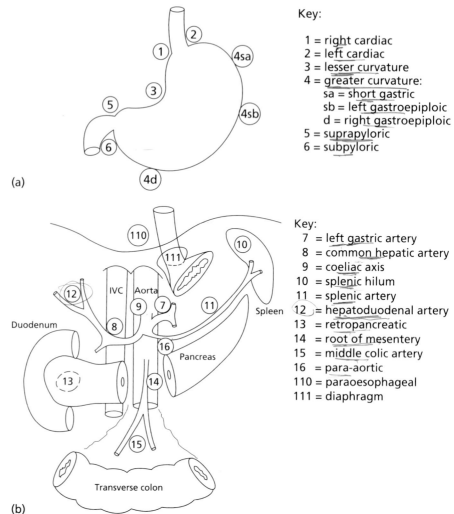

Key:

1 = right cardiac
2 = left cardiac
3 = lesser curvature
4 = greater curvature:
    sa = short gastric
    sb = left gastroepiploic
    d = right gastroepiploic
5 = suprapyloric
6 = subpyloric

Key:

7 = left gastric artery
8 = common hepatic artery
9 = coeliac axis
10 = splenic hilum
11 = splenic artery
12 = hepatoduodenal artery
13 = retropancreatic
14 = root of mesentery
15 = middle colic artery
16 = para-aortic
110 = paraoesophageal
111 = diaphragm

and also on histological assessment. Depth of invasion of the cancer can only be determined accurately by histological analysis and is designated the symbol pT. There are five layers of the stomach wall – mucosa (m), submucosa (sm), muscularis propria (pm), subserosa (ss) and serosal (s). Early gastric cancer (m or sm) is pT1, deeper invasion without breach of the serosa is pT2 and confirmed serosal involvement is pT3. Invasion of an adjacent structure is pT4.

The completed PHNS staging process allows each case to be allocated to a stage of the disease as shown in **Table 3.4**. The staging is refined on the basis of the microscopic findings (**Table 3.5**). It should be noted that the final staging also takes account of resection margins and if malignant cells are detected histologically within 10 mm of the proximal and distal margins then the cancer is downstaged.

Stage	Peritoneal metastases	Liver metastases	Nodal metastases	Serosal invasion
I	P_0	H_0	N_0	S_0
II	P_0	H_0	N_1	S_1
III	P_0	H_0	N_2	S_2
IV	P_1, P_2, P_3	H_1, H_2, H_3	N_3, N_4	S_3

Table 3.4 *Stage classification based on gross findings in gastric cancer (PHNS system)*

Stage	Macroscopic or histological			Histological
	Peritoneal metastases	Liver metastases	Nodal metastases	Depth of invasion
I	P_0	H_0	N_0	ps
II	P_0	H_0	N_1	ssy
III	P_0	H_0	N_2	se
IV	P_1, P_2, P_3	H_1, H_2, H_3	N_3, N_4	si,sei

ps, deepest layer invaded is muscularis mucosa, border distinct; ssy, deepest layer invaded is subserosa, border ill-defined; se, serosa involved; si, infiltration of neighbouring tissue; sei, coexistence of se and si.

Table 3.5 *Staging based on histopathology in gastric cancer (PHNS system)*

AJC and WCC modifications of the TNM system

These two systems are modifications of Kennedy's original description of the TNM system.[3] The American Joint Committee on Cancer Staging Systems and the UICC staging systems were widely adopted in the USA and Europe.[4,5] The AJC system has gained more popularity in the United Kingdom and is outlined in **Table 3.6**. In this system R is used to indicate whether there is evidence of residual cancer after the resection; R0 indicates complete resection, R1 microscopic evidence of residual cancer and R2 is macroscopic residual cancer. This R factor should not be confused with the Japanese use of R for the level of nodal resection which has now been changed to D to avoid confusion.

T factor	T_1	confined to the mucosa and submucosa
	T_2	involving the muscularis propria and the subserosa
	T_3	spread to involve the serosa
	T_4	spread to contiguous structures
N factor	N_0	no nodal metastases
	N_1	perigastric nodes within 3 cm of primary tumour
	N_2	nodes greater than 3 cm from tumour involved
	N_3	non-excised nodes involved
M factor	M_0	absence of metastatic disease
	M_1	presence of metastatic disease

Table 3.6 *Clinical staging of gastric cancer – AJC*

Internationally unified TNM system

The use of three different staging systems for gastric cancer, even though all are based on TNM, has led to considerable confusion. In order to try and eliminate this confusion and to introduce the most recent progress in diagnosis and treatment the Japanese have proposed an acceptable unified staging system. The concept is that of TNM, i.e. there are only three basic prognostic variables, with the proviso that in patients who are M0 the pT and pN factors have almost equal significance. M1 includes distant lymph nodes, peritoneal seedlings, liver and distant metastases. Stages 1 and 3 have been subdivided into A and B to allow tighter grouping of prognostic groups.

The unified TNM staging system is shown in **Table 3.7**. This system was approved by the UICC and AJC in 1985 and in Japan in 1986. Table 3.7 illustrates the 1997 update of the unified TNM staging system.[6] Use of this system is strongly recommended.

T Factor

Tx	Primary tumour cannot be assessed
T0	No evidence of primary tumour
Tis	Carcinoma *in situ*: Intraepithelial tumour without invasion of the lamina propria
T1	Tumour invades lamina propria or submucosa
T2	Tumour invades muscularis propria or subserosa
T3	Tumour penetrates serosa (visceral peritoneum) without invasion of adjacent structures
T4	Tumour invades adjacent structures

N Factor

Nx	Regional lymph nodes cannot be assessed
N0	No regional lymph node metastasis
N1	Metastasis in 1 to 6 regional lymph nodes
N2	Metastasis in 7 to 15 regional lymph nodes
N3	Metastasis in more than 15 regional lymph nodes

M Factor

Mx	Distant metastasis cannot be assessed
M0	No distant metastasis
M1	Distant metastasis

Stage Grouping

Stage 0	Tis	N0	M0
Stage Ia	T1	N0	M0
Stage Ib	T1	N1	M0
	T2	N0	M0
Stage II	T1	N2	M0
	T2	N1	M0
	T3	N0	M0
Stage IIIa	T2	N2	M0
	T3	N1	M0
	T4	N0	M0
Stage IIIb	T3	N2	M0
Stage IV	T4	N1, N2, N3	M0
	T1,T2,T3	N3	M0
	Any T	Any N	M1

Table 3.7 *Internationally unified TNM staging system for gastric cancer*

Fujii *et al.*[7] compared the prognostic accuracy of the 1997 fifth edition of the TNM lymph-node metastases classification system with that of the anatomical classification of the Japanese Research Society of Gastric Cancer in 1489 cases of gastric cancer. Both systems performed well; the new TNM staging was, however, a better index of prognosis for regional lymph nodes. The new system classifies more patients as N1 and fewer as N2 or N3. This does not alter the prognosis for N1 tumours but gives the N2 and N3 tumours a worse prognosis.[8]

Oesophageal cancer

The TNM classification for oesophageal cancer has evolved since 1976. The Japanese Society for Esophageal Diseases system is used to define the anatomical location of the tumour.[9] The TNM staging system then classifies the primary tumour, nodal spread and distant metastases.

Anatomical description

The Japanese Society published the original description of anatomical subsites in 1976. In this description the oesophagus was divided into four parts.
  1. Cervical oesophagus (Ce) between the cricopharyngeus muscle and the upper border of the sternum.
  2. Intrathoracic oesophagus is further subdivided into three parts:
    (a) *Upper intrathoracic (Iu)* extends from thoracic inlet to the level of the tracheal bifurcation, approximately 24 cm from the upper incisor teeth.
    (b) *Middle intrathoracic (Im)* proximal half of the oesophagus between the tracheal bifurcation and the oesophago-gastric junction. The lower level is approximately 32 cm from the upper incisor teeth.
    (c) *Lower intrathoracic (Ei)* This lower part of the oesophagus includes the abdominal oesophagus (Ea) and the distal half of the oesophagus between the tracheal bifurcation and the oesophago-gastric junction. It is about 8 cm long and the lower level is about 40 cm from the upper incisor teeth.

The Japanese Society only classified squamous cell carcinomas. As a result the TNM classification, which was unified to include the UICC and AJC classifications, has included adenocarcinomas. Adenocarcinomas arising in the region of the oesophago-gastric junction pose a problem for classification. They may arise in one of three ways:

1. From metaplastic columnar epithelium in the lower oesophagus.
2. Glandular epithelium of the cardia of the stomach.
3. Fundus of the stomach with proximal spread.

The tumour is described as Ec when the major portion is in the oesophagus, E = C where there are equal lengths in the oesophagus and stomach and Ce when the bulk of the tumour is in the proximal stomach. The major problem with this classification is the inability to identify the true oesophago-gastric junction in patients with circumferential cancers in this area.

The 1997 edition of the unified TNM staging has redefined the anatomical subsites of oesophageal cancer.[6] This is the system that is currently recommended in the West.

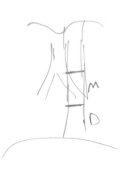

1. Cervical oesophagus From the lower border of the cricoid cartilage to the thoracic inlet at the suprasternal notch, approximately 18 cm from the upper incisor teeth.

2. Intrathoracic oesophagus

(a) *Upper thoracic portion* from the thoracic inlet to the level of the tracheal bifurcation, approximately 24 cm from the upper incisor teeth.

(b) *Mid-thoracic portion* The proximal half of the oesophagus between the tracheal bifurcation and the oesophago-gastric junction. The lower level is approximately 32 cm from the upper incisor teeth.

(c) *Lower thoracic portion* The distal half of the oesophagus between the tracheal bifurcation and the oesophago-gastric junction. The lower level is approximately 40 cm from the upper incisor teeth. This portion is approximately 8 cm in length and includes the abdominal oesophagus.

The anatomical sites of the regional lymph nodes that are involved in oesophageal cancer are listed according to the TNM classification:

Cervical – scalene, internal jugular, upper cervical, paraoesophageal, supraclavicular and cervical.

Intrathoracic – internal jugular, tracheobronchial, superior mediastinal, paratracheal, perigastric (excluding coeliac), carinal, pulmonary hilar, perioesophageal, left gastric, paracardial, nodes of the lesser curve of the stomach and posterior mediastinal nodes. These nodes differ slightly from the nomenclature as described by the Japanese Society in 1976 (**Fig. 3.3**). However, the groups are broadly similar.

The most common metastatic sites are the liver, lungs, pleura and less commonly the kidneys and brain. Tumour may extend directly into mediastinal structures before distant spread is evident.

Rules for classification of oesophageal cancer

Clinical staging

This depends on the anatomical extent of the tumour that can be determined prior to treatment. Assessment includes physical examination, endoscopic biopsies, laboratory studies and imaging as previously described. The location of the tumour, depth of invasion and evidence of nodal and distant spread should be described.

Histopathological staging

This is based on the findings at surgical exploration and on resection of the oesophagus and resected en bloc tissues and other tissue biopsies. Extension of the tumour into adjacent structures and evidence of distant spread should be carefully documented. A single classification serves all regions of the oesophagus for both clinical and histopathological staging. The adjacent structures invaded depends on the location of the primary tumour. Involved structures should be specified in the description.

TNM definition

Primary tumour (T factor) Depth of invasion is shown in **Table 3.8**.

Figure 3.3
Lymph node groups.

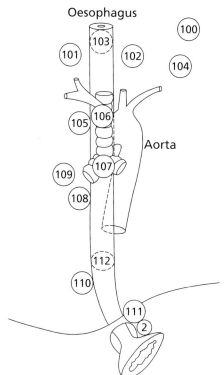

Oesophagus

Aorta

Key:
100 = lateral cervical
101 = cervical paraoesophageal
102 = deep cervical
103 = retropharyngeal
104 = supraclavicular
105 = upper thoracic paraoesophageal
106 = paratracheal
107 = tracheal bifurcation
108 = middle thoracic paraoesophageal
109 = pulmonary hilum
110 = lower thoracic paraoesophageal
111 = diaphragmatic
112 = posterior mediastinal
  2 = left cardiac

Regional lymph nodes (N factor) The definition of regional node metastases has been revised since the original description by the Japanese Society. Any lymph node involved in the regions that have been described already were classified as N1 disease. Any nodes outwith the specific regional nodes are defined as distant metastases (M1). (See the list above and **Table 3.8** for further details.)

Distant metastases This is subdivided into M0, where no distant metastases are detected and M1 where there is evidence of distant metastases. Although the Japanese have added pleural dissemination as a separate category (PL), this is included in the M factor in the unified TNM classification where pleural metastases are recorded as M1.

Clinico-pathological staging

The preoperative and intraoperative findings are refined after histological examination of the resected specimen to allow the cancer to be classified into one of four stages (**Table 3.9**). As with gastric cancer there are three staging systems currently in use. The Japanese PHNS system is again the most meticulous, but is not widely used outside Japan. It is important to use an agreed unified staging system so that results can be easily compared. The UICC and AJC system, which is easier to use, is shown in **Table 3.9**. These definitions are taken from the latest TNM classification.[6] It must be emphasised that the N factor in the staging system is not the same as the extent of lymphadenectomy. Three fields of lymphadenectomy are described and defined for lymph node clearance during oesophageal resection (see Chapter 5).

T Factor

Tx	Primary tumour cannot be assessed
T0	No evidence of primary tumour
Tis	Carcinoma *in situ*
T1	Tumour invades lamina propria or submucosa
T2	Tumour invades muscularis propria
T3	Tumour invades adventitia
T4	Tumour invades adjacent structures

N Factor

Nx	Regional lymph nodes cannot be assessed
N0	No regional lymph node metastasis
N1	Regional lymph node metastasis

M Factor

Mx	Distant metastasis cannot be assessed
M0	No distant metastasis
M1	Distant metastasis

For tumours of the lower thoracic oesophagus

M1a	Metastasis in coelic lymph nodes
M1b	Other distant metastasis

For tumours of the upper thoracic oesophagus

M1a	Metastasis in cervical lymph nodes
M1b	Other distant metastasis

For tumours of the mid-thoracic oesophagus

M1a	Not applicable
M1b	Non-regional lymph node or other distant metastasis

Table 3.8 *Internationally unified TNM clinical classification for oesophageal cancer*

Stage 0	Tis	N0	M0
Stage I	T1	N0	M0
Stage IIA	T2	N0	M0
	T3	N0	M0
Stage IIB	T1	N1	M0
	T2	N1	M0
Stage III	T3	N1	M0
	T4	Any N	M0
Stage IV	Any T	Any N	M1
Stage IVA	Any T	Any N	M1a
Stage IVB	Any T	Any N	M1b

Table 3.9 *Internationally unified TNM staging grouping for oesophageal cancer*

Preoperative staging

The decision-making algorithm demonstrated in **Fig. 3.4** takes the reader through the investigation pathway of a patient with histological confirmation of either oesophageal or gastric cancer for whom surgical intervention with curative intent is the primary objective.

Figure 3.4
Algorithm for the investigation of patients with oesophago-gastric carcinoma.

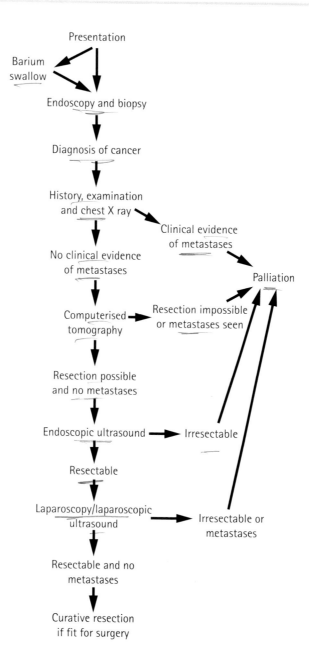

Clinical assessment and routine investigations

In the age of spiral computed tomography (CT) and endoscopic ultrasound (EUS) it is easy to forget the importance of a careful history, examination and simple investigations in the assessment of patients with cancer of the oesophagus and stomach. Clinical evidence of disseminated disease early in a patient's staging process can prevent further unnecessary, expensive, invasive and distressing investigations.

Cancer cachexia implies disseminated disease in most gastrointestinal malignancies and this is certainly true for oesophageal and gastric cancer. However one must not forget that weight loss in oesophageal cancer may also be related to a reduced oral intake secondary to a malignant stricture and not necessarily always due to widespread disease. If in doubt a short period of preoperative enteral feeding, with associated weight gain, may help identify which patients may still benefit from surgical resection.

A recent history of hoarseness of voice raises the possibility of malignant invasion of the recurrent laryngeal nerve that, if proven, is a contraindication to curative resection.

However a hoarse voice can also be caused by chronic aspiration of oesophageal contents secondary to obstruction. Direct or indirect laryngoscopy will identify cord paralysis or laryngeal oedema.

Advanced local disease can also result in an oesophago-tracheal or oesophago-bronchial fistula – the patient presenting with a chronic cough and aspiration pneumonia. Bronchoscopy or barium swallow confirms the diagnosis, thus avoiding further unnecessary staging investigations. If direct invasion is seen it can be biopsied. If rigid bronchoscopy is used then significant compression of the trachea or the carina, in addition to local fixity, can also be assessed.

Palpable supraclavicular nodes may indicate disseminated disease and again, if metastatic tumour is confirmed on needle aspiration cytology, curative resection will not be possible. However as lymphadenopathy can also be caused by chronic aspiration pneumonia from an oesophageal stricture, cytological or histological confirmation is essential. Although clinical examination on the ward will reveal the majority of enlarged cervical lymph nodes, the opportunity to undertake a further examination of the neck under general anaesthesia, for either rigid bronchoscopy or laparoscopy, should be taken.

In advanced disease, hepatomegaly usually indicates the presence of liver metastases and can be confirmed by abdominal ultrasonography.

Chest radiograph

A plain chest radiograph should be taken in all patients. A paralysed hemidiaphragm secondary to malignant invasion of the phrenic nerve or a malignant pleural effusion are again contraindications to curative surgery, and if present will prevent further investigations. A chest radiograph also supplies the surgeon with a crude but valuable assessment of cardiopulmonary function when it is combined with an electrocardiograph, cardiopulmonary history and examination.

Contrast radiology

Although endoscopic fibreoptic examination of the upper gastrointestinal tract remains the first-choice diagnostic procedure for both oesophageal and gastric cancer, barium radiology can still provide useful information in some patients. It is particularly useful for those with strictures when the full extent of the tumour cannot always be assessed at endoscopy. Increasingly CT, discussed below, will provide the missing information but on occasions barium studies can still be of use.

Oesophagus

Double contrast barium radiology should initially be taken with the patient erect with at least one film including the pharynx and one including the open lower oesophageal sphincter. Further films should then be taken in both supine and erect positions. Carcinoma of the oesophagus starts as an intramucosal lesion, with advancement of growth either in an infiltrative or polypoidal manner with possible ulceration accompanying the former. The radiological length of the tumour as seen on this examination provides good correlation with the depth of extension and with curability.[10] With oesophageal cancers under 5 cm in length, 40% are localised, 35% have evidence of distant metastases or are unresectable and 25% are locally advanced. When the tumour is greater than 5 cm in length 75% have evidence of metastases or are unresectable, 25% are locally advanced and only 10% are localised. Another useful sign of local mediastinal invasion is deviation of the axis of the lumen of the oesophagus within the lesion in relation to the expected luminal axis of the oesophagus. This information is also useful before endoscopic or radiological intubation for palliation. When this criterion is used alone there is a false-positive rate for mediastinal invasion of 10% and a false-negative rate of 8%.[10] When the barium flow through the stricture is completely outside the projected axis of the oesophagus then the lesion is almost always unresectable.

Detection of early oesophageal cancer

Four macroscopic types of early oesophageal carcinoma, occurring in the high incidence area of China, have been reported;[11] congested, erosive, plaque-like and polypoidal. Erosive lesions are the most common and account for 45% of early lesions. The earliest radiological abnormality is an area of mucosa that is a little flattened or nodular and rigid with incomplete distensibility that is best seen tangentially. An 'en face' view will usually show an oesophageal fold stopping at the upper limit of the tumour associated with mucosal irregularity and nodularity. These areas usually persist as an area of incomplete collapse when a peristaltic wave passes down the oesophagus. The presence of a mound or plaque suggests submucosal invasion.[12] Minor surface irregularities should be reported in detail so that a careful endoscopic examination can be carried out with biopsy and/or cytology. In high-risk areas such as China, comparative studies of balloon cytology, radiology and endoscopy show detection rates of 98%, 38% and 85%, respectively.[13] In these areas of high incidence concomitant oesophagitis is almost universal in the adult population and these figures may not be directly transferable to the situation in Western countries.

Stomach

Advanced carcinomas are characterised by malignant invasion into or beyond the muscularis propria and manifest radiologically as polypoidal, ulcerating or infiltrating lesions. This produces the characteristic fluoroscopic findings of rigidity and absent peristalsis at the site of the tumour. Polypoidal carcinomas on double contrast examination produce striking luminal defects, frequently with irregular advancing tumour margins. With ulcerating carcinomas the most common radiological feature is an irregular nodular tumour mass which is sharply demarcated from the surrounding normal mucosa. The associated irregular ulcer crater usually fails to penetrate the normal gastric contour. Diffuse infiltrating carcinomas or linitis plastica result in an abrupt circumferential narrowing of the gastric lumen with various abnormalities of the mucosal surface pattern. Mucosal folds will be absent, being replaced by a featureless surface or one that exhibits nodularity due to submucosal tumour infiltration.

Detection of early gastric cancer

Advances in the diagnosis of gastric adenocarcinoma have resulted from extensive Japanese experience with double contrast barium meals. This is especially true of early gastric cancer which accounts for approximately 35% of all cancers seen in Japan.[14] Classification of early gastric cancer (EGC) refers to the macroscopic appearance applicable to both radiology and endoscopy and is shown in **Fig. 3.5**. A common misconception is that early lesions are always small; they can be sizeable tumours with either extensive mucosal involvement or prominent intraluminal masses. Approximately 70% are of the superficial depressed type (IIc). Contrast radiological diagnosis is based on an analysis of the depression and the associated radiating folds. Depressions are irregular and uneven due to proliferation of the malignant tissue. Radiating folds extending to the malignant area reveal characteristic changes such as abrupt tapering, clubbing, interruption or fusion. Excavating (type III) cancers differ from the superficial depressed types by virtue of a greater depth of erosion. Early polypoidal carcinomas (type I) exhibit radiological features similar to those of benign tumours.

Endoscopy

Upper gastrointestinal endoscopy and biopsy, with or without cytological examination, is the most important investigation in the diagnosis of oesophageal and gastric carcinoma and should be performed on any patient in whom the disease is suspected.

Oesophagus

The appearances of early squamous cell carcinoma at endoscopy vary widely. The most common appearance is that of a superficial erosive cancer consisting of a slightly depressed lesion with grey erosions in a reddish mucosa. Early squamous carcinomas have also been described as whitish elevated plaques, slight depressed erythematous areas or as erosions suggestive of gastro-oesophageal reflux disease.

Figure 3.5
Early gastric cancer.

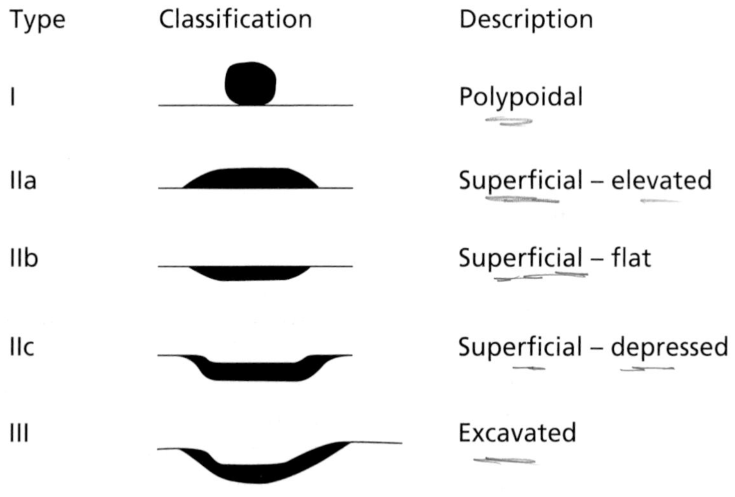

Type	Classification	Description
I		Polypoidal
IIa		Superficial – elevated
IIb		Superficial – flat
IIc		Superficial – depressed
III		Excavated

Superficial polypoidal lesions also occur and when present are more likely to be associated with symptoms than other macroscopic types. In a Japanese study it was shown that endoscopy permitted a correct diagnosis of early oesophageal carcinoma in 100% of patients but contrast radiology only detected 47% of lesions.[15] The majority of lesions missed were of the superficial type. Endoscopic biopsy and brush cytology are complementary investigations and if facilities are available both should be performed. Several factors influence the accuracy of endoscopic biopsy including the number of biopsy specimens taken. When 6 to 10 specimens are obtained the diagnostic accuracy exceeds 80%.[16]

With advanced carcinoma prebiopsy dilatation may be necessary to enable biopsies to be taken from the central portion of the tumour rather than from the proximal limit of the tumour which may only reveal non-neoplastic mucosa due to submucosal tumour infiltration. This is especially true of adenocarcinoma around the cardia. Dilatation should also be performed where possible in order to examine the distal limit of the tumour. The accuracy of endoscopic brush cytology or cytological examination using the balloon technique is reported to exceed 70%.[16,17] By combining the results of cytology and multiple endoscopic biopsies an accuracy approaching 100% can be obtained.[16]

In vitro dye staining is being used increasingly in some centres to facilitate detection of early oesophageal cancer.[18] The stains most commonly used are 1–2% Lugol's iodine, 1–2% toluidine blue and 1–2% methylene blue. Lugol's solution stains non-keratinised squamous epithelium in proportion to its intracellular glycogen content. Early oesophageal cancer consistently shows negative staining allowing more accurate biopsies to be undertaken. Lugol's solution is not useful for isolating dysplastic epithelium because about 50% of such areas are stained positively. Using toluidine blue, dysplastic epithelium usually stains blue. Methylene blue can be used to stain columnar epithelium as it is taken up by goblet cells but not by the squamous epithelium. Methylene blue may also accentuate mucosal relief making differentiation of columnar and squamous epithelium more obvious at endoscopy.

Advanced cancer is macroscopically classified into three main types: (1) exophytic or polypoidal; (2) ulcerative; and (3) diffusely infiltrative. Many forms may coexist within any single tumour and the tumour usually involves a major part of the circumference of the oesophageal lumen. A diffusely infiltrative carcinoma manifests itself as an obvious thickening and rigidity of the oesophageal wall of variable length with fixation of the irregularly thickened, coarsely nodular, usually non-ulcerated mucosa to the deeper layers of the oesophageal wall. Luminal narrowing is also common. A peculiar form of oesophageal cancer described as 'superficial spreading cancer' is defined as a lesion with intramucosal extension of the tumour at least 2 cm from the main bulk of the tumour.[19] The boundary between involved and uninvolved mucosa may be indistinguishable. It is therefore extremely important when considering surgical resection to realise that oesophageal cancers have a tendency to spread submucosally and to establish satellite lesions at some distance from the obvious primary tumour. Small mucosal elevations, especially proximal to the main lesion, should be given special attention and accurate biopsies taken. Whether these lesions represent intramural metastases from the submucosal spread or primary intramucosal carcinomas (so-called 'field change') remains controversial.

The goal of endoscopic surveillance in patients with Barrett's metaplasia is to detect neoplastic lesions that may not be apparent on gross endoscopic examination. A systematic series of endoscopic biopsies should be carried out as high-grade dysplasia and early adenocarcinoma can be detected in mucosa that is endoscopically unremarkable.[20] Early cancers are sometimes associated with friability of the mucosa, superficial erosions, ulcerations, nodularity, plaques, polyps or early strictures. Endoscopic cytology is considered a complement but not an alternative to biopsy.[21]

Stomach

It is possible at endoscopy to define the nature of gastric cancer, its situation and its dimensions. From the tumour's size and cell type the possibility of spread can be predicted. All endoscopists should be acutely aware of various macroscopic appearances of early gastric cancer (Fig. 3.5) with multiple biopsies being taken from any mucosal gastric abnormality. This is especially true of patients at risk of gastric carcinoma, such as those with pre-existing gastric ulcers, patients who have undergone previous gastric surgery for benign disease, those with a family history of carcinoma of the stomach, those with atrophic gastritis and patients with pernicious anaemia.

The sensitivity of brush cytology of suspicious gastric lesions has recently been shown to be almost as high as that of oesophageal cytology. In a study of 903 patients with gastric carcinoma, cytology yielded positive results in 785 (sensitivity 87%) and biopsies were positive in 826 (sensitivity 92%). When the two techniques were combined a positive diagnosis was established in 886 patients (sensitivity 98%).[22] Cytology was positive in 52 patients with negative biopsies and a further 8 patients in whom biopsies had not been obtained had positive cytology. Cytology therefore added 60 positive results to the overall diagnostic yield (6.7%). In this study, brushings were done after the biopsy had been taken which may lead to difficulty in retrieving precise samples from the bleeding abraded surface. Improvement in the accuracy of cytology might have been obtained if the cytological sampling had been carried out before the biopsy as has been advocated.[23] Better results are obtained if the brush used for cytology is immersed in saline and stirred vigorously, with centrifugation of the resulting fluid rather than direct application onto slides.[24] Cytology, however, does add to the expense and requires an experienced endoscopist and cytopathologist. However it is important for the surgeon to know which histological type of gastric carcinoma is present – diffuse or intestinal – as they possess different biological behaviours.[25] Patients with the diffuse type of tumour usually have a worse prognosis.

Ultrasonography

The role of ultrasound in detecting liver metastases is well established, but there has been increasing interest more recently in the ultrasonographic assessment of cervical lymph nodes, with needle aspiration for cytology if abnormal or enlarged nodes are seen.

Computed tomography (CT)

CT is commonly used for preoperative staging of tumours in both the oesophagus and stomach, but its ability to stage these tumours accurately remains controversial. There is no doubt that the more recent spiral scanners are significantly better than the previous generation of machines, but recent data comparing spiral CT with other techniques such as endoscopic ultrasound and laparoscopic ultrasound have been disappointing (see below).

Oesophagus

Post-mortem studies have shown invasion of mediastinal structures to be present in almost 20% of cases, with 12% invading the trachea or bronchi and 2% invading the heart and aorta respectively.[26] The main sites of distant metastases are to liver, lung, bone and kidney, and occur respectively in 19%, 11%, 5% and 4% of patients. Although in the past many retrospective studies reported CT to be accurate in the preoperative staging of oesophageal carcinoma, in addition to evaluating resectability,[27–32] many of these studies lacked precise correlations to surgery and pathology (**Table. 3.10**) and this level of accuracy has been refuted by recent prospective studies.[33–35]

One area of controversy is the loss of the perioesophageal fat plane. When present, invasion is highly unlikely but when absent, even in well-nourished patients, it cannot be taken as absolute evidence of invasion. This may account for the overestimation of tracheal, bronchial, aortic and cardiac invasion in many studies. Extraoesophageal tumour extension, in particular to the tracheobronchial tree, aorta and heart can be determined using the following signs: (a) the presence of an intraluminal bud; (b) obvious displacement and deformation of the tracheobronchial tree, aorta or pericardium; (c) increased thickness of the membranous trachea, bronchus, wall of the aorta or left atrium; (d) growth extending beyond the posterior wall of the trachea at the level of the aortic arch. Invasion of the aorta is more difficult to ascertain and although it occurs very infrequently, its presence is of great importance to the surgeon. It has been suggested that aortic invasion is considered indeterminate with contact of 45–90% between the aorta and tumour and that invasion can only be predicted with accuracy if there is more than 90% contact. However this is not universally accepted, and one study found 6 patients with almost total circumferential tumour growth around the aortic circumference seen on CT scanning in whom aortic invasion at surgery was not found.[35] A recently introduced criterion for aortic invasion is based on the loss of the paravertebral fat space present in the triangle formed by the aorta, oesophagus and vertebral body.[36] If this fat space is completely obliterated by soft tissue in a patient with an oesophageal cancer then invasion of the aorta is usually present.

		Incidence of invasion of		
		trachea/bronchus	**aorta**	**heart**
Retrospective studies[7–12]	286	35% (20–46)	27% (17–49)	13% (0–18)
Autopsy study[6]	2240	12%	2%	2%

Table 3.10 *Incidence of local spread of oesophageal carcinoma (CT versus autopsy)*

Owing to the variability of the normal anatomy at the gastro-oesophageal junction the findings on CT in patients with carcinoma of the gastro-oesophageal junction should be interpreted with caution.[37,38,39] A coexisting hiatus hernia may mimic or obscure both oesophageal and gastric invasion. CT is inaccurate in predicting diaphragmatic invasion although this in itself is unlikely to influence surgical resection. Diaphragmatic invasion can be considered present on CT when the crura are surrounded by a tumour mass. The close relationship of the oesophagus, gastro-oesophageal junction and diaphragm and the absence of an intervening fat plane are the main reasons for the difficulty in assessing diaphragmatic involvement.

Preoperative staging of carcinoma of the cardia using CT varies in accuracy from 68–86% and the presence of lymph-node metastases cannot be reliably predicted. It is impossible to differentiate abnormally enlarged nodes that contain tumour from those that are enlarged as a result of benign reactive hyperplasia. The size of the lymph node regarded as a criterion for malignant involvement varies with different authors from 5 to 15 mm.[35] However, lymph nodes of more than 1 cm in diameter can be seen within the mediastinum in healthy people.[40] It is also well known that nodes of normal size may contain metastatic deposits. The sensitivity for the detection of mediastinal lymph nodes is about 48% with a specificity of 90% and an accuracy of 70%.[37] Subdiaphragmatic lymphadenopathy can be detected with a sensitivity of 61%, a specificity of 94% and an accuracy of 82% but lower figures are found in prospective studies.[38] Malignant cervical or supraclavicular lymphadenopathy occurs in about 60% of patients with upper third carcinomas. In one study of 100 patients with oesophageal carcinoma who underwent transcutaneous sonography of the neck, lymph nodes were considered abnormal if greater than 5 mm in diameter along the short axis.[41] Ultrasonography detected enlarged supraclavicular lymph nodes in 22 patients whereas CT (obtained in 90 of the 100 patients) detected enlarged nodes in only 15. A total of 23 patients underwent fine needle aspiration biopsy under ultrasound guidance, 16 of whom had proven metastases histologically. In only three of the patients were the lymph nodes palpable.

CT scanning is, however, of value in the detection of distant metastases and several studies have demonstrated the overall accuracy in detecting liver metastases to be between 80–98%.[37,38,42] Comparison of the accuracy of scintiscan, ultrasound and CT in patients with a variety of primary tumours with potential hepatic involvement found little difference between the three techniques.[42] Scintigraphy and ultrasound had an accuracy of 80% with CT 84% and the authors concluded that lesions less than 3 cm in diameter were liable to be missed by all three techniques. Advances in technique and the evolution of newer CT scanners have brought the size of lesions easily seen down to about 1 cm. The results of isotope scanning for detecting liver metastases remain conflicting. One study[43] reported that both liver scintigraphy using technetium sulphur colloid and ultrasound were 97% accurate in determining the presence or absence of liver metastases in 100 patients with colorectal cancer. Whereas other studies have only reported accuracies of the order of 64–80% for hepatic scintiscans.[42,44,45] When used to enhance the diagnostic scintigraphy, grey-scale ultrasound has been shown to have an accuracy of 93%.[46] Most authors have not been able to reproduce this level of accuracy and figures of 75–80% are reported in the literature.[42,47] Pulmonary metastases are shown more frequently on CT than on simple chest radiography. Peritoneal metastases are rarely detected by CT.

Stomach

Early hopes that conventional CT would provide accurate staging for gastric carcinoma were disappointing and results from spiral CT have not been much better. This is partly because of the problem of nodal status as mentioned earlier. The CT appearances of gastric carcinoma are variable and usually present with focal or diffuse wall thickening, frequently projecting into the lumen of the stomach with or without ulceration. In the presence of a carcinoma the thickness of the stomach wall when distended is greater than 5 mm and a thickness of over 2 cm usually correlates with transmural extension.[48] Assessment of extension into adjacent organs is unreliable unless a large bulk of tumour is present within the involved structure. Peritoneal spread is rarely detected and often moderate amounts of ascites can go unrecognised. In one study using conventional CT in a series of 75 patients with gastric adenocarcinoma 47% of patients were incorrectly staged by CT with 31% under-staged and 16% over-staged.[49] Understaging was due to the factors described above and over-staging was due to overdiagnosed malignant lymphadenopathy and invasion of contiguous organs as predicted by a loss of the fat plane. As with oesophageal carcinoma this sign is unreliable as patients are often emaciated and the fat plane may also be lost due to inflammatory adhesions. Furthermore pancreatic invasion has been described when the fat plane is intact. The sensitivity of CT to detect invasion of the pancreas is only 27%.[49]

Technical improvements with high-resolution dynamic two-phase CT with intravenous contrast and oral ingestion of water to distend the stomach have certainly improved the diagnostic accuracy in detecting the primary tumour: up to 88% in one study.[50] In this study 5 of the 9 early gastric cancers and 41 of the 43 advanced cancers were diagnosed. The uninvolved gastric wall showed a two- or three-layer pattern on the dynamic CT scan, corresponding to the inner mucosal layer showing marked enhancement, the outer submucosal layer with lower attenuation and another outer muscular-serosal layer showing moderate enhancement. The four early cancers were missed because of their small size and a partial volume effect. The advanced cancers showed moderate to marked heterogeneous enhancement in the early phase and homogeneous enhancement of the entire lesion in the equilibrium phase of the dynamic CT. This is thought to be due to the neovascularity of gastric cancer. The authors of this study were, however, unable to differentiate between EGC involving the mucosa or submucosa and more advanced carcinoma involving the muscular or subserosal areas of the gastric wall. The overall accuracy of dynamic CT in determining the T category was 65% and the accuracy in determining the degree of serosal invasion was 83%; others have reported similar figures.[51]

A study from Japan which assessed high-resolution CT and adjacent organ invasion showed that an absence of fat plane or an irregularity of the border between the tumour and the adjacent organ was not significantly related to invasion.[52] However, when the mean densities at the region of interest were measured they were found to be significantly greater at invasion sites than at non-invasion sites. Although this allowed invasion of the pancreas, liver and colon to be assessed with an accuracy of 75%, 61% and 78% respectively, these authors still found that CT had a limited value in differentiating inflammatory adhesions with fibrosis or oedema from true invasion.

Dynamic CT is also associated with improved detection of metastatic regional lymph nodes, with a sensitivity of 74%, a specificity of 65% and an accuracy of 70%.[50] Detection of involved perigastric nodes close to the primary tumour was much lower as these lymph nodes often appear confluent with the primary tumour. Following the change of TNM staging, identification of regional nodal involvement no longer reflects N2 status and therefore CT will continue to struggle for accurate nodal staging.

CT scanning to detect distant metastases produces accuracy figures similar to those seen in oesophageal cancer, but despite the increasing accuracy of dynamic spiral CT, assessment of the primary tumour remains disappointing and cannot be used to plan surgery.

Magnetic resonance imaging (MRI)

Magnetic resonance imaging is an alternative to CT and prediction of mediastinal invasion is similar between the two investigations. The accuracy of CT and MRI in the detection of tracheal or bronchial invasion is 89% and 90% respectively.[37] Accuracy rates of 75% for aortic invasion and 88% for pericardial invasion have been reported for MRI.[53] However there are drawbacks to the use of MRI which, when combined with its more limited availability and higher cost, makes CT the preferred investigation for staging of both oesophageal and gastric tumours. MRI is limited in its ability to examine more than one organ system or one area of the body during a single examination, is not as good as CT for evaluation of pulmonary metastases and a high quality study of the entire mediastinum and the upper abdomen in one sitting is difficult to obtain due to movement artefacts.

Endoscopic ultrasonography (EUS)

Although first reported in 1980, it has taken the recent technical advances seen over the last few years for EUS to become the established diagnostic tool for the local staging of oesophageal and gastric carcinoma.[54,55]

Instruments for EUS

There are three techniques for imaging upper gastrointestinal cancer using endoscopic ultrasonography.

- There are two types of echo endoscope, both with an oblique forward viewing tip. One contains a radial transducer and the accessory channel of the endoscope can be used for fine needle aspiration of lesions. The other contains a rotating transducer that provides a complete circumferential view but cannot be used for targeted biopsies. It is also possible for colour doppler to be used with some transducers, allowing blood vessels to be visualised more accurately.
- A smaller diameter (9 mm) non-optical flexible oesophagoscope which is positioned over a guide-wire can be used to negotiate strictures through which the larger echo endoscopes cannot pass.

● A catheter miniature higher frequency echo probe is now available. This is inserted through the accessory channel of an ordinary gastroscope. The tip of the probe is positioned on the lesion and a balloon attached to the probe is filled with water to create an acoustic window.

EUS of primary tumour

Using 7.5–12 Mhz frequency, the wall of the oesophagus and stomach can be seen as five layers of alternating bright (hyperechoic) and dark (hypoechoic) bands (**Fig. 3.6**). From inside out these layers correspond to the wall of the balloon, the mucosa, the submucosa, the muscularis propria and finally the adventitia (oesophagus) or serosa (stomach). The presence of thickening through these layers as caused by a carcinoma can clearly be seen (**Fig. 3.7**).

EUS of lymph nodes

Unlike CT which can only assess lymph node size, EUS provides additional information regarding shape, border demarcation, echo intensity and echo texture. Although nodes greater than 8 mm have often been considered to be malignant, size is an unreliable guide and other criteria are now used. In general it is thought that rounded, sharply demarcated, homogeneous, hypoechoic features indicate malignancy whereas elongated, heterogeneous, hyperechoic lymph nodes with indistinct borders are more likely to be benign or inflammatory. However, these endosonographic features may not be evident in cases of micrometastases and evaluation of these features is subjective and may vary between different observers – possibly even between the same observer on different occasions. In a study of

Figure 3.6
EUS of oesophagus showing the five different layers. Note the small T1 tumour at 12 o'clock.

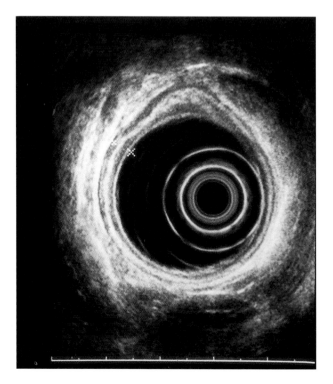

Figure 3.7
EUS of oesophagus showing a T4 tumour with extension into the mediastinum and aortic fascia (seen at 4 o'clock).

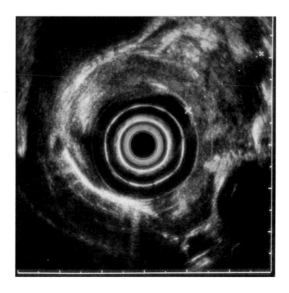

100 patients with oesophageal carcinoma, one study found an overall sensitivity of 89% for the detection of malignant lymph nodes.[56] When EUS identified any lymph nodes the likelihood of NI disease was 86%, whereas when lymph nodes were not seen the chance of N0 disease was 79%. When at least one of the above-predicted features of malignancy was present, specificity increased from 75% to 92%, and when all four features were present, metastases were found histologically in 100%. The features most sensitive for discriminating benign from malignant lymph nodes appears to be the central echo pattern followed, in order, by border, shape and size.

As already mentioned, EUS can be used to perform fine needle aspiration of mediastinal masses or lymph nodes. Although tumour involvement of local lymph nodes is not in itself a contraindication to resection, it does allow the surgeon to discuss more accurately the risks and benefits of resection with the patient. In future it may also help identify patients for neo-adjuvant therapy. EUS-guided FNA can also be used to evaluate recurrence following resection.

EUS staging of oesophageal carcinoma

The transducer is introduced into the stomach and then withdrawn at 1 cm intervals through the oesophagus. The clinician should determine the extent of maximal tumour penetration and the relationship of the tumour to surrounding structures. Lymph nodes should be classified as described above and the layers of the oesophagus can be studied.

EUS is more accurate at staging depth of tumour invasion and lymph-node metastasis than CT.[57] **Table 3.11** illustrates the accuracy of EUS in staging oesophageal cancer.[58,59,60,61] Extension of tumour outside the wall of the oesophagus and possible extension into heart, aorta, vertebrae and pulmonary vessels can be readily assessed (**Fig. 3.8**), although invasion of the airways is more difficult due to the artefact produced by the air.

The main problem with EUS is failure to pass through the stricture leading to an incomplete assessment of the tumour, which in the Bristol series can occur in

Histology	Catalano[58]	Rosch[59]	Grimm[60]	Dittler[61]
T1	33	50	90	81
T2	75	78	86	77
T3	82	91	93	89
T4	89	80	83	88
N0	94	42	85	70
N1	89	89	88	74

Table 3.11 *Accuracy of EUS in oesophageal carcinoma [T + N stage] [%]*

as many as 1 in 5 patients.[62] However this same group went on to demonstrate that adequate information can still be provided by these incomplete examinations in relation to surgical decision making.[63] This problem can be circumvented by using the non-viewing smaller probe which is passed over a guide-wire passed under gastroscopic vision.

Another alternative is to pass the smaller catheter miniature echo probe. Recent small trials have shown that this has a similar sensitivity and specificity for staging oesophageal cancer and superficial oesophageal carcinoma to a standard EUS examination.[64,65] The miniature probe has the additional advantage of being able to evaluate tight strictures through which the normal ultrasound endoscope cannot pass although it is technically more difficult to use than its larger counterpart.

EUS staging of gastric carcinoma

When compared to CT, EUS has consistently been shown to be superior for the staging of gastric carcinoma.[66] Although the results of EUS in assessing T stage of gastric tumours is not quite as good as for the oesophagus due to the distensibility of the stomach, accuracies of 83% in T1, 61% in T2, 87% in T3 and 76% in T4 have been reported in one large series of 403 patients with an overall accuracy of 81%.[67] These results confirm those of previous studies (**Table 3.12**).[58,59,68,69] In the light of recent developments in endoscopic treatment for early gastric cancer, accurate staging is essential and figures from several studies suggest that EUS has an overall accuracy for staging early gastric cancer of around 77%.[67,70,71,72,73]

Histology	Rosch[59]	Grimm[60]	Dittler[68]	Ziegler[69]
T1	71	90	81	91
T2	64	79	71	81
T3	83	62	87	86
T4	64	89	79	89
N0	75	85	93	88
N1	86	50	65	64

Table 3.12 *Accuracy of EUS in gastric carcinoma [T + N stage] [%]*

Figure 3.8
(a) CT and (b) EUS of the same patient with a T3 N1 tumour in the mid-oesophagus.

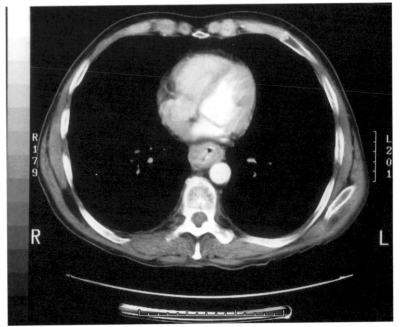

(a)

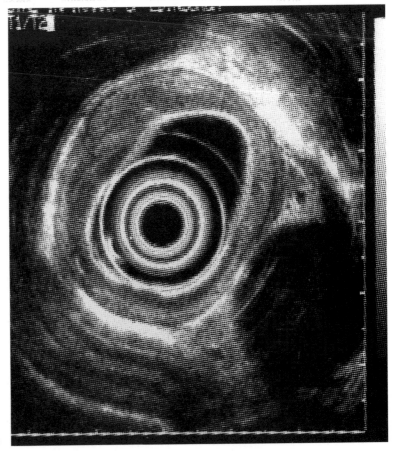

(b)

The presence of peptic ulceration complicates interpretation of EUS due to distortion of the normal layers of the stomach wall.[71] Furthermore, fibrous proliferation in reaction to benign peptic ulcer disease is often indistinguishable from the fibrotic reaction induced by malignant invasion.[74] The ultrasonographic appearances of oedema around a tumour are similar to those of tumour itself and can lead to over-staging, whereas microinfiltration of tumour cannot be visualised with EUS, resulting in under-staging. Reports of the detection of malignant lymph nodes in gastric cancer vary from 55% to 87%,[68,75,76,77,78,79,80,81] with accuracy highest for the perigastric nodes of the lesser curve. EUS assessment of nodes in other locations is significantly less accurate.

Laparoscopy

EUS combined with CT scanning is now accepted as being the most accurate method for T staging primary gastroesophageal malignancy.[82]

Unfortunately both modalities are poor at staging distant lymph nodes, small hepatic metastases and peritoneal metastases with sensitivities of 58% and 33% for oesophageal and gastric cancer respectively.[82] It is in these patients that laparoscopy is of particular value.

Even before the introduction of EUS, a group of surgeons in Glasgow had shown laparoscopy to be significantly more sensitive at demonstrating these modes of metastasis than either CT or percutaneous ultrasound for lower oesophageal and gastric cancer.[38] Further data from the same group demonstrated that as a result of laparoscopy 21% of the 179 patients studied avoided unnecessary surgery. However 21% of the patients going forward to surgery were discovered to have inoperable tumours, primarily due to disease above the diaphragm.[83]

In another large study of 369 patients with carcinoma of the oesophagus and gastric cardia, metastases to liver, peritoneum, omentum, stomach and intra-abdominal lymph nodes was found in 52 (14%) patients.[84] Laparoscopic false-negative results in patients subjected to laparotomy was only 4% (3% to the liver, 1% to peritoneum and 0.4% to the omentum). In a comparative study of laparoscopy, percutaneous ultrasound scanning and scintigraphy in patients with oesophageal and gastric carcinoma others have again demonstrated laparoscopy to be more accurate in detecting hepatic metastases and these modalities combined removed the need for surgery in 58% of the patients studied.[47] Although these authors concluded that laparoscopy was useful in patients with oesophageal carcinoma, they were less convinced that such information on liver metastases would alter decision making for gastric carcinoma, considering these patients would still require palliative procedures.

As mentioned earlier in this chapter such decisions must be made for each individual patient, but with many more non-surgical palliative options now available, laparoscopy has an equally important role in gastric cancer.

Laparoscopic ultrasonography (lapUS)

Following the rapid improvements in laparoscopic instrumentation over the last decade, combined with the better understanding and increased use of intra-operative ultrasound for staging tumours at open surgery, it was not surprising that this technology would be combined to produce laparoscopic ultrasound probes. In addition to providing visual information regarding overt peritoneal, serosal and liver metastases, lapUS also demonstrates tumour depth (**Fig. 3.9**), associated lymphadenopathy (**Fig. 3.10**) and small metastases deep within the liver parenchyma (**Fig. 3.11**). Early reports comparing the staging of gastric cancer by laparoscopy,

Figure 3.9
Laparoscopic ultrasound examination of the lower (intra-abdominal) oesophagus in (a) a normal patient and (b) a patient with a T3 carcinoma of the lower oesophagus extending across the oesophago-gastric junction.

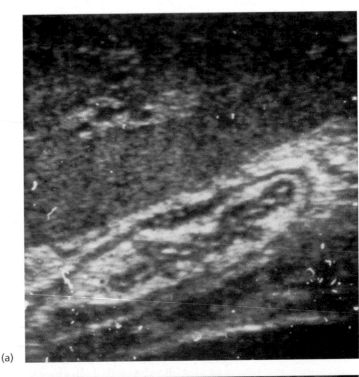

(a)

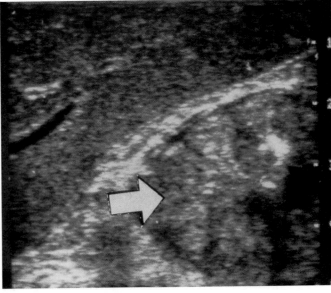

(b)

Figure 3.10
Laparoscopic ultrasound examination of the coeliac axis in two patients with lower oesophageal carcinoma showing (a) an enlarged left gastric lymph node in one patient (N1 disease) and (b) extensive malignant lymphadenopathy around the coeliac axis in the other (M1 disease).

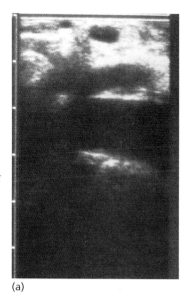 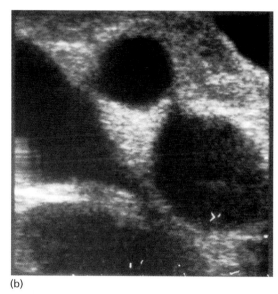

(a) (b)

Figure 3.11
Laparoscopic ultrasound of a patient with gastric carcinoma showing a 6 mm liver metastasis deep within the right lobe of the liver.

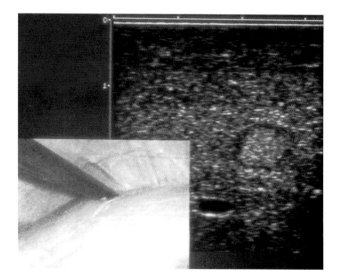

lapUS and CT showed that for overall TNM staging lapUS (82%) was more accurate than laparoscopy alone (67%) and conventional CT alone (47%).[85]

 Other studies using lapUS in patients with both gastric and oesophageal cancer have shown even better figures with accuracies of 91% for T staging and N staging.[86] The stomach needs to be distended with water for accurate T staging, particularly if assessment of pancreatic invasion is required (**Fig. 3.12**).

Although these early studies of lapUS were promising, there remained doubt as to the overall influence of lapUS over and above the proven value of laparoscopy. Indeed one study of 60 patients concluded that laparoscopy was not effective in staging oesophageal cancer and the inclusion of laparoscopic ultrasound was of

Figure 3.12
Laparoscopic ultrasound of the stomach showing (a) a small T2 carcinoma and (b) an extensive T4 tumour with invasion of the pancreas. Note the disrupted plane between the posterior surface of the tumour and the anterior surface of the pancreas.

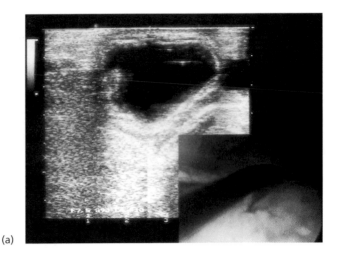

(a)

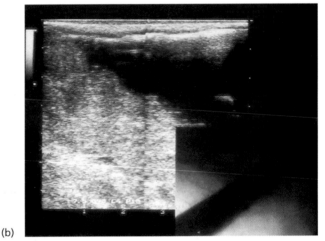

(b)

little benefit.[87] Of course much depends on the overall surgical philosophy regarding indications for resection. When influence on decision making is specifically examined, and the surgical philosophy is only to resect potentially curable oesophageal and gastric cancers, or for specific palliation of gastric tumours which cannot be achieved using non-surgical means, laparoscopy (after clinical assessment and CT scanning) prevented 'unnecessary surgery' in 18 of 93 (19%) patients.[88] The addition of lapUS after laparoscopic inspection in the remaining 75 patients prevented unnecessary surgery in a further 7 (8%).

 Not only does laparoscopy and lapUS improve staging for both oesophageal and gastric carcinoma, it also can identify those patients with advanced disease who will not benefit from surgery and therefore prevents unnecessary laparotomy.

In addition to permitting more appropriate treatment to be offered to individual patients in whom surgery will not produce any hope of cure, valuable operating time set aside for major resectional surgery can be conserved. This assumes of course that the diagnostic laparoscopy is carried out on a separate list. With the mini-laparoscopes now available there is potential in the future for carrying out these procedures on an outpatient basis. One additional benefit of the short diagnostic laparoscopy is the assessment of the response to general anaesthesia of a frail elderly patient who would require major abdominal/thoracic surgery.

Bronchoscopy

Rigid bronchoscopy used to be considered essential for all patients with upper and middle third oesophageal carcinomas to assess invasion of the tracheobronchial tree. With the improvements in other staging modalities already discussed, this is no longer always the case. However if EUS demonstrates a bulky tumour in the middle third of the oesophagus that extends outside the adventitial layer and a good view of the interface between tumour and airway cannot be seen, bronchoscopy is indicated. Although flexible bronchoscopy can identify actual tumour spread into the airway, rigid bronchoscopy has the additional ability to assess significant compression of the trachea or carina, as well as fixity.

Cervical ultrasound and fine needle aspiration biopsy of cervical lymph nodes in oesophageal cancer

Ultrasound evaluation of cervical lymph nodes in patients with oesophageal cancer has been shown to reveal lymph node metastases in between 10–28% of patients.[89,90,91] The accuracy of ultrasound in the detection of cervical lymph node metastases is improved if the size, heterogeneity of internal echoes, morphology of the margins and the deformation caused by compressive instrumental manipulation of the node are evaluated. In one study ultrasound scanning revealed that 7 out of 37 patients with oesophageal cancer had cervical lymph node metastases and of these 2 patients had no other evidence of metastatic spread.[90]

Most of the studies have examined patients with squamous cell cancer, and aggressive surgery in those patients with cervical nodal metastases appears to be of some value. In one study of 23 patients with squamous cell carcinoma of the thoracic oesophagus who underwent bilateral cervical lymphadenectomy in addition to oesophagectomy (three-field lymphadenectomy), 4 (16.5%) patients survived 5 years.[92] Long-term survival was only achieved in those patients with upper third or middle third tumours. Similar data are very unlikely to be produced for adenocarcinoma.

Other investigations

Further investigations on patients with oesophageal and gastric cancer should be carried out if there are any other suggestions of potential metastatic disease, depending on clinical assessment and the results of other investigations. These might include isotope bone scanning, CT of the brain and echocardiography. Echocardiography not only provides valuable information on cardiac function in patients with a history of ischaemic heart disease, but can also assess the possibility of pericardial invasion in bulky middle and lower oesophageal tumours.

Possible future prognostic indicators

There are a variety of prognostic indicators for gastrointestinal tract malignancies including tumour markers, acute-phase proteins and cytokine genotypes.

Numerous studies have shown that acute-phase proteins and tumour markers correlate well with both tumour stage and prognosis for pancreatic and gastric cancer.[93,94] Recent work which examined the polymorphisms of IL-1b and their relationship with survival in pancreatic cancer found a positive association between one of these genotypes and reduced survival from pancreatic cancer.[95] There has however been very little work in this field in oesophageal cancer although one study has shown that fibrinogen levels appear to correlate with stage of disease.[96] Results from a recent study that examined polymorphism within the tumour necrosis factor locus showed that these correlated with survival in patients with oesophageal cancer.[97] This suggests that the patient's immunological response to oesophageal cancer may influence survival and appears to be genetically predetermined rather than secondary to tumour phenotype.

Currently the decision to proceed to curative resection is determined by the fitness of the patient for surgery and how far the disease has spread. In the future additional independent prognostic indicators such as cytokines may enable clinicians to reduce the number of failed curative resections.

Summary of preoperative staging

The appropriate management of patients with oesophageal and gastric cancer depends on accurate preoperative staging of the disease. Conventional preoperative staging based on physical examination, barium swallow and meal, endoscopy, bronchoscopy and CT often under-stages the disease. The reasons for the inaccuracy are the inability to determine the depth of oesophageal or gastric wall involvement, the extent of infiltration to other organs and failure to identify lymph-node metastases.

Staging is significantly improved by the addition of EUS, although in lower oesophageal and gastric cancer information on peritoneal metastases can only be obtained from laparoscopy, with or without lapUS. These opinions are based on the premise that surgery is only considered for potentially curative lesions. If surgery is the preferred method of palliation, irrespective of staging investigations, neither EUS nor laparoscopy will alter the clinical decision.[98] However there can be no doubt that in considering surgical resection for patients with oesophageal and gastric cancer all possible preoperative information should be obtained in order that a fully informed discussion can take place between the patient, the relatives and the clinician regarding the treatment options. Involvement of multidisciplinary teams that include surgeons, interventional endoscopists, radiation oncologists and palliative care physicians greatly enhance this process and allow the most appropriate management to be provided for each patient. Furthermore every patient with oesophageal and gastric cancer has a right to expect this information. If selective neo-adjuvant treatment is to be considered, accurate preoperative staging is essential.

Intraoperative assessment and staging

With the current preoperative staging techniques already discussed, there should not be unexpected findings at operation and thus it should be possible to undertake surgery with a clear plan on type of procedure and extent of resection.

However, occasionally surprises do occur and before embarking on resection careful operative staging of the cancer must be carried out. This has two objectives: firstly, to confirm preoperative staging and in particular ensure that the cancer has not been under-staged; and secondly to reassess whether the planned operative procedure remains appropriate in the light of any revised staging.

The presence of hepatic metastases not detected on preoperative scanning or laparoscopy should be looked for and if present biopsied and submitted for frozen section. If necessary intraoperative ultrasound can be used to help clarify any dubious abnormality.

The presence and extent of peritoneal deposits should also be biopsied and submitted for frozen section, particularly if a positive result might change operative strategy to a lesser procedure, such as bypass, or no procedure at all.

The extent of the primary tumour and in particular the proximal and distal palpable margins must be carefully examined. The lateral margins must also be evaluated to stage the depth of invasion and the presence of fixity to adjacent structures. It is also important to decide whether adherence to another organ is inflammatory or neoplastic although this is often difficult to determine with certainty and without a full trial dissection.

The extent of lymph node involvement may also alter the surgical procedure. If enlarged nodes are within the planned extent of the en bloc resection then it is not vital to decide whether they are malignant. However enlarged nodes that either cannot be safely resected or lie outside the margins of the resection should be regarded as distant metastases and sampled for frozen section. If positive for metastases, the surgical decision can be altered as appropriate.

Final histopathological staging

The final staging of oesophageal and gastric cancer is important for a number of reasons: firstly, it allows an accurate prediction of prognosis and may indicate the need for adjuvant therapy; secondly, when results are compared to preoperative and intraoperative staging it provides ongoing quality control and educational feedback; and thirdly, it allows the results from different centres to be compared. The different staging classifications have already been discussed.

 In the light of the data discussed in this chapter, patients with oesophago-gastric cancer now have a right to expect their clinicians to undertake careful and meticulous attention to detail in all three areas of staging, which can only be provided by incorporating many of the investigative techniques described here into their routine practice.

Acknowledgements

This chapter, in the first edition of *Upper Gastrointestinal Surgery*, was written by John Anderson. Although we have revised and updated the text, much of the background data remains and we wish to acknowledge his contribution to this revised chapter.

References

1. Blazeby JM, Alderson D, Farndon JR. Quality of life in patients with oesophageal cancer. In: Recent results in cancer research – Esophageal carcinoma, vol. 55 J Lange J and JR Siewert (eds.). Berlin: Springer-Verlag, 2000, pp. 193–204.

2. Japanese Research Society for Gastric Cancer. The general rules for the gastric cancer study in surgery and pathology. Jpn J Surg 1981; 11:127–39.

3. Kennedy BJ. TNM classification for stomach cancer. Cancer 1970; 26:971–83.

4. Beahrs OH, Henson DE, Hunter RVP, Kennedy BJ (eds.) Manual of staging of cancer. Philadelphia: JB Lippincott, 1992.

5. Hermanek P, Sobin LH (eds.) UICC:TNM classification of malignant tumours, 5th edn. Berlin: Springer-Verlag, 1996.

6. UICC:TNM classification of malignant tumours, 5th edn. Berlin: Springer-Verlag, 1997.

7. Fujii K, Isozaki H, Okajima K et al. Clinical evaluation of lymph node metastases in gastric cancer defined by the fifth edition of the TNM classification in comparison with the Japanese system. Br J Surg 1999; 86:685–9.

8. Alderson D. Gastrointestinal cancer abstracts. The Stomach 1999; 2:7–8.

9. Japanese Society for Esophageal Diseases. Guide for the clinical and pathological studies on carcinoma of the esophagus. Jpn J Surg 1976; 6:69–78.

10. Rosenberg JC, Roth JA, Lichter AS et al. Cancer of the oesophagus. In: Devita VT, Hanman S, Rosenkerg SA (eds.) Cancer: principles and practice of oncology. London: JB Lippincott, 1985, pp. 621–57.

11. Yang G, Huang H, Sungliang Q et al. Endoscopic diagnosis of 115 cases of early oesophageal carcinoma. Endoscopy 1982; 14:157.

12. Sata T, Sakai Y, Kajita A et al. Radiographic microstructures of early oesophageal carcinoma: correlation of specimen radiography with pathologic findings and clinical radiography. Gastrointest Radiol 1986; 11:12–19.

13. Zhang DW. Fiberesophagoscopic diagnosis. In: Huang GJ, K'ai WY (eds.) Carcinoma of the esophagus and gastric cardia. Berlin: Springer-Verlag, 1984, pp. 217–36.

14. White RM, Levine MS, Enterline HT et al. Early gastric cancer – recent experience. Radiology 1985; 155:25–7.

15. Adachi Y, Kitamura K, Tsutsui S et al. How to detect early carcinoma of the esophagus. Hepato Gastroenterol 1993; 40:207–11.

16. Witzel L, Halter F, Gretillat PA et al. Evaluation of specific value of endoscopic biopsies and brush cytology for malignancies of the oesophagus and stomach. Gut 1976; 17:375–7.

17. Hanson JT, Thoreson C, Morissey JF. Brush cytology in the diagnosis of upper gastrointestinal malignancy. Gastrointest Endosc 1980; 26:33–5.

18. Kawai K, Takemoto T, Suziki S et al. Proposed nomenclature and classification of the dye-spraying techniques in endoscopy. Endoscopy 1979; 11:23–5.

19. Soga J, Tanaka O, Sasaki K et al. Superficial spreading carcinoma of the esophagus. Cancer 1981; 50:1641–5.

20. Reid BJ, Weinstein WM, Lavin KJ et al. Endoscopic biopsy can detect high grade dysplasia or early adenocarcinoma in Barrett's oesophagus without grossly recognizable neoplastic lesions. Gastroenterology 1988; 94:81–90.

21. Levine DS, Reid BJ. Endoscopic diagnosis of esophageal neoplasms. Gastrointest Endosc Clin North Am 1992; 2:395–413.

22. Cusso X, Mones J, Ocana J et al. Is endoscopic gastric cytology worthwhile? An evaluation of 903 cases of carcinoma. H Clin Gastroenterol 1993; 16:336–9.

23. Chambers LA, Clark WE. The endoscopic diagnosis of gastroesophageal malignancy: a cytologic review. Acta Cytol 1986; 30:110–4.

24. Waldron R, Kerrin M, Ali A et al. Evaluation of the role of endoscopic biopsies and cytology in the detection of gastric malignancy. Br J Surg 1990; 77:62–3.

25. Miwa K. Cancer of the stomach in Japan. Gann Monogr Cancer Res 1979; 22:61.

26. Postlethwait RW. Surgery of the esophagus. New York: Appleton-Century-Crofts, 1979.

27. Daffner RH, Halber MD, Postlethwait RW et al. CT of the esophagus. II carcinoma. Am I Roentgenol 1979; 133:1051–5.

28. Coulomb M, Lebas JF, Sarrazin R et al. L'apport de la tomodensitometric an bilan d'extension des cancers de l'oesophage. J Radiol 1981; 62:475–87.

29. Moss AS, Schnyder P, Thoeni RF et al. Esophageal carcinoma, pre-therapy staging by computed tomography. Am Roentgenol 1981; 136:1051–6.

30. Picus D, Balfe DM, Koelher RE et al. Computed tomography in the staging of esophageal carcinoma. Radiology 1983; 146:433–8.

31. Thompson WM, Halvorsen RA, Foster WL et al. Computed tomography for staging esophageal and gastro-esophageal cancer: reevaluation. Am J Roentgenol 1983; 141:951–8.

32. Schneekloth G, Terrier F, Fuchs WA. Computed tomography in carcinoma of esophagus and cardia. Gastrointest Radiol 1983; 8:193–206.

33. Samnelsson L, Hambraeus GM, Melcke CE et al. CT staging of oesophageal carcinoma. Acta Radiol (Diagn) 1984; 25:7–11.

34. Quint LE, Glazier GM, Orringer MB et al. Esophageal carcinoma: CT findings. Radiology 1985; 155:171–5.

35. Fekete F, Gayet B, Frija J. CT scanning in the diagnosis of oesophageal disease. In Jamieson GG (ed.) Surgery of the oesophagus. Edinburgh: Churchill Livingstone, 1988, pp. 85–9.

36. Halvorsen RA, Thompson WM. Gastrointestinal cancer, diagnosis staging and the follow-up role of imaging. Semin Ultrasound, CT, MRI 1989; 10:467–80.

37. Thompson WM, Halverson RA. Staging esophageal carcinoma II: CT and MRI. Semin Oncol 1994; 21:447–52.

38. Watt I, Stewart I, Anderson D et al. Laparoscopy, ultrasound and computed tomography in cancer of the oesophagus and cardia: a prospective comparison for detecting intra-abdominal metastases. Br J Surg 1989; 76:1036–9.

39. Halvorsen RA, Thompson W. Computed tomographic staging of gastrointestinal tract malignancies. Part I. Esophagus and stomach. Invest Radiol 1987; 22:2–16.

40. Schnyder PA, Gamsu G. CT of the pretracheal-retrocaval space. Am J Roentgenol 1981; 136:303–8.

41. Overhagen IT, Lameris JS, Berger MY et al. Improved assessment of supraclavicular and abdominal metastases in oesophageal and gastro-oesophageal carcinoma with the combination of ultrasound and computed tomography. Br J Radiol 1993; 66:203–8.

42. Smith IJ, Kemeny MM, Sugarbaker PH et al. A prospective study of hepatic imaging in the detection of metastatic disease. Ann Surg 1982; 195:486–91.

43. Lamb G, Taylor I. An assessment of ultrasound scanning in the recognition of colorectal liver metastases. Ann R Coll Surg Engl 1982; 64:391–3.

44. Castagna J, Benefield JR, Yamada H et al. The reliability of liver scans and function tests in detecting metastases. Surg Gyencol Obstet 1972; 134:463–6.

45. Lunia S, Partnasarathy KL, Bakshi S et al. An evaluation of 99mTc-sulful-colloid liver scintiscans and their usefulness in metastatic workup: a review of 1424 studies. J Nucl Med 1975; 16:62–5.

46. Sullivan C, Taylor KJW, Gattschalk A. The use of ultrasound to enhance the diagnostic utility of the equivocal liver scintigraph. Radiology 1978; 128:727–52.

47. Shandall A, Johnson C. Laparoscopy or scanning in oesophageal and gastric cancer. Br J Surg 1985; 72:449–51.

48. Hada M, Hihara T, Kakishita M. Computed tomography in gastric carcinoma: thickness of gastric wall and infiltration to serosa surface. Radiat Med 1984; 2:27–30.

49. Sussman SK, Halvorsen RA, Illescas FF et al. Gastric adenocarcinoma: CT versus surgical staging. Radiology 1988; 167:335–40.

50. Cho JS, Kim JK, Rho SM et al. Pre-operative assessment of gastric carcinoma: value of two-phase dynamic CT with mechanical i.v. injection of contrast material. Am J Roentgenol 1994; 163:69–75.

51. Minami M, Kawawucni N, Itai Y et al. Gastric tumours: radiologic-pathologic correlation and accuracy of T staging with dynamic CT. Radiology 1992; 185:173–8.

52. Tsubnraya A, Naguchi Y, Matsumoto A et al. A preoperative assessment of adjacent organ invasion by stomach carcinoma with high resolution computed tomography. Jpn J Surg 1994; 24:299–304.

53. Quint LE, Glaziel GM, Orringer MB et al. Esophageal imaging by MR and CT: study of normal anatomy and neoplasms. Radiology 1985; 156:727–31.

54. Classen M et al. Ultrasonic tomography by means of an ultrasonic fiberendoscope. Endoscopy 1980; 12:241–4.

55. Terada M, Tsukaya T, Saito Y. Technical advances and future developments in endoscopic ultrasonography. Endoscopy 1998; 30 (Suppl 1):a3–a7.

56. Catalano MF, Sivak MV, Rice T et al. Endosonographic features, predictive of lymph node metastasis. Gastrointest Endosc 1994; 40:442–6.

57. Chak A, Canto M, Gerdes H et al. Prognosis of oesophageal cancers preoperatively staged to be locally invasive (T4) by endoscopic ultrasound (EUS): a multicentre retrospective cohort study. Gastrointest Endosc 1995; 42:501–6.

58. Catalano MF, Van Dam J, Sivak MV. Malignant esophageal strictures: staging accuracy of endoscopic ultrasonography. Gastrointest Endosc 1995; 541:535–9.

59. Rosch T, Lorenz R, Zehker K et al. Local staging and assessment of resectability in carcinoma of the esophagus, stomach and duodenum by endoscopic ultrasonography. Gastrointest Endosc 1992; 38:460–7.

60. Grimm H, Binmoeller KF, Hamper K et al. Endosonography for preoperative locoregional staging of esophageal and gastric cancer. Endoscopy 1993; 25:224–30.

61. Dittler HI, Siewert JR. Role of endoscopic ultrasonography in esophageal carcinoma. Endoscopy 1993; 25:156–61.

62. Vickers J, Alderson D. Influence of luminal obstruction on oesophageal cancer staging using endoscopic ultrasonography. Br J Surg 1998; 85:999–1001.

63. Vickers J, Alderson D. Oesophageal cancer staging using endoscopic ultrasonography. Br J Surg 1998; 85:994–8.

64. Kim CY, Thomson A, Bandres D et al. Endoscopic ultrasound (EUS)-guided fine needle aspiration (FNA) biopsy using radial scanning endosonography: results of diagnostic accuracy [abstract]. Gastroenterology 1997; A3341.

65. Tio TL, Fleischer DEF, Wang GQ et al. High-frequency balloon catheter ultrasound (CUS) in assessing oesophageal dysplasia and cancer in Lin-Xian, China: a comparison with 20-MHz EUS [abstract]. Gastroenterology 1997; A3352.

66. Botet JF, Lightdale CJ, Zaiber AG et al. Preoperative staging of gastric cancer: comparison of endoscopic US and dynamic CT. Radiology 1991; 181:426–32.

67. Shim CS. Role of endoscopic ultrasonography for gastric lesions. Endoscopy 1998; 30 (Suppl 1):A55–A59.

68. Dittler HJ, Siewert JR. Role of endosonography in gastric carcinoma. Endoscopy 1993; 25:162–6.

69. Ziegler K, Sanft C, Zimmer T et al. Comparison of computed tomography, endosonography, and intraoperative assessment in the TN staging of gastric carcinoma. Gut 1993; 34:604–10.

70. Abe S, Lightdale CJ, Brennan MF. The Japanese experience with endoscopic ultrasonography in the staging of gastric cancer. Gastrintest Endosc 1993; 39:586–91.

71. Shimizu S, Tada M, Kawai K. Endoscopic ultrasonography for early gastric cancer. Endoscopy 1994; 26:767–8.

72. Kida M, Yamada Y, Sakaguchi T et al. The diagnosis of gastric cancer by endoscopic ultrasonography. Stomach Intestine 1991; 26:61–70.

73. Yasuda K, Mukai H, Eisai C et al. Evaluation of the degree of gastric cancer invasion by endoscopic ultrasonography (EUS) for endoscopic treatment of early gastric cancer. Stomach Intestine 1992; 27:1167–74.

74. Ohashi S, Nakazawa S, Yoshino J. Endoscopic ultrasonography in the assessment of invasive gastric cancer. Scand J Gastroenterol 1989; 24:1039–48.

75. Caletti GC, Brocchi E, Gibilaro M. Sensitivity, specificity and predictive value of endoscopic ultrasonography in the diagnosis and assessment of gastric cancer. Gastrointest Endosc 1990; 36:194–5 [abstract].

76. Grimm H. EUS in gastric carcinoma. 10th International Symposium on Endoscopic Ultrasonography 1995; 109–11.

77. Caletti G, Ferrari F, Brocchi E et al. Accuracy of endoscopic ultrasonography in the diagnosis and staging of gastric cancer and lymphoma. Surgery 1993; 113:14–27.

78. Akahoshi K, Misawa T, Fujishima H et al. Preoperative evaluation of gastric cancer by endoscopic ultrasound. Gut 1991; 32:479–82.

79. Heintz A, Mildenberger P, Georg M et al. Endoscopic ultrasonography in the diagnosis of regional lymph nodes in esophageal and gastric cancer – results of studies in vitro. Endoscopy 1993; 25:231–5.

80. Akahoshi K, Misawa T, Fujishima H et al. Regional lymph node metastases in gastric cancer: evaluation with endoscopic US. Radiology 1992; 182:559–64.

81. Hildebrant U, Feifel G. Endosonography in the diagnosis of lymph nodes. Endoscopy 1993; 25:243–5.

82. Lightdale CJ. Endoscopic ultrasonography in the diagnosis, staging and follow-up of esophageal and gastric cancer. Endoscopy 1992; 24:297–303.

83. Molloy RG, McCourtney JS, Anderson JR. Laparoscopy in the management of patients with cancer of the gastric cardia and oesophagus. Br J Surg 1995; 82:352–4.

84. Dagnini G, Caldironi MW, Marin G et al. Laparoscopy in abdominal staging of esophageal carcinoma. Report of 369 cases. Gastrointest Endosc 1986; 32:400–2.

85. Finch MD, John TG, Garden OJ et al. Laparoscopic ultrasonography for staging gastroesophageal cancer. Surgery 1997; 121:10–7.

86. Anderson DN, Campbell S, Park KG. Accuracy of laparoscopic ultrasonography in the staging of upper gastrointestinal malignancy. Br J Surg 1997; 84:580.

87. Romijn H, Van Overhagen H, Spillenaar Bilen EJ et al. Laparoscopy and laparoscopic ultrasonography in staging of oesophageal and gastric carcinoma. Br J Surg 1998; 85:1010–2.

88. Smith A, Finch MD, John TG et al. Role of laparoscopic ultrasonography in the management of patients with oesophagogastric cancer. Br J Surg 1999; 86:1083–7.

89. Bressani Doldi S, Lattuada E, Zappa MA et al. Ultrasonographic evaluation of the cervical lymph nodes in preoperative staging of eosphageal neoplasms. Abdom Imaging 1998; 23:275–7.

90. Van Overhagen H, Lameris JS, Zonderland HM et al. Ultrasound and ultrasound-guided fine needle aspiration biopsy of supraclavicular lymph nodes in patients with esophageal carcinoma. Cancer 1991; 67:585–7.

91. Bonvalot S, Bouvard N, Lothaire P et al. Contribution of cervical ultrasound and ultrasound fine-needle aspiration biopsy to the staging of thoracic oesophageal carcinoma. Eur J Cancer 1996; 32A:893–5.

92. Nishimaki T, Tanaka O, Suzuki T et al. Clinical implications of cervical lymph node metastasis patterns in thoracic esophageal cancer. Ann Surg 1994; 220:775–81.

93. Lundin J, Roberts PJ, Kuusela P *et al*. Prognostic significance of serum CA 242 in pancreatic cancer. A comparison with CA 19-9. Anticancer Research 1995; 15 [5B]: 2181–6.

94. Kodera Y, Yamamura Y, Torii A *et al*. The prognostic value of preoperative serum levels of CEA and CA 19-9 in patients with gastric cancer. Am J Gastroenterol 1996; 91 [1]:49–53.

95. Barber MD, Lynch SF, Powell JJ *et al*. Interleukin-1b gene polymorphisms correlate with survival in pancreatic cancer. Br J Surg 1998; 85:1564.

96. Wayman J, O'Hanlon D, Hayes N *et al*. Fibrinogen levels correlate with stage of disease in patients with oesophageal cancer. Br J Surg 1997; 84:185–8.

97. O'Mahony L, Jackson J, Feighery C *et al*. Polymorphisms within the tumour necrosis factor region affect survival of patients with oesophageal cancer. Surgical Research Society Abstracts, Br J Surg 1998; 85:687.

98. Fok M, Chong SWK, Wong J. Endosonography in patient selection for surgical treatment of esophageal carcinoma. World J Surg 1992; 16:1098–103.

4 Anaesthetic assessment and perioperative care

Ian H. Shaw

INTRODUCTION

The likely benefit derived from a particular therapy depends not only on the stage of the gastric or oesophageal disease but also on the fitness of the patient. Hence accurate preoperative assessment of the patient is essential before assigning him or her to a particular therapeutic option. Upper gastrointestinal surgery is a challenge for all the professionals involved. It is major surgery which impinges on the cardiorespiratory system. Early communication and dialogue between the surgical and anaesthetic teams are essential to identify potential problems and ensure comprehensive preanaesthetic investigation and preparation. The quality of perioperative care is an important determinant in the outcome for these patients. The time facilitated by the preoperative staging period should be used efficiently to render the patient optimally fit before surgery. Attention to detail is important.

The preoperative assessment should be clearly recorded and the results presented in a manner that makes them readily accessible and understandable.

Clinical assessment

The preoperative physiological state of the patient is one of the most important factors in determining outcome following major surgery. Meticulous preoperative evaluation and investigation are a prerequisite to successful surgical outcome.

The aim of preoperative evaluation and assessment before major surgery is to optimise the patient's physiological status in order to make some evaluation as to the likely outcome following the intended surgery. To achieve the latter Copeland et al.[1] proposed a Physiological and Operative Severity Score for the enUmeration of Mortality and morbidity (POSSUM). POSSUM amalgamates a physiological score with an operative severity score to give an estimation of the risk of mortality and morbidity. Cardiorespiratory signs, symptoms and examination together with biochemical, haematological and operative factors are all taken into consideration. The operative severity is determined with reference to surgical complexity, estimated blood loss and the presence or absence of malignancy. The value of such a system is that it acknowledges the significance of both the patient's physiological parameters and the magnitude of surgical intervention to surgical outcome.

As a result of the over-prediction of mortality, a modified system, P-POSSUM has been proposed.[2] Regardless, both identify the patient's pre-existing medical condition as a major determinant of postoperative outcome.

Past medical history

At a very early stage details should be sought of the patient's past medical history. Any condition which may be of perioperative consequence must be identified. Enquiries should also be made regarding any significant family history.

Patients undergoing major elective surgery who have a pre-existing physiological impairment of one or more of the major organ systems have a higher risk of postoperative complications and mortality.[3] In this respect, particular attention should be paid to the cardiovascular and respiratory systems.

Cardiorespiratory disease has been identified as the commonest coexisting disease in patients presenting for oesophagectomy.[4] Some of the most useful information about cardiorespiratory function and perioperative risks can be obtained by meticulous history taking. Pre-existing ischaemic heart disease, poorly controlled hypertension and pulmonary dysfunction are all associated with increased operative morbidity. This is especially pertinent when the surgery involves the upper abdomen and thorax.[5]

The patient should be questioned as to the presence of any of the following symptoms: Chest or arm pain, palpitations, shortness of breath on exertion, paroxysmal nocturnal dyspnoea, orthopnoea, syncope, intermittent claudication, cough, wheeze and expectoration. A useful pointer is some measure of the patient's exercise tolerance. Having identified any of these symptoms, further specialised referral and investigation may be necessary. All patients should have their blood pressure measured and recorded at the first opportunity together with a physical examination of the cardiorespiratory system looking for evidence of cardiomegaly, jugular venous distension, ventricular failure, abnormal heart sounds and inadequate chest expansion and air entry. Evidence of cerebrovascular disease should be sought such as vertebrobasilar insufficiency, dizziness, transient ischaemic attacks and carotid bruits excluded.

Any previous thoracic or upper abdominal surgery should be noted. Previous thoracic surgery can impede the collapse of the non-dependent lung during a thoracotomy as a result of adhesions. Any previous lung resection of the dependent lung can preclude the use of one-lung anaesthesia thereby making surgical access difficult.

Perioperative cardiorespiratory reserve can be influenced by other systemic disorders. In particular symptoms related to renal or hepatic dysfunction should be sought. Endocrine disease, especially thyroid dysfunction and diabetes mellitus, should be evaluated – the latter frequently being associated with significant cardiovascular and renal impairment, both of which are associated with an increased perioperative risk.

Some neurological and musculoskeletal diseases can influence the perioperative course particularly where respiratory function and reserve are affected as the result of a thoracotomy. In such patients careful evaluation of any disability and

Grade	Definition
ASA 1	Normal healthy patient
ASA 2	Patient with mild systemic disease
ASA 3	Patient with a severe systemic disease that limits activity but is not incapacitating
ASA 4	Patient with incapacitating disease that is a constant threat to life
ASA 5	Moribund patient not expected to survive 24 hours with or without surgery

Table 4.1 *The American Society of Anesthesiologists assessment of physical status*

neurological impairment is important. This is also of relevance if epidural analgesia is being considered.

Having carefully evaluated the patient an indication of perioperative risk can be made. The American Society of Anesthesiologists classification of physical status (**Table 4.1**) is well recognised and familiar to all anaesthetists. Although its correlation with perioperative risk has some limitations it does provide a useful global assessment and its use is advocated.

As might be expected perioperative risk increases with increasing ASA score,[6,7] in particular postoperative pulmonary complications.

Upper gastrointestinal surgery may be contraindicated in those patients who present as ASA 4.

Past anaesthetic history

Where possible, details of previous anaesthetics should be made available in order to identify any past anaesthetic complications. Relying on the patient's account of previous anaesthetics may give rise to incomplete or erroneous information; indeed the patient may be unaware of earlier problems such as difficulties with endotracheal intubation, perioperative cardiovascular instability and bronchospasm.

A family history of malignant hyperthermia or pseudo-cholinesterase deficiency should be excluded. Malignant hyperthermia is associated with a considerable mortality and requires very specific anaesthetic management. On the very rare occasions when either of these two conditions have been identified the anaesthetic team must be involved at a very early stage.

Medication and allergies

It is important to establish what medication, if any, a patient is taking. There are many potential interactions between the drugs used during surgery and a patient's regular medication. In practice however few actually warrant discontinuation and all medication should be continued up until the time of surgery.[8] If there is any doubt the anaesthetic team should be consulted in good time. There are however a few notable exceptions to this rule.

Depending on the specific drug, oral hypoglycaemics should be discontinued either on the day before or the day of surgery. Anticoagulated patients should be managed with reference to the local hospital guidelines. Patients on regular aspirin need careful consideration, particularly if epidural analgesia is a consideration. Although rare, patients on first-generation monoamine oxidase inhibitors must be brought to the anaesthetists' attention early as the medication may have to be discontinued four weeks prior to surgery under psychiatric supervision. The *British National Formulary* guidelines relating to those patients taking the oral contraceptive pill should be followed.

A history of allergic reactions to drugs, surgical preparations, dressings and latex should be sought and clearly recorded. Any previous blood transfusions should also be noted.

The efficacy of medication prescribed for cardiorespiratory conditions should be evaluated at an early stage. This is particularly important in patients with known ischaemic heart disease, poorly controlled hypertension and chronic obstructive pulmonary disease (COPD). Suboptimal treatment of these conditions can add appreciably to the perioperative risks in a patient undergoing thoracic or upper abdominal surgery.[9]

Social habits

Smoking has long been regarded as a major aetiological factor in perioperative morbidity. Some studies have suggested a 4-fold increase in postoperative pulmonary complications in patients who smoke. Smoking is associated with COPD, emphysema, ischaemic heart disease, peripheral and cerebrovascular disease. Pulmonary complications include mucus hypersecretion, impaired bronchial clearance, poor lung compliance, hypersensitivity of the airways, enhanced coagulability and blood viscosity, and impaired oxygen transport (**Table 4.2**).

Abnormality	Time to return to normal
Nicotine	3–4 hours
Carboxyhaemoglobin	1–3 half-lives
Ciliary function	4–6 days with some improvement over months
Sputum production	2–6 weeks
Small airway function	6 weeks minimum
Laryngeal hypersensitivity	5–10 days
Platelet function	3 days
Hb, RBC, Hct, WBC	24 hours
Immune function	6 weeks minimum
Microsomal enzyme induction	6–8 weeks
Postoperative pulmonary morbidity	8 weeks

Table 4.2 *Effects of stopping smoking prior to surgery (from Erskine and Hanning)*[22]

Following upper abdominal and thoracic surgery the inability to clear bronchial secretions proficiently can result in atelectasis and subsequent hypoxia. Smoking has been identified as one of several predisposing factors in the aetiology of post-operative adult respiratory distress syndrome following oesophagectomy.

Chronic excessive alcohol consumption can result in acute withdrawal symptoms in the postoperative period. The patient's response to some anaesthetic drugs can be less predictable. Associated hepatic, upper gastrointestinal and neurological dysfunction can also add to the anaesthetic risks.

The social misuse of addictive drugs can also have implications for the conduct of the anaesthesia and surgery.

Gastro-oesophageal reflux

Gastro-oesophageal reflux (GOR) is a major predisposing factor in pulmonary aspiration and a potentially lethal complication of general anaesthesia.[10] The greatest risk of aspiration and regurgitation is during induction prior to endo-tracheal intubation and following extubation in a semiconscious patient.

Apart from a preoperative history of symptomatic regurgitation, other predisposing factors include obesity, hiatus hernia, delayed gastric emptying, difficulty with bag-and-mask ventilation and difficulty with endotracheal intubation. Patients undergoing oesophageal and abdominal surgery are known to be at greater risk of aspiration, in particular those with dysphagia.

The presence of GOR has a significant influence on the conduct of the anaesthetic and prophylactic measures to protect the airway have to be considered.

Evaluation of the airway

Any anatomical or pathological factors which may impede endotracheal intubation should be noted. Early communication with the anaesthetic team is important. The position of the trachea, temporo-mandibular joint and neck movement should be assessed. Prominent or irregular dentition, a receding mandible, limited mouth opening or tongue protrusion and obesity can make visualisation of the larynx difficult. These difficulties can be especially problematic when endo-bronchial intubation is required.

The nasal airway should be checked for patency.

Preoperative investigations

The value of preoperative investigations in patients undergoing oesophageal surgery is two-fold. Firstly they provide a reference baseline for the anaesthetic and postoperative management of these often complex patients. The interference with normal oxygenation and ventilation, the potential for haemodynamic instability and the appreciable operative and postoperative fluid requirements make oesophageal surgery a major insult on the body's normal physiological processes. Maintaining homeostasis with reference to preoperative values is essential.

Secondly, preoperative investigations aim to identify any remediable abnormality as well as any abnormality that will contribute to an accurate evaluation

Haematological	Haemoglobin
	Full blood count
	Coagulation screen
Biochemical	Urea and electrolytes
	Blood glucose
	Liver function tests
	Arterial blood gases on air
Electrocardiogram	Resting 12 lead
Pulmonary function tests	Before and after bronchodilation
Radiology	Chest radiology
Exercise test	

Table 4.3 *Minimum routine preoperative investigations for a patient presenting for upper gastrointestinal surgery*

of the patient's physical status and operative risks. Optimisation of the patient's physical status within the limits of any coexisting disease is the goal.

The minimum preoperative investigations for all patients undergoing upper gastrointestinal surgery are given in **Table 4.3**. Further investigations are undertaken as dictated by the individual patient's results, past medical history and clinical findings.

Haematological and biochemical investigations

The main value of haematological and biochemical investigations is to establish a reference baseline for perioperative care and to a lesser degree identify any remediable factors in the preoperative stage.

Although the minimum acceptable preoperative haemoglobin concentration remains controversial it would seem prudent to have a circulating haemoglobin concentration of approximately 10 g/dl. As well as operative blood loss oesophageal surgery can involve appreciable fluid loads resulting in a haemodilution. While this is acceptable to a degree it depends on an adequate preoperative haemoglobin. Where preoperative blood transfusion is regarded as necessary then this should be performed at least 24 hours before any proposed surgery in order to allow the oxygen-carrying capacity of the transfused blood to reach optimal levels.

Interestingly a recent randomised controlled trial of blood transfusion in the critically ill found that tolerating a haemoglobin in the range 7–9 g/dl did not adversely affect mortality when compared to the more liberal use of blood transfusion.[11] All of the patients did have serious pre-existing acute illness and consequently the situation may not be directly comparable to optimally fit patients undergoing elective surgery. Unlike previous studies, even patients with known ischaemic heart disease appeared to tolerate a more restrictive transfusion regime, the exceptions being patients with acute myocardial ischaemia and angina.

Where time permits, patients with confirmed deficiency anaemias should be treated appropriately with iron, folate or vitamin B12 to promote erythropoiesis rather than be subjected to the risks of a blood transfusion.[12]

Any abnormality in coagulation should be further investigated and referred to a haematologist. Apart from any surgical risk, abnormal clotting or platelet function contraindicates the use of epidural analgesia.

Renal and hepatic function must be evaluated. Hypokalaemia should be corrected early. A low serum albumin may reflect an inadequate nutritional status and should prompt the assessment of serum iron, calcium, essential and trace elements and other indices of nutritional status. Blood sugar should be measured. The end-organ complications of diabetes can be multiple and associated with an increased perioperative risk.

Electrocardiogram (ECG)

The history, physical examination and ECG are critical for a rational assessment of the risk of perioperative myocardial infarction.[13] All patients presenting for oesophageal surgery, regardless of age, should have a preoperative ECG. The ECG should be evaluated in the context of any clinical findings and symptomatology the patient may experience.

Previous myocardial infarction, ischaemia, ventricular hypertrophy, conduction and rhythm disturbances may add appreciably to the operative risks.[14,15] In one study[16] the preoperative ECG was found to be a better predictor of cardiac risk than exercise testing.

A normal resting ECG does not exclude ischaemic heart disease. The resting ECG is normal in 25–50% of patients with coronary artery disease. Conversely, 5–10% of asymptomatic patients have been shown to have an abnormal ECG of relevance to anaesthesia.[17] Silent myocardial ischaemia, which can be associated with significant decreases in coronary blood flow, is recognised as a frequent and potentially serious marker of morbidity.[18]

Arterial blood gases

Arterial blood gases at rest on room air should be assessed. Evaluation of any abnormality must be considered in relation to the clinical findings and any other investigations, in particular pulmonary function tests.

Hypoxia suggesting an intrapulmonary shunt may be of greater significance during any subsequent one-lung anaesthesia. Low preoperative oxygen saturation has been correlated with postoperative hypoxaemia following thoracotomy for non-pulmonary surgery[19] and also a higher incidence of pulmonary complications.[20]

Nunn et al.[21] reported that in patients with COPD undergoing non-thoracic surgery the preoperative arterial PO_2, and whether they were dyspnoeic at rest, were the best predictors of the need for postoperative ventilatory support. Entwistle et al.[19] reported that in patients who had a thoracotomy for non-pulmonary surgery, the patients who were hypoxic preoperatively remained hypoxaemic 4 days after surgery.

Hypercarbia is indicative of ventilatory impairment and as a consequence the patient may be at risk of increased postoperative morbidity. However current evidence suggests that, in the absence of impaired exercise tolerance hypercarbia alone is not a good predictor of complications although this data relates primarily to pulmonary surgery.

Pulmonary function tests

It is generally recognised that owing to the number of variables a precise indication of the pulmonary risks for the individual patient cannot be reliably predicted by pulmonary function tests alone.

Much of the evidence relating preoperative pulmonary function to postoperative outcome after thoracotomy concerns pulmonary surgery involving lung resection. The collapse of one lung during oesophageal surgery is a temporary measure to facilitate surgical access only, and does not involve a permanent reduction in lung volume. With the patient's ventilated lung in the dependent position, the use of high inspired oxygen concentrations and other manoeuvres, the predictive value of preoperative pulmonary function tests is open to debate.

Regardless, all patients should have simple pulmonary function tests performed before and after therapeutic bronchodilation. The forced vital capacity (FVC), the forced expiratory volume in 1 second (FEV_1) and the FEV_1/FVC ratio determined.

It is to be anticipated that significantly impaired pulmonary function will result in difficulties in maintaining adequate oxygenation during one-lung anaesthesia and the postoperative period. An inability to clear retained bronchial secretions, as might be implied by a measured peak expiratory flow rate of less than 65% predicted, has been shown to correlate with an increase in the incidence of post-oesophagectomy pulmonary complications.

The FEV_1 has some predictive value in those patients undergoing lung resection but its significance in those undergoing transient one-lung anaesthesia for non-pulmonary surgery is less clear. Wong et al.[7] who acknowledge that both pre-existing pulmonary and non-pulmonary factors are important in postoperative pulmonary complications, identified an FEV_1 <1.2 l or an FEV_1/FVC ratio of < 75% as an important risk factor in non-cardiothoracic surgery. A post-bronchodilator FEV_1 of >2 l is regarded as satisfactory for a pneumonectomy, and > 1.5 l for a lobectomy. By contrast Nagawa et al.[23] found that the FVC was the most important predictor of postoperative pulmonary complications following an oesophagectomy.

Pulmonary function test results must be considered in relation to those appropriate for the patient's height and weight. In evaluating the test results, consideration must be given to the fact that setting a strict 'cut off' as regards acceptable pulmonary function may deny the patient their only chance of curative surgery. The results of pulmonary function tests must therefore be considered in relation to the clinical findings and the arterial blood gas analysis, particularly the PaO_2.[19,20]

Where further investigation is deemed necessary this should be conducted under the supervision of a chest physician.

Radiology

The chest X-ray taken during the staging of oesophageal cancer should be made available to the anaesthetist. Any abnormalities in tracheal and bronchial anatomy being noted. Heart size and lung fields should be viewed with reference to any coexisting cardiorespiratory disease. Normal heart size does not preclude abnormal function.

Further information about cardiorespiratory anatomy and function may be obtained from the preoperative CT scan and ultrasound examination. In selected patients, where oxygenation during one-lung anaesthesia is regarded as doubtful, any imbalance of pulmonary ventilation and perfusion may be demonstrated by V/Q scanning.

Exercise testing

Although the patient's exercise capacity is a subjective estimation it can be a very useful measure of cardiorespiratory reserve. If the patient experiences chest pain or dyspnoea on minimal exertion they are unlikely to be tolerant of the haemodynamic changes often associated with oesophageal surgery.

Any patient who remains asymptomatic after climbing several flights of stairs, walking up a steep hill, running a short distance, cycling, swimming or performing heavy physical exercise should tolerate the rigours of oesophageal surgery. However it is important to appreciate that an apparent ability to perform these activities does not exclude cardiorespiratory disease and indeed this is a major criticism of exercise testing performed in the absence of cardiovascular monitoring. Cohn[24] demonstrated that 20–30% of asymptomatic post–infarction patients had silent ischaemia on exercise testing.

Desaturation during exercise, equivalent to climbing three flights of stairs, suggests a limited pulmonary reserve and appears to have some predictive power as regards postoperative complications in patients undergoing a pneumonectomy.[25]

The value of preoperative exercise testing remains debatable and is probably of limited value in asymptomatic healthy individuals. Carliner et al.[16] concluded that exercise testing was not reliable in predicting perioperative cardiac risk.

Regardless, symptomatic patients will require further detailed investigation. Formal treadmill testing in patients with symptomatic ischaemic heart disease can be helpful. If the cardiovascular parameters at which ischaemia occurs can be identified, then attempts can be made to control these variables peroperatively.

Bronchoscopy

Preoperative bronchoscopy is desirable in any patient with oesophageal disease who has symptoms or radiological evidence of carinal or bronchial involvement. The correct placement of a double lumen endobronchial tube may be impeded by tumour compression or airway displacement. Any variations of the normal anatomy of the upper airway can also be noted.

Other investigations

Patients with an audible murmur or significant symptomatic ischaemic heart disease should have an echocardiogram. Those with a history of transient ischaemic attacks (TIA) and carotid bruits should have Doppler studies.

Preoperative preparation

Cardiovascular system

The thoracic stage of an oesophagectomy is associated with surgical manipulation of the hiatus and mediastinum and can result in sudden life-threatening hypotension in a patient with limited cardiopulmonary reserve or cerebrovascular disease.

Although all past medical history needs to be considered prior to oesophageal surgery, particular emphasis is placed on any past or present cardiorespiratory symptoms and disease. Patients presenting with several cardiovascular risk factors need careful assessment and preparation. All patients should be rendered optimally fit in the preoperative period before undertaking anaesthesia and oesophageal surgery.

Goldman et al.[5] are credited with being the first to critically evaluate pre-existing risk factors with perioperative outcome and the cardiac risk index they formulated remains widely quoted (**Table 4.4**). Numerous subsequent studies supported and added to their findings. All concluded that pre-existing cardio-respiratory disease was a major contributory factor in perioperative morbidity and mortality. Subsequent studies particularly highlighted angina and heart

Criteria	Points
History	
Age over 70 years	5
Myocardial infarction within 6 months	10
Physical examination	
S3 gallop or jugular venous distension	11
Significant aortic stenosis	3
Preoperative electrocardiogram	
Rhythm other than sinus or premature atrial contractions	7
More than 5 premature ventricular contractions/minute	7
General status	
$PaO_2 < 8$ kpa or $PaCO_2 > 6.6$ kPa	
potassium < 3 mmol/l or $HCO_3 > 20$ mmol/l	
blood urea nitrogen > 50 mg/dl	
creatinine > 3 mg/dl	
Abnormal aspartate aminotransferase	
Signs of chronic liver failure	
Bedridden from non-cardiac disease	3
Operation	
Intraperitoneal or thoracic	3
Emergency	4
Total possible	**53**

Of the patients scoring greater than 26 points 56% died from a cardiac disease and 22% sustained life-threatening complications.

Table 4.4 *Computation of the Goldman risk index*[5]

failure[15] as a major contributory risk factor. Advanced age, a history of cerebrovascular accident (CVA) and diabetes mellitus also appear to contribute to the perioperative cardiovascular risk. Evidence relating to these risk factors has been comprehensively reviewed by Mangano[14] and Juste et al.[26]

In addition to the risk factors identified by Goldman et al. uncontrolled or poorly controlled hypertension may be associated with an increased perioperative morbidity.[9,27] Inadequately controlled hypertension can result in operative cardiovascular instability with associated myocardial ischaemia. Exaggerated responses to surgical stimulation and manipulation, changes in posture, hypovolaemia and anaesthetic agents can occur. There is evidence that major intraoperative deviations of heart rate and blood pressure, from preoperative levels, correlate with the occurrence of myocardial ischaemia.

It is important that hypertension is identified early and full use made of the preoperative period to attain a blood pressure appropriate to the patient's age. Where uncertainty exists the resting patient should be placed on 4-hourly overnight blood pressure measurements. Sustained hypertension, including during sleep, or a widely fluctuating blood pressure, may be indicative of hypertension.

Patients with known or symptomatic ischaemic heart disease need very careful evaluation. All the evidence confirms that ischaemic heart disease is a major perioperative risk factor. Myocardial infarction within 6 months of any proposed surgery represents an appreciably increased operative risk, the risk of reinfarction being greatest within the first 3 months. Reinfarction following surgery has a substantial mortality. Goldman et al.[28] identified upper abdominal and thoracic surgery as adding to the risk. This was confirmed by Steen et al.[9] who specified non-cardiac thoracic and upper abdominal surgery lasting over 3 hours as contributory factors.

Patients who have had a recent CABG or angioplasty do not appear to be at an increased risk provided they have good residual ventricular function, remain asymptomatic and have no other cardiac risk factors.[9,29] There is, however, an opinion that believes conclusive evidence is still wanting.

Patients with symptomatic ischaemic heart disease, angina, valvular disease and evidence of heart failure, in whom surgery is proposed as a therapeutic option, should be investigated further. Angina which is increasing in frequency and intensity, occurring at rest, less responsive to standard therapeutic measures and associated with disturbances of rhythm must be followed up promptly. Prompt referral to a cardiologist is desirable as treadmill testing, echocardiography and angiography may be necessary.

Respiratory system

The surgical site has long been identified as a predictor of pulmonary risk. Upper abdominal and thoracic surgery carries the greatest risk of postoperative pulmonary complications. Patients over the age of 65 years with operable oesophageal cancer are known to be at a higher risk of postoperative complications,[20] as are patients with pre-existing chronic obstructive pulmonary disease; the risks being compounded by prolonged surgery and anaesthesia.[7] Consequently optimal respiratory function is particularly important in patients being considered for a curative resection in which a thoracotomy and peroperative one-lung ventilation is required.[23]

Where the results of pulmonary function tests suggest suboptimal function, any reversibility of airflow obstruction identified after bronchodilator therapy, should be followed up with vigorous preoperative physiotherapy and regular bronchodilator administration. Expert advice from a chest physician should be sought at an early stage as a short course of steroids may be necessary. Deep-breathing exercises, chest physiotherapy and incentive spirometry have been shown to reduce the risk of postoperative pulmonary complications.[30]

Endobronchial intubation in asthmatics can precipate bronchospasm secondary to carinal and bronchial stimulation. Known asthmatics should be on optimal therapy with reference to their *best* measured peak expiratory flow rates.

Intercurrent chest infections must be treated aggressively. One of the commonest causes of postoperative complications following oesophageal cancer surgery is pulmonary infection[20] and in one study accounted for 30% of the deaths following oesophagectomy.[31]

All patients who smoke should be encouraged to stop immediately. Smoking is a well-recognised aetiological factor in perioperative morbidity, in particular pulmonary complications. All the evidence to date suggests that it is beneficial for patients to stop smoking preoperatively. Optimal recovery from the reversible effects of smoking (**Table 4.2**) ideally takes about 8 weeks.[22]

Oral and dental hygiene should be addressed as this can be a source of chronic sepsis that could disseminate infection to the tracheobronchial tree during intubation.

Nutritional status

Patients should have their weight (in kilograms) and height (in metres) recorded at the first opportunity. Body Mass Index (BMI) may then be deduced by the weight divided by the height squared (kg/m^2). Serum total protein and albumin should be determined.

Malnourishment may be indicated by a low BMI (< 18.5), a body weight less than 90% predicted, 20% weight loss and a low serum albumin. A falling BMI and serum protein may be associated with an increased risk of postoperative complications.[20,23]

Marked weight loss may reflect advanced disease and requires careful evaluation of nutritional status. Malnourished patients are prone to infection and delayed wound healing. Hypoalbuminaemia preoperatively will be exacerbated by haemodilution and starvation in the postoperative period and can lead to an increase in pulmonary and extravascular water.

Consideration should be given to preoperative nutritional support in those operable patients who are debilitated and wasted. Dietetic advice should be sought in this respect.

Obesity has been associated with increased operative risks,[32] and there is evidence that patients at their ideal body weight do better after surgery.

Psychological function

A specialist nurse familiar with the care of patients after gastrointestinal surgery should carefully assess patients informally as should the consultant in charge. A judgement should be made as to the level of understanding in a particular case and the appropriateness of the therapeutic options proposed. Counselling should be made readily available to all patients and carers at the time of diagnosis before interventional decisions are made.

The provision of printed information, which the patient and the family can consider in their own time, is one way to aid understanding of the disease and the proposed treatment. A relationship and an environment should be created in which patients and relatives are given the time and opportunity to freely ask questions relating to the disease and treatment. Specialist nursing staff have an important role to play in this respect.

Every effort should be made to familiarise the patient with the hospital environment, including the intensive care unit, in order to minimise fear and misunderstanding.

Patient cooperation is crucial and can be enhanced by reassurance and good communication. Descriptions of the methods of pain relief, oxygen and intravenous fluid administration, the awareness of intercostal, nasogastric and bladder drainage and the likelihood of prolonged periods without oral intake, must be adequately explained. All patients and their relatives should be counselled about the treatment options, paying particular attention to the results and limitations of surgery.

Thromboembolic prophylaxis

Patients undergoing oesophagectomy are at risk of thromboembolic complications. Watson[33] reported that serious thromboembolic complications occur in less than 10% of patients undergoing oesophageal cancer surgery.

To reduce the incidence of thromboembolic complications prophylactic low-dose heparin together with anti-thromboembolism stockings (TED) should be provided preoperatively. Low-dose molecular weight heparin and unfractionated heparin are equally efficacious prophylactic agents in major general surgical operations.[34] Pneumatic calf compression should be applied preoperatively and care taken in positioning the patient during surgery.

Where postoperative extradural analgesia is being proposed, unfractionated heparin and low molecular weight heparins should be discontinued 6 and 12 hours respectively before the insertion of the extradural catheter.

Patients on aspirin represent a particular problem. The decision to discontinue such therapy is a matter of choice for the individual surgeon. Where extradural analgesia is being considered, current opinion is that any patient taking 300 mg or more each day should have the drug discontinued 2 weeks prior to surgery. Those on low-dose therapy (75 mg) may remain on the medication. Intermediate-dose regimens should be discussed with the anaesthetist. Many non-proprietary over-the-counter medicines contain aspirin: it is therefore important to establish if the patient is taking any such medicines regularly, of which their general practitioner may be unaware.

Antibiotic prophylaxis

There is good evidence that the prophylactic administration of antibiotics can decrease morbidity, shorten hospital stay and reduce infection-related costs in general surgical operations. Broad-spectrum antibiotic prophylaxis against respiratory and wound infections should be administered immediately preoperatively or on induction of anaesthesia in accordance with locally agreed antibiotic policies.

Blood cross-match

Provided the haemoglobin is optimal preoperatively, 4 units of blood should be crossed-matched prior to surgery. Although immunosuppression has been described following transfusion, there is still no strong evidence that autologous or allogenic blood transfusion alters the prognosis in malignant disease. Consequently blood should never be withheld if there is a clinical indication (see Chapter 5).[35]

Peroperative management

Preoptimisation

Recently, evidence has been presented suggesting that admission to an intensive care unit (ICU) prior to major surgery, including oesophagectomy, may have a benefical effect on postoperative outcome. During a period of preoptimisation, Wilson et al.[36] ensured an adequate circulating haemoglobin concentration and administered various regimens of fluids and inotropes to patients in an attempt to enhance oxygen delivery. They demonstrated a reduction in mortality and length of stay in hospital as a consequence. Preoperative fluid loading was regarded as the most important factor. The study design has however been criticised and further evaluation of this interesting concept is awaited. The preoperative admission of high-risk patients to intensive care for cardiovascular optimisation has been shown to bring about a reduction in mortality and morbidity.[37] The demands on intensive care resources may limit preoptimisation to high-risk patients only.

Anaesthesia

The choice of anaesthetic technique for upper gastrointestinal surgery is largely one of individual preference taking into account the medical status of the patient. A technique utilising nitrous oxide and oxygen, and a volatile anaesthetic agent supplemented by opiate analgesics, neuromuscular paralysis and intermittent positive pressure ventilation is by far the most common. Total intravenous anaesthesia is another, although less popular, alternative. Combined techniques using general and regional anaesthesia are also popular.

Where given, premedication is again a matter of individual preference. Where dysphagia is troublesome soluble and liquid preparations should be used. H2 antagonists should be administered to those patients felt to be at risk from aspiration. With few exceptions, the patient's current medication should be given up until and including the day of surgery. This is especially important for cardiorespiratory therapeutic agents.

Rapid sequence induction

Where there is an appreciable risk of pulmonary aspiration the anaesthetist will elect to perform a rapid sequence induction and intubation in order to protect the airway during the induction of anaesthesia. A rapid sequence induction involves washing the nitrogen out of the lungs by preoxygenation with 100% oxygen for 3 minutes or more. This reservoir of oxygen allows the induction and intubation – after the administration of a short-acting depolarising muscle relaxant – to be performed in the apnoeic patient. An assistant protects the airway by gently pushing the cricoid ring against the adjacent cervical vertebral body so occluding the oesophageal lumen. Oesophageal occlusion is maintained until the trachea has been isolated by endotracheal intubation.

Endobronchial intubation

Anaesthesia for oesophageal surgery should only be undertaken by anaesthetists familiar with the complexities of one-lung ventilation.

Both gastric and oesophageal surgery can be performed in a patient intubated with a standard endotracheal tube. However, since oesophageal surgery usually involves a thoracotomy, unilateral lung deflation to facilitate surgical access is preferred. An appropriate double lumen endobronchial tube is selected. To facilitate the peroperative collapse of the right lung, as during a two-stage oesophagectomy, a left-sided endobronchial tube is used (**Fig. 4.1**). When a left

Figure 4.1
A Robertshaw double lumen endobronchial tube for isolating the left lung during the thoracic stage of an oesophagectomy. Photo by courtesy of Phoenix Medical Ltd.

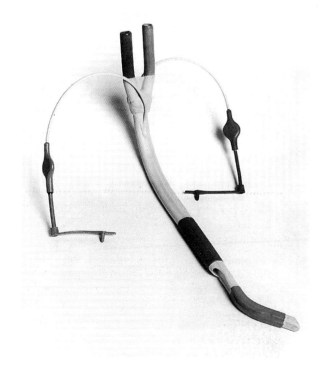

thoracoabdominal surgical approach is intended a right-sided endobronchial tube will allow collapse of the left lung. Irrespective of the side of the intended thoracotomy, a left-sided double lumen tube is the most popular as many maintain it is easier to position correctly. The right upper lobe bronchus is particularly susceptible to occlusion during right-sided endobronchial intubation owing to its close proximity to the carina.

Malposition of the endobronchial tube is excluded by auscultation of the chest and demonstration that both lung fields can be isolated from each other and ventilated adequately. During auscultation it is important to confirm that the left upper lobe bronchus is not compromised by the tube, otherwise one-lung anaesthesia will be associated with severe hypoxaemia. There is published evidence that shows malposition is less likely if the position of the double lumen tube is confirmed by fibreoptic bronchoscopy. However, the lumen of many of the smaller double lumen tubes are too small to allow the passage of some fibreoptic bronchoscopes and this limits its use in practice. Having correctly positioned the endobronchial tube the tracheal cuff is inflated immediately in order to isolate the lungs from the contents of the upper gastrointestinal tract should regurgitation occur.

Double lumen tubes are bulky and can interfere with the passage of a nasogastric tube. Some anaesthetists advocate passing the nasogastric tube before intubation, although in a patient with dysphagia this may increase the risk of pulmonary aspiration.

During a two-stage oesophageal operation when lung deflation will not be required for several hours, it is desirable to deflate the endobronchial cuff in order to minimise the risk of mucosal damage as a consequence of prolonged cuff inflation. After repositioning the patient in the lateral position for the second thoracic stage of the procedure it is essential to recheck the function of the double lumen tube.

Peroperative monitoring

The peroperative monitoring of patients undergoing oesophageal and gastric surgery should be comprehensive taking into consideration the patient's medical status (**Table 4.5**). Thoracotomy and one-lung anaesthesia will necessitate

Vital functions
  Electrocardiogram
  Blood pressure: non-invasive or invasive
  Central venous pressure
  Hourly urine output
  Oximetry
  Core temperature

Ventilation
  End tidal carbon dioxide
  Inspired oxygen concentration
  Airway pressure
  Tidal volume

Table 4.5 *Minimum peroperative monitoring of a patient during upper gastrointestinal surgery*

invasive cardiovascular monitoring. Invasive blood pressure and central venous pressure monitoring allows the anaesthetist to detect instantaneously cardiovascular instability associated with one-lung anaesthesia and surgical manipulation of mediastinal and hiatal structures.

Heat conservation

Heat conservation is an important aspect of anaesthetic management during major surgery. Hypothermic patients are more intolerant to pain and discomfort postoperatively and exhibit cardiovascular instability particularly as they vasodilate on rewarming. Shivering causes a substantial increase in oxygen consumption which can lead to hypoxaemia unless adequate supplementary oxygen is given.

Oesophageal surgery

The anaesthetic management of the first stage of a two-stage oesophagectomy is identical to the management of an abdominal gastrectomy. Most of the difficulties for the anaesthetist arise from the need for one-lung anaesthesia during the second stage of the procedure.

Cardiovascular instability

Surgical manipulation of the hiatus and mediastinum is often associated with sudden cardiovascular instability. Excessive peritoneal traction can cause an increase in vagal tone that is manifest as a profound bradycardia. Manipulation of the heart can precipitate unstable dysrhythmias. A misplaced retractor, hand or surgical pack can result in a sudden reduction in venous return and a fall in cardiac output and blood pressure. Delivering the stomach through the hiatus into the chest is especially hazardous in this respect. There is some evidence that the more extensive the hiatal dissection and diaphragmatic resection during the abdominal stage of a two-stage oesophagectomy, then the less disruption there is to the cardiovascular system during the delivery of the stomach into the thorax during the second stage. If this cardiovascular instability is associated with a period of relative hypoxia during one-lung anaesthesia the situation can become potentially life threatening if uncorrected. Again, good communication between the surgeon and the anaesthetist is of paramount importance.

One-lung anaesthesia

With the patient in the left lateral position the dependent lung is ventilated through the longer endobronchial limb. To aid surgical access to the oesophagus the non-dependent right lung is collapsed by occluding the gas flow through the tracheal limb and opening the lumen to the atmosphere. Adequate ventilation must be delivered to the dependent lung to avoid hypoxaemia. The endobronchial portion of the tube in the dependent bronchus is especially prone to displacement during surgical manipulation of any tumour adjacent to the carina and excessive movement of the tube can have an effect on the ventilation delivered to the dependent lung.

In consequence, by collapsing the non-dependent lung, the area available for respiratory exchange is substantially reduced. In adopting the lateral position gravity allows the less compliant dependent lung to be preferentially perfused. Blood perfusing the collapsed lung is no longer oxygenated and will mix with oxygenated blood from the ventilated dependent lung in the heart causing venous admixture and a fall in arterial oxygen tension.

The aetiology of hypoxia during one-lung anaesthesia is multifactorial (**Table 4.6**). and not exclusively due to the collapse of one lung (**Fig. 4.2**). Hypoxia during one-lung anaesthesia for oesophageal surgery can be of a greater magnitude than during surgery for primary lung disease. Diseased lung is often poorly perfused and the ensuing hypoxia activates the hypoxic pulmonary vasoconstrictor response, an important homeostatic mechanism that serves to direct blood flow to better oxygenated parts of the lungs. In a patient undergoing an oesophagectomy a healthy lung is suddenly deflated and a substantial imbalance of ventilation and perfusion occurs (i.e. V/Q mismatch). Pulmonary hypoxic vasoconstriction counteracts the effects of non-ventilated alveoli on gas exchange by the redistribution of capillary blood towards the oxygenated lung.

However the hypoxic pulmonary vasoconstrictor response is known to be rendered less responsive by hypocarbia ($PaCO_2$ < 4.0 kPa), increased FiO_2 and inhalational anaesthetic agents. This latter observation does not appear to be significant at the inhaled anaesthetic concentrations commonly used during surgery. For a more detailed discussion of the hypoxic pulmonary vasoconstrictor response the reader should consult the review by Eisenkraft.[38]

One-lung anaesthesia does not appear to impair the efficiency of the lungs to remove carbon dioxide from the body. This is reflected by the observation that no major compensatory adjustments of the minute ventilation are necessary when switching from two-lung ventilation. During an oesophagectomy the ventilated lung is subjected to compressive forces which can result in a degree of pulmonary atelectasis. Surgical manipulation, the effects of gravity on mediastinal structures, the weight of the abdominal contents acting through a paralysed diaphragm and the weight of the patient lying on the dependent lung all contribute in this respect. A fall in functional residual capacity and compliance in the dependent ventilated lung ensues. In consequence patchy atelectasis within the dependent lung is not an uncommon finding on a postoperative chest radiograph.

The second stage of an oesophagectomy involves the collapse of the non-dependent lung to facilitate surgical access.

One-lung anaesthesia in a patient with healthy lungs

Pre-existing disease in the dependent ventilated lung

Displaced endobronchial tube

Partly occluded endobronchial tube

Low cardiac output due to hypovolaemia, mediastinal manipulation or compression of the inferior vena cava

Peroperative deterioration of the dependent lung

Massive blood transfusion

Table 4.6 *Aetiology of peroperative hypoxia during one-lung anaesthesia for oesophageal surgery*

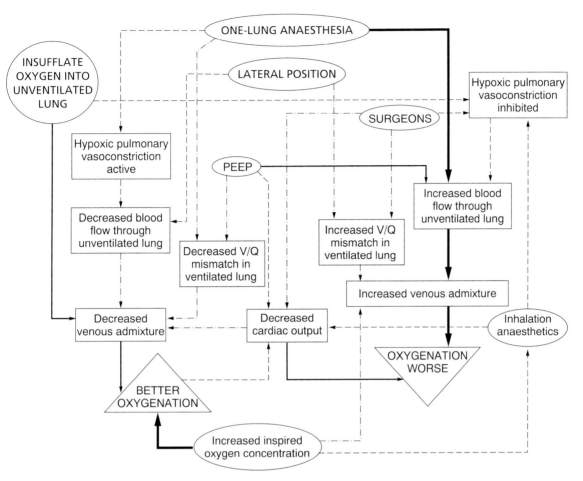

Figure 4.2
Interactions between various factors which can affect arterial oxygenation during one-lung anaesthesia for an oesophagectomy. Physiological influences are placed in oblong boxes in the centre and the resultant effect on oxygenation indicated by the orientation of the triangles. Relevant extrinsic factors are placed in ovals round the periphery. The thickness of the connecting arrow indicates the relative importance of the effect. Most of these factors can have both beneficial and detrimental effects and the difficulty in predicting the behaviour of an individual patient lies in the varying balances between these effects. During an oesophagectomy in particular, surgical manipulation can be of major significance. After Kerr[45] with permission.

Anaesthetic techniques during one-lung anaesthesia

One of the anaesthetist's primary objectives during the thoracic stage of an oesophagectomy is to match ventilation with perfusion in the dependent lung. With this in mind several manoeuvres have been proposed (**Table 4.7**).

Provided the double lumen tube is correctly positioned and cardiac output maintained, adequate oxygenation can often be achieved simply by increasing the fractional inspired oxygen concentration to 0.5. If hypoxia persists increasing the oxygen concentration further to 100% is often sufficient.

Dependent lung ventilation
  Increasing the inspired oxygen concentration
  Positive end expiratory pressure (PEEP)

Non-dependent deflated lung
  Oxygen insufflation
  Continous positive end expiratory pressure (CPAP)

Both lungs
  Intermittent two-lung ventilation
  Continuous two-lung ventilation with lung retraction

Circulation
  Maintenance of an adequate cardiac output
  Temporary interruption of arterial blood flow to non-dependent lung

Table 4.7 *Manoeuvres to reduce the ventilation/perfusion mismatch during the thoracic stage of an oesophagectomy*

If hypoxia persists the anaesthetist has several options available not all of which have been fully substantiated as totally beneficial. The application of 5–15 cm H_2O positive end expiratory pressure (PEEP) to the dependent ventilated lung has been advocated as a means of preventing atelectasis. PEEP increases the area available for gas exchange and improves the functional residual capacity by recruiting collapsed alveoli so reducing any existing shunt. PEEP cannot however be regarded as free of risk. It increases the pulmonary vascular resistance within the ventilated lung and can redirect blood through the non-ventilated lung and thus the risk of barotrauma is ever present. Combined with any detrimental effects PEEP might have on cardiac output there can in some circumstances be an exacerbation of the hypoxia. It has been postulated that the beneficial effects of PEEP can be enhanced by applying continuous end expiratory pressure (CPAP) to the collapsed lung. In practice however this combined manoeuvre is often associated with a reduction in cardiac output.

The insufflation of 2–5 l/min of 100% oxygen to the collapsed non-dependent lung is a simple and often effective way of maintaining adequate oxygenation during one-lung anaesthesia. Too high a flow can result in reinflation of the lung and obscure the surgical field. Insufflation of oxygen into the collapsed lung can also obtund the homeostatic hypoxic pulmonary vasoconstrictor response. The application of less than 10 cm H_2O CPAP to the collapsed lung is said to have a similarly beneficial effect. Provided that adequate anaesthesia is maintained awareness is not a problem.

An important aspect of the anaesthetic management of the second stage of an oesophagectomy is the maintenance of an adequate cardiac output, blood pressure and organ perfusion. Changes in cardiac output will affect arterial oxygenation even in the presence of optimal pulmonary ventilation. Where an appreciable shunt already exists (> 30%) a fall in cardiac output will exacerbate any systemic hypoxia. Surgical behaviour is an important factor in the wellbeing of the patient. During an oesophagectomy inadvertent surgical compression of the inferior vena cava or the right atrium can precipitate a sudden reduction in cardiac output with deleterious effects on oxygenation and organ perfusion.

When the anaesthetist is unable to maintain adequate oxygenation despite the above measures then two-lung ventilation, either intermittently or continuously with retraction of the non-dependent lung, will have to be adopted. Unquestionably this will make the surgery considerably more difficult and re-identifying the surgical plane after deflation can be difficult (S. M. Griffin, personal communication). Temporary occlusion of the pulmonary artery supplying the non-ventilated lung has been advocated in the past where the hypoxia is persistent and unresponsive to the above measures. In practice this is almost never necessary.

On completion of the surgery the collapsed lung is aspirated and reinflated by hand ventilation under direct vision. Failure to reinflate the lung fully can be a major cause of postoperative hypoxia. Difficulty in reinflation, although uncommon, may be encountered if endobronchial secretions are especially tenacious and suction bronchoscopy is then indicated. The anaesthetist has to be vigilant when moving the patient from the lateral to the supine position as this can be associated with a sudden fall in blood pressure due to improved perfusion of the non-dependent tissues. The nasogastric tube should be stitched securely into position.

Postoperative care

Appropriate postoperative facilities for the patient's aftercare must be available prior to undertaking upper gastrointestinal surgery.

The postoperative care of these patients must be of a high standard if the skills of the anaesthetist and surgeon are to be consolidated. The aim of postoperative monitoring is to facilitate prompt intervention so as to prevent complications arising which increase morbidity or mortality. Where a patient is nursed will depend on the nature of the surgery, the medical status of the patient and the facilities available within the hospital. The options are generally on a surgical ward familiar with upper gastrointestinal surgery, in a High Dependency Unit (HDU) or an Intensive Care Unit (ICU). These last two have the advantage of a higher nurse to patient ratio and the facilities to monitor the patient invasively. The patient should be adequately monitored during the period of transfer from the operating theatre to the HDU or ICU.

The major concerns during the immediate postoperative period after upper abdominal or thoracic surgery are hypoxia, thermoregulation, cardiovascular stability, renal function and analgesia. Baseline postoperative haematological and biochemical profiles, an arterial blood gas and a chest X-ray should be obtained.

The first 48 hours postoperatively are extremely important. Thoracoabdominal and upper abdominal surgery are known to have a higher incidence of postoperative hypoxaemia and desaturation, particularly during the early postoperative period.[39]

All patients who have undergone an uncomplicated gastrectomy can usually be extubated in theatre and then nursed in a ward or HDU. Where a period of postoperative ventilation is indicated then transfer to an ICU is mandatory. The criteria for extubation under these latter circumstances should include a stable cardiovascular system, less than 50 ml/hour blood loss from the surgical drains, the absence of hypercarbia and an adequate oxygen saturation on an FiO_2 of less than 0.4 while breathing spontaneously, an active cough and gag reflex, the ability to respond to commands and the absence of distressing pain and confusion.

Postoperative hypoxia

Postoperative hypoxia is a common sequel to upper gastrointestinal surgery. At an arterial oxygen tension of less than 8 kPa or 90% oxygen saturation, end organ hypoxia can ensue if left uncorrected. All patients must receive humidified oxygen appropriate to their needs postoperatively and have their oxygen saturation monitored as provision of oxygen by a face mask alone may be insufficient.

Advanced age, smoking, pre-existing cardiorespiratory disease and obesity can further exacerbate hypoxia. In the immediate postoperative period the residual effects of anaesthesia can cause hypoxia. Diffusion hypoxia is a well-recognised transient short-lived phenomenon observed at the cessation of anaesthesia. When nitrous oxide is discontinued this highly diffusible gas enters the alveoli and dilutes the alveolar air resulting in a fall in PaO_2 unless supplementary oxygen is administered. Opiate analgesia and inhalational anaesthetics also depress the ventilatory response to carbon dioxide and hypoxia.

Upper abdominal and thoracic operations are detrimental to ventilatory mechanisms and gas exchange. The aetiology of postoperative hypoxia is multifactorial and typically lasts for several days. Both the vital capacity and functional residual capacity (FRC) are reduced. As the FRC falls it encroaches on the closing volume such that airway closure occurs during tidal ventilation in the dependent parts of the lungs. The resultant pulmonary shunt gives rise to hypoxia. Among the contributory factors are persistent pain, supine posture, inadequate expectoration and subsequent atelectasis, a decrease in thoracic compliance, diaphragmatic and intercostal muscle dysfunction and pleural collections.

Several measures to minimise postoperative hypoxia and pulmonary complications following upper gastrointestinal surgery have been advocated. These include adequate analgesia, a semi-erect posture (particularly in the obese) that increases FRC, continuous humidified oxygen for 4 consecutive days and regular physiotherapy. Some clinicians prefer a brief period of postoperative ventilation on ICU for patients who have undergone an oesophagectomy. This can be of value in allowing for the vital functions to be optimised to aid lung expansion for efficient endobronchial suction and for physiotherapy to be performed without distress.

Cardiovascular instability

Fluid and blood requirements have to be carefully monitored during the immediate postoperative period. Patients who have undergone a prolonged oesophagectomy often require appreciable volumes of fluid in the immediate postoperative period. Central venous pressure monitoring can be useful in the evaluation of the patient's fluid requirement. A fall in systemic vascular resistance coinciding with rewarming after prolonged surgery can be associated with systemic hypotension and an inadequate urine output. An acceptable haemoglobin concentration must be maintained for adequate oxygen transport.

Although common practice, blood transfusion is a potentially hazardous procedure and blood should only be given when absolutely necessary. Stored blood has a high affinity for oxygen as a result of a decrease in electrolyte 2,3-diphosphoglycerate. The oxygen dissociation curve (ODC) is displaced to the left and impaired tissue oxygen delivery can result. This effect is further exacerbated by hypothermia and alkalosis. Apart from the risk of transfusion reactions and transmission of infection, blood transfusion can also be associated with electrolyte disturbances, coagulopathies and impaired gas exchange secondary to pulmonary microaggregate deposition. Provided the patient is kept normovolaemic and pulmonary gas exchange is unimpeded a degree of postoperative haemodilution will be tolerated by most patients. Adequate tissue oxygenation can be maintained at a haematocrit of 25–30%. Tissue blood flow will be maintained by a combination of increased stroke volume and cardiac output and a fall in viscous flow resistance.

Maintaining normovolaemia is very important as hypovolaemic patients can demonstrate an exaggerated hypotensive response to opiate analgesics. New dysrhythmias in the postoperative period must be evaluated carefully. Atrial fibrillation in particular may herald early mediastinitis and an anastomotic leak. Chest drains which have been inserted too far can also precipitate atrial fibrillation. There is no evidence that prophylactic digitalisation is of any value in patients who have undergone an oesophagectomy.

Postoperative pain

Pain can be considerable after upper abdominal and thoracic surgery. Pain inhibits movement and coughing leading to sputum retention, atelectasis and chest infection. Effective pain relief has been consistently shown to improve pulmonary function postoperatively as assessed by measured improvements in FEV_1 and vital capacity. The elected method of pain relief after gastrectomy and oesophagectomy will depend on the expertise and facilities available. Most commonly this involves either systemic patient-controlled analgesia (PCA) or epidural analgesia. Both techniques can be supplemented by non-steroidal analgesia (NSAID) provided there are no contraindications to their use.

Although the main source of pain will be the surgical site, discomfort can arise from elsewhere. Inability to move around freely in the immediate postoperative period, shoulder pain arising from an unfamiliar posture during thoracotomy, difficulties with micturition, gastrointestinal distension and hypothermia can all exacerbate existing pain.

Parenteral patient-controlled analgesia (PCA)

A small bolus of intravenous morphine delivered on patient demand by a preprogrammed syringe driver is considerably more efficacious than as-required intramuscular injections. The system allows the size and rate of the bolus injection to be altered. Inadvertent overdosage is avoided by limiting the size of the boluses, the total dose administered and the timed interval between doses. For safety the control panel should be locked and out of reach of the patient and relatives.

The technique is flexible, painless and well received by patients who can attain more consistent analgesia largely because any individual variation in opiate pharmacokinetics and pharmacodynamics is compensated for by the patients themselves. The most suitable opiate analgesics are those with relatively short half-lives. The infusion should be administered through a dedicated cannula or a one-way valve to avoid retrograde accumulation of opiate when administered in conjunction with an intravenous infusion. A constant background infusion of opiate is associated with a higher incidence of complications and is best avoided particularly outwith an area of high dependency nursing. Concomitant treatment with antiemetics is usually necessary.

A prerequisite of PCA following surgery is adequate monitoring of respiratory function and the conscious state. PCA is only effective if the patient has the ability to cooperate and comprehend. Although a safe technique, before using any PCA system staff training is mandatory as technical errors can be fatal.

Epidural analgesia

Epidural analgesia using either a continuous infusion of opiate, local anaesthetic, or a combination of both, can provide extremely effective postoperative analgesia following upper gastrointestinal surgery. Efficacy can be further enhanced by employing patient-controlled delivery devices to provide supplementary extradural boluses. A reduction in postoperative respiratory complications, hospital stay and mortality has been attributed to the use of epidural analgesia after oesophagectomy.[40]

Provided a patient with an epidural receives appropriate skilled care the technique, although not without side effects, is relatively safe.[41]

Whether the epidural catheter is sited before or after the induction of anaesthesia is currently a matter of much debate. Serious morbidity related to regional anaesthesia is extremely uncommon but the risk of inflicting unrecognised neural damage has led some clinicians to propose that they should only be inserted in the awake patient. Others argue that there is little evidence of any increased risk of neural damage in the anaesthetised patient, that commonly patient preference is to be anaesthetised first, that this is the technique used in children, and that under some circumstances it is not an option. In one study of epidural analgesia after oesophagectomy all catheters were sited in anaesthetised patients without complication.[40] The choice rests with the individual anaesthetist after obtaining informed consent from the patient.

The vertebral level at which an epidural catheter is inserted will depend upon the dermatomes to be rendered analgesic. Ideally this should represent a central dermatome of the surgical incision. However the effective placement of an epidural catheter in the lower thoracic region is advocated by some clinicians who maintain that it is easier and safer to identify the epidural space at the lower vertebral level. Conversely an epidural sited in the lower vertebral region may necessitate the use of higher doses of local anaesthetics and opiates, increasing the risk of central side effects.

Epidural analgesia offers a number of advantages: there is a lower incidence of respiratory morbidity compared with systemic opiates, it may facilitate early postoperative extubation particularly when it is combined intraoperatively with general anaesthesia, and it appears to allow the more rapid return of normal gastrointestinal function. Of these, the reduced respiratory morbidity is invariably quoted as the most advantageous.[40,42] Any beneficial effects from thoracic epidural analgesia on lung volumes, respiratory mechanics and gas exchange are dependent on the extent of the segmental block. A fuller discussion of the patho-physiology of thoracic epidural analgesia can be found in the recent review by Van Aken and Rolf.[43]

Epidural analgesia is a potentially hazardous technique and requires a high degree of skill, particularly in the thoracic region. The patient must be closely observed by trained and competent staff thereafter. Both medical and nursing staff have to be totally familiar with possible side effects especially in recognising an excessively high block, hypotension, central nervous system and respiratory depression. Parenteral opiates are contraindicated in the presence of a function-ing epidural.

In a recent prospective study of epidural analgesia[41] catheter-related complica-tions were identified as the most common and avoidable, in particular catheter dislodgement. The same audit reported that 75% of the insertion sites exhibited local inflammation 4 days postoperatively. Other complications associated with epidural analgesia include failed, incomplete or inadequate analgesia, lower limb motor weakness, pruritus, nausea, headache as a consequence of inadvertent dural puncture and hallucinations. Although ward-based epidural analgesia is becoming more common with the deployment of dedicated pain teams, consideration should always be given to nursing these patients in an ITU, HDU or appropriate ward environment with adequate staff and monitoring.

Bilateral sympathetic autonomic blockade and subsequent hypotension is common after extradural bupivacaine particularly in the thoracic region. Hypotension is exacerbated by hypovolaemia, head-up posture and limited cardiovascular reserve. Consequently patients unable to tolerate fluid loads may not be ideal candidates for epidural analgesia employing local anaesthetics. Epidural opiates are devoid of these cardiovascular effects but can be associated with central respiratory depression of an unpredictable and insidious onset. The risk of respiratory depression by cephalad spread of the epidural opiate appears to be related to the lipid solubility of the drug. Morphine, an opiate of low lipophilicity, can cause respiratory depression of late onset in contrast to highly soluble fentanyl which can precipitate the early onset of respiratory depression. The central depressant effects of epidural opiates are potentiated by systemic opiates and the two should never be administered concurrently. Diamorphine may be used as an alternative to morphine.

In an attempt to reduce the risks of these side effects combinations of opiates and local anaesthetics have been used with some success. However the sympathetic block does not seem to be readily amenable to changes in drug combination.

Epidural analgesia may be administered by bolus or by continuous infusion. Although effective, the latter has a higher incidence of CNS depression when opiates alone are given. The choice of therapeutic agent for epidural analgesia after upper gastrointestinal surgery should be made only after consideration of all the potential side effects (**Table 4.8**).

Local analgesia

Infiltration of the wound with local anaesthetic at the end of surgery is more effective for somatic pain than visceral pain but may help to reduce the patient's

	Opiates	**Local anaesthetics**
Cardiovascular	Usually no effect	Frequently causes hypotension secondary to sympathetic block
Respiratory Depression	**Early** from systemic absorption	Unusual unless block involves depression of the intercostal muscles and diaphragm
	Late from rostral spread in the CSF augmented by age/dose/posture/ aqueous solubility /additional systemic opiate	An excessively high block
Nausea and vomiting	Similar to i.m. administration	Only as a sequelae to hypotension
Itching	Most common with morphine than fentanyl or diamorphine. Relieved by naloxone or an antihistamine	Nil
Urinary retention	Variable. Improved by naloxone	Common with lower blocks
Sedation	Excessive sedation can be associated with severe respiratory depression	Occasionally mild as a result of decreased input to the reticular activating system

Table 4.8 *Comparison of opiates and local anaesthetics when given via the epidural route (from Wilson and Smith, with permission)*[44]

opiate requirement. Bupivacaine (0.25% without adrenaline) to a maximum dose of 2 mg/kg is the most popular.

Summary

Upper gastrointestinal surgery and particularly for carcinoma, presents the anaesthetist with a challenge. Good communication between the surgeon and the anaesthetist is important for the wellbeing of the patient. During the preoperative period the patient's cardiopulmonary status should be optimised, if necessary recruiting specialist advice. Upper abdominal and thoracic surgery have significant effects on respiratory mechanics which have implications for the postoperative care. During one-lung anaesthesia surgical manipulation of an oesophageal tumour and adjacent mediastinal structures can have a major impact on cardiovascular stability and oxygenation. Successful surgery can only be consolidated by a high standard of appropriate postoperative care. Effective postoperative analgesia is necessary to improve pulmonary function.

References

1. Copeland GP, Jones D, Walters M. POSSUM: a scoring system for surgical audit. Br J Surg 1991; 78:355–60.

2. Prytherch DR, Whiteley B, Higgins B et al. POSSUM and Portsmouth POSSUM for predicting mortality. Br J Surg 1998; 85:1217–20.

3. Shoemaker WC, Appel PL, Kram HB et al. Prospective trail of supranormal values of survivors as therapeutic goals in high-risk surgical patients. Chest 1988; 94:1176–86.

4. CEPOD 1992: The Report of the National Confidential Enquiry into Perioperative Deaths. 1990. Campling EA, Devlin HB, Hoile RW, Lunn JN (eds.).

5. Goldman L, Debra MPH, Caldera RN et al. Multifactorial index of cardiac risk in noncardiac surgical procedures. New Engl J Med 1977; 297:845–50.

6. CEPOD 1995: The Report of the National Confidential Enquiry into Perioperative Deaths. 1992/93. Campling EA, Devlin HB, Hoile RW, Lunn JN (eds.).

7. Wong DH, Weber EC, Schell MJ et al. Factors associated with postoperative pulmonary complications in patients with severe chronic obstructive pulmonary disease. Anaesthesia and Analgesia 1995; 80:276–84.

8. Drug and Therapeutic Bulletin. Low molecular weight heparins for venous thromboembolism. 1998; 36:25–9.

9. Steen PA, Tinker JH, Tarhan S. Myocardial reinfarction after anaesthesia in surgery. JAMA 1978; 239:2566–70.

10. Black GW. Aspiration pneumonitis and its prevention. Hospital Update 1994; 20:1S–7S.

11. Hebert PC, Wells G, Blajchman MA et al. A multicenter randomised controlled clinical trial of blood transfusion in the critically ill. New Engl J Med 1999; 340:409–17.

12. Gombotz H. Preoperative anaemia and polycythaemia. Baillère's Clinical Anaesthesiology 1998; 12:451–69.

13. Goldman L. Assessment of perioperative cardiac risk. New Engl J Med 1994; 330:707–09.

14. Mangano DT. Preoperative assessment of the patient with cardiac disease. Baillière's Clinical Anaesthesiology 1989; 3:47–102.

15. Detsky AS, Abrams HB, McLauchlin JR. Predicting cardiac complications in patients undergoing non-cardiac surgery. J Gen Int Med 1986; 41:211–19.

16. Carliner HN, Fisher ML, Plotnick GD et al. Routine preoperative exercise testing in patients undergoing major non-cardiac surgery. Am J Surg 1985; 56:51–8.

17. Dick WF. Preoperative screening for elective surgery. Baillière's Clinical Anaesthesiology 1998; 12:349–71.

18. Deanfield JE, Shea M, Ribiero P et al. Transient ST-segment depression as a marker of myocardial ischaemia during daily life. Am J Cardiol 1984; 54:1195–1200.

19. Entwhistle MD, Roe PG, Sapsford DJ et al. Patterns of oxygenation after thoracotomy. Br J Anaesth 1991; 67:704–11.

20. Fan ST, Lau WY, Yip WC et al. Prediction of postoperative pulmonary complications in oesophagogastric surgery. Br J Surg 1987; 74:408–10.

21. Nunn JF, Milledge JS, Chen D et al. Respiratory criteria of fitness for surgery and anaesthesia. Anaesthesia 1988; 43:543–51.

22. Erskine RJ, Hanning CD. Do I advise my patient to stop smoking preoperatively? Current Anaesthesia and Critical Care 1992; 3:175–80.

23. Nagawa H, Kobori O, Mutto T. Prediction of pulmonary complications after transthoracic oesophagectomy. Br J Surg 1994; 81:860–2.

24. Cohn PF. Silent ischaemia as a manifestation of asymptomatic coronary artery disease. Am J Cardiol 1985; 56:28D–34D.

25. Ninan M, Sommers KE, Landreneua RJ et al. Standardised exercise oximetry predicts post pneumonectomy outcome. Ann Thorac Surg 1997; 64:328–33.

26. Juste RN, Lawson AD, Soni N. Minimising cardiac anaesthetic risk. Anaesthesia 1996; 51:255–62.

27. Prys-Roberts C, Meloche, R. Foex P. Studies of anaesthesia in relation to hypertension. I: Cardiovascular responses of treated and untreated patients. Br J Anaesth 1971; 43:122–27.

28. Goldman L, Caldera DL. Risks of general anaesthesia and elective operation in the hypertensive patient. Anaesthesiology 1979; 50:285–90.

29. Hiber KC, Evans MA, Bresnahan JF et al. Outcome of noncardiac operations in patients with severe coronary artery disease successfully treated preoperatively with coronary anagioplasty. Mayo Clin Proc 1992; 67:15–20.

30. Brooks-Brunn JA. Postoperative atelectasis and pneumonia. Heart Lung 1995; 24:94–115.

31. CEPOD 1993: The Report of the National Confidential Enquiry into Perioperative Deaths.

1991/1992. Campling EA, Devlin HB, Hoile RW, Lunn JN (eds.).

32. Shenkman Z, Shir Y, Brodsky JB. Perioperative management of the obese patient. Br J Anaesthesia 1993; 70:349–59.

33. Watson A. Operable oesophageal cancer. Current results from the West. World J Surg 1994; 18:361–67.

34. Drug and Therapeutic Bulletin. Drugs in the perioperative period. Stopping or continuing drugs around surgery. 1999; 37:62–4.

35. Busch ORC, Hop WCJ, van Papendrecht MAW et al. Blood transfusion and prognosis in colorectal cancer. New Engl J Med 1993; 328:1372–6.

36. Wilson J, Wood I, Fawcett J et al. Reducing the risk of major elective surgery: Randomised controlled trial of preoperative optimisation of oxygen therapy. BMJ 1999; 7191:1099–103.

37. Curran JE, Grounds RM. Ward versus intensive care management of high risk surgical patients. Br J Surg 1998; 85:956–61.

38. Eisenkraft JB. Anaesthesia and hypoxic pulmonary vasoconstriction. In: Atkinson RS, Adams AP (eds). Recent Advances in Anaesthesia vol. 18. Edinburgh: Churchill Livingstone, 1994, pp. 103–22.

39. Xue FS, Bai WL, Zhang GS et al. The influence of surgical sites on early postoperative hypoxaemia in adults undergoing elective surgery. Anaesthesia and Analgesia 1999; 88:213–9.

40. Watson A, Allen PR. Influence of thoracic epidural analgesia on outcome after resection of oesophageal cancer. Surgery 1994; 115:429–32.

41. Burstal R, Wegener F, Hayes C et al. Epidural analgesia: prospective audit of 1062 patients. Anaesthesia and Intensive Care 1998; 26:165–172.

42. Ballantyne JC, Carr DB, de Ferranti S et al. The comparative effects of postoperative analgesic therapies on pulmonary outcome; cummulative meta-analyses or randomised, controlled trials. Anaesthesia and Analgesia 1998; 86:598–612.

43. Van Aken H, Rolf N. Clinical anaesthesiology: Thoracic epidural anaesthesia. Baillière's Best Practice and Research 1999; 13:2–109.

44. Wilson IG, Smith G. Management of acute pain. Hospital Update 1993; April:214–22.

45. Kerr JH. Physiological aspects of one-lung anaesthesia. International Anaesthesiology Clinics 1972; 10:61–78.

5 Surgery for cancer of the oesophagus

S. Michael Griffin

INTRODUCTION

Oesophageal cancer is well recognised as being one of the most challenging pathological conditions confronting the surgeon. This is not only due to the versatility required in surgical reconstruction but also the magnitude of the surgical procedure, dealing with wide areas of the neck, mediastinum and abdomen. No other modality to date has consistently been shown to provide a chance of cure in this increasingly common cancer. Many efforts have been made to increase the cure rate while maintaining the safety of the procedure, but despite this, the overall survival for oesophageal cancer remains around 10% in most countries. Whereas treatment for cancer of the oesophagus is multidisciplinary, surgery, whenever possible, is the primary mode of therapy. The surgical procedure required may need to differ in individual cases, depending on the nature of the tumour and the condition of the patient and, therefore, the method of approach and the extent of resection and dissection.

The disease often presents late when increasing dysphagia has developed over several months and the tumour has been present for many months or years. Patients with oesophageal cancer have to be considered either for radical treatment or simply for palliative therapy in those who are too elderly or unfit or whose tumours are too far advanced. Although surgery for advanced tumours (T3N1) is unlikely to lead to long-term survival, it nevertheless provides symptomatic relief for the patient suffering from progressive dysphagia, loss of weight and increasing retrosternal discomfort. As the disease predominantly affects the elderly, treatment must be associated with a low morbidity and mortality. Although surgical intervention may not be tolerated well in very elderly people, neither indeed are radiotherapy or chemotherapy regimens, both of which can cause debilitating systemic effects and have their own morbidity and mortality.

Several modalities of therapy are available to the clinician dealing with oesophageal cancer. A combination of these modalities may well have to be used in the future management of these patients. While randomised multicentred clinical trials are essential in assessing future therapeutic regimens the lead clinician in the multidisciplinary team must exercise judgement in the choice of the appropriate combination of therapies available at the present time. These will depend on patient age, fitness, symptoms, prognosis and the stage and histopathology of the malignancy itself.

Surgical pathology

The majority of oesophageal neoplasms are epithelial in origin. They arise from the squamous lining of the mucosa, but increasingly also from metaplastic columnar epithelium, resulting in glandular carcinomas affecting specialised epithelium in the lower oesophagus. Tumour site and histology are two crucial factors requiring assessment: tumours arising from different sites in the oesophagus vary in their behaviour. Squamous cell carcinoma and adenocarcinoma arising from the cervical oesophagus, thoracic oesophagus and cardia, differ in their mode of spread and response to therapeutic modalities. This has been discussed in detail in Chapter 1. It is essential, therefore, that the anatomical regions of the oesophagus are described such that the different therapeutic surgical procedures adopted for tumours at each site can be understood.

Surgical anatomy

The oesophagus is a midline hollow viscus, starting at the cricopharyngeal sphincter at the level of the 6th cervical vertebra, entering the chest at the level of the suprasternal notch and traversing the posterior mediastinum and entering the abdomen through the oesophageal hiatus in the diaphragm to join the stomach at the cardia. It bears a close relationship to the trachea and pericardium in front and the vertebral column posteriorly. The vagus and its branches are in close proximity over its entire length. There is no serosal covering. The thoracic duct enters the posterior mediastinum through the aortic opening in the diaphragm. It lies on the bodies of the thoracic vertebrae posterolateral to the oesophagus and between the aorta and the azygos vein. The left atrium and the inferior pulmonary veins lie in intimate contact with the left wall of the lower third of the oesophagus.

The TNM classification has been proposed and revised in 1997[1] to combine the salient features of the staging process. This classification has divided the oesophagus into discrete anatomical regions (see **Fig. 5.1**).

Hypopharynx and cervical oesophagus

The region between the level of the pharyngo-epiglottic fold and the inferior border of the cricoid cartilage is known as the hypopharynx; that above, as the oropharynx. The cervical oesophagus begins at the lower border of the cricoid cartilage and terminates at the level of the thoracic inlet or jugular notch. Surgical management of carcinomas in these regions differs from that of other parts of the oesophagus, because tumour extension in these two areas commonly overlap. This is considered separately later in the chapter.

Figure 5.1
Anatomical regions of the hypopharynx, oesophagus and gastric cardia.

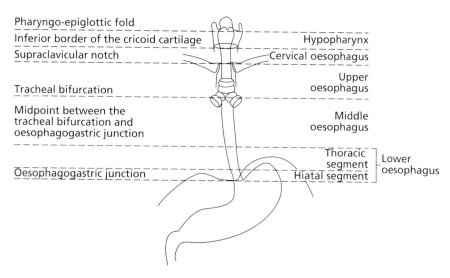

Upper oesophagus

This segment of the oesophagus extends between the level of the jugular notch and the carina.

Middle oesophagus

This section of oesophagus extends from the tracheal bifurcation to the midpoint between the tracheal bifurcation and the oesophago-gastric junction.

Lower oesophagus

This is comprised of both the lower thoracic oesophagus and the hiatal segment of the oesophagus. The latter segment is often termed the 'abdominal oesophagus'. The oesophago-gastric junction is a somewhat nebulous term and the anatomy depends on the differing view points of surgeons, endoscopists, radiologists, pathologists and anatomists. It is further complicated by the presence or absence of a hiatal hernia and the presence or absence of a columnar lined oesophagus.

Blood supply and lymphatics

The blood supply is derived directly from the aorta in the form of oesophageal vessels together with branches adjacent to or from organs such as the pulmonary hilum, trachea, stomach and thyroid gland. The venous drainage is through tributaries draining into the azygos and hemiazygos system in the chest, via the thyroid veins in the neck and the left gastric vein in the upper abdomen.

The lymphatics of the oesophagus are distributed predominantly in the form of a submucous plexus and a paraoesophageal plexus. Both plexi receive lymph from all parts of the respective layers of the oesophageal wall. The plexi communicate through penetrating vessels which traverse the longitudinal and circular muscle walls. The paraoesophageal plexus drains into the paraoesophageal lymph nodes which are situated on the surface of the oesophagus and also into perioesophageal lymph nodes, situated in close proximity to the oesophagus. Lymphatics also drain from the perioesophageal nodes to the lateral oesophageal nodes or directly from the para to the lateral oesophageal nodes, skipping the perioesophageal group (see **Table 5.1** and **Fig. 3.3,** Chapter 3).[2]

Preoperative surgical preparation

Meticulous preoperative evaluation and estimation of surgical risk is a prerequisite to successful surgical outcome in this disease. Postoperative complications may be either patient or surgeon related. Patient-related factors include extreme age, malnutrition secondary to malignancy in general or to dysphagia, immunosuppression secondary to bone-marrow depression that may result from adjuvant chemo- or radiotherapy and lastly, associated systemic diseases which are more common with increasing age.

Nutritional support

Significant malnutrition as well as dehydration are frequently seen in patients with oesophageal narrowing and should be corrected preoperatively. Malnutrition is associated with loss of tissue function leading to many potential complications during the postoperative period, such as wound breakdown, respiratory failure secondary to poor respiratory mucle function as well as deep vein thrombosis and infective complications.[3,4] Nutritional deficiency can be corrected either enterally or parenterally. Enteral feeding is simpler and safer, using high calorie and protein liquid feeds of known volume and composition, given either by mouth or via a fine-bore tube placed endoscopically.

 The routine use of parenteral feeding (TPN) is controversial on general and immunological grounds and should be avoided in order to minimise nosocomial infections and associated sepsis. There is evidence that increased nosocomial infections occur when the GI tract is not used for nutrition in the pre- and postoperative periods.[5]

Paraoesophageal nodes (on the wall of the oesophagus)
Cervical (101) [a]Upper thoracic (105) Middle thoracic (108) Lower thoracic (110)

Perioesophageal nodes (in immediate apposition to the oesophagus)
Deep cervical (102) Supraclavicular (104) Paratracheal (106) Subcarinal (107) Para-aortic or posterior mediastinal (112) Diaphragmatic (111) Left gastric (7) Lesser curvature (3) Coeliac (9) Right cardiac (1) Left cardiac (2)

Lateral oesophageal nodes (located lateral to the oesophagus)
Posterior triangle of the neck (100) Hilar (109) Suprapyloric (5) Subpyloric (6) Common hepatic (8) Greater curvature (4)

---

[a] For location see Chapter 3, Fig. 3.3

Table 5.1 *Lymph nodes of the oesophagus*

In those patients who have failed to show satisfactory improvement, it may be necessary to construct a feeding jejunostomy, either before or at the time of routine surgery, in order to continue hyperalimentation via the enteral route. Nevertheless, preoperative and postoperative feeding by jejunostomy in every patient cannot be recommended on current evidence.[6,7]

Respiratory care

Optimisation of respiratory function is vital in preventing the serious pulmonary complications associated with prolonged surgery and thoracotomy.[4] Smoking ought to be discouraged as early as possible. Preoperative physiotherapy with coughing exercises and effective use of the diaphragm by restoration of muscle strength through ambulation is encouraged. High-risk patients should also be provided with vigorous physiotherapy with or without bronchodilators prior to surgery. Orodental hygiene is also relevant in preventing a source of chronic sepsis that could disseminate infection to the tracheobronchial tree during intubation.

To reduce the incidence of thromboembolic complications, prophylactic low-dose heparin together with anti-thromboembolism stockings, must be provided as soon as the patient comes into hospital.

Mental preparation

To minimise fear and apprehension, every effort must be made to familiarise the patient with the hospital environment, including the intensive care unit. Patient cooperation is crucial and can be enhanced by reassurance and good communication. Descriptions of the methods of pain relief, oxygen and intravenous fluid administration and the awareness of intercostal tube drainage and the likelihood of prolonged periods without oral intake, must be adequately explained. All patients and their relatives should be counselled about the treatment options, paying particular attention to results and limitations of surgery.

Perioperative preparation and anaesthetic details are highlighted and explained in depth in Chapter 3.

Surgical objectives

Curative surgical resection of oesophageal malignancy is based on the principle that if all neoplastic tissue can be removed, then resection and reconstruction could lead to a worthwhile period of survival and possible cure, but only if operative mortality is low and the life expectancy of the patient is not shortened for other reasons. An extended radical procedure to resect the oesophagus and draining lymph nodes can be justified even if the tumour has invaded the perioesophageal tissues as well as the local lymph nodes in a fit patient. A similar argument would be untenable in an elderly patient in whom a decreased chance of long-term survival would be preferred to the high morbidity and mortality that would ensue from such an extended radical operation.

Surgical therapy still remains the only treatment that has consistantly been shown to provide prolonged survival, albeit in only 10–20% of cases.[8,9]

Resection, therefore, must be the chosen method of therapy in fit patients with T1 and T2 tumours of the middle and lower thirds of the oesophagus. Survival is related to the stage of disease and with Stage I disease, 5-year survivals of greater than 80% have been achieved[10,11] emphasising the importance of early detection. In Stage III disease, surgery alone produces poor results and trials of neo-adjuvant therapies must be completed in order to outline the optimal therapeutic strategy.

An attitude of pessimism has prevailed over many years owing to poor surgical results achieved in small series by non-specialised units. The overall results of surgical resection for all stages of tumour have improved over the past 20 years with falling morbidity and mortality associated with the procedure. The reasons for this are listed in **Table 5.2**.

Among these is an increased tendency to concentrate the management of such cases in specialist units with the numbers treated allowing the development of a multidisciplinary approach that involves surgeons, gastroenterologists, clinical oncologists, anaethetists, radiologists and intensivists as well as physiotherapists and nursing staff. Studies have confirmed that improved results parallel experience in managing this condition[12] and poor results occur when experience is limited.[13,14] There is now overwhelming evidence to confirm the influence of surgeon case-volume on the outcome of site-specific cancer surgery.[14,15] Other reasons for improved outcome include better patient selection, earlier diagnosis by open access endoscopy, screening of Barrett's oesophagus and improved preoperative, operative and postoperative management.

Principles of oesophagectomy

Resection of primary tumour

Oesophageal cancer spreads longitudinally in the submucosal lymphatics. The incidence of positive resection margins reported in the literature is high.[16,17,18] Fortunately, with new advances in endoscopic and radiological techniques such as endoscopic ultrasound, the tumour extent and spread, together with the diagnosis of synchronous lesions, can now be accurately assessed. It is crucial to obtain accurate information concerning these tumours by careful examination using videoendoscopy, endoscopic ultrasound and spiral CT in the preoperative staging process. This will help to determine the exact level of resection. It is still often difficult to ascertain the length for clear surgical margins, particularly in high lesions, despite exhaustive preoperative investigations.

1.	Increase in specialist units
2.	Multidisciplinary approach
3.	Earlier diagnosis
4.	Better patient selection
5.	Improved perioperative management

Table 5.2 *Reasons for improved results for oesophageal resection*

Rules on resection margins

Much discussion has centred around how many centimetres of macroscopically normal oesophagus should routinely be removed either side of the palpable primary lesion. Skinner et al.[19] advocated that a minimum resection margin of 10 cm from the palpable edge of the tumour was essential to minimise the risk of anastomotic recurrence and positive resection margins. This figure, however, does not take into account the nature, pattern and location of the primary cancer. It also fails to discriminate between in vivo margins of resection and resection margins measured by the histopathologist when a considerable degree of shrinkage has occurred after fixation in formalin. This shrinkage has been clearly documented in an elaborate study by Siu et al.[20] who demonstrated a significant difference between the length of resection margin obtained in vivo, and that achieved after fixation with formalin. They also demonstrated that the tumour itself contracted very little in size, even after fixation.

Many studies have also demonstrated that localised tumours require shorter lengths of clearance for safe surgical margins.[21] Not infrequently, primary tumours with multicentric lesions are encountered which require more extensive lengths for safe surgical margins. In squamous cancers, three representative patterns of presentation are encountered (see **Fig. 5.2**).[22] Failure to take this into account may explain the finding of positive resection margins in nearly 40% of specimens when the oesophageal resection margin is limited to only 4 cm and still of 17% when the margin is 10 cm.[17,18] Therefore, 10 cm is a reasonable resection margin to attain in both directions if at all possible. In practice, this rule of perfection can rarely be achieved. A 10-cm margin on both sides of a tumour measuring an average of 5.5 cm would require an overall length of specimen exceeding that of the normal human oesophagus. Under these circumstances it would be necessary, in tumours with an upper margin of less than 10 cm from the cricopharyngeus, for a resection of the distal pharynx and larynx. The choice between a safe margin and the preservation of a patient's voice needs to be carefully considered. In general, preservation of the patient's voice would be the preferred option, especially if resection were deemed likely to be palliative and a macroscopically clear margin had been obtained. Much of the published evidence is conflicting and it has been suggested that a resection margin of 4 cm or more results in anastomotic recurrence in less than 15% of cases.[23] This particular study also showed that if patients were given radiotherapy to the anastomotic site after the operation they

Figure 5.2
(a) A single cancer;
(b) multifocal cancer
(c) intramural vascular
spread. There is a
high risk of positive
resection margins in
(b) and (c). Shaded
areas represent
sub-mucosal spread.

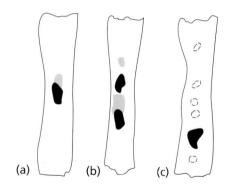

(a)　(b)　(c)

did not subsequently develop recurrence. None of those with recurrence had been treated with radiotherapy postoperatively.

It is the author's opinion that when only a short resection margin can be obtained through the thoracic exposure, a cervical phase with total oesophagectomy is advisable. If resection margins of less than 4 cm are obtained, consideration should be given to using supplementary adjuvant intraluminal or external beam radiotherapy.[24] Adenocarcinoma of the lower oesophagus commonly infiltrates the gastric cardia, fundus and lesser curve. Extensive sleeve resection of the lesser curve and fundus is necessary to minimise positive distal resection margins. Other studies have demonstrated that patients with microscopically positive margins undergoing palliative resection died of other manifestations before clinical evidence of locoregional recurrence.[25,26] A tumour-free surgical margin is, therefore, not the only important factor to be considered in radical surgery. Nevertheless, it should be the main goal of every operation. Most authors would agree that in order to make allowance for intramural submucosal spread of squamous and adenocarcinomas a subtotal oesophagectomy should be carried out in patients with tumours of the mid and lower oesophagus.

Resection of lymph nodes

Early experiences of lymphadenectomy for oesophageal cancer[27] have been further reinforced by the results of the Japanese in the treatment of gastric cancer[28] which are now being reproduced in the UK.[29] The evidence for radical lymph node dissection in squamous and adenocarcinoma of the oesophagus is less extensive, and the extent of lymphadenectomy continues to be an area of considerable controversy.

There is little doubt that some patients with oesophageal cancer who have lymph-node involvement could be cured by surgical clearance.[30] The identification of those patients who would benefit is one aspect that provides the preoperative staging process with its greatest challenge. Early experience of endoscopic ultrasonography has suggested that this technique is both highly sensitive and specific in detecting lymph-node metastases, in both the paraaortic and paraoesophageal regions. Recent experience with this technique suggests that patients for radical lymph-node dissection can be selected more accurately.[31]

Many reports describe retrospective series of differing extents of lymph adenectomy in squamous and adenocarcinoma of the oesophagus.[19,32,33,34,35] These include no formal lymph node dissection as well as one-field, two-field and three-field lymphadenectomies.

 Unfortunately, very few prospective randomised trials are available for analysis.[36,37,38]

The description of the tiers of lymph nodes in oesophageal cancer has been designed according to the anatomy of the lymphatic draining system of the oesophagus.[2,39,40,41]

The extent of lymphadenectomy is demonstrated in **Fig. 5.3**. Many surgeons do not practise a formal lymphadenectomy during either transhiatal or transthoracic approaches to oesophagectomy.

Formal one-field lymph node dissection would involve the dissection of the diaphragmatic, right and left para-cardiac, lesser curvature, left gastric, coeliac, common heaptic and splenic artery nodes.

Figure 5.3
Extent of resection and fields of lymph node dissection routinely carried out for cancer of the oesophagus.

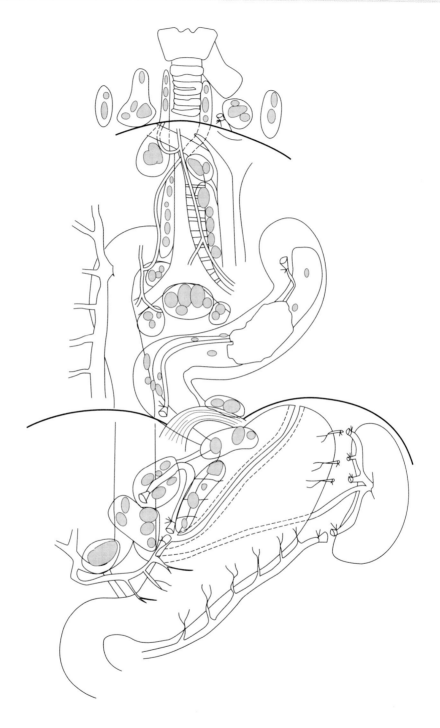

Two-field dissection includes the paraaortic (mediastinal nodes) together with the thoracic duct, the right and left pulmonary hilar nodes, the paraoesophageal nodes, tracheal bifurcation and the right paratracheal nodes.

Three-field dissection includes the first and second fields as well as a dissection in the neck to clear the brachiocephalic, deep lateral and external cervical nodes and including the right and left recurrent nerve lymphatic chains (deep anterior cervical nodes).

The fields of nodal dissection should not be confused with the histopathological staging of nodal involvement (see Chapter 3, Tables 3.8 and 3.9). Much of the data available on lymph–node dissection in oesophageal cancer suffers from poor definition of the terms oesophagectomy and oesophagectomy with lymph–node dissection. It is essential, therefore, that all surgical techniques are standardised such that meaningful data can be derived in the future.

There seems little justification for oesophagectomy to be performed with intent to cure without any attempt to clear the first level of lymph nodes. According to the literature 80% of all squamous oesophageal malignancies have lymph node metastases at the time of surgery.[33] Patients with either squamous or adenocarcinoma of the oesophagus affecting the upper, middle and lower regions, have lymph node metastases in the mediastinal nodes in over 70% of cases.[26,33,35,42] Many personal series of oesophageal cancer surgery have confirmed that over three-quarters of patients presenting with lower-third tumours had positive lymph nodes in the coeliac trunk, left gastric and common hepatic territories. To perform a potentially curative resection for carcinoma in the middle and lower thirds, a dissection of abdominal and mediastinal lymph nodes is essential. Series from Japan as well as Europe have confirmed that systematic nodal dissection employing meticulous surgical technique can be performed with acceptable operative morbidity and mortality. Despite these advances in lymph–node dissection during the last few decades, there is currently a mode of scepticism as to whether this really contributes to an improvement in survival. It is the author's opinion that two-field lymph–node dissection is justified on the grounds of the histopathological and surgical data presented by both Japanese and European groups.[30,32,33,35,43,44,45]

The role of extensive three-field dissection in oesophageal malignancy is less clear. The difference in tumour spread between squamous cell carcinoma and adenocarcinoma needs to be better reported and understood. Many reports combine these quite separate tumours and, therefore, confuse the results. Akiyama reports nearly a quarter of lower-third squamous tumours presenting with metastases in the neck. Five-year survival rates showed no significant difference between two-field and three-field dissection in this group of patients.[33] In adenocarcinoma of the lower oesophagus, dissection of the cervical nodes cannot be justified, as there is no evidence that three-field nodal dissection provides any survival benefit. Although abdominal nodal dissection for cancer of the upper thoracic oesophagus (third field) has not been shown to be beneficial, dissection in the neck for these upper-third tumours does appear to have some justification.[30,33]

As for many other solid organ tumours controversy persists as to the value of lymphadenectomy in oesophageal cancer. There are two predominant attitudes: first, there is the concept that lymph–node metastases are considered simply as markers of systemic disease and the removal of involved nodes will confer no benefit. Some surgeons advocate removal of the primary lesion alone and claim the same survival as with more extensive resections.[46] Second, there is the belief that in some patients with positive nodes cure can be obtained by an aggressive surgical approach focusing on wide excision and extended lymphadenectomy using a transthoracic approach. As described earlier the results of different extents of surgery are difficult to compare. Nevertheless, optimal staging, locoregional control and improved cure rates are strong arguments for more extensive surgery including lymphadenectomy.

Optimal staging

There can be no doubt that lymph–node dissection contributes to the accuracy of the final staging of the disease.[32,33,44]

Locoregional tumour control

More extensive surgery produces prolonged tumour-free survival. In recent years overwhelming evidence has accumulated that R0 resection (no residual tumour left behind) is a very important prognostic variable after surgical excision.[47] To consistently achieve an R0 resection, organ dissection and lymphadenectomy must be radical. Roder et al.[48] showed in a series of 204 resections, a statistically significant difference between R0 and R1 or R2 (Residual disease left behind) resections for squamous cell carcinoma with a five year survival rate of 35% and below 10% respectively. Lerut et al.[45] demonstrated a 20% 5-year survival for R0 versus zero 5-year survival for R1 and R2 resections in advanced Stage III and Stage IV adeno- and squamous cell carcinomas.

Locoregional disease-free survival is a difficult yet important goal to achieve in oesophageal carcinoma as the majority of patients present with advanced disease. Furthermore, recurrent locoregional mediastinal disease can be very difficult to palliate. Dresner and Griffin[32] described mediastinal and abdominal local recurrence in 21% of patients after two–field nodal dissection in 176 patients. Clark et al.[49] found that nodal recurrence occurred within the area of dissection in only 20% of a small group of 43 patients. In addition Lerut demonstrated a 4-year survival of 22% in patients with Stage IV disease as a result of distant lymph–node metastases. This further endorses the apparent beneficial effect of adequate lymphadenectomy in reducing local recurrence.[45]

Improved cure rate

The third argument for extended lymphadenectomy is the contribution to an improved survival. Unfortunately, this argument suffers from a lack of definite evidence from randomised trials as already discussed. Although many questions relating to surgical technique remain unanswered, several groups accept the value of lymphadenectomy when treating oesophageal carcinoma. It is not yet clear, however, which patients will benefit from such systematic nodal dissection. There is some evidence that patients with early stage oesophageal carcinoma, in whom up to 50% have nodal involvement, would also benefit from extensive resection with lymphadenectomy.[50] Nevertheless some series have described T1 disease as having a zero rate of nodal metastases.[32] The role of radical lymphadenectomy in early-stage disease remains in question.

Method of reconstruction of the oesophagus

Route of reconstruction

After resection of the cervical, thoracic or abdominal oesophagus, one of three main paths can be used for reconstruction (see Fig. 5.4).

Figure 5.4
*Three routes of
oesophageal
reconstruction.
(1) Presternal route;
(2) retrosternal route;
(3) posterior
mediastinal route.*

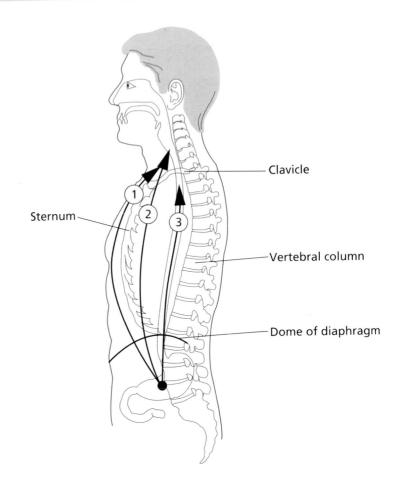

Clavicle

Sternum

Vertebral column

Dome of diaphragm

Presternal route

Historically the presternal route was the preference of many surgeons. This is approximately 2 cm longer than the retrosternal route which in turn is approximately 2 cm longer than the posterior mediastinal route. As a result, the popularity of this route of reconstruction has declined over recent years. There seems little indication for using this route unless the thorax is of extremely small capacity such that a bulky oesophageal substitute could compromise effective respiration.

Retrosternal route (Anterior mediastinal)

The space between the sternum and the anterior mediastinum is easily created with good dissection. There is reported to be a lower incidence of cervical anastomotic dehiscence compared with that of the presternal route. Unfortunately its major disadvantage stems from the somewhat unnatural position of the cervical oesophagus in front of the trachea which results in an unpleasant sensation on swallowing.

A major indication of the use for this extra anatomical route of reconstruction is in the emergency treatment of anastomotic dehiscence or the dehiscence of a gastric substitute which has caused posterior mediastinal sepsis. After incomplete resection (R1 and R2) there is some evidence that a retrosternal conduit would be preferable to the posterior mediastinal route.[51]

The retrosternal route is created by blunt finger dissection through the abdominal and cervical incisions and further developed by insertion of a malleable intestinal retractor. The tip of this instrument is passed up to the neck in direct contact with the back of the sternum. Care is taken not to deviate from the midline. The sternohyoid and sternothyroid muscles are divided in the neck and this allows the passage of the oesophageal substitute easily into the left or right side of the neck.

Posterior mediastinal route

This route provides the shortest distance between abdomen and the apex of the thorax and also the neck.

This is the preferred route of reconstruction in the primary surgical excision of oesophageal cancers.[51,52]

Gastric or colonic substitutes are easily passed through the posterior mediastinum after completion of the oesophageal dissection in the thorax. No attempt is made to close the pleura after this route of reconstruction.

Organ of reconstruction

Reconstruction with stomach

The method of reconstruction should be kept as simple as possible, to minimise complications. Oesophageal replacement is determined by the site of the primary lesion. The stomach is the preferred option as this organ is easy to prepare and involves only one anastomosis.

The patient is positioned supine and exposure obtained using an upper midline incision. There are five broad principles and practices which must be observed in the preparation of the stomach as an oesophageal substitute.

1. *The use of isoperistaltic stomach and vascular integrity.* The right gastroepiploic and the right gastric artery and veins are vital in the maintenance of viability of the stomach when used as an oesophageal substitute. The greater omentum is opened and the entire course of the right gastroepiploic artery is carefully identified and preserved. The vascular arcade is interrupted at the junction where the right gastroepiploic artery meets the left. The short gastric vessels are divided and ligated (see **Fig. 5.5**).

2. *Excision of the lesser curvature.* Cancers of the lower two-thirds of the oesophagus require complete clearance of the lesser curve lymph nodes as well as the left gastric, coeliac trunk, splenic artery and common hepatic lymph nodes. The left gastric artery should be ligated at its origin and resection of the proximal half of the lesser curvature of the stomach, including the cardia, is performed. The right gastric artery contributes to the maintenance of the gastric intramural vascular network and should be preserved if possible. In carcinoma of the cervical oesophagus the entire arterial arcade along the lesser curvature of the stomach can be preserved. In this situation, all of the stomach is used for reconstruction.

3. *Preservation of the intramural vascular arcade.* Extensive intramural arterial anastomoses between the vascular arcades of the lesser and greater curvatures exist.

Figure 5.5
*Main arteries of the
stomach and points of
division of vessels and
stomach for
oesophageal sub-
stitution.*

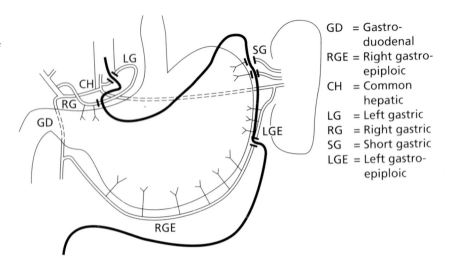

GD = Gastro-
         duodenal
RGE = Right gastro-
          epiploic
CH = Common
         hepatic
LG = Left gastric
RG = Right gastric
SG = Short gastric
LGE = Left gastro-
         epiploic

This has been well demonstrated by El–Eishi and Thomas.[53,54] This extensive vascular network must be preserved during resection of the left gastric area of the lesser curvature and the cardia of the stomach. The extent of the resection of the lesser curvature is determined by a line connecting the highest point of the fundus (see **Fig. 5.6**) and the lesser curvature at the junction of the right and left gastric arteries. This allows the removal of all potentially involved lymph nodes, yet preserves the arterial network to the fundus. There is no evidence to suggest that the trunk and descending branches of the left gastric artery running along the lesser curve need to be preserved and from an oncological view point it is essential that these are excised with the specimen. Care should be taken to ligate the short gastric vessels away from the greater curvature of the stomach so as not to damage the intramural network. The right gastroepiploic artery provides an adequate blood flow to maintain vascularity in the region of the fundus which is the area used for anastomosis.

    4. *The high point of the stomach.* The stomach is a flexible and capacious organ; its high point is the logical and sensible place at which to fashion an anastomosis with the remaining oesophagus. It is easily identified by applying traction with the surgeon's fingers in an upward direction after all preparations have been completed. The stomach is transected as described previously (see **Fig. 5.6**).

    5. *Gastric drainage.* The role of pyloroplasty and/or pyloromyotomy after gastric reconstruction is contentious. As truncal vagotomy is inevitable, pyloroplasty should be required because of the resulting gastric stasis. Many surgeons believe that a pyloroplasty is essential following an oesophago–gastric resection but the situation is not identical to truncal vagotomy for duodenal ulcer disease, because the pyloro–duodenal area is almost always normal and the pylorus comes to lie vertically after the operation, aiding gastric emptying. Nevertheless, delay in gastric emptying has been reported in patients not undergoing pyloroplasty.[55]

 As complications of pyloroplasty are minimal, it is the author's view that this should be performed routinely to prevent the life-threatening complications of early gastric stasis and aspiration and the less serious ones of late vomiting and bloatedness.[56,57]

Figure 5.6
The high point of the stomach.

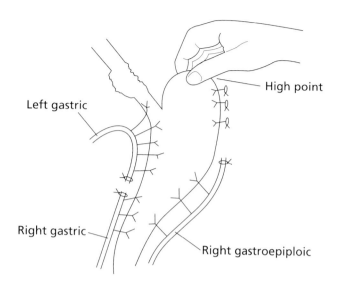

On occasions the upper anastomosis may need to be as high as the back of the tongue, so methods of stomach lengthening must be considered.

Methods of lengthening the stomach

1. *Kocher manoeuvre*: This manoeuvre is essential and allows the distance between the first part of the duodenum and the hiatus to be reduced.
2. *Excision of lesser curve of stomach*: When the lesser curve of the stomach is unusually short, an increase in length of the gastric substitute can be obtained, by dividing the lesser curve between curved clamps, before its resection. If absolutely necessary, a tense right gastric artery may be sacrificed by division at the level of the pylorus. The right gastroepiploic artery can maintain an adequate blood flow along the greater curvature.
3. *Incision of the serosa on the gastric wall*: Multiple incisions placed in the gastric serosa may lengthen the stomach. A longitudinal incision placed along the resection line allows this to occur. The indications for this procedure are extremely rare.
4. *Reversed gastric tube:* This method was originally described by Gavriliu but is very rarely necessary.[58]

Reconstruction with colon

The principal indication for the use of colonic interposition is for tumours close to the gastro-oesophageal junction which need an extensive oesophageal as well as gastric resection. A small proportion of patients presenting with oesophageal malignancy will have had a previous gastric resection for peptic ulcer disease, precluding the use of stomach as the oesophageal substitute. The choice of an oesophageal replacement under these circumstances lies between colon and jejunum. The colon is often recommended because of its advantage in having a greater capacity as a reservoir than the jejunum. Rarely, it may be used in an emergency after failed gastric interposition.

Indications for colonic reconstruction (see **Table 5.3**)

It is preferable to use the colon in an isoperistaltic fashion. Unfortunately, the vascular pattern of the colon varies and careful selection of the correct vascular pedicle to ensure viability of the transverse colon is essential. Each case requires evaluation on its own merit because of variations in anatomy. Not infrequently, the marginal artery is found to be of insufficient calibre to maintain viability of the transposed colon. Although the vascular appearance determines the appropriate colonic segment for use in each individual, the two possibilities for effective use of isoperistaltic colon are: a) Transverse colon based on the left colic vessels; b) Right colon based on the middle colic vessels.

The disadvantage of transverse colon is that an abnormally narrow marginal artery may exist at the splenic flexure, thus compromising the blood supply of the proximal colonic segment. Preoperative assessment by angiography of the colonic vascular pathway has been suggested,[59] but careful intraoperative observation of the vascular anatomy with temporary occlusion of vessels before division is a simple manoeuvre which is effective in most cases.

Surgical technique

Preoperative mechanical bowel preparation is necessary as is oral antibiotic cover to sterilise the bowel for 48 hours prior to surgery. The omentum is freed from the transverse colon and the hepatic and splenic flexures, while the entire colon is mobilised so that it can be placed outside the abdominal cavity for inspection of its vascular blood supply. Mobilising the sigmoid colon provides additional length so that the transverse colon can be tunnelled into the chest, to reach the neck. The proximal colon should be divided and, after anastomosis to the oesophagus, placed on sufficient stretch to prevent redundancy within the chest or in the substernal area. The colon should then be anchored in the straightened position by sutures to the crural margin of the hiatus, although not circumferentially. Continuity of the large bowel is re-established by end-to-end anastomosis, which is conveniently performed before the colo-jejunostomy or colo-gastrostomy for anatomical reasons. Excellent technical descriptions for the use of various segments of colon have been described by Demeester[60] and Belsay.[61]

Reconstruction with jejunal

Replacement of the lower oesophagus is accomplished using either a Roux-en-Y technique or by segmental interposition. Replacement of the upper oesophagus is accomplished by free jejunal transfer with microvascular anastomosis of the jejunal pedicle to neck vessels. It is sometimes possible to create a long loop for replacement of the entire thoracic oesophagus. The jejunum should be considered the third choice, after colon and stomach, and chosen only when the other two organs are unsuitable or absent.

---

1. Previous gastric resection

2. Tumours with extensive gastric involvement

3. Failed gastric transposition

Table 5.3 *Indications for colonic reconstruction*

No specific measures are required to prepare the small bowel preoperatively other than to ensure that patients are not known to have small bowel pathology. A loop of jejunum is identified in the upper segments within the first 25 cm after the duodeno-jejunal flexure. Typical jejunal vascular pattern of arterial arcades are encountered in this area and the veins and arteries are close together but bifurcate at separate levels making individual division of the veins and arteries essential. Transillumination of the mesentery helps identify the jejunal vascular tree precisely. It is important to appreciate that during the creation of a jejunal loop, it is the length of the free edge of the mesentery which will determine the length of the loop created rather than the length of the jejunum itself. The jejunum is usually longer than the mesentery and will, therefore, have a tendency to become redundant.

The technique of microvascular free jejunal transfer for reconstruction of the upper oesophagus is well described elsewhere.[62] The specific indications for such a reconstruction are usually after pharyngo-laryngectomy performed for carcinoma of the hypopharynx, post-cricoid region and cervical oesophagus. The operation is usually performed with a radical neck dissection as part of the primary treatment programme or as palliative surgery following recurrence after radiotherapy.

Method of surgical approach

The preceding discussion has described the method and rationale underpinning the surgical objectives in treating oesophageal cancer. The aims of resecting the primary tumour together with the lymph nodes and producing the oesophageal reconstruction, must be achieved safely and effectively and with ease of access. The method of surgical approach to obtain these objectives must be considered in each individual case. The choice of the surgical approach is dependent on the tumour location, the extent of spread, the fitness, age and build of the individual patient and whether surgical intervention is intended to be curative or palliative.

Carcinoma of the hypopharynx and cervical oesophagus pharyngolaryngo-oesophagectomy

Resection of squamous lesions in this area is achieved by removal of the larynx, the lower pharynx, cervical trachea, one or both lobes of the thyroid gland and cervical oesophagus. If the tumour is located in the hypopharynx only (post-cricoid region), the thoracic oesophagus may be conserved and a free graft of jejunum transferred by microvascular anastomosis, as previously described. If tumour has extended to the lower part of the cervical oesophagus, a total pharyngolaryngo oesophagectomy and gastric transposition, with immediate pharyngogastric reconstruction, is the treatment of choice.

The patient is placed in the supine position with the neck hyperextended; a U-shaped incision provides excellent access. It allows the construction of a permanent tracheostomy with ease and may be extended into a Y-shaped incision ready for a median sternotomy if required. The resection includes a radical lymph-node dissection in the neck. The thyroid and parathyroid glands are also removed en bloc with the internal jugular vein and the deep internal cervical nodes. The common carotid artery, vagus nerve and the sympathetic trunk are carefully protected.

Two-phase subtotal oesophagectomy via a right thoracotomy for carcinomas of the middle and lower thirds of the oesophagus

There has been much disagreement concerning the ideal approach to the thoracic oesophagus. The left thoracotomy was used for the first oesophagectomy and remained a standard approach until the 1960s.[63] The advantage of the left thoracotomy is that it provides better access to the lower few centimetres of oesophagus, but satisfactory exposure of the upper and middle thoracic oesophagus, trachea and surrounding tissue is restricted by the intervening aortic arch and descending aorta. It has been argued that access to the left paratracheal nodes and hilum of the left lung is restricted in the right thoracotomy approach. Experienced oesophageal surgeons have encountered no difficulty in dissecting the left mediastinum from the right side. Two-phase right thoracotomy (initially described by Lewis and Tanner) is now becoming accepted as the approach of choice to the thoracic oesophagus.[33,55] A right thoracotomy and laparotomy through an upper midline incision are performed for carcinomas situated in the thoracic oesophagus. Both resection and reconstruction of the oesophagus are carried out at one stage but in two phases the abdominal mobilisation of the stomach being the first of these. After completion of the second phase of mediastinal dissection through a right thoracotomy, the stomach is delivered into the chest and an anastomosis fashioned at the thoracic inlet.

The procedure begins with exploration of the abdomen to exclude the presence of gross distant metastases and to determine whether or not resection is indicated. After performing routine gastric mobilisation, which has been described earlier, the coeliac trunk together with its branches, namely the common hepatic and the roots of the splenic and left gastric arteries, are then skeletonised by complete removal of the surrounding lymph nodes. The left gastric artery is divided and ligated at its origin and each nodal group marked with a suture to help identification when the stomach is delivered into the chest. The patient is then placed in the left lateral decubitus position and is held firmly in place by a moulding mattress. Two sandbags are placed under the axilla and thorax to facilitate elevation of the ribcage. The pelvis is strapped to the operating table. The right arm is fixed on an armrest while the left is stretched out on an arm-support. All pressure points must be protected by padding.

The incision is made in line with the 5th intercostal space, beginning at the lower angle of the scapula and extending to the border of the sternum. The 4th intercostal space may be preferred for tumours of the middle third. The superior mediastinal pleura is incised along the course of the right vagus nerve and is extended upwards towards the brachiocephalic and subclavian arteries. The right recurrent laryngeal nerve is preserved and meticulous dissection is then applied to the lymph node chain alongside it. The pleura is incised along the border of the superior vena cava and the right paratracheal lymph nodes located between the trachea and the vein are then dissected free. Care is taken not to dissect circumferentially around the trachea, as this may prejudice its blood supply. Routine division and/or resection of the arch of the azygos vein is crucial for adequate exposure. The azygos vein marks the line of dissection caudally to the hiatus. The incision through the pleura is deepened to expose the adventitia on the descending aorta. The thoracic duct through which the lymph flows is rarely the site of metastases, except in extensive disease. There are, however, numerous lymph nodes scattered along the length of the duct in the para-aortic region. To remove these an en bloc resection together with the duct is necessary. The duct is easily identified after minimal sharp dissection in the inferior mediastinum on the adventitia of the right aspect of the descending thoracic aorta. The duct is ligated at this point and the proximal end after resection in the superior mediastinum, along the posterior border of the oesophagus. Chylothorax secondary to inadvertent and undetected damage to the thoracic duct is therefore prevented. Dissection continues on to the right pulmonary hilium where there is almost always a small anthracotic lymph node. The right bronchial, carinal and left bronchial nodes are dissected. It is advisable to avoid monopolar diathermy in this region because of the vulnerability of the membranous part of both the trachea and bronchi.

The oesophagus is then transected at the thoracic inlet. The stomach is delivered into the chest and the specimen removed after careful sleeve resection of the lesser curvature en bloc with the coeliac, left gastric, lesser curve, splenic artery and hepatic artery nodes. Oesophago-gastric anastomosis is fashioned in the apex of the thorax.

Combined synchronous two-team oesophagectomy

Modification of the standard access for oesophagectomy has been described wherein mobilisation of the stomach and abdominal oesophagus proceeds synchronously with mobilisation of the thoracic oesophagus via a right thoracotomy using a second operating team.[64,65] A reduction in operating and anaesthetic time was suggested as a possible reason for decreased operative morbidity and mortality rates in Hong Kong Chinese patients. Patients in the study had a lower incidence of pulmonary and cardiovascular disease than those with oesophageal cancer in the West. A comparison of the synchronous two-team approach with conventional two-stage subtotal oesophagectomy was performed in Western patients.

Not only was there a higher incidence of complications and a higher mortality rate but nodal dissection in larger, more obese patients was technically very difficult because of more limited surgical access.[66]

Three-phase subtotal oesophagectomy for tumours of the upper middle third of the oesophagus

Some surgeons prefer to expose and divide the oesophagus in the neck. This certainly provides excellent access for a relatively easy anastomosis, although it often does not allow resection of much more oesophagus than can be removed by the two-phase approach. This is because the cervical oesophagus is relatively short and it is difficult to perform an anastomosis unless a stump of oesophagus is left, hence the term subtotal oesophagectomy. McKeown[67] recommended cervical anastomosis on the grounds that a leak in the neck is less catastrophic than a thoracic leak. This is probably an overstatement and is now of limited significance as overall oesophageal anastomotic leakage is uncommon approximately 1–2% in practised hands. The three-phase operation takes longer to complete and is also associated with early postoperative difficulty in swallowing. This is probably because of the extensive proximal mobilisation of the cervical oesophagus. Proponents of the three-phase operation claim that a more complete oesophagectomy is achieved. The need for a subtotal oesophagectomy regardless of the site of the primary tumour was justified by pathological studies, which apparently indicated extensive proximal submucosal spread of tumour. If the tumour cannot be resected with adequate longitudinal margins then the three-phase technique ought to be employed.

The first phase of this operation is routine gastric mobilisation with dissection of the nodal groups as described before. The second phase should mirror the dissection described in the preceding section but adding the mobilisation of the oesophagus in the apex of the thorax. The right thorax is closed and the patient turned supine once again. Through either a left- or right-sided cervical incision, the whole of the thoracic oesophagus can be removed and the stomach delivered into the neck and an oesophago–gastrostomy fashioned.

Left-sided subtotal oesophagectomy for middle and lower third oesophageal cancers

For many years the left thoracotomy has been adopted, not only for carcinoma of the lower oesophagus and cardia, but also for carcinoma of the upper and mid-thoracic oesophagus. The left thoraco-abdominal approach continues to maintain an established position as an appropriate surgical approach to resection of tumours at the cardia. Although many thoracic surgeons continue to use the left approach to lesions of the lower and mid-oesophagus, the access to perform a formal abdominal nodal dissection through a diaphragmatic incision is thought to be inadequate. Advocates of the left thoractomy approach have failed to quote data about nodal status, or incidence of mucosal resection margins.[68,69] Randomised studies comparing the left approach to the right have never been performed and so a clear survival advantage has not emerged for either operative technique. Nevertheless Molina et al.[70] compared a 10-year experience of both the left and right approaches and clearly showed a higher incidence of residual tumour at the line of resection in patients undergoing a left thoracotomy. Others have reported a high incidence of residual tumour at the line of resection when performing a standard left thoracotomy when compared with a more extensive subtotal oesophagectomy.[71,72]

The left-sided approach was modified by Matthews and Steel.[42] They described a two-stage procedure with a left thoraco-laparotomy followed by a left-neck approach. Much more extensive access was achieved by dividing the costal margin of the diaphragm peripherally for 15 cm close to its origin on the ribs. Although this more extensive resection should decrease positive resection margins, no data on the incidence of positive margins was quoted. This left-sided approach is nevertheless absolutely contraindicated if the tumour is situated at or above the aortic arch, for which a standard three-stage right-sided approach is necessary. Although data are few on the incidence of respiratory complications in the left-sided approach, Molina et al.[70] and Earlam's comprehensive review suggest an increased incidence of serious chest infections following the left-sided approach.[73]

Transhiatal oesophagectomy for upper and lower third tumours of the oesophagus

Controversy still exists about the role of oesophagectomy without thoracotomy in oesophageal cancer surgery. Proponents of the technique argue that most cancers are already locally advanced at the time of surgery and that 'cures' are fortuitous and dependent on the stage at presentation rather than the operative technique employed. Opponents claim improvements in survival for a small proportion of patients undergoing radical en bloc resection for a more favourable tumour stage.[44,74] The safety and benefits of this approach may be questioned if applied inappropriately. The original technique was described as a blind procedure, which therefore defied one of the most fundamental principles of surgery, that surgical procedures should always be carried out under direct vision.[75,76,77] Nevertheless refinements to the technique have been made and the operation has developed and gained many advocates.[78]

A modified technique of transhiatal oesophagectomy under direct vision has been described[79] using a modification of the transhiatal technique described by Pinotti.[80] In this technique almost the entire procedure is undertaken under direct vision and the anastomosis performed in the neck as a combined synchronous operation. The operation attempts to ensure adequate local clearance by avoiding direct contact with the tumour as well as carrying the majority of the procedure out under direct vision. The authors demonstrated no evidence of proximal or distal resection margin involvement with the tumour and an acceptable morbidity and mortality. Details of the surgical procedure are clearly described elsewhere.[80] At present there are only selected indications for transhiatal oesophagectomy.

Carcinoma of the hypopharynx and cervical oesophagus. If the tumour is well localised the incidence of mediastinal metastases is low and the thoracic oesophagus remains morphologically normal. Oesophagectomy without thoracotomy can, therefore, be safely performed by blunt dissection. Radical neck dissection with pharyngo-laryngo oesophagectomy is carried out at the same time and reconstruction fashioned using the stomach through the posterior mediastinal route. A further advantage to this technique is that it ensures that no synchronous early lesions within the oesophagus are left behind, as would happen if a free jejunal graft were used in the neck. Some authors describe transhiatal oesophagectomy as the procedure of choice in *intraepithelial squamous carcinoma of the oesophagus.* These tumours rarely disseminate via the lymphatics.[22] With substantial progress being made in endoscopic techniques using epithelial dye-staining and endoscopic ultrasonography, early tumours can be more accurately staged. When tumour penetration is confined to the epithelial layer, resection by transhiatal oesophagectomy is entirely feasible. A few enthusiasts have even advocated transhiatal oesophagectomy for *middle-third tumours,* although most would consider these tumours to represent a contraindication. Nevertheless, *advanced adenocarcinoma of the lower oesophagus* has been successfully treated for many years by blunt transhiatal oesophagectomy.[34]

The debate over which operative procedure is most appropriate for the treatment of lower third oesophageal carcinoma will continue. Randomised studies have never been performed and no clear survival advantage has emerged for any particular operative technique.[8] Alderson *et al.*[79] confirm that radical transhiatal oesophagectomy is not as radical a procedure as that proposed by Skinner.[19] The dissection does not include the thoracic duct and para-aortic nodes. A number of retrospective audits have been published comparing disparate groups of transhiatal and transthoracic approaches.[81,82]

These have failed to demonstrate meaningful differences between the two approaches; in a very small comparative randomised study, no statistical differences were encountered.[83]

Randomised controlled trials of radical transhiatal oesophagectomy against two-field lymph-node dissection for lower-third tumours would need to be performed to establish the role of each in the surgical treatment of cancer of the oesophagus.

 It is of interest to note that one of the randomised studies comparing transthoracic with transhiatal approaches has demonstrated no difference in cardiopulmonary dysfunction in the two groups. The numbers in each group were small.[84]

Endoscopically assisted oesophagectomy for cancer

A number of techniques have been described aimed at reducing the severity of the surgical insult and complications produced by formal thoracotomy. These include thoracoscopic dissection within the chest,[85,86] laparoscopic mobilisation of the stomach for oesophageal replacement,[87] a combined laparoscopic and thoracoscopic approach[88] and a mediastinoscopic technique.[89] Although endoscopic mobilisation is entirely possible, the length of time for the procedure appears prohibitive. Experience with thoracoscopically assisted oesophagectomy has not been uniformly encouraging. Although this technique avoids thoracotomy, and dissection and haemostasis are performed under direct vision, prolonged deflation of the right lung contributes to the frequency of postoperative respiratory problems. The hospital stay has not been shown to be shortened and respiratory complications overall were increased when compared with the open technique.[85] Extent of lymphadenectomy was compromised and respiratory complications were unchanged in a Hong Kong series. Widespread adoption of this technique cannot be recommended at present.

The mediastinoscopic technique allows the entire operation to be performed without changing the position of the patient, but dissection of the lower third of the oesophagus is extremely difficult. Lymph-node dissection cannot accurately be performed and the technique has not achieved widespread acceptance. Some encouraging reports from Japan of endoscopic mucosal resection for mucosal squamous cancers limited to the lamina propria have been achieved, but this technique is not at present common practice in the West.

Overall, preliminary results from endoscopically assisted techniques do not show a clear benefit over open surgery in terms of mortality and morbidity although as yet it is too early to evaluate overall survival. If the technique of thoracoscopic and laparoscopic surgery is to contribute to the management of oesophageal cancer, then all efforts should be made to restrict these operations to those centres with extensive experience of open surgery and with sufficient expertise in minimally invasive surgery.

Technique of anastomosis

There have been no major changes in suturing techniques of the intestinal tract for many years. Meticulous technique is essential in achieving good results after oesophageal anastomosis. Morbidity and mortality were for many years related to anastomotic leakage.[90] The surgical principles relating to oesophageal anastomoses are the same as those in other parts of the alimentary tract. Emphasis is placed on (a) adequate blood supply; (b) absence of tension in the anastomosis; (c) accurate approximation of epithelial edges and (d) precise layer to layer suturing with primary healing. One-, two- and three-layer anastomoses have been described, but no conclusive randomised controlled studies have been reported. A two-layer oesophago-gastric anastomosis is advocated by Akiyama[22] who emphasises the importance of the absence of a serosal layer, which he believes would reinforce strength at the anastomotic site. He therefore advocates a carefully preserved adventitia, which provides sufficient strength to support sutures.

Stapling devices were introduced into GI surgery by Ravitch and Steichen.[91] These instruments have been further developed for ease of introduction and application; the latest adopts a low profile head which permits a larger diameter anvil to be introduced into the oesophageal stump. A larger diameter anastomosis is thereby fashioned, reducing the main drawback to stapled oesophageal anastomoses – that of benign anastomotic stricture.[30,92,94] These anastomotic fibrotic strictures are frequent after both manual and mechanical anastomosis but a higher rate of benign stricture is seen using the mechanical stapler.[93] Strictures are particularly associated with anastomoses constructed with a staple ring diameter of 25 mm or less.[94] The author routinely uses stapling instruments for intrathoracic oesophageal anastomoses but continues to use a hand suture in the anastomosis of the cervical oesophagus and in circumstances where mechanical instruments are impractical.

Anastomotic leakage is more frequent in the neck than in the chest although the related mortality rate has not been shown to be different. The incidence of leakage does not depend on any suture material, or on technical modalities used to perform the anastomosis. Indeed the anastomosis is a technical procedure and suture healing is independent of the patient's biological condition.

No significant difference has been demonstrated between leakage rates using hand sewn and mechanical anastomoses.[95]

Higher overall incidence of leak rates is found in collective reviews rather than in reports from specialist units.

Postoperative management

A detailed account of immediate postoperative care after oesophageal cancer surgery is described in Chapter 4 and a summary is given in **Tables 5.4** and **5.5**. Meticulous attention to the maintenance of fluid balance and respiratory care are essential in the immediate postoperative period. Pain control and physiotherapy are crucial. As complications of feeding jejunostomy can occur, it is difficult, based on current evidence, to recommend it for every patient.[6] Most patients will commence feeding on the 5th or 6th postoperative day. Only if respiratory or surgical complications develop should early provision of enteral nutrition become essential. A feeding jejunostomy by either an open or percutaneous route is the preferred mode of administration under these circumstances. Early mobilisation is important in preventing venous thrombosis and pulmonary embolus. It also enhances ventilation, clearance of sputum and early bowel movement. It is the author's practice to remove the chest drains on the 5th and 6th postoperative days once oral feeding has recommenced, although some surgeons remove them 48 hours after surgery.

The role of routine postoperative radiological imaging of the oesophageal anastamosis is an important issue, but evidence of extravasation in a patient who

1.	Fluid balance
2.	Intensive physiotherapy
3.	Analgesia
4.	Anti-thromboembolic measures
5.	Nutrition

Table 5.4 *Routine postoperative measures*

1.	25 ml water/hour from day 1
2.	4 × daily intensive physiotherapy from day 1 to day 4
3.	Antibiotics days 0–2
4.	Mobilisation at day 2
5.	Nasogastric suction for days 1–5
6.	Chest drains removed days 5 and 6

Table 5.5 *Routine sequence of events after extubation*

is not sick may not have clinical relevance.[96] Non–ionic contrast media may pick up gross leaks, but if normal should be followed up by barium investigations to exclude small ones. Patients who are clinically well should be started on oral feeding while contrast radiology should be reserved for patients showing signs of sepsis, pleural effusion or haemodynamic instability.

Routine nasogastric decompression is continued for 5–6 days until gastro-intestinal activity is restored. Patients are allowed 25 ml of water every hour soon after extubation. Subcutaneous low–dose heparin is administered routinely until the patient is discharged. Chest physiotherapy is commenced in Intensive Care and continued 4-hourly for the first three days. Systemic antibiotics are commenced on the morning of surgery and continued for 48 hours as a prophylactic measure. All patients should be counselled by the surgeon, an oesophageal cancer nurse practitioner and a dietician prior to discharge.

Postoperative complications

Postoperative complications may be subdivided into those that are common to any major surgical procedure in an elderly population, and those specific to oesophageal resection. The complication rate of oesophageal surgery is relatively high. Early recognition of such complications and rapid proactive management is essential to achieve good results.

General complications

These complications (see also Chapter 4) may be minimised by improved patient evaluation preoperatively and adopting prophylactic measures to counteract the predisposing factors. Respiratory complications constitute the largest proportion of this group.[4,97] Pain from the extensive incisions is the major contributor to decreased ventilation and atelectasis which leads to bronchopneumonia and respiratory failure. Mucous plugs may result in lobar collapse. Impaired diaphragmatic movement is caused by incisions placed on the diaphragm and extensive lymphadenectomy can cause poor lymphatic drainage of the pulmonary alveoli, leading to parenchymal fluid retention and a consequent acute pulmonary oedema. Significant respiratory complications occur in between 25–50% of cases following subtotal oesophagectomy.[98]

Thromboembolic complications are not uncommon in malignant disease in the elderly age groups. These complications are comparatively rare in Oriental patients but not infrequent in Western series. Serious thromboembolic complications in oesophageal cancer surgery occur in less than 10% of all procedures.[98]

Myocardial ischaemia and cerebral vascular episodes are specific to the age group undergoing surgery and are precipitated by hypoxia, hypotension and underlying vascular occlusive disease.

Haemorrhage is relatively uncommon and blood loss during surgery should range from 250–1500 ml. Acute primary bleeding from major vessels is uncommon. Secondary hemorrhage is also rare and is almost always associated with a mediastinal infection from a specific complication such as an anastomotic leakage. The value of minimisation of surgical blood loss should not be underestimated. Perioperative blood transfusion, although not associated with an increase in complications or mortality, was a significant predictor of decreased overall survival. Stage for stage two studies have suggested that blood transfusion is associated with early and late recurrence of disease.[96,99] Wound infections are uncommon because of perioperative antibiotic prophylaxis and in particular when meticulous aseptic technique is used during surgery.

Specific complications

The second group of complications following oesophageal surgery for cancer is specific to the procedure.

Anastomotic leakage and leakage from the gastric resection line

Early disruption (within 48–72 hours) is the result of a technical error. If early disruption occurs and the general condition of the patient is good and the diagnosis confirmed, then the patient should be re-explored for correction of the technical fault. Later disruptions manifest themselves between the 5th and 10th postoperative day and are due to ischaemia of the tissues or tension on the anastomotic line. Further operative intervention is likely to be hazardous and detrimental. Conservative treatment with nasogastric suction, persistent chest drainage, therapeutic antibiotic regimens and early enteral nutrition via a jejunostomy are all essential. Late anastomotic leakage should not result in a high mortality, if it is aggressively managed. Dehiscence of the gastric resection line is more unusual and usually dramatic. Re-exploration is essential as the extent of leakage is frequently large.[100] The incidence of anastomotic leakage is influenced by a variety of factors including cancer hypermetabolism, malnutrition, anastomotic vascular deficit, anastomotic tension and surgical technique. The incidence of anastomotic leakage has decreased significantly over the last ten years and rates of well under 5% should be expected.[8,100] Total gastric necrosis can occur with catastrophic consequences. The condition must be diagnosed early, resuscitation immediate and the patient returned to theatre for the formation of a cervical oesophagostomy and closing off the gastric remnant. The establishment of a feeding jejunostomy is essential. At a later date when the patient has stabilised, a colonic interposition is used to restore intestinal continuity.

Chylothorax

The thoracic duct can often be damaged during mobilisation of advanced oesophageal cancers, whether via a right thoracotomy or through the transhiatal route. A comprehensive review[101] reports chylothorax occurring in up to 10% of patients after blunt transhiatal oesophagectomy. An incidence of 2–3% during open resection is commonly reported.[98,101] Accidental damage to the thoracic duct can be prevented by identification during dissection as previously described and ligating the duct low in the inferior mediastinum on the right lateral aspect of the descending thoracic aorta. Chylothorax usually presents in the first 7 days after surgery when the patient has commenced oral intake, especially of fat-containing nutrients. A massive increase in chest drainage occurs that results in malnutrition and significant immune suppression from the subsequent white-cell loss. Monitoring of lymphocytes aids a swift diagnosis with a markedly decreased CD4 count being the main finding. Immediate re-exploration is recommended, as the damaged thoracic duct is easily identified at the time of re-exploration.[102] It is difficult to predict whether a chylous leak will spontaneously heal despite attempts to quantify the size of the leak.[103] In view of this and in order to prevent the progressive weakening of the patient's general health re-exploration is mandatory. Pre-exploratory intake of enteral fat can help to locate the leaking duct. Prolonged total parenteral nutrition has been used but patients rapidly become malnourished and frequently require a long hospital stay. Prior to surgical ligation, enteral feeding using medium-chain triglycerides helped to decrease the chylous loss. *Prophylactic antibiotic cover for pneumocystis is essential for the lymphopoenic patient.*

Recurrent laryngeal palsy

The incidence of recurrent layngeal palsy has increased over recent years due to the increase of cervical oesophago-gastric anastomoses. It is often unilateral and can be transient. Recurrent layngeal nerve palsy is extremely rare when the anastomosis is constructed in the apex of the chest via the thoracotomy route for subtotal oesophagectomy. If the palsy is transient but unilateral, the opposite cord may well compensate. The use of a percutaneous tracheostomy or a temporary formal tracheostomy may be required to safeguard the airway. If the palsy is permanent, teflon injection of the cord or a formal thyroplasty can restore adequate voice volume and a satisfactory cough.[104]

Gastric outlet obstruction

Gastric outlet obstruction is prevented by the routine use of a pyloroplasty. In the author's experience there have been no cases of perioperative gastric outlet obstruction following subtotal oesophagectomy and pyloroplasty in over 300 consecutive resections. Acid or alkaline reflux is common but not troublesome provided the anastomosis is in the apex of the thorax. Procedures which leave part of the stomach as an abdominal organ and part of the stomach as a thoracic organ predispose to gastro-oesophageal reflux. Prokinetic agents can improve gastric emptying and minimise these complications. Dumping after oesophago-gastric reconstruction is relatively common but usually resolves in the 12 months following surgery. It is adequately treated by the avoidance of high carbohydrate loads.

Benign anastomotic stricture

Benign anastomotic stricture is a late complication following any form of anas-tomosis – either mechanical or handsewn. These strictures are extremely easy to treat and respond to a single dilatation performed with the flexible endoscope under sedation.[94] Stenoses after stapled anastomosis are becoming increasingly rare, now that larger diameter staple guns are being routinely used.

Overall results of single modality resectional therapy

Overall results of surgical therapy in oesophageal cancer can be analysed in terms of hospital mortality and patient survival. Assessment of quality of life during this period is essential, but available data at present, although interesting, are preliminary.[105,106]

Hospital mortality

Two comprehensive reviews during the last two decades shed some light on trends in both hospital mortality and overall survival.[8,73] Although individual units have achieved considerably better results, the analysis of the literature on oesophageal carcinoma during the 25-year period from 1953–78 can be compared with an analysis of 1201 papers of surgical treatment for oesophageal carcinoma from 1980–1988.

 Müller's review[8] confirmed that the average hospital mortality rate following resec-tion had halved during the following decade when compared with the figures reported by Earlam and Cunha-Melo in 1980.[73]

The overall mortality rate was quoted as 13% and this decrease from Earlam's report of 28% was attributed to the introduction of prophylactic antibiotics, peri-operative parenteral and enteral nutrition and by improvements in anaesthesia, surgical technique and intensive care medicine. Some authors have differentiated their results for oesophageal resection relating to changes in operative technique and perioperative management over a certain time span. Hospital mortality rates in these units dropped from a median of 22% to a median of 5% from their first descriptions to their latest series. No evidence has been provided to relate tumour biology to mortality rate following oesophageal resection. There was also no difference in mortality rates between resections for squamous cell carcinoma and adenocarcinoma. Overall mortality rates in many series can be confusing because of variations in definitions. 'In hospital' and not 30-day mortality rates should be quoted in all papers, but unfortunately this continues not to be the case. Mortality rates of 10% and above in the present decade are no longer acceptable for the continued practice of this complicated and demanding surgical procedure. Series from specialist centres in the last few years cite operative hospital mortality rates of less than 5%.[30,32,96] There is certainly no place for the occasional oesophagectomist in the management of this serious disease.[12,107]

Comparisons of hospital mortality rates for different resection techniques reveal only minor differences. In the review by Müller the lowest mortality rate was found with transhiatal oesophagectomy with a median figure of 8%. These data, however, are not strictly comparable because transhiatal resection was the most recent surgical development and, therefore, benefitted from the experience of recent advances in perioperative care.

Nevertheless, preoperative risk analysis using a composite scoring system to predict operative risk decreased mortality in a large series from 9.4% to 1.6%.[108]

Rigorous preoperative assessment will continue to reduce hospital mortality from this major thoracoabdominal operation (see Chapter 4).

Survival figures

In a review of the 1980s, Müller et al. found that 56% of all resected patients survived the first postoperative year, 34% the second, 25% the third, 21% the fourth and 20% the 5th year after resection. These figures were very similar to those collected by Earlam and Cunha-Melo, revealing that despite improved hospital mortality overall, long-term prognosis had remained unchanged. No differences in the 5-year survival rates were noted between different techniques of resection but en bloc resections showed a significantly better long-term prognosis.[43,74] The primary determinants of overall outcome appear to be the stage of the tumour and the cell type. Prognosis is excellent with tumours invading the lamina propria or submucosa only; 32% of the patients with these tumours described in Müller's review survived 5 years if the tumour was confined to the muscularis propria at the time of presentation. If lymph-node involvement was confirmed, the 5-year survival rate reduced to 13%. Better results with resection and two-field lymphadenectomy for node-positive tumour have been achieved in specialist units.[9,19,30,32,36,37,38,43,44] Considerable evidence exists to suggest that adenocarcinomas within Barrett's epithelium tend to fare worse than squamous lesions, although this may simply reflect the more advanced stage at which these lesions tend to present.[42] Indeed with increasing numbers of early tumours being diagnosed on surveillance programmes for Barrett's oesophagus, the preponderance of early tumours presenting may reverse this trend.

Summary and future research

Cancer of the oesophagus is a depressing condition which is rapidly increasing in incidence and has a poor overall survival rate. At present there is no ideal treatment and each patient requires treatment strategies designed to suit their specific problems. At present surgical resection provides the only prospect of long-term survival. It is nevertheless still associated with significant risk, although this has dramatically decreased over the last 20 years. During the same time period, however, the cure rate of both squamous and adenocarcinoma of the oesophagus have failed to improve significantly. There is now overwhelming evidence to suggest that early cancer of the oesophagus (that is, the primary tumour confined to the oesophageal wall without lymph-node metastases) is associated with a much better prognosis than more advanced tumours. These patients have a good chance of cure with radical surgery. Any operation for carcinoma in the gastrointestinal tract must be designed to minimise the risk of anastomotic and locoregional recurrence. Subtotal oesophagectomy with two-field lymph-node dissection seems to satisfy these criteria. Nevertheless, other surgical approaches including radical transhiatal oesophagectomy may well achieve the same goal.

The majority of patients will still die of their disease and genuine efforts must be made to determine if those with a short survival time can be identified and spared unnecessarily aggressive attempts at cure and palliation. Referral of all patients with oesophageal malignancy to centres with a specialist interest in highly intensive staging investigations should be encouraged, as these centres can take part in large prospective trials, focusing on both attempted curative and palliative treatments. Clinical research must concentrate on randomised trials incorporating:

1. The separate assessment of squamous and adenocarcinomas. The rapid increase in incidence of adenocarcinomas in the West requires urgent assessment of other therapeutic modalities prior to surgery.
2. The standardisation of surgical procedures, histopathological examination and treatment protocols.
3. The further assessment of nodal staging and value of biopsy by linear array endoscopic ultrasonography.

Scientific research should focus on molecular biological techniques and the development of effective and less toxic preoperative neo-adjuvant regimens. Future clinical research must focus on prospective studies assessing the role, extent and timing of different therapeutic modalities. Until these studies are concluded, however, the data suggest that the best option for a patient with an oesophageal cancer is to have a surgical resection performed safely and effectively.

References

1. Sobin LH, Wittekind CH (eds.) UICC Classification of malignant tumours, 5th edn. New York: John Wiley, 1997.

2. Japanese Society for Oesophageal Diseases. Guidelines for the clinical and pathological studies on carcinoma of the oesophagus. Part 1: Clinical Classification. Jpn J Surg 1976; 6:64–78.

3. Tetheroo GWM, Wagenboort JHT, Castelei A et al. Selective decontamination to reduce Gram negative colonization and infections after oesophageal resection. Lancet 1990; 335:704–7.

4. Nagawa H, Kobori O, Muto T. Prediction of pulmonary complications after transthoracic oesophagectomy. Br J Surg 1994; 81:860–2.

5. Moore FA, Feliciano DV, Adrassy RJ et al. Early enteral feeding compared with parenteral, reduces post operative septic complications. The results of a meta-analysis. Ann Surg 1992; 216:172–83.
    This meta-analysis emphasises the benefits of enteral feeding in the perioperative period.

6. Watters JM, Kirkpatrick SM, Norris SB et al. Immediate post-operative feeding results in impaired

respiratory mechanics and decreased mobility. Ann Surg 1997; 226:369–77.

 7. Heslin MJ, Latkany L, Leung D *et al*. A prospective randomised trial of early enteral feeding after resection of upper gastrointestinal malignancy. Ann Surg 1997; 226:567–77.
This small trial questions routine feeding jejunostomy in all operative patients.

 8. Muller JM, Erasmitt T, Stelzner M, Zieren U *et al*. Surgical therapy of oesophageal cancer. Br J Surg 1990; 77:845–57.
This large trial reviewed oesophageal surgical publications in the 1980s, demonstrated improvements in operative mortality from the previous decade, but no better overall survival.

9. Lerut T. Oesophageal cancer – past and present studies. Eur J Surg Oncol 1996; 22:317–25.

10. Bonavina L. Early oesophageal cancer: results of a European multicentre study. Br J Surg 1995; 82:98–101.

11. Holscher AH, Bollschweiler E, Schneider PM *et al*. Early adenocarcinoma in Barrett's oesophagus. Br J Surg 1997; 84:1470–73.

12. Sutton DN, Wayman J, Griffin SM. Learning curve for oesophageal cancer surgery. Br J Surg 1998; 85:1399–1402.

13. Miller JD, Jain MK, de Gara CJ *et al*. Effect of surgical experience on results of oesophagectomy for oesophageal cancer. J Surg Oncol 1997; 65:20–21.

14. Patti MG, Corvera CU, Glasgow RE *et al*. A hospital's annual rate of oesophagectomy influences the operative mortality rate. J Gastro Surg 1998; 2:186–92.

15. Begg CB, Cramer LD, Hoskins WJ *et al*. Impact of hospital volume on operative mortality for major cancer surgery. JAMA 1998; 280 (20):1783–4.

16. McKeown KC. Trends in oesophageal resection for carcinoma. Ann R Coll Surg Engl 1972; 51:213–39.

17. Hill S, Cahill J, Wastell C. The right approach to carcinoma of the cardia, preliminary results. Eur J Surg Oncol 1992; 18:282–6.

18. Giuli R. Surgery for squamous carcinoma of the oesophagus – an overview. In: Jamieson GG (ed.) Surgery of the oesophagus. Edinburgh. Churchill Livingstone 1988; pp. 585–95.

19. Skinner DB. Enbloc resection for neoplasms of the esophagus and cardia. J Thorac Carciovasc Surg 1983; 85:59–71.

20. Siu KF, Cheung HC, Wong J. Shrinkage of the oesophagus after resection of carcinoma. Ann Surg 1986; 203:173–6.

21. Akiyama H, Tsurumaru M, Watonabe G *et al*. Development of surgery for carcinoma of the oesophagus. Am J Surg 1984; 147:9–16.

22. Akiyama H. Surgery for cancer of the oesophagus. Williams and Wilkins, 1990; pp. 43–4 and pp. 223–24.

23. Tam PC, Siu KF, Cheung HC *et al*. Local recurrences after subtotal oesphagectomy for squamous cell carcinoma. Ann Surg 1987; 205:189–94.

24. Wong J. Esophageal resection for cancer: The rationale of current practice. Am J Surg 1987; 153:18–24.

25. Mandard AM, Chasle J, Marnay J *et al*. Autopsy findings in 111 cases of esophageal cancer. Cancer 1981; 48:329–35.

26. Sons HU, Borchard F. Cancer of the distal oesophagus and cardia. Incidence, tumourous infiltration and metastatic spread. Ann Surg 1986; 203:188–95.

27. Moynihan B. Abdominal operations, vol. 1. Philadelphia and London: WB Saunders, 1916; pp. 285–317.

28. Maruyama K. Results of surgery correlated with staging in cancer of the stomach. In: Preece PE, Cuschieri A, Wellwood JM (eds.) Cancer of the stomach. London: Grune and Stratton. 1986, pp. 145–163.

29. Sue Ling H, Johnstone D, Martin IG *et al*. Gastric cancer – a curable disease in Britain. Br Med J 1993; 307:591–96.

30. Lerut T, Coosemans W, de Leyn P *et al*. Is there a role for radical oesophagectomy. Eur J Cardiothorac Surg 1999; 16 (Suppl.1) S44–S47.

31. Vickers J, Alderson D. Influence of luminal obstruction on oesophageal cancer staging using endoscopic ultrasonograpy. Br J Surg 1998; 85:999–1001.

32. Dresner SM, Griffin SM. Pattern of recurrence following radical oesophagectomy with two field lymphadenectomy. Br J Surg 2000; 87:1426–33.

33. Akiyama H, Tsurumaru M, Udagawa H, Kajiyama Y. Radical lymph node dissection for cancer of the thoracic oesophagus. Ann Surg 1994; 22:364–73.

34. Orringer M. Transthoracic versus transhiatal esophagectomy. What difference does it make? Ann Thorac Surg 1987; 44:116–18.

35. Siewert JR, Roder JD. Lymphadenectomy in oesophageal cancer surgery. Dis Esoph 1992; 2:91–7.

 36. Goldminc M, Maddern G, Le Prise E *et al*. Oesophagectomy by a transhiatal approach or thoracotomy: a prospective randomised study. Br J Surg 1993; 80:367–70.

 37. Kato H, Watanabe H, Tachimore Y, Izuka T. Evaluation of neck lymph node dissection for thoracic carcinoma. Ann Thorac Surg 1991; 51:931–5.

 38. Hagen JA, Peter JH, Demeester TR. Superiority of extended en bloc esophagogastrectomy for carcinoma of the lower esophagus and cardia. J Thorac Cardiovasc Surg 1993; 106:850–59.
These three randomised studies add weight to the argument that radical surgery is safe and has limited survival benefit.

39. Haagensen DC. The lymphatics in cancer. Philadelphia: WB Saunders, 1972; pp. 245–9.

40. Sato T, Sacamoto K. Illustrations and photographs of surgical oesophageal anatomy, specially prepared for lymph node dissection. In: Color atlas of surgical anatomy for oesophageal cancer. Tokyo and Berlin: Springer–Berlhe, 1992; pp. 25–90.

41. Tanabe G. Clinical evaluation of oesophageal lymph flow system based on the R1 uptake of removed regional lymph nodes following lymphoscintigraphy (written in Japanese). J J Surg Soc 1986; 87:315–23.

42. Matthews HR, Steel A. Left sided sub total oesophagectomy for carcinoma. Br J Surg 1987; 74:1115–17.

43. Altorki NK, Girardi L, Skinner DB. En bloc oesophagectomy improved survival for Stage III Oesophageal Cancer. J Thorac Cardiovasc Surg 1997; 114(6):948–55.

44. Lerut TE, De Leyn P, Coosemans W *et al.* Advanced esophageal carcinoma. World J Surg 1994; 18:379–87.

45. Lerut T, De Leyn P, Coosemans W *et al.* Surgical strategies in esophageal carcinoma with emphasis on radical lymphadenectomy. Ann Surg 1994; 216:583–90.

46. Orringer MB, Marshall B, Stirling MC. Transhiatal oesophagectomy for benign and malignant disease. J Thoracic Cardiovasc Surg 1993; 105:265–77.

47. International Union against Cancer (UICC) Hermanek P, Henson T, Hutter RVP, Sobin LH, eds, Suppl 1993, Berlin/Heidelberg, New York.

48. Roder JD, Bucsh R, Stein JH *et al.* Ratio of invaded to removed lymph nodes as a predictor of survival in sqaumous cell carcinoma of the oesophagus. Br J Surg 1994; 81:410–13.

49. Clark GWB, Peters JH, Ireland AP *et al.* Nodal metastasis and sites of recurrence after enbloc oesophagectomy for adenocarcinoma. Ann Thorac Surg 1994; 58:646–54.

50. Kato H, Tachimori Y, Mizobuchi S *et al.* Cervical, mediastinal and abdominal lymph node dissection (three field dissection) for superficial carcinoma of the thoracic oesophagus. Cancer 1993; 72:2879–82.

51. Gawad KA, Hosch SB, Bumann D *et al.* How important is the route of reconstruction after oesophagectomy: a prospective randomised study. Am J Gastroenterol 1999; 94(6):1490–96.

52. Bartels SH, Thorbon S, Siewert JR. Anterior versus posterior reconstruction after transhiatal oesophagectomy: a randomised controlled trial. Br J Surg 1993; 80:1141–44.
These trials confirm that the mediastinal route is the preferred route for reconstruction after curative resection.

53. El Eishi HI, Ayoob SF, Abet el Khalek M. The arterial supply of the human stomach. Acta Anat 1973; 86:565–80.

54. Thomas DM, Langford RM, Russell RCG *et al.* Anatomical basis for gastric mobilization in total oesophagectomy. Br J Surg 1979; 166:23–233.

55. Cheung HC, Siu KF, Wong J. An exclusive right thoracic approach for cancer of the middle third of the oesophagus. Ann Thorac Surg 1974; 18:1–15.

56. Cheung HC, Siu KF, Wong J. Is pyloroplasty necessary in oesophageal replacement by stomach? A prospective randomised controlled trial. Surgery 1987; 102:19–24.
This randomised trial failed to show significant differences in morbidity and mortality between pyloroplasty and no drainage after gastric transposition.

57. Law S, Cheung MC, Fok M *et al.* Pyloroplasty and pyloromyotomy in gastric replacement of the oesophagus after oesophagectomy: a randomised controlled trial. J Am Coll Surgeons 1997; 184(6):630–36.

58. Gavriliu D. Aspects of oesophageal surgery: current problems in surgery. Chicago Year Book, 1974; pp. 36–44.

59. Ventemigala R, Caleal KG, Frazier OH *et al.* The role of pre-operative mesenteric arteriography in colon interposition. J Thorac Cardiovasc Surg 1977; 74:98–104.

60. Demeester TR. Indications of surgical technique in long term functional results of colon interposition or bypass. Ann Surg 1988; 208:460.

61. Belsay RHR. Reconstruction of the oesophagus with left colon. J Thorac Cardiovasc Surg 1965; 49:33.

62. Sasaki TM. Free jejunal graft re-construction after extensive head and neck surgery. Am J Surg 1980; 139:650.

63. Logan A. The surgical treatment of carcinoma of the oesophagus and cardia. J Thoracic Cardiovasc Surg 1963; 46:150–61.

64. Nansen EN. Synchronous combined abdomino-thoracocervical oesophagectomy. Aust N Z J Surg 1975; 45:340–48.

65. Chung SCS, Griffin SM, Woods SDS *et al.* Two team synchronous esophagectomy. Surg Gynaecol Obstet 1990; 170:68–9.

66. Hayes N, Shaw I, Raimes SA *et al.* Comparison of conventional Lewis Tanner two stage oesophagectomy with the synchronous two team approach. Br J Surg 1995; 82:95–7.
This small randomised trial demonstrated higher complication and mortality rates in Western patients operated upon by the synchronous technique.

67. McKeown KC. The surgical treatment of carcinoma of the oesophagus. A review of the results in 478 cases. J Royal Coll of Surg Edin 1985; 30:1–14.

68. Graham JN, Eng JB, Sabanathan S. Left thoracotomy approach for resection of cancer of the oesophagus. Surg Gynaecol Obstet 1989; 168:49–53.

69. Lu YK, Li YM, Gu YZ. Cancer of the oesophagus at the oesophago-gastric junction. Analysis of results of 1025 resections after 5–20 years. Ann Thorac Surg 1987; 43:176–81.

70. Molina JE, Lawton BR, Myers WO et al. Oesophago-gastrectomy for adenocarcinoma of the cardia. Ann Surg 1982; 195:146–51.

71. Papachristou DN, Fortner JG. Anastomotic failure complicating total gastrectomy and esophagogastrectomy for carcinoma of the stomach. Am J Surg 1979; 138:399–402.

72. Hankins JR, Cole FN. Attar S et al. Adenocarcinoma involving the oesophagus. J Thoracic Cardiovasc Surg 1974; 68:148.

73. Earlam R, Cunha Melo JR. Oesophageal squamous cell carcinoma 1: A critical review of surgery. Br J Surg 1980; 67:381–90.

74. Skinner DB, Little AG, Ferguson MK. Selection of operation for oesophageal cancer based on staging. Ann Surg 1986; 204:391–401.

75. Turner GG. Excision of thoracic oesophagus for carcinoma with construction of an extra thoracic gullet. Lancet 1933; 1:1315–16.

76. Lequesne LP, Ranger D. Pharyngo-larygectomy with immediate pharyngo-gastric anastomosis. Br J Surg 1966; 53:105–9.

77. Ong GB. Carcinoma of the hypo-pharynx and cervical oesophagus. In: Smith R (ed.) Progress in clinical surgery. London: J & A Churchill, 1969, series 3, pp. 155–78.

78. Orringer M, Sloan H. Esophagectomy with thoracotomy. J Thorac Cardiovasc Surg 1978; 5:643–54.

79. Alderson D, Courtney SP, Kennedy RH. Radical transhiatal oesophagectomy under direct vision. Br J Surg 1994; 81:404–7.

80. Pinotti HW. A new approach to the thoracic oesophagus by the abdominal transdiaphragmatic route. Langenbeck Arch Chir 1983; 359:229–35.

81. Pommier RF, Vetto JT, Ferris BL et al. Relationships between operative approaches and outcomes in oesophageal cancer. Am J Surg 1998; 175(5):422–5.

82. Boyle MJ, Franceschi D, Livingstone AS. Transhiatal versus transthoracic oesophagectomy: complications and survival rates. Am J Surg 1999; 65(12):1137–41.

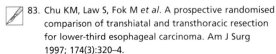
83. Chu KM, Law S, Fok M et al. A prospective randomised comparison of transhiatal and transthoracic resection for lower-third esophageal carcinoma. Am J Surg 1997; 174(3):320–4.

84. Jacobi CA, Zierenti U, Muller JM et al. Surgical therapy of oesophageal carcinoma. The influence of surgical approach and oesophageal resection on cardiopulmonary function. Eur J Cardiothorac Surg 1997; 11(1):32–7.
These two small randomised studies failed to demonstrate differences in cardiopulmonary complications between the transhiatal and transthoracic approaches.

85. McAnena OJ, Roger J, Williams NS. Right thoracoscopic assisted oesophagectomy for carcinoma. Br J Surg 1994; 81:236–8.

86. Law S, Fok M, Chu CM, Wong J. Thoracoscopic oesophagectomy for oesophageal cancer. Surgery 1997; 122:8–14.

87. Jagot P, Sauvanet A, Berthoux I et al. Laparoscopic mobilization of the stomach for oesophageal replacement. Br J Surg 1996; 83:540–2.

88. Nguyen NT, Schauer P, Luketich JD. Minimally invasive oesophagectomy for high grade dysplasia. Surgery 2000; 127(3):284–90.

89. Buess G, Kipfmuller K, Nahrun M et al. Endoskopis chemikro chirurgische dissektion des osophagus. In: Buess G (Ed.) Endoskopie. Koln: Arzte, 1990; pp. 358–75.

90. Hernreck S, Crawford DG. The oesophageal anastomotic leak. Am J Surg 1976; 132:794–8.

91. Ravitch MM, Steichen FM. A stapling instrument for end to end inverting anastomoses in the gastro-intestinal tract. Ann Surg 1979; 189:791–7.

92. Dresner SM, Lamb PJ, Wayman J et al. Benign anastomotic stricture following oesophagectomy and stapled intra-thoracic oesophago gastrostomy: risk factors and management. Br J Surg 2000; 87:370–1.

93. Bardini B, Asolati M, Ruol A et al. Anastomosis. World J Surg 1994; 18:373–8.

94. Griffin SM, Woods SDS, Chan A et al. Early and late surgical complications of sub-total oesophagectomy for squamous carcinoma of the oesophagus. J Royal Coll Surg Edin 1991; 36:170–3.

95. Law S, Fok M, Chu K et al. Comparison of hand-sewn and stapled oesophago-gastric anastomosis after oesophageal resection for cancer. A prospective randomised controlled trial. Ann Surg 1997; 226:169–73.
This small study showed no difference in anastomotic integrity between stapled and hand-sewn anastomosis but confirmed a higher rate of strictures using the stapler for anastomosis.

96. Karl RC, Schreiber R, Boulware D et al. Factors affecting morbidity, mortality and survival in patients undergoing lvor Lewis Oesophago-gastrectomy. Ann Surg 2000; 231:635–43.

97. Fan ST, Lau WY, Yip WC et al. Prediction of post operative pulmonary complications in oesophago-gastric cancer surgery. Br J Surg 1987; 74:408–10.

98. Watson A. Operable oesophageal cancer. Current results from the West. World J Surg 1994; 18:361–7.

99. Dresner SM, Hayes N, Griffin SM. The effect of blood transfusion on outcome following two field node dissection for oesophageal cancer. Eur J Surg Oncol 2000; 26:492–7.

100. Paterson IM, Wong J. Anastomotic leakage: an avoidable complication of Lewis Tanner oesophagectomy. Br J Surg 1989; 76:127–9.

101. Bolger C, Walsh TN, Tanner WA *et al*. Chylothorax after oesophagectomy. Br J Surg 1991; 78:578–87.

102. Merigliano S, Molena D, Ruol A *et al*. Chylothorax complicating oesophagectomy for cancer: A plea for early thoracic duct ligation. J Thorac Cardiovasc Surg 2000; 119:453–7.

103. Dugue L, Sauvenet A, Farges O *et al*. Output of chyle as an indicator of treatment for chylothorax complication oesophagectomy. Br J Surg 1998; 85:1147–9.

104. Griffin SM, Chung SCS, Van Hasselt CA *et al*. Late swallowing problems after oesophagectomy for cancer. Malignant infiltration of the recurrent laryngeal nerves and its management. Surgery 1992; 112:533–5.

105. Blazeby JM, Williams MH, Brooks ST *et al*. Quality of life measurement in patients with oesophageal cancer. Gut 1995; 37:505–8.

106. O'Hanlon D, Harkin M, Hayes N *et al*. Quality of life assessment of patients undergoing treatment for oesophageal cancer. Br J Surg 1995; 82:1682–5.

107. Bancewicz J. Cancer of the oesophagus. BMJ 1990; 303:3–4.

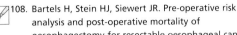108. Bartels H, Stein HJ, Siewert JR. Pre-operative risk analysis and post-operative mortality of oesophagectomy for resectable oesophageal cancer. Br J Surg 1998; 85:840–4.
This prospective study has tested out a composite scoring system based on pre-operative physiological status and found it cost-effective.

6 Surgery for cancer of the stomach

Simon A. Raimes

INTRODUCTION

There can now be genuine grounds for optimism in treating gastric cancer even in Western countries. On one hand the incidence of the disease is decreasing and on the other, increased efforts to diagnose it at a treatable stage and the recognition that the results of treatment are best for those that specialise in managing the disease has led to improving cure rates. Specialist centres in the UK, Europe and the USA are now reporting significant improvements in survival rates, apparently as a result of trying to emulate Japanese practice, which remains the 'gold standard' for the treatment of gastric cancer. Historically, 5-year survival figures for similar stages of the disease reveal results that are up to 20% better in Japan than in the West.[1] In striving to achieve similar results it is important to understand the evolution of Japanese gastric cancer treatment to determine whether Western surgeons who adopt this practice can realistically expect to achieve similar results.

Development of gastric cancer treatment in Japan

Stomach cancer is the most common cause of cancer death in Japan. Thirty years ago the survival rates were little different to those reported in the West. There are three important changes that have occurred subsequently:

National screening programme for gastric cancer

Mass survey of the population by mobile X–ray units began in 1960. Barium meal screening of the population over 40 years of age has been a massive undertaking. In 1988 5.2 million people were screened, of whom 13% required further investigation but only 0.12% were diagnosed with gastric cancer. The programme has proved to be cost-effective in those over 65 years of age. Success may be measured by the fact that in 1988 62.4% of cancers detected by screening were early mucosal or submucosal lesions.

Japanese Research Society for Gastric Cancer (JRSGC)

This was established in 1961 to promote basic research and the management of gastric cancer. The initial objective was to collect standardised data on clinical (macroscopic) staging at the time of surgery and subsequent pathological (microscopic) staging to allow accurate comparison of results. Recommended surgical techniques and rules for documentation of surgery were published and are regularly updated. Pathological assessment is rigidly standardised and similarly updated. The JRSGC and the National Cancer Center in Tokyo started a nationwide collection of data in 1963. Around 10 000 cases are registered annually, though it should be emphasised that this is less than 20% of gastric cancers treated each year in Japan – it is highly selective and certainly represents the very best practice in the country.

Radical gastric cancer surgery

Radical excision of the stomach and the related lymphatic drainage had previously been practised in specialist centres in both Japan and the West. Publication by the JRSGC of precise definitions of radicality and a standardisation of operations in the 'General Rules' reinforced this concept and led to the widespread adoption of radical gastric surgery in Japan. It has been proposed that this surgical attitude has been a major factor in the improvement in results. Remarkably, this has never been tested in a randomised trial and Japanese surgeons claim that to try and do so now would be unethical.

The real question is to what extent has each of the above factors contributed to the overall improvement in survival. These measures were introduced concurrently and the Japanese have not been able to separate the respective contributions of earlier diagnosis, improved pathological staging and radical surgery. This analysis is very important in understanding how practice is evolving in the West.

Development of gastric cancer treatment in the West

Screening for gastric cancer

A UICC Workshop held in the UK in 1990 concluded that asymptomatic screening of the population for gastric cancer was only cost effective in countries with a high incidence of the disease. It could not be recommended as a public health policy in the West.

Screening of symptomatic 'dyspeptic' patients does increase the proportion of early gastric cancers diagnosed.[2] Increased availability of endoscopic services, including open and direct access endoscopy, is improving the stage at which cancers are diagnosed.[3] However, it must be emphasised that there is a significant difference in outcome between symptomatic cancers diagnosed at an earlier stage and that of screen-detected asymptomatic cancers included in Japanese series. In Japan there is a significantly improved long-term survival after surgery in asymptomatic screened cancer cases when compared with those presenting with symptoms.[4]

Shift to the left phenomenon. The presentation of gastric cancer can be considered to produce a spectrum of disease with the worst stages to the right. Asymptomatic screening and, to a lesser extent, symptomatic screening not only increase the proportion of early cancers at the far left end of the spectrum, but also shift the whole spectrum to the left. Staging simply divides the spectrum of the disease into four sections. The shift-to-the-left phenomenon may mean that all stages contain a higher proportion of patients in the more favourable left side of the stage. This may partly explain why the survival of all stages of gastric cancer is better in screened populations. It is also postulated that increased population awareness of the risk of gastric cancer, such as has occurred in Japan, also contributes to a shift-to-the-left phenomenon even in the non-screened population as more patients recognise the potential significance of their symptoms and report them earlier. Increased awareness of Western populations to significant gastrointestinal symptoms linked to the increased availability of diagnostic services should shift the spectrum of disease to the left, though this will never have the same impact as asymptomatic screening.

It may be more meaningful to compare Western results with those of symptomatic Japanese patients only – this would allow a more accurate prediction of the likely effects of the widespread adoption of radical surgery in the West.

Effects of radical surgery and improved pathology on staging

The staging systems used in the West have not been as clearly defined or standardised as those in Japan. Accurate comparison of results was not possible until 1985 when the UICC and AJCC agreed a unified staging system (see Chapter 3).

It should be realised that there are also other, more subtle, effects on the process of staging that affect a comparison of Western and Japanese practice.

Stage migration phenomenon The extent of lymph-node involvement (N factor) is an important aspect of staging. The Japanese Rules for Pathology require very detailed sampling of each defined node group and multiple sections of each node. The detection of nodal micrometastases by this type of detailed sampling is more likely than in standard Western pathological assessment. If the same principles were applied in the West a proportion of cancers would be allocated to a worse stage on the basis of the true N factor (see Chapter 3). Present Western pathological analysis produces an over-optimistic staging of cancers and this is one reason why long-term survival is not as good as the comparable Japanese figures for the same stage. Many specialist centres have already addressed this shortcoming and nodal staging is now much more accurate.

Another very important factor in the accurate staging of cancers on the basis of lymph-node involvement is the extent of the lymphadenectomy. If only the first tier of nodes is excised then the N factor could not be more than N1. In the best Japanese centres all second-tier and possibly some third-tier nodes are also excised en bloc and so if there are metastases in these nodes the cancer will be correctly staged N2 or N3. Examination of 5-year survival figures (5YSR) in Japan reveals the importance of correctly determining the N factor by more radical lymphadenectomy:

T2N1M0 71% 5YSR   T2N2M0 52% 5YSR
T3N1M0 46% 5YSR   T3N2M0 23% 5YSR[5]

It is interesting to note that correct staging of a node-positive cancer may decrease the 5-year survival expectancy by about 20%. It is still not clear what proportion of the 'benefit' of radical lymphadenectomy is due to removal of nodal tissue as opposed to that attributable to the correct pathological staging of the cancer. This not only affects a comparison of Japanese and Western results, but is also an important factor that should be allowed for in randomised studies comparing D1 and D2 lymphadenectomy.

Different disease in the West?

It has been suggested that gastric cancer in the West may be a different disease to that in Japan.[6] There is, however, little evidence to support this hypothesis. Comparison of the results of gastric cancer treatment in racially similar Tokyo and Honolulu Japanese shows poorer results for those treated by Western methods.[7] The natural course of the disease, the modes of spread and areas of recurrence are similar. If early gastric cancers are excluded then most prognostic factors are also similar.[8] However, there are two factors that may be of some significance:

Lauren histological type Many studies show a higher proportion of intestinal-type cancer in Japan. This type has a better prognosis than the diffuse type that is more commonly seen in the West.

Proximal cancers Cancers of the proximal third of the stomach have a worse prognosis than those in the distal two-thirds.[9] Results of surgery are significantly worse in cancers of the proximal third in Japan. Recent Western series report a 40–50% incidence of proximal cancers compared with 20–30% in Japan. The incidence of proximal cancers is increasing more rapidly in the West and it is possible that this will negate the beneficial effects of other factors that are being improved.

Perioperative mortality of radical surgery in the West

While the Japanese specialist centres report mortality rates of 1–3% for radical gastric surgery, this is considerably higher in the West and particularly for total gastrectomy.[10] Even centres of excellence in the West report a mortality rate of 5–10% for curative surgery and this is even higher for palliative procedures.[11] The results are improving, but are unlikely ever to equal the Japanese figures because Western patients are, on average, 10 years older and have a higher incidence of cardiovascular disease than those with gastric cancer in Japan. Japanese patients are thinner and have a very low incidence of postoperative thromboembolic complications. The higher incidence of proximal cancers in the West means that the proportion of total gastrectomies is higher; it should be remembered that this operation is associated with a mortality of about twice that of a subtotal resection.

Role of radical surgery in Western practice

It is apparent from the previous analysis that the results obtained in gastric cancer treatment in Japan are superior to those in the West for multiple and complex reasons. It has to be accepted that comparison of overall survival rates is of little meaning. Even now that there is a uniform staging system there are subtle reasons why Japanese patients may do better, related to the 'stage migration' and 'shift-to-the-left' phenomena and the higher incidence of proximal cancers in the West.

Past experience with radical gastric resection in the West produced variable and usually disappointing results, with any therapeutic gain being negated by the higher mortality of more extensive surgery. Only a few specialist centres have pursued the concept of radical excision as practised by the Japanese, while most gastric cancer surgery has remained within the remit of the 'general surgeon'. Most non-specialist surgeons have restricted their surgical effort to limited resections that can be achieved with a lower operative mortality. The Leeds General Infirmary experience is presently closest to Japanese practice in the UK (**Table 6.1**). They have reported stage-specific survival rates nearer to those of best Japanese practice, at least for the earlier stages, and with an acceptable mortality.[11] Unfortunately the actual contribution of radical surgery remains uncertain because, in addition to adopting this surgical policy, they have concurrently introduced pathology reporting along Japanese lines and an enhanced endoscopy service for the rapid investigation of symptomatic patients. Despite this reservation the Leeds practice is now the 'gold standard' in the UK. Other centres in the USA and Europe are now reporting similarly impressive results for a radical surgical approach.[12,13] On the basis of this analysis of the differences between Japanese and Western practice, it is more meaningful to compare Western results with those of the specialist centres such as Leeds.

It seems reasonable to assume that radical gastric cancer surgery does produce some survival benefit, but that this may be variable depending on the stage of the disease. However if that advantage is only small for Western patients then it could be offset by the increased mortality of more radical surgery. In addition, more extensive resections are associated with increased postoperative morbidity, long-term sequelae and nutritional consequences.

Summary

It is apparent that the common 'nihilistic' approach to gastric cancer in the West is no longer acceptable. Modern radical gastric cancer surgery is still evolving and only when the benefits of this approach outweigh the increased risks of more extensive resection will this become standard practice. While surgery will require greater subspecialisation, the role of improved pathological assessment and most importantly, earlier detection of the disease must not be overshadowed by concentrating on radical surgery alone. Our understanding of the potential benefits

	Comparison of Results from Leeds (11) and Tokyo (37) Cumulative 5-year survival as %	
	TOKYO	**LEEDS**
All potentially curative resections	75	54
Early gastric cancer	91	91
Stage I	91	87
Stage II	72	65
Stage III	44	18

Table 6.1 *5-year survival after potentially curative gastric cancer surgery*

of radical surgery is developing rapidly, but must primarily be based on the pathology of the disease and how surgery has failed in the past to control gastric cancer in most patients.

Areas of failure after gastric cancer surgery

A rational approach to surgery for gastric cancer requires an understanding of the modes of spread of this cancer and how it recurs after surgery. This knowledge is essential in defining the aims and limitations of radical surgery.

Metastatic pathways

Direct extension

Into adjacent organs or structures that may be excised en bloc with the stomach as part of a potentially curative resection.

Lymphatic spread

Lateral spread occurs in the submucosal and subserosal lymphatic plexuses depending on the depth of penetration of the cancer. Drainage is then to the perigastric nodes and subsequently along the lymphatics that accompany the arteries to the stomach back to the coeliac trunk. This is discussed in detail in the section on lymphadenectomy (p. 166). Lymphatic spread can occur at any stage, but becomes more common the deeper the invasion through the stomach wall. Between 60–80% of patients with evidence of intra-abdominal metastatic spread will have lymph-node involvement.[15] Lymphatic spread is the most common mode of dissemination in both intestinal and diffuse types of gastric cancer, emphasising the potential importance of adequate nodal excision.

Peritoneal spread

This should only occur once the cancer has breached the serosal surface when cells can be shed into the peritoneal cavity. There is evidence that the likelihood of retrieving viable shed cells is proportional to the area of serosa that is invaded.[16] There is experimental evidence that shed cells can adhere to and infiltrate intact peritoneum.[17] Presently up to 75% of cancers in the West are serosa-positive and thus a large number of patients have the potential for intraperitoneal recurrence by cell implantation in the gastric bed or elsewhere in the peritoneal cavity. Peritoneal seedling is much more common in diffuse-type cancers (45–75% versus 10–30% for the intestinal-type).[15] Surgery that includes removal of the intact lesser sac peritoneum may possibly be of value for a localised cancer with only posterior wall serosal invasion, but in general, surgery has no curative role in treating this mode of spread. In the West, it is very important to appreciate this limitation in treating the majority of patients with gastric cancer.

Haematogenous spread

Despite the rich vascular supply of the stomach, liver metastases at the time of diagnosis are relatively uncommon, even in advanced cancers. It has been postulated that gastric cancer is inefficient in metastasising via the haematogenous route and this may apply to the diffuse type in particular. The alternative explanation is that diffuse-type cancers spread rapidly by other routes and that while haematogenous spread may occur, the patient dies of other metastatic disease before liver and distant metastases become clinically apparent.

Concept of gastric cancer as a locoregional disease

It has been observed that even in cancers that are locally advanced at the time of diagnosis the disease is still confined to the area of the stomach, the retroperitoneum and peritoneal cavity liver and distant metastases are frequently not detected. Wangensteen and his colleagues' study of reoperation data in patients who had previously undergone 'curative' gastric resection supports this concept. This was reported in a paper by Gundersen and Sosin that should be regarded as essential reading.[18] The reoperations were mainly elective procedures in patients thought to be at high risk of recurrence. On second look over 80% had evidence of recurrence. Looking at those with recurrence, the most important finding was that while 29.3% had haematogenous spread, in just 6.1% was this the only mode of recurrence – all the other patients had additional gastric bed or peritoneal disease. In total 87.8% had disease in the gastric bed and anastomosis and a third of these patients had distant peritoneal seedlings. Importantly, virtually all those who had serosa-positive (T3 and T4) cancers at the time of their first resection had intra-abdominal recurrence. It was apparent that the extent of resection had little effect on the incidence or type of recurrence. Wangensteen concluded that radical surgery had produced little benefit in this group of patients. These findings have subsequently been confirmed in other studies.[19,20]

The pattern of recurrence is quite different in serosa-negative (T1 and T2) cancers and especially early gastric cancers. Unlike serosa-positive cancers that tend to recur early (within 2 years), if recurrence does occur it does so later and more frequently, as haematogenous metastases without local recurrence.

The high incidence of serosa-positive cancers in the West explains why the overall outlook after gastric resection is still poor. Recurrence occurs early and within the abdomen – most of these patients probably do not live long enough to show evidence of blood-borne metastases. It is possible that improved locoregional control of serosa-positive cancers will not prevent patients dying later of distant metastases. However, control of locoregional recurrence would improve the prognosis in a large number of patients even if cure were not achieved. The value of the symptom-free interval in those patients who cannot be cured by surgery should not be underestimated.

It has been postulated that there is a biphasic pattern of recurrence in gastric cancer. There is a first early phase of local failure in the gastric bed, anastomosis and peritoneal surfaces most commonly seen in serosa-positive cancers and diffuse-type cancers in particular. The second later phase of failure is caused by haematogenous metastases to the liver or distant organs. This is more commonly seen in earlier cancers and intestinal-type cancers that have not recurred locally in the first phase.

The role of surgery is limited to complete removal of curable lesions that have not disseminated at the time of diagnosis and to minimising the early phase of locoregional recurrence.

Strategies to minimise locoregional failure

Local or gastric bed recurrence

There are three factors to consider:

1. Complete resection of the primary lesion to ensure that all resection margins are free of malignant cells. This includes extending the resection line in continuity to adjacent structures and organs if feasible and safe.
2. En bloc resection of all potentially involved lymph nodes within the normal lymphatic pathways from the stomach.
3. Prevention of implantation of free cancer cells in the gastric bed. Sugarbaker and colleagues have proposed a 'Tumour cell entrapment hypothesis' which suggests that cells shed before or during surgery can implant on and remain viable in the deperitonealised resection site. These cells may already be present in the peritoneal cavity at the time of surgery in serosa-positive cancers or may be shed during resection from the tumour surface and cut lymphatics and blood vessels.[21]

It is apparent that appropriate radical surgery has a definite role in the control of the first two factors. However, it will have only a minimal effect in preventing cell implantation on the gastric bed, especially in serosa-positive and more advanced cancers with lymphatic spread into the second tier of nodes or beyond. Analysis of survival benefit from radical lymphadenectomy shows a statistically insignificant advantage for T3 and T4 cancers.[22] A benefit is most apparent in stage II and IIIa cancers, producing a decrease in the incidence of local recurrence and an increased rate of cure.[23,24,25]

Peritoneal dissemination

Viable cancer cells may be shed preoperatively and during or soon after surgery. Meticulous surgical technique with en bloc resection of the stomach, affected adjacent organs and intact gastric lymphatic chains is important to prevent 'iatrogenic' cell spillage into the peritoneal cavity. Measures to destroy free cells in the perioperative period will be required in addition to surgery in patients who have serosal involvement and/or metastases in the second lymph-node tier. There is increased interest in intraperitoneal chemotherapy in the West – it is already commonly utilised in Japan as part of the multimodality treatment of advanced cancers.[26,27] This treatment is of most value if started during or immediately after surgery. Delayed postoperative treatment does not improve survival. This is thought to be because cells have already implanted in the gastric bed and are protected by a fibrinous coagulum.[28]

Summary

The most important objective for the surgeon is to define the point of diminishing returns in gastric cancer surgery. Radical surgery has a place in controlling local disease and in some patients this will lead to cure, particularly for serosa-negative cancer. In others radical surgery can prolong symptom-free survival time.[32,33] However it is important to realise that in the future surgery will probably be only one part of the multimodality treatment of advanced gastric cancer: the potential roles of chemotherapy and radiotherapy are discussed in more detail in Chapter 7. A recent review of multimodality treatment of resectable gastric cancer by Averbach and Jacquet is recommended.[15]

Principles of gastric cancer resection

There are certain basic principles that should be adhered to when resecting gastric cancer, and there is now considerable evidence on which to base standardised procedures. However each case is different and there are multiple factors that affect the operative tactics. The stage of the cancer, evidence of spread, mode of spread and the patient's health, age and build all have to be taken into account in 'designing' the appropriate procedure for each patient. We can now talk in terms of a 'rational gastric resection' based on the standardised procedures but taking these other factors into account. The components of a gastric cancer resection are considered under the following headings:

1. Extent of the gastric resection
2. Lymphadenectomy
3. Splenectomy
4. Distal pancreatectomy
5. Extended resections
6. Lesser resections.

Extent of gastric resection

The most fundamental aim of gastric cancer surgery is to excise the primary lesion adequately. The type of gastrectomy required to achieve this depends on the position of the cancer and the margin necessary to be certain not to leave malignant cells at the anastomotic line.

Lateral spread in the gastric wall occurs by direct invasion and by spread within the submucosal and subserosal lymphatics. Once the submucosa has been penetrated there may be extensive lateral spread within the abundant lymphatic plexus. Diffuse-type cancers are particularly prone to spread in this way; in their most aggressive forms most or all of the submucosa may be infiltrated thus producing a linitis plastica. It is important to realise that both the oesophagus and duodenum can be infiltrated by spread in the mural lymphatics – in the former via the submucosal channels and the latter via the subserosal channels. This must be taken into account when planning the extent of resection if there is palpable tumour at either end of the stomach.

It often stated that diffuse-type cancers require a wider resection margin than the intestinal type.[29] Some European surgeons recommend a total gastrectomy for any diffuse-type lesion.[1] This concept is debatable, as examination of resection margins has shown that a 5 cm margin from the palpable edge of the tumour is sufficient for both intestinal and diffuse types.[30] Cancers that have penetrated the serosa require a wider margin and 6 cm from the palpable edge of the tumour or infiltrated wall has been recommended.[31]

Serosa-negative cancers, particularly of the intestinal type, may be resected with a smaller margin in elderly or high-risk patients. The place of limited resections is discussed later.

Type of gastrectomy (**Fig. 6.1**)

Distal third cancer (A and AM)

A subtotal (80%) gastrectomy with resection of the first part of the duodenum is recommended.[34] A total gastrectomy is only indicated for large tumours or when there is submucosal infiltration to within 7–8 cm of the oesophago-gastric junction.

Middle third cancer (M and MA)

In many cases a total gastrectomy will be necessary, but this depends on the amount of stomach remaining below the oesophago-gastric junction after excising an adequate margin of stomach proximal to the palpable edge of the tumour. A minimum of 2 cm is needed and so for a serosa-negative cancer there must be a 7 cm margin from the oesophago-gastric junction and at least 8 cm for a serosa-positive cancer. A smaller margin could be accepted in elderly patients and particularly for intestinal-type cancers.

Proximal third cancer (C, CM and MC)

The choice of resection here is between a proximal subtotal or a total gastrectomy. Anastomosis of the distal stomach to the oesophagus produces a poor functional result; alkaline reflux in particular can be very troublesome and difficult to

Figure 6.1
Extent of gastric resection.

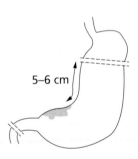

Antral carcinoma
Subtotal gastrectomy and resection of first part of duodenum

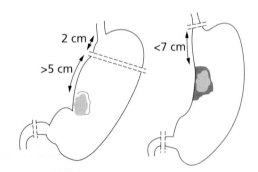

Carcinoma of middle third
Subtotal or total gastrectomy depending on proximal margin of resection

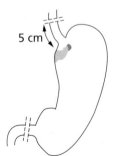

Carcinoma of cardia
Total gastrectomy and resection of lower oesophagus

control.[35] This is not the experience of all specialist centres and some routinely use a proximal subtotal resection without apparently compromising survival rates or producing unacceptable side effects.[36] Cancer of the proximal third of the stomach tends to be more advanced for both T and N stages when compared with distal cancers.[37] In the absence of a prospective randomised study total gastrectomy is presently recommended as a better cancer operation and with fewer significant side effects. Nutritional problems are, however, more common than after proximal gastrectomy.

Cancer of the cardia poses a particular problem in terms of surgical approach, extent of resection and lymph-node excision.[38] If an adequate proximal margin can be obtained then the preferred approach is a total gastrectomy with excision of the crural muscles around the hiatus and transhiatal excision of the lower mediastinal nodes.[39] The alternative approaches to cancer around the oesophago-gastric junction have been discussed in more detail in Chapter 5.

Extensive cancers (CMA)

Total gastrectomy is indicated provided there is a chance of worthwhile palliation in this type of advanced cancer, which is usually of the linitis plastica type. In this situation there is often distant spread, usually as peritoneal seedlings. In cases where there is no detectable distant spread surgical resection is probably indicated even if invaded adjacent organs have to be removed as well. Importantly, wide resection margins have to be incorporated as there are malignant cells in the submucosal lymphatic plexuses well away from the palpable edge of the cancer. It has been argued that surgery is not worthwhile for this type of gastric cancer and certainly the poor results suggest that resection is only providing limited palliation.[40] In the absence of any other effective treatment then resection, possibly combined with intraperitoneal chemotherapy, is indicated in younger patients with disease confined to the stomach and perigastric tissues.

Total gastrectomy de principe for distal cancers

The absolute indications for removal of the whole stomach have been listed above – in these circumstances this is termed a 'total gastrectomy de necessite'. There are surgeons who argue that all cancers of the stomach, even those in the distal third, should be treated in the same way – 'total gastrectomy de principe'. It is important to understand the arguments for and against such a policy.

1. *Less risk of positive proximal resection margin*
    Provided the rules on safe margins of resection are adhered to this is rare. If the margins are still positive despite an adequate margin then this usually indicates an aggressive malignancy and anastomotic recurrence as the only site of recurrence is unusual.[41]
2. *Multicentric cancer and gastric mucosal 'field change'*
    The incidence of stump cancer, even in long-term survivors, is low. However, an important part of the preoperative work-up before a subtotal gastrectomy is careful endoscopic examination and biopsy of the proximal stomach. If this shows evidence of a premalignant field change, there are multiple gastric polyps or the patient has pernicious anaemia then total gastrectomy is advised.[42]

3. *Adequacy of lymphadenectomy*

It has been argued that total gastrectomy allows a more certain D2 lymphadenectomy. The only difficult nodes to remove en bloc in a subtotal gastrectomy are the left paracardial group. While it is still possible to resect these nodes, since they are positive in less than 5% of distal cancers, there is no real significant therapeutic advantage in doing so. Survival of patients with positive left paracardial nodes is very poor and there is no demonstrable therapeutic advantage in doing so for distal cancers.

There are no studies that prove a significant survival benefit for total gastrectomy *de principe* – a recently completed randomised study has shown no survival benefit.[43] Against this is a higher mortality for total gastrectomy which in most Western reports is about twice that of subtotal gastrectomy. Even in the best hands the mortality of total gastrectomy is up to 5% and is on average nearer 10%. There is an increased risk of long-term nutritional problems after total gastrectomy, particularly in older patients and even when a jejunal pouch is constructed.[44] Quality of life assessments also show a significant benefit for subtotal gastrectomy in the long term.[45]

On the basis of the available data there is no support for the concept of total gastrectomy de principe for cancers in the lower half of the stomach.

Lymphadenectomy

Lymph-node metastasis is the most common mode of spread in gastric cancer. It is now recognised that lymphatic spread can occur in the absence of haematogenous spread and that gastric cancer may remain a localised disease even when nodes are involved. This underlies the concept of lymphadenectomy as a surgical method for curing gastric cancer. The pattern of spread should in theory divide into four zones based on the arterial blood supply of the stomach. Detailed pathological studies show that lymphatic involvement is not this predictable, mainly due to the abundant blood and lymphatic plexuses in the submucosal layer of the stomach.[46]

The patterns of lymph-node involvement have been extensively investigated by the Japanese. As described in Chapter 3 the nodes have been grouped into 16 stations (see Fig. 3.2 in Chapter 3) and these are listed in **Table 6.2**. Studies of large numbers of patients treated at the National Cancer Centre in Tokyo have shown the likelihood of involvement of each node station for cancers in different parts of the stomach[47] – see **Table 6.3**.

In planning the extent of lymphadenectomy three factors have to be considered:

1. The likelihood of metastasis at each node station.
2. The possible survival benefit of removing all nodes at that station.
3. The additional risk of mortality and serious morbidity in removing the nodes.

The JRSGC database has shown that resection of stations 1 to 12 only produces any worthwhile benefit in terms of 5-year survival. The improvement in survival after removal of stations 13 to 16 is so small that any possible benefit is almost certainly negated by the increased mortality and morbidity associated with the extended radical resection. The station 12 hepato-duodenal ligament nodes are in the third tier for all thirds of the stomach. These nodes are involved in 9% of

1.   Right cardiac nodes
2.   Left cardiac nodes
3.   Nodes along the lesser curvature
4.   Nodes along the greater curvature
        4sa – nodes along short gastric arteries
        4sb – nodes along left gastroepiploic artery
        4d – nodes along the right gastroepiploic artery
5.   Suprapyloric nodes
6.   Infrapyloric nodes
7.   Nodes along left gastric artery
8.   Nodes along the common hepatic artery
9.   Coeliac artery nodes
10. Splenic hilum nodes
11. Nodes along the splenic artery
12. Nodes in the hepatoduodenal ligament
13. Nodes on the posterior of pancreas
14. Nodes at the root of the mesentery
15. Nodes on the middle colic artery
16. Para-aortic nodes
110. Lower thoracic paraoesophageal nodes
111. Diaphragmatic nodes

Table 6.2 *Lymph node stations: Names and locations of the regional lymph nodes of the stomach*

Data from the National Cancer Center Hospital in Tokyo[33] **Percentage risk of nodal metastases for advanced gastric cancers**		
Node Station	**Distal (A)**	**Middle (M)**	**Proximal (C)**
1	7	16	31
2	0	1	13
3	38	40	39
4	35	31	11
5	12	3	2
6	49	15	3
7	23	22	19
8	25	11	7
9	13	8	13
10	0	2	10
11	4	4	12
12	8	2	1
13–16	(0–5% for all)		

Table 6.3 *Incidence of metastasis at each node station for cancers in the proximal, middle and distal thirds of the stomach*

lower third and 4% of middle third cancers. Five-year survival rates of up to 25% have been reported in Japan for patients who have had positive station 12 nodes resected. This manoeuvre is probably worthwhile in distal cancers where N2 nodes appear involved. Some surgeons resect these nodes routinely as part of a D2 resection.

Definition of extent of lymphadenectomy

The Japanese introduced the concept of tiers of lymph nodes with lymphatic spread occurring progressively through the tiers. The tiers are allocated an N number:

N1 Perigastric nodes closest to the primary lesion
N2 Distant perigastric nodes and the nodes along the main arteries supplying the stomach.
N3 Nodes outside the normal lymphatic pathways from the stomach. Involved in advanced stages or by retrograde lymphatic flow due to blockage of normal pathways.

The tiers are different for each third of the stomach – see **Table 6.4**.

It is important to understand the nomenclature as all too often the extent of nodal dissection is wrongly described in the literature.

D1 *Limited lymphadenectomy*: all N1 nodes removed en bloc with the stomach.

Location	AMC,MAC MCA,CMA	A AM	MA, M MC	C CM
1st Tier (N1)	1 2 3 4 5 6	3 4 5 6	3 4 5 6 1	1 2 3 4s
2nd Tier (N2)	7 8 9 10 11	7 8 9 1	2 7 8 9 10 11	4d 7 8 9 10 11 5 6
3rd Tier (N3)	12 13 14 110 111	2 10 11 12 13 14	12 13 14	12 13 14 110 111

Notes: 1. Stations 2 and 10 should be excised in a D2 resection for an MC cancer but are optional for M and MA.
2. Station 5 and 6 resection is optional for C and CM and if not resected the operation is still classified as a D2 resection.

Table 6.4 *Lymph node tiers according to the rules of the JRSGC*

D2 *Systematic lymphadenectomy:* all N1 and N2 nodes removed en bloc with the stomach. If any of the second tier stations are not resected then this is technically a D1 resection, but is sometimes represented as a D1/D2 resection.

D3 *Extended lymphadenectomy:* a more radical en bloc resection including the third tier nodes. This more commonly includes only some stations, such as the station 12 nodes, and should be represented as a D2/D3 resection.

In the Japanese Rules for Gastric Cancer Surgery the minimum requirement for an effective resection of gastric cancer is a systematic D2 lymphadenectomy.

Lymphadenectomy and cure of gastric cancer

This concept is strictly defined in the Japanese Rules:

Absolute curative resection The surgical D number is greater than the pathological N number e.g. D2 lymphadenectomy for N0 or N1 disease.

Relative curative resection The D number equals the N number.

Effect of the International Unified TNM Staging System on definition of lymphadenectomy

As explained in Chapter 3 the introduction of the agreed staging system has been important in allowing direct comparison of results of treatment. It has to be recognised that this introduces certain problems with describing the extent of lymphadenectomy in the precise way practised by the Japanese. It is recommended that the JRSGC Rules are still used for describing the *extent of the lymphadenectomy* and the Unified TNM Staging System for *pathological staging* of the cancer.

The case for D2 systematic lymphadenectomy

No other aspect of gastric cancer surgery has proved more controversial in recent years. While the Japanese continue to advocate this as a basic requirement of surgery, surgeons in most other countries have been reluctant to adopt this radical approach, although there is increasing recognition among surgeons specialising in the treatment of gastric cancer that D2 lymphadenectomy has a role in the surgical cure of this disease. The factors to consider are the potential improvement in survival and local control of the disease set against the additional mortality and morbidity of more radical surgery.

The evidence can be divided into that from Japanese sources and that from other countries.

Japanese evidence

The widespread adoption of systematic lymphadenectomy in Japan was based on a comparison of the results of this type of resection with that of historical control data. There are published results of uncontrolled studies comparing different levels of node resection, but no randomised controlled studies. The Japanese medical profession are so convinced of the value of radical lymphadenectomy that no trials have been performed and none are presently in progress.

The value of D2 lymphadenectomy is stated to be reduction in gastric bed recurrence leading to a longer disease-free interval and increased survival rate.

The extent of lymphadenectomy correlates well with survival in Japanese studies. Multivariate analysis has shown that this is an independent positive variable for survival.[48] On the basis of historical data it has been claimed that the inclusion of a D2/D3 lymphadenectomy in the surgical treatment of 'curable' gastric cancer has doubled the survival rate.[49] There are many other Japanese reports of improved survival after D2 compared with lesser resections.[50,51,52] As shown in **Table 6.5** this applies for all stages of the disease, although as previously explained this simple type of analysis does not take into account the more accurate pathological staging that is inevitable with more extensive nodal resections.

One of the ways to extract information about the benefit of systematic lymphadenectomy from these Japanese studies is to compare the survival difference for patients with N1 node involvement only. An incomplete D1 (D0) resection produces a 4% 5YSR, rising to 46% for a D1 resection and with a further 10% benefit for a D2 resection.[53] Importantly this emphasises the value of complete resection of the first node tier. It also reveals a modest, but definite advantage in removing the second tier if only first tier nodes are involved. Again this is with the proviso of the effect of understaging with resections less than D2. It is possible to calculate the likely level of error by looking at the proportion of patients with N1 disease only in those undergoing a D2 resection and comparing this with the proportion of N1 cases in those undergoing a D1 resection – this provides a fairly crude correction factor for under-staging/stage migration. However this factor often accounts for most of the apparent gain from a D2 resection.

Perhaps more convincing evidence can be obtained from examining the outcome of patients with N2 disease who have undergone a D2 lymphadenectomy. It is apparent from Table 6.5 that for each T stage some patients do survive 5 years. It is reasonable to assume that they would not have survived as long after a lesser resection that would have left malignant nodes in the gastric bed. While

Stage	TNM	5YSR (%)
Ia	pT1 pN0 M0	99
Ib	pT1 pN1 M0	90
	pT2 pN0 M0	88
II	pT1 pN2 M0	79
	pT2 pN1 M0	71
	pT3 pN0 M0	69
IIIa	pT2 pN2 M0	52
	pT3 pN1 M0	46
	pT4 pN0 M0	52
IIIb	pT3 pN2 M0	23
	pT4 pN1 M0	26
	pT4 pN2 M0	16
IV	M1	10

Table 6.5 *5-year survival related to stage of gastric cancer*

only a very small proportion of T1 cancers have spread to N2 nodes (*vide infra*), up to 31% of T2 cancers and more than 40% of T3 cancers have second tier nodal spread.[54] Turning back to Table 6.5 it can be seen that a 5YSR of 52% for T2N2 should equate to an improvement of up to 15% for T2 disease if a D2 lymphadenectomy rather than a lesser resection is performed for T2 cancers. The improvement for T3 cancers is less as the 5YSR is only 23% for T3N2, but this still equates to about a 10% improvement for T3 disease over a lesser lymphadenectomy. The improvement in Japanese patients is mainly seen in those with small areas of serosal involvement and there was no benefit for Borrmann type IV cancers.[55] There are now non-Japanese series showing a similar trend for the survival of N2 patients,[56] although radical lymphadenectomy has not proved as beneficial for those with serosal invasion.[57]

Further evidence for a benefit of systematic lymphadenectomy comes from studies of the effects of different operative strategies for node-negative cancers. There is now evidence of an improvement in survival of node-negative (N0) patients after D2 compared with D1 lymphadenectomy.[58] This seems to be explained by the failure of standard histological stains to identify micrometastases in nodes.[59] It is likely that a proportion of node-negative cases should be classified as having node-positive disease with malignant cells identified in first tier nodes. There are now similar reports from specialist Western units.[60] It is likely that on the same basis a proportion of N1 cancers do actually have N2 disease and so this may partly explain the benefit of a D2 against a lesser lymphadenectomy.

It must also be realised that specialist Japanese units report a mortality of less than 2% for gastrectomy with D2 lymphadenectomy. Morbidity is also low, though increased significantly with complete removal of node stations 10 and 11 if this requires splenectomy and distal pancreatectomy.

Non-Japanese evidence

Many Western surgeons have been unable to reproduce the beneficial effects of radical lymphadenectomy. In attempting to emulate Japanese practice they have encountered higher mortality and morbidity rates than for less radical operations. However, there are now reports from specialist centres in the USA, UK and Europe of D2 lymphadenectomy results that are much closer to those reported from Japan.[12,23,61] More importantly, there are a number of prospective controlled studies comparing the different operative strategies. These provide valuable evidence for the role of radical node dissection in gastric cancer surgery.

German Gastric Cancer Study[62]

A prospective but non-randomised study of the practice of D1 and D2 lymphadenectomy took place in specialist German surgical units between 1986 and 1989. The definition of a level of lymphadenectomy was based on the number of nodes retrieved from the specimen rather than the surgeon's description or analysis of node stations. This definition is obviously open to question. The overall survival results are shown in **Table 6.6**.

Multivariate analysis revealed that D2 lymphadenectomy was an independent positive factor for survival. More detailed analysis showed that this only applied for those patients who were N0 or N1 and not N2 – this also explains why a significant survival benefit was only detected for stages II and IIIa. Interestingly

	D1 Group Standard node dissection (n = 558)	D2 Group Extended node dissection (n = 1096)
Morbidity and mortality		
30-day mortality	5.2%	5.0%
Anastomotic leak	8.2%	8.0%
Serious sepsis	3.2%	4.7%
Cardiopulmonary complications	9.5%	9.3%
5-year survival		
Stage Ia	86%	86%
Stage Ib	72%	69%
Stage II	27%	55%*
Stage IIIa	25%	38%**
Stage IIIb	25%	17%

All results statistically insignificant except: *p < 0.001
**p < 0.03

Table 6.6. *Results of the German Gastric Cancer Study (Siewert et al. 1993[63])*

the Japanese have produced very similar results from the same type of analysis.[47] Ten-year results have shown a statistically significant independent effect of D2 resection for the subgroups of Stage II disease only. This effect appeared to be independent of the stage migration factor.[63]

There was no significant difference in mortality and morbidity between the two types of resection, though the results were not as good as those from Japan. As previously discussed this is at least partly due to the greater age and higher incidence of concomitant disease in European patients.

Cape Town D1 versus D2 Study[64]

This was a small prospective randomised study comparing the results of 21 patients undergoing a D1 resection with 22 having a D2 resection for potentially curable gastric cancer. There was no survival difference between the groups at 3.1 years. There was a significantly higher incidence of complications, greater transfusion requirement and longer hospital stay in the D2 group.

Chinese University of Hong Kong D1 versus D3 Study[44]

A small prospective randomised trial of 55 patients undergoing either D1 subtotal or D3 total gastrectomy with distal pancreatectomy and splenectomy for resectable cancer in the distal half of the stomach. There was no survival advantage for those undergoing the more radical operation. As with the Cape Town study there was a significantly higher complication rate (particularly related to the splenic and pancreatic resection), greater transfusion requirement and longer hospital stay in the D3 group. It should be noted that the Japanese do not recommend routine resection of the spleen and pancreas for node stations 10 and 11 in distal cancers.

Both this and the Cape Town study involved too few patients to demonstrate a statistically significant difference in survival for more radical surgery. However, both confirmed the increased dangers of radical surgery.

The Dutch Gastric Cancer Trial[66]

A multicentre prospective randomised trial comparing D1 and D2 lymphadenectomy. It involved 33 surgical departments coordinated by Leiden University Hospital and recruited 380 patients in the D1 group and 331 in the D2 limb. Because most Dutch surgeons were not familiar with the D2 operation a Japanese surgeon from the National Cancer Center in Tokyo taught and supervised 8 coordinating surgeons who then continued the supervision of the other participating surgeons.

The main findings were:

	D1	D2	
Perioperative mortality (%)	4	10	p = 0.004
Significant complications (%)	25	43	p < 0.001
Median hospital stay (days)	18	25	p < 0.001
5-year survival (%)	45	47	p = NS

Pathological assessment of resected lymph nodes demonstrated the difficulty in adhering rigidly to the JRSGC Rules. Unfortunately 81% of patients who had undergone D2 resection had absence of node groups that should have been resected ('non-compliance') and in 48% of the D1 patients there were nodes present that should not have been resected ('contamination').[67] It is likely that these technical protocol violations have affected the survival results – it seems that the two randomised groups were eventually not greatly different. Importantly many of the participating surgeons contributed only relatively small numbers of patients at a time when they were still in their 'learning curve' for the D2 operation. This factor may have affected the completeness of the nodal resection and is also likely to have contributed to the increased mortality and morbidity of the more radical operation. This has been refuted by the coordinating surgeons, but nevertheless must be taken into account and is still being debated.

What is accepted is that the improvements in survival with D2 resection detected in the subgroups Stages II and IIIa are largely attributable to stage migration. It is also recognised that the increased mortality and morbidity of the D2 resections was largely due to the 3-fold increase in splenectomy and 10-fold increase in distal pancreatectomy in this group compared to the D1 group. Analysis of risk factors showed that splenectomy was an important risk factor for overall complications, while pancreatectomy and type of gastrectomy were the only factors significantly influencing the occurrence of major surgical complications.[68]

MRC Gastric Cancer Surgical Trial (STO1)[69]

A prospective randomised multicentre study comparing D1 and D2 lymphadenectomy and with 200 patients in each limb. Uniformity of surgical technique was ensured by the use of standardised descriptions and videos and by monitoring the surgeons' reports. This quality control was not nearly as rigorous as that employed in the Dutch trial. It should be noted that the definition of a

D1 resection was not that of the JRSGC, but that of the unified TNM staging system (for pathological staging) and so this does confound the aims of the trial to some degree.

The mortality and incidence of adverse events are remarkably similar to the Dutch trial and also largely related to resection of the spleen and pancreas. It was also accepted that many of the surgeons were in their 'learning curve' for the D2 operation. Patients who had both pancreas and spleen resected had a significantly poorer survival than those who had neither organ resected (though in some cases this reflected a more advanced proximal cancer rather than adherence to the trial protocol requiring resection of the tail of pancreas and spleen for middle and proximal third cancers). The hazard ratio for those having only their spleen removed fell just below the significance level.[70] In a subgroup analysis patients undergoing a D2 lymphadenectomy without resection of their spleen or distal pancreas had the best long-term survival, though these were mainly patients with distal cancers.

	D1	D2	
Perioperative mortality (%)	6.5	13	p = 0.04
Overall morbidity (%)	28	46	p < 0.001
Median (range) hospital stay (days)	14 (6–101)	14 (10–147)	p = NS
5-year survival (%)	35	33	p = NS

Summary

1. At present there is no evidence from randomised trials that D2 resection confers a survival benefit over D1 resection. None of these trials are from Japan and a major criticism is the lack of experience of the participating surgeons in the D2 technique and subsequently the high rates of serious complications, mortality and trial protocol violations. Most participating surgeons only performed small numbers of cases and it is now recognised that there is a significant learning curve for radical gastric cancer surgery.[71] Two of the studies were too small to demonstrate a statistical difference in survival. There has been much criticism of the two larger trials, but both have conclusively failed to show a benefit for the *routine* use of D2 resections. Both have shown the detrimental effects on postoperative complications and long-term survival of resecting the distal pancreas and spleen as part of a D2 operation. This has also been recognised in Japan where there has been a change in practice away from pancreatic and splenic resection in recent years (*vide infra*).

2. Results of large non-randomised studies from Japan and other countries, including Germany, support a significant survival benefit for D2 resection. Analysis of results suggests that the benefit is largely confined to those with N0 and N1 disease. A small subgroup with N2 disease should also theoretically benefit. The increase in 5-year survival is most obvious for Stages II and IIIa.

3. Comparison of results for the TNM stages does not allow for the 'stage migration phenomenon' related to more extensive nodal resection. The relative contributions of the surgical effort and correct pathological staging have been tested in hypothetical models and suggest that perhaps half the apparent improvement is related to correct staging/stage migration.

4. It is believed that resection of second tier nodes should decrease the incidence of local recurrence in the gastric bed in node-positive patients. This benefit is more likely to be apparent when the cancer has not penetrated the serosal layer. Series from Japan and the West show that a significant proportion of patients with N2 disease survive for more than 5 years after a D2 resection – it is unlikely that they would survive as long after a lesser lymphadenectomy.

5. The mortality and morbidity of D2 resection is higher than D1 resection. In all countries this is particularly related to removal of the spleen and distal pancreas. In the West there are the additional factors of the age and general health of gastric cancer patients.

Conclusions

Gastrectomy with D2 lymphadenectomy should not be used *routinely* in the surgical treatment of gastric cancer in Western patients.

Gastrectomy with D2 lymphadenectomy should presently only be performed by surgeons with proven experience of this type of radical surgery.

The added risks of D2 lymphadenectomy over a lesser nodal dissection are minimal for cancers in the distal half of the stomach and in the absence of any evidence of distant spread (including evidence of third tier nodal involvement) this is the operation of choice. This is supported by a large number of non-randomised studies from Japanese and Western specialist centres and from subgroup analysis of the randomised MRC trial.

The situation for cancers in the proximal half of the stomach is more complicated. There is some evidence to support the use of a D2 or modified D2 lymphadenectomy in Stages II and IIIa, but probably only in those with no or minimal serosal involvement. Those who are serosa-positive or have N2 nodal involvement will require adjuvant (or preferably neo-adjuvant) chemotherapy and nodal resections that are modified to minimise morbidity and mortality.[15]

The role of radical surgery in Stages IIIb and IV disease has yet to be defined. It may achieve a decrease in local recurrence in the gastric bed and thus a prolonged symptom-free interval, but almost certainly does not significantly improve the chance of cure.

The place of D2 resection in patients with Stage I disease is not proven, but given the higher incidence of node-positive early cases in the West, rational use in younger and fitter patients is recommended at present.[3,72] The continued use of radical surgery in apparently node-negative cases is also supported by recent research and clinical studies.[59]

The future trend will be towards radical node resections that are tailored to the pre-operative and operative staging of each case.[73] Improvements in staging techniques should allow a more rational approach to specific node station resections based on the likelihood of involvement and the potential benefit of en bloc removal of each station and balanced against the age and general health of the patient. The place of splenic and pancreatic removal as part of a radical lymphadenectomy is now doubtful and is discussed at length in the next two sections.

Splenectomy

The addition of a splenectomy increases the rate of septic and thromboembolic complications after a gastrectomy.[68,74] It also affects the immunological response to certain bacteria and possibly to gastric cancer.[75] However, this is controversial and a recent study has found that splenectomy is not an independent variable for postoperative septic problems.[76] The evidence for a lasting adverse immunological effect in cancer patients is theoretical rather than proven. There are both univariate and multivariate analyses that suggest lack of survival benefit or even a negative prognostic effect in all stages of gastric cancer except possibly stage IV.[77,78] However, there are also studies that have not confirmed an independent effect on survival.[79] In view of these concerns there is an increasing trend to avoid splenectomy unless specifically indicated.

Indications for splenectomy

Direct invasion of spleen or tail of pancreas

If all macroscopic disease can be resected and the operation is potentially curative then en bloc splenectomy or pancreato-splenectomy is worthwhile. If the operation is obviously palliative then the likely benefit of splenectomy has to be weighed against the increased risk of morbidity and mortality.

Removal of splenic hilum (station 10) lymph nodes

There are two factors to consider:

1. *The likelihood of station 10 nodal metastases* There are several excellent Japanese papers documenting the incidence of splenic nodal metastases in advanced gastric cancer.[47,77,80] The summarised mean incidence for the different parts of the stomach are:

Distal third (A)	< 1%
Middle third (M)	10%
Upper third (C)	15–20%
Whole stomach	25%

   This analysis can be further refined for proximal cancers by taking into account whether the cancer involves the greater curve, in which case positive nodes are more likely.[47] The incidence of nodal involvement is also related to the depth of invasion and is significantly lower in T1 and T2 cancers. The incidence of positive nodes in proximal third cancers may be higher in Western patients due to there being a greater proportion of more advanced cancers – in the MRC trial 25% of cases with C or CM cancers had positive station 10 nodes.[70]

2. *The likely survival benefit of removing all station 10 nodes* Even if the splenic nodes are removed the survival of patients with distal cancers and positive station 10 nodes is minimal. In proximal cancers with positive nodes the 5-year survival is up to 25% in the National Cancer Center in Tokyo.[47]

It is simple to calculate that if the spleen was removed in all Western patients with proximal third cancer then the survival benefit, without sub-group analysis, is only 6% even if Japanese results can be reproduced.

The indications for splenectomy to allow complete removal of station 10 lymph nodes have been tightened in recent years. This should only be considered for cancers in the upper stomach and possibly even then restricted to cancers involving the greater curve and fundus of the stomach. There is a need to test this recommendation in a randomised trial.[70] In view of the suspected adverse immunological effects of splenectomy in the earlier stages of gastric cancer there is now a good case for not removing the splenic hilar nodes in T1 or T2 cancers. Further evidence is required.

 The spleen should not be removed for cancers confined to the distal half of the stomach.

Clearance of station 10 nodes with splenic preservation

This was previously thought not to be feasible. The Japanese have reported a technique of dissecting out the splenic hilar nodes and have confirmed removal of all lymphatic tissue.[81] This procedure is still controversial in Japan and there are doubts that the technique can be consistently performed in Western patients. At present splenic hilar dissection should only be attempted by specialists with training in the technique, until of proven value in Western patients.

Distal pancreatectomy

En bloc pancreatic resection is associated with a significant increase in morbidity and mortality when compared with gastrectomy with or without splenectomy. This has been consistently demonstrated in studies of radical gastric surgery in the West. Complications include pancreatic leakage, abscess formation, fistula and acute pancreatitis. A few patients will become diabetic after distal pancreatectomy. The complications of the associated splenectomy have to be added to those of the pancreatic resection.

Indications for distal pancreatectomy

In view of the high complication rate the indications for resection of the left side of the pancreas have to be carefully analysed.

Direct invasion of tail of pancreas

As previously discussed this should only be contemplated if all macroscopic disease can be removed.

Removal of splenic artery (station 11) lymph nodes

There are two factors to consider:

1. *The likelihood of station 11 nodal metastases* About 10% of patients with proximal cancers have positive splenic artery nodes. As with station 10 nodes the highest incidence is seen with greater curve and advanced cancers. In some patients only the nodes closest to the coeliac trunk are involved, this being due to retrograde lymphatic spread rather than antegrade spread along the normal lymphatic pathway. This type of involvement is seen in advanced

cancers affecting any part of the stomach. In such cases resection of the nodes around the origin of the artery may reduce local gastric bed recurrence and increase the disease-free interval, but there is no evidence that it will improve the chance of cure.

2. *The likely survival benefit of removing all station 11 nodes* The 5-year survival of patients undergoing resection of positive splenic artery nodes is reported to be 15–20% in Japan.[47]

The decision to resect station 10 and 11 nodes, necessitating distal pancreatectomy and splenectomy, has to be made with the realisation that in Western gastric cancer practice the cost:benefit ratio is at best only marginal. The benefit for proximal third cancers can be calculated to be only about 2% if all patients had a distal pancreatectomy – less than the increased risk of mortality. The Japanese have now confirmed that there is no survival benefit even for localised proximal third cancers.[82] This procedure is not indicated for cancers in the distal half of the stomach, though nodes along the proximal part of the splenic artery (11p nodes) are excised as part of a radical D2 excision of the coeliac trunk nodes.[82] En bloc pancreatic excision should now only be considered in the younger and fitter patient with an advanced proximal cancer where a lesser procedure is anticipated to leave residual cancer.

There is no place for *routine* resection of the distal pancreas in gastric cancer surgery.

Pancreas-preserving gastrectomy

This has been described in Japan for excision of station 11 nodes in patients with proximal cancers.[84] It requires splenectomy as the splenic artery and accompanying nodes are dissected off the pancreas and the artery ligated just distal to the branching of the dorsal pancreatic artery. Lymphangiographic studies show that the splenic artery lymphatics lie within the subserosal space on the upper and posterior aspect of the pancreas and never within the parenchyma. The arterial supply to the distal pancreas is adequate after ligation of the distal splenic artery. Preservation of the pancreas significantly reduces the incidence of postoperative complications. There is increasing experience with this technique in Japan. It is contraindicated if there is direct invasion of the pancreas. There is concern that this type of dissection is difficult to consistently perform in Western patients. At present only those with specialist training should attempt this procedure.

Extended resections

The concept of gastric cancer remaining a locoregional disease with relatively late distant spread has already been discussed. It is possible that in some patients with locally advanced disease it is still possible to produce prolonged survival and perhaps cure by radical surgery, though such cases have to be carefully selected.[85] Extended resection is defined as any dissection beyond a D2 subtotal or total gastrectomy. It is advocated by the Japanese for resectable advanced cancers with no evidence of distant spread.

There are two categories of extended resection to consider.

En bloc resection of involved adjacent organs

Spread into adjacent organs can occur in two different ways:

1. *Intramural spread* either by direct growth or via lymphatics into the oesophagus or duodenum. Extending the resection margin either proximally or distally is certainly worthwhile as cure is still possible.
2. *Transmural spread* into adjacent organs e.g. pancreas, spleen, left lobe of liver and transverse mesocolon. Pathological assessment in cases of apparent invasion show that in about one-third the adherence to another organ is inflammatory rather than neoplastic. Trial dissection and intraoperative biopsy must not be attempted as there is a risk of disseminating malignant cells. Resection of the adjacent organ is thus recommended provided the patient is fit enough to undergo the extended procedure. If the patient is unfit or too elderly for a radical excision then gastrectomy is still worthwhile as about a third will still have a clear lateral resection margin.

The results of surgical series of extended resections must be interpreted with care. Transmural spread has a much worse prognosis than intramural spread and series may include different proportions of each.[86] It is also important to determine whether the paper includes only patients with pathological confirmation of transmural invasion or all patients with adherence to adjacent organs. It is not entirely surprising that late analysis of the results of extended resection has produced conflicting results. Overall it appears that there is a small survival advantage, but this is only realised if operative mortality is minimised in what are usually very major operations.[87] The 5YSR for resections where two adjacent organs are invaded is only 4% and thus lower than the increased mortality risk. The risks in older patients and those with concomitant diseases must be carefully weighed up against the potential survival benefit.[88] Extended resection should only be considered when there will be no evidence of macroscopic residual disease (R0 – no residual disease; R1 – microscopic residual disease; R2 – macroscopic residual disease) after the resection. It must be remembered that these more advanced gastric cancers are almost inevitably node-positive and the minimum level of node dissection in an extended resection should be a D2 lymphadenectomy.[62]

Extended lymphadenectomy

Removal of node stations 13–16 has only been reported to be of benefit in Japan.[52] Resection of third and fourth tier para-aortic nodes does potentially decrease the risk of gastric bed recurrence and prolong the symptom-free interval. It is uncertain whether this potential benefit is worthwhile in Western patients because of the increased risks of radical resection. It is unlikely that D3 or D4 resections are of any benefit except perhaps in younger patients with T4 disease. Such patients are more likely to benefit from adjuvant therapy and so at present the place of extended lymphadenectomy remains uncertain. At the time of writing there is a multicentre randomised trial in Japan comparing D2 and D4 lymphadenectomy for advanced cancer.

Super-extended radical gastrectomy

Appleby's operation

The concept of 'en bloc' resection of gastric cancer is taken a step further with Appleby's operation. This involves total gastrectomy with splenectomy and distal pancreatectomy together with resection of the coeliac trunk and common hepatic artery to the point where it branches into the hepatic and gastroduodenal arteries. Blood supply to the liver is from the superior mesenteric artery via the pancreatico–duodenal arcade. Even in the most experienced hands there is a mortality of 7.2% and it is now rarely performed, even in Japan.[89]

Left upper quadrant evisceration

Addition of a transverse colectomy to a standard D2 resection is known as a left upper quadrant evisceration (LUAE). It has been advocated for advanced cancers in the proximal stomach and in cancers with invasion of adjacent organs in an attempt to minimise the risk of local recurrence and improve survival.[90]

There are limited indications for extended surgery in Western patients. The differentiation between curative and palliative surgery for locally advanced cancers is often blurred. It is likely that extended resections do improve symptom-free survival in some patients even if cure is not achieved.[91] However this surgery has to be performed with low mortality and morbidity to produce a positive cost:benefit ratio.

Limited gastric resections

In the elderly or unfit patient it is reasonable to consider a less radical gastric resection, accepting that while the chance of cure may be reduced there is a lower mortality and serious morbidity rate and a lower incidence of nutritional sequelae.

In Japan the concept of a reduced or limited resection with curative intent is much more important because of the high incidence of screened early gastric cancers (EGC). Early cancers have a much lower rate of nodal metastasis and resection without lymphadenectomy may be a 'relative curative' procedure. In Japan the incidence of positive nodes is 3–5% for cancers confined to the mucosa, but rises to 16–25% for cancers invading the submucosa.[90] The rates are lower for smaller lesions and if there is no mucosal ulceration.[92] However the superficial spreading type of EGC has a positive node rate of over 30% and there may be remote nodes. This is becoming more important in the West as the rate of EGC detection is now over 20% in many studies, though over half are type IIc or III (see Chapter 1) that may not be suitable for limited surgery.

In Japan only 1.1% of mucosal cancers and 5.4% of submucosal cancers have positive N2 nodes and the 5YSR rates are 90% and 78% respectively for T1mN2 and T1smN2.[47] It could be argued that the benefit of a D2 resection is minimal for mucosal cancers and marginal for submucosal cancers and it has been proposed that a limited D1 resection is as effective. While this is a rational argument for mucosal cancers it does rely on the accurate endoscopic identification of suitable lesions. The improved survival of 4% for submucosal cancer with a D2 resection means that mortality of the procedure has to be considerably less than 4% and so should be restricted to fitter and younger patients and avoiding pancreatic and splenic resection. Higher rates of N2 involvement have been reported in some Western studies.[72] In addition there is evidence from studies of nodal micrometastases that the rate of node involvement is higher than estimated by standard histology and it is these under-staged patients who die of recurrence – this changes the cost:benefit analysis.[93]

 This issue remains contentious, but at present limited gastric and nodal resections are not routinely recommended in the West.[94]

The accurate identification of mucosal lesions is now possible with endoscopic ultrasound and so a sub-group of patients can be selected for limited resection who may be cured. Those patients with small non-ulcerated lesions confined to the mucosa and who would be considered to be at higher risk from surgery can be considered for limited resection even in Western practice.[95]

A detailed description of the many different operations described for limited resection of early cancers is not necessary, but they can be simply classified under the following headings:

Endoscopic resection

This is only used for mucosal cancers that can either be destroyed by laser or resected via the endoscope. The latter technique has the advantage that resection margins can be assessed. Laser treatment is easier and quicker and is recommended for the elderly and particularly those with multifocal disease (5–15%) who may need repeated treatments. Careful endoscopic monitoring is mandatory after this type of treatment and it remains controversial. It is stated that all mucosal lesions of <10 mm diameter and all type I protruding early cancers of <20 mm diameter may be safely resected endoscopically.[96] While the mortality of such procedures is extremely low, even in the elderly and unfit, it has been emphasised that the long-term results are not yet known and have yet to be compared with radical surgery in younger patients.

Gastric resection

This includes wedge excision and partial gastrectomy with or without nodal dissection. Various pylorus-preserving procedures have been described for middle third and proximal cancers.[97] Recently there have been a considerable number of reports of laparoscopic-assisted limited resections.[98,99] These operations still require an abdominal incision and advocates of minimal incision surgery argue that open limited surgery can be achieved more rapidly and safely and at a lower cost.

There is no doubt that quality of life is better after limited gastric resections and particularly in terms of post-prandial symptoms and nutritional sequelae. It is important to remember the cost:benefit ratio for elderly patients is very different from that of a younger patient – at NCCH in Tokyo the 5YSR rate in those over 80 with EGC was only 53.8% with most dying of other diseases rather than recurrent cancer.[100] In addition the time course for the progression of early gastric cancer is long even when untreated and if recurrence occurs after surgery this may be many years later and usually as distant metastases.[101] Comparative studies with radical surgery are in progress in some centres in Japan. A recent survey showed that the majority of cancer centres in Japan now use some form of limited resection for older and less fit patients. Use of these procedures in the West may be limited by the lower incidence of early gastric cancer and the higher incidence of nodal spread in such cases. The increasing use of endoscopic ultrasound may open up this treatment option for older Western patients with both early and advanced cancers.

Technique of gastric resection with D2 lymphadenectomy

The aim of this section is not to provide a detailed operative manual, but to summarise the basic steps of the main procedures. More detailed descriptions that can be recommended are those by McCulloch[102] and Craven.[103] Both are strongly influenced by the work of Keiichi Maruyama from the National Cancer Center in Tokyo.

Incision

Gastric cancers below the cardia can be resected via an upper midline incision. In obese or heavily built patients it is usually necessary to extend the incision below the umbilicus to gain adequate exposure and room to operate. Some surgeons use a left thoraco-abdominal approach for radical excision of the upper stomach, but there is an increased morbidity and mortality associated with disrupting the left costal margin and diaphragm and entering the left chest. This type of approach should be reserved for cancers in the cardia where it is necessary to resect more than 5 cm of the lower oesophagus to obtain adequate proximal clearance. Increasingly those with specialist experience are using the abdominal transhiatal approach.[39] This involves excision of the crura and oesophagophrenic ligament en bloc with the cardia. In addition, the diaphragm is divided anterior to the hiatal opening thus allowing a wide exposure of the lower mediastinum. With appropriate retraction it is possible to resect 6–8 cm of lower oesophagus together with associated lymphatic tissue. The bilateral subcostal or 'rooftop' incision also provides excellent exposure of the upper stomach and hiatus.

Intraoperative staging

This has been discussed in detail in Chapter 3. Meticulous staging is essential in deciding the appropriate type of resection and lymphadenectomy. Evidence of serosal invasion, invasion of an adjacent organ, peritoneal seedlings, apparent nodal involvement beyond the second tier and liver metastases must be sought. If any of these are found then radical surgery alone may not cure the patient and a decision has to be made about whether to proceed with the planned dissection, modify the operation with a view to adjuvant therapy or to opt for a lesser palliative procedure. Some additional intraoperative investigations may be helpful in making this decision:

Peritoneal cytology

This is widely used in Japan. The finding of free malignant cells in the absence of macroscopic peritoneal seedlings is now an indication for the additional use of intra and postoperative intraperitoneal chemotherapy in Japan. This treatment modality is now being investigated in the West where, in view of the higher incidence of T3 and T4 cancers, it is likely to become more widely used. Washings are taken from the pelvis before any dissection is started (or preferably at staging laparoscopy). Cells are not detected pre- or intraoperatively when the serosa is intact. More than a third of patients with macroscopic evidence of serosal penetration will have malignant cells detectable in their peritoneal washings.[104] Survival is significantly shorter in the positive cases and this finding is an indication for the use of adjuvant early postoperative intraperitoneal chemotherapy.

Frozen-section histology of lymph nodes

It must be stressed that if a D2 resection is being contemplated then no node in the first or second tier should be sampled as all lymphatic tissue must be taken en bloc. If there are nodes in the third or fourth tiers that appear involved these should be sampled as this level of spread is now regarded as distant metastasis and may be a contraindication to D2 resection.

The trend towards splenic and pancreatic preservation has led to the dilemma of deciding whether to sample enlarged nodes at stations 10 and 11 – in the younger fitter patient it is probably best to proceed with an en bloc radical resection rather than disrupt the lymphatic pathways. In the older or less fit patient the additional risks of splenectomy and distal pancreatectomy make node sampling worthwhile if these organs do not need to be resected as part of the lymphadenectomy.

Frozen-section histology of other tissue

As previously stated apparent direct invasion from the stomach into another organ should not be sampled for fear of disseminating cancer cells. In some diffuse cancers there may be concern about the proximal or distal resection margin and histological assessment may be helpful. In elderly or unfit patients undergoing potentially curative limited resections of the stomach, sampling of the resection margin may be necessary. Any lesions or seedlings found at distant sites in the peritoneal cavity should be sent for histology.

Liver biopsy

Any lesions palpated in the liver or detected with intraoperative ultrasound should be sampled before progressing to a radical operation.

Operative strategy after staging

Three types of resection are considered:

1. Subtotal D2 gastrectomy
2. Total D1/D2 gastrectomy without splenectomy and distal pancreatectomy
3. Total D2 gastrectomy with splenectomy and distal pancreatectomy.

Variations on these procedures and extended or limited versions may all be indicated in certain circumstances. These three operations fulfil the requirements for radical treatment of gastric cancer in the majority of patients and are the basic armaments of the specialist gastric cancer surgeon. The initial part of the dissection is common to all three procedures.

Initial dissection

1. Mobilise hepatic flexure of colon and fully Kocherise the duodenum and head of pancreas. This allows examination of retropancreatic and para-aortic nodes.
2. Mobilise splenic flexure of colon and carefully divide any adhesions between omentum and spleen so that the capsule is not torn during the dissection.
3. Separate the greater omentum from the transverse colon along a bloodless line about 1 cm from the bowel. This plane of dissection is continued onto the anterior leaf of the transverse mesocolon. This leaf can be completely separated from the posterior leaf so that the lesser sac remains intact. This is not always an easy dissection in Western patients and requires some patience. It is especially important for cancers that breach the serosa of the posterior wall of the stomach. The line of dissection continues between the peritoneum over the pancreas and the gland itself and care must be taken not to damage the parenchyma.
4. At the right side this line of dissection leads onto the right gastroepiploic vessels and subpyloric nodes. These nodes are swept up on the vessels which are bared and ligated at their origins.
5. The lesser omentum is divided along the line of the reflection on the liver capsule. There is usually an accessory left hepatic artery in the omentum and this should be ligated close to the liver. The line of dissection is continued upwards proximally over the oesophagogastric junction to include the oesophagophrenic ligament and, in cancers of the cardia, part of the diaphragm. Distally the line of dissection passes down the peritoneum over the hepatoduodenal ligament to the upper border of the duodenum.
6. At this stage the surgeon should perform the optional dissection of the lymphatic tissue in the hepato-duodenal ligament (station 12) nodes. This is only done for cancers in the lower half of the stomach and particularly if there is evidence of involvement of the suprapyloric or common hepatic nodes. The dissection starts at the reflection of the peritoneum in the porta hepatis and includes the peritoneum and all lymphatic tissue from both front and back of the bile ducts, common and right and left hepatic arteries and the portal vein down to the neck of the pancreas. The gallbladder may be removed as part of this dissection.
7. Whether or not the hepato-duodenal ligament has been dissected out, the line of dissection brings the surgeon down onto the common hepatic artery and the origin of the often insubstantial right gastric artery. This is ligated at its origin taking care not to damage or occlude the hepatic artery.
8. The first part of the duodenum is now freed from the head of the pancreas. There are several small vessels running between the gastroduodenal and superior pancreato-duodenal arteries and the duodenal wall. It is important

to ligate these individually and not use diathermy in this area as both the pancreas and duodenum can suffer damage leading to leakage. The duodenum should be divided at least 2 cm distal to the pylorus – a wider margin is needed for cancers in the distal stomach. The duodenal stump should be as short as possible and whether closed by suture or staples it is a wise step to invert the closure line with interrupted seromuscular sutures.

9. Lifting the distal stomach up and to the left, the dissection of the lymphatics and peritoneum on the posterior wall of the lesser sac is continued to the left. This includes the tissue on the upper border of the body of the pancreas, along the common hepatic artery and to the left of the portal vein. Troublesome bleeding is often encountered near the pancreas and the left gastric vein sometimes passes down behind the upper border of the pancreas to the splenic vein. Great care is needed in this area and again vessels should be ligated or transfixed rather than diathermised close to pancreatic parenchyma. The retroperitoneal nodes to the left of the portal vein tend to bleed quite profusely and dissection of these nodes should only be contemplated for upper third cancers – in other cases the peritoneal dissection is continued up onto the posterior aspect of the proximal lesser curve thus exposing the right crus of the diaphragm. Inferiorly the dissection reaches the junction of common hepatic and splenic arteries on the upper border of the pancreas.

10. The lymphatic tissue around the origin of the splenic artery is divided and swept up towards the left gastric artery if the operation is for a distal cancer or if the spleen and pancreas are not to be removed. The nodal tissue around the coeliac trunk is carefully dissected off the artery trying to avoid entering the tough neural and fibrous tissue around the origin of the trunk on the anterior aorta. All this tissue is swept upwards with the lymphatic tissue on the left gastric artery. The left gastric artery is then ligated at its origin leaving the distal coeliac trunk and the origins of the common hepatic and splenic arteries bared completely. The left gastric vein is variable and there may be more than one – it is ligated as found.

At this point the operation strategy depends on the extent of the planned resection.

Subtotal gastrectomy

All the tissue on the proximal lesser curve from the oesophago-gastric junction downwards should be removed with the left gastric pedicle. This starts with ligation of the ascending branch of the artery and vein at the hiatus. Small vessels passing to the stomach wall are individually ligated. If involved nodes are detected in this tissue it is preferable to do a total gastrectomy. There is debate about the left cardial nodes, but the author's view is that when the patient with a distal cancer has involvement of this node group the resection has no chance of being curative. The effort needed and the small chance of damaging the proximal short gastric vessels during the dissection make it not worthwhile.

The final part of the dissection involves separating the left side of the greater omentum from the splenic flexure of the colon and following the line of resection up to the lower pole of the spleen. The dissection of the anterior leaf of the mesocolon is completed between the middle colic vessels and the splenic flexure.

This continues over the distal pancreas up towards the hilum of the spleen. At this point the left gastroepiploic vessels are identified with the artery being the first branch of the splenic artery visible at the hilum. The inferior two or three short gastric arteries are also ligated nearer to the stomach to allow full mobilisation of the greater curve. The blood supply of the stomach remnant is entirely from the proximal short gastric arteries (**Fig. 6.2**).

Total gastrectomy without splenectomy and distal pancreatectomy

The resection is the same thus far. The ligation of the short gastric arteries should be as close to the hilum as is safe. In order to achieve this it is best to divide the peritoneum (lienorenal ligament) lateral to the spleen and mobilise the spleen and tail of pancreas. If there appear to be involved nodes in the hilum, the splenic artery and vein should be dissected off the tail of the pancreas, transfixed and divided so removing the spleen with the stomach.

The nodal dissection is continued up the front of the aorta from the coeliac trunk up into the hiatus, the assistant lifting the stomach up to allow a good view of this area. Two significant vessels are encountered in removing this tissue en bloc with the stomach. The first is the posterior gastric or short gastric artery that passes to the posterior proximal stomach from the splenic artery. The other is the left phrenic artery that should be divided near the upper border of the left adrenal gland to allow the left cardial nodal tissue to be dissected completely off the left crus. The left subphrenic branch of this vessel is divided as it reaches the diaphragm so freeing the lymphatic tissue on the left aspect of the oesophago-gastric junction. It is often not appreciated that the cardia is retroperitoneal in this area and the resection must include all the tissue in the triangle between the upper border of the tail of the pancreas, the left crus and the upper pole of the spleen. Both vagi and the other small vessels around the lower oesophagus are divided so that only the oesophagus attaches the stomach. The length of oesophagus mobilised depends on the resection margin required. The transhiatal approach for cardia cancers has already been described (**Fig. 6.2**).

Total gastrectomy with splenectomy and distal pancreatectomy

Resection of the spleen and pancreas via an abdominal incision is not technically easy because of limited space. One commonly used manoeuvre is to divide the peritoneum laterally and mobilise the spleen and distal pancreas to the right. The alternative is to mobilise the pancreas where the splenic artery joins it and to divide the pancreas, artery and vein at this point. The dissection is then continued to the left posterior to the pancreas until the lienorenal ligament is divided so freeing the spleen. The dissection is then continued up in the retroperitoneum above the tail of the pancreas as described. When the decision has been made to do a complete D2 resection for a proximal cancer the author finds this latter manoeuvre easier and less bloody than mobilisation of the spleen and pancreas to the right with the limited exposure provided by an abdominal approach. An essential step in the distal pancreatectomy is ligation of the pancreatic duct.

This completes the description of a D2 resection. The next section describes the principles and techniques of reconstruction.

Figure 6.2
*(a) D2 Subtotal
gastrectomy; (b) D2
total gastrectomy
with preservation of
spleen and pancreas.*

D2 subtotal gastrectomy

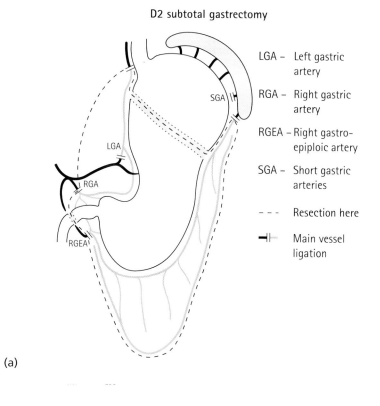

LGA – Left gastric
           artery

RGA – Right gastric
           artery

RGEA – Right gastro-
            epiploic artery

SGA – Short gastric
           arteries

– – –   Resection here

⊣⊢   Main vessel
         ligation

(a)

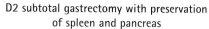

D2 subtotal gastrectomy with preservation
of spleen and pancreas

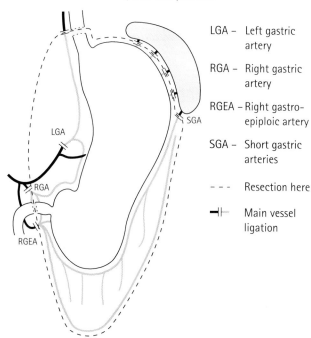

LGA – Left gastric
           artery

RGA – Right gastric
           artery

RGEA – Right gastro-
            epiploic artery

SGA – Short gastric
           arteries

– – –   Resection here

⊣⊢   Main vessel
         ligation

(b)

Reconstruction after gastric resection

The stomach is a complex organ that functions as a reservoir for ingested food and is involved in digestion and absorption. One of the most important functions is the ability to accommodate a meal without a marked rise in intraluminal pressure. However, the most important function is the release of food to the small intestine at a controlled rate that allows adequate mixing with bile and pancreatic juices and does not overwhelm the digestive and absorptive capacity of the small intestine. Control of the rate of delivery of the stomach contents to the small intestine requires an intact and innervated pylorus. Gastric emptying is regulated by a complex neurohumoral feedback from the small intestine. Any gastric resection interferes with all of these functions – the aim of the reconstruction is to minimise the disturbance to the upper gastrointestinal physiology.

The two main dangers for a patient undergoing a major gastric resection for cancer are recurrence of the cancer and significant malnutrition. There is a tendency to concentrate mainly on the former and to forget that weight loss and inadequate absorption of essential nutrients can severely affect quality of life after a gastrectomy.

In recognising that many patients will not be cured by radical surgery it is most important to maximise quality of life while the patient is free of symptomatic recurrence. This is achieved by appropriate reconstruction of the upper gastrointestinal tract and then close follow-up of nutritional status.

Aims of reconstruction

1. The construction of the least complex anastomosis to allow adequate nutritional intake.
2. The procedure should be safe and not add to the mortality and morbidity of the gastric resection.
3. The alteration in upper gastrointestinal physiology should be minimised.
4. It should not be prone to long-term complications such as bacterial overgrowth.
5. Reconstruction prevents the reflux of bile and alkaline duodenal juices into the oesophagus.
6. It will not obstruct at an early stage if there is gastric bed recurrence.

Reconstructions can be broadly divided into two groups:

Duodenal bypass

The duodenal stump is closed and the proximal jejunum used to provide continuity. This results in a less physiological mixing of food with bile and pancreatic enzymes and a significant alteration in neurohumoral feedback from the duodenum. This latter abnormality is not so important after excision of the antrum and pylorus and in any case is probably more important in theory than in reality. The best clinical results are obtained using the Roux-en-Y technique with a 40–60 cm limb of proximal jejunum. There are many variations on this technique, but the important thing is that all prevent the reflux of duodenal contents into the gastric remnant and oesophagus. The disadvantage of a Roux reconstruction is that this segment of proximal jejunum is important for optimum digestion and absorption, but food passing through it has not mixed with bile and pancreatic enzymes. Use of a long jejunal loop instead of a Roux limb 'wastes' even more proximal jejunum and, unless a very long loop is used, is associated with a high incidence of bile reflux problems.

Duodenal continuity

This is maintained by either joining the gastric remnant to the duodenal stump or interposing a segment of proximal jejunum between the oesophagus or gastric remnant and the duodenal stump. It allows a more physiological mixing of food with bile and enzymes, though this is by no means normal because of the rapid passage of unprepared food through the duodenum. The main disadvantages are an increased risk of symptomatic bile and alkaline reflux and a higher rate of postoperative complications, particularly with the more complex interposition procedures. This type of procedure is not advisable for locally advanced cancers that tend to recur in the gastric bed and may lead to early obstruction of the anastomoses or interposed jejunum. Cuschieri gives a very good account of these procedures which is recommended.[105]

Examples of the various reconstruction procedures for subtotal and total gastrectomy are shown in **Fig. 6.3**.

Jejunal pouch reconstruction

The most common symptom after total gastrectomy is early satiety. This restricts food intake and makes it difficult for patients to maintain an adequate calorie intake. Various operations have been devised to increase the reservoir capacity of the proximal jejunum. Initially such operations were used as remedial procedures in patients with severe restriction of intake or with disabling post-prandial symptoms, but they are now used routinely by some gastric cancer surgeons, either as modifications of the Roux limb or as formal jejunal pouches, supported by the results of randomised trials.[106,107] Despite the theoretical advantages of these operations there is no good evidence that they significantly improve nutrition.[107] Most quality of life studies have failed to show a significant or clinically important improvement with intestinal pouches.[108,109] Rigorous dietetic surveillance is probably of more value than the actual type of reconstruction in ensuring optimal nutrition after a gastrectomy.[110,111]

 Conflicting and in some cases inconclusive evidence from randomised trials means that no firm recommendation can be made for jejunal pouch construction after total gastrectomy.

Early postoperative complications

As with any abdominal surgical procedure complications can be divided into those of a general nature and those specifically associated with gastric resection and reconstruction. The general complications of major gastric surgery are covered in Chapter 4. The complication rate is higher after total gastrectomy and

Figure 6.3
Reconstruction after gastrectomy.

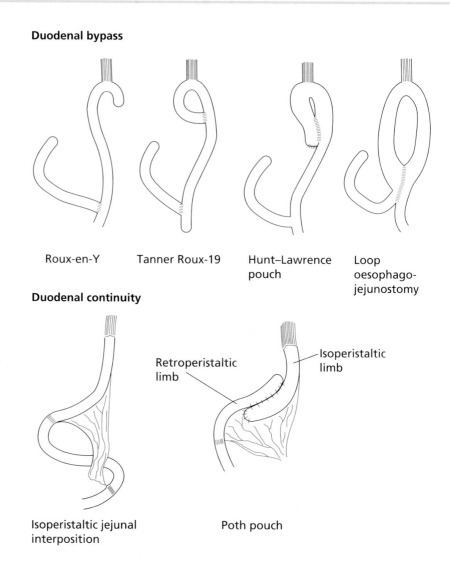

Duodenal bypass

Roux-en-Y   Tanner Roux-19   Hunt–Lawrence pouch   Loop oesophago-jejunostomy

Duodenal continuity

Retroperistaltic limb   Isoperistaltic limb

Isoperistaltic jejunal interposition   Poth pouch

particularly if the spleen and distal pancreas have been resected. A basic principle in radical gastric surgery is to recognise complications early and deal with them in a proactive way. This is especially important for intra-abdominal complications within the first few days of surgery. One of the important lessons to learn is to 'look and see' rather than 'wait and see'. A second-look laparotomy when the patient is still stable is considerably safer than waiting until the condition of the patient has deteriorated and sepsis has developed. An early operation may allow correction of the problem while a delay may make this impossible.

The following are the more common intra-abdominal complications specific to gastrectomy for cancer.

Haemorrhage

This may be either reactive, within the first few hours of surgery, or secondary, caused by partially or inadequately treated intra-abdominal sepsis. Early relaparotomy is advocated for definite or even suspected reactive haemorrhage. It must be remembered that drains can occlude with blood clot and the clinical suspicion of bleeding in a haemodynamically unstable patient is sufficient indication to operate. Even if the bleeding stops spontaneously the presence of blood clot in the gastric bed acts as a potential site for secondary infection and it is preferable to remove this.

Secondary haemorrhage is truly life threatening and the old adage that prevention is better than treatment could not be more true for this complication. Any intra-abdominal sepsis must be treated aggressively and in particular collections around the coeliac trunk as erosion of the main arteries in this area is extremely dangerous. If the radiological facilities are adequate then embolisation may be attempted. The author's experience is that in full-blown secondary haemorrhage there is little time to take definitive action and immediate laparotomy is a safer option. This is not to say that surgical control of secondary haemorrhage is easy, but temporary control may save the patient's life while preparation is made for definitive control. Haemorrhage from the coeliac trunk vessels may require cross-clamping of the aorta. Since the hiatus is filled by the reconstruction it is often safer to clamp the aorta above the diaphragm using a left thoracic or thoracoabdominal approach and so avoid damage, or further damage, to the anastomoses. This complication most commonly occurs about 2 or more weeks after the gastrectomy when postoperative adhesions are dense and maturing – in the heat of the moment significant damage can occur. Suture of the eroded vessels is often difficult in the presence of infection and a non-adsorbable monofilament material is recommended. It is most important that the infected area is adequately debrided and drained prior to closure.

Duodenal stump leak

This may be due to technical error, afferent limb obstruction or ischaemia of the duodenal margin. The role of drains in abdominal surgery is always debatable, but a silastic tube drain to the duodenal stump is strongly recommended. In early leaks the appearance of bile-stained fluid in the drain is an indication for re-exploration and it is frequently possible to correct the problem completely. Conservative management of early leaks produces a less predictable outcome and so intervention is far safer.

Delayed leaks can often be treated conservatively if the duodenal contents come out through the drain and the patient is not obviously septic. In this situation it may be safer to apply gentle suction to the drain for the first few days to ensure the leak remains localised and a fistulous tract is established. Parenteral nutrition is not necessary if the leak is controlled as it is preferable to give an enteral elemental-type diet and to suppress pancreatic secretion with a subcutaneous somatostatin-analogue infusion. Drainage should be continued for at least 14 days and the drain then gradually pulled back from the duodenum. Provided the tract has matured, the resistance in the tract will be greater than that in the duodenum and the fistula should close rapidly. If the fistual output is greater than 200 ml/24 hours without suction then drainage should be continued for longer, and contrast studies obtained to determine whether there is a technical problem with the reconstruction. In delayed leakage that does not appear in the drain the patient usually presents with a subhepatic abscess. In this situation percutaneous radiological drainage may be sufficient provided the patient's clinical condition responds to drainage. Drainage is continued until the fistula dries up and although this may take weeks it is worthwhile persevering. The patient can continue on enteral nutrition, with or without a subcutaneous somatostatin-analogue, and need not stay in hospital if otherwise well.

Any patient who remains septic and unwell despite drainage requires surgical exploration, debridement of the cavity and placement of a drain close to the point of leakage. If there is a major defect then a Foley-type catheter can be placed in the duodenum with a plan to form a controlled fistula. It is unwise to try and suture the duodenum if the presentation is delayed because of the poor tissue condition due to associated sepsis.

Anastomotic leak

This may occur because of technical error, ischaemia of the tissues or tension on the anastomotic line; in fact all these causes are 'technical errors'. If identified within the first 72 hours then reoperation is advised. At worst this will allow placement of a drain right up against the point of leakage and also the construction of a more distal feeding jejunostomy. At best the anastomosis can be repaired or patched before sepsis is established in the surrounding tissues. Early leakage in more complex reconstructions may be from any of several suture lines and, even more importantly, may be due to jejunal ischaemia. This must be dealt with before complete disruption occurs when the chance of survival diminishes rapidly.

The management of a delayed presentation anastomotic leak is more controversial. If the leak is contained and only identified on a contrast study prior to beginning enteral feeding then it is wise to keep the patient on a liquid diet and repeat the contrast study every 7 days to confirm resolution of the cavity. If the patient is septic, however, then a drain must be placed in the cavity. The dilemma is whether to do this radiologically and risk incomplete drainage or to explore the cavity surgically and risk a very difficult operation. Surgical exploration has the advantage that a feeding jejunostomy can be constructed and the septic area debrided, but the whole upper abdomen is often 'glued up' with new adhesions at this time – it is not an operation for the inexperienced surgeon. There is no doubt that with appropriate surgical action, modern antibiotics, expert radiological assistance and enteral feeding techniques anastomotic leakage is no longer a surgical disaster; it is still the most common surgical cause of death, however, and can be avoided by adhering to basic surgical principles.

Intra-abdominal sepsis

This may present at any time in the first 2 weeks after a gastrectomy. It may be caused by anastomotic or duodenal leakage, pancreatic necrosis due to pancreatic parenchymal damage during the resection or leakage from the pancreatic stump. Sepsis is statistically more common after splenectomy, although whether this is an immunological effect or simply reflects damage to or resection of the pancreas as part of the operation is unclear.

Computerised tomography with both intravenous and intraluminal contrast is important in defining the site and cause of the sepsis. The choice between radiological and surgical drainage has already been discussed. The dangers of incompletely drained sepsis with deterioration of the patient's condition and the risk of secondary haemorrhage makes adequate drainage essential.

It is not unreasonable to start with radiological drainage unless there is significant tissue necrosis identified on the scans. Percutaneous drainage may be only a temporising measure while the patient's condition is improved and the surgeon must always be prepared to abandon this method of drainage and opt for surgical debridement. It should also be remembered that sepsis after gastrectomy is usually in the gastric bed or high up under the left diaphragm and in both situations there are bowel loops between the abdominal wall and the cavity. Safe drainage of this type of abscess is often difficult and there is a serious risk of damage to the intervening structures. Surgical exploration and drainage through a left subcostal incision is often safer and avoids interfering with the reconstruction or having to dissect through adherent loops of jejunum and transverse colon. It also allows reasonable access to the pancreatic tail or stump.

Pancreatic fistula

Whenever the tail of the pancreas is resected it is advisable to place a drain in the vicinity. Minor pancreatic leaks are relatively common and can be controlled by the drain. Uncontrolled leakage usually presents as a left upper quadrant abscess. It may occur after damage to the tail of the pancreas during splenectomy or following distal pancreatectomy. There is often associated necrosis of the pancreatic and peripancreatic tissue. The principle of treatment is as outlined above – surgical drainage with debridement of necrotic tissue and placement of a silastic tube drain to the point of leakage is recommended. Since the proximal pancreatic duct is not obstructed this type of leak will close spontaneously. Subcutaneous infusion of a somatostatin–analogue is usually helpful in reducing the volume of the leaked juice more quickly.

Post-splenectomy infections

Left subphrenic abscess after splenectomy has already been discussed. There is increasing evidence that splenectomy predisposes the patient to an increased risk of bacterial infections in both the early postoperative period and for at least 2 years after surgery. Immediate prophylaxis with twice daily oral penicillin is now recommended for patients of all ages. The patient should also be immunised with vaccines against pneumococci, meningococcus and *Haemophilus influenzae*. If the splenectomy has been planned as part of a radical procedure these vaccines are most effective if administered preoperatively. The patient should have an annual influenza vaccine and an updated pneumococcal vaccine every 2 or 3 years.

Late sequelae and complications

The place of follow-up clinics after cancer surgery is a subject that generates considerable discussion and debate. In this section it should become apparent that methodical follow-up of patients who have had a gastrectomy for cancer is mandatory if they are to realise their maximum quality of life, even if survival is likely to be limited. Quality of life is a difficult concept to define. While there are several 'tools' for the measurement of quality of life after surgery, these are mainly useful in the research setting. Regular follow-up by the surgeon and other trained personnel is the best way of identifying and solving problems that affect the patient's physical and psychological wellbeing after major cancer surgery.

The main long-term problems and complications may be divided into three groups:

1. Side effects and post-prandial sequelae
2. Nutritional problems
3. Recurrence of cancer.

Side-effects and post-prandial sequelae

Early fullness

Loss of the reservoir function of the stomach results in a feeling of early satiety and upper abdominal pain in some patients. Although the proximal jejunum dilates after a gastrectomy it can never completely replace the gastric reservoir and all patients have to limit their meal size to some extent. Good dietary advice is important to ensure an adequate calorie intake in more frequent, smaller meals. The role of gastric pouches has already been discussed and they do apparently decrease the incidence of early satiety. Early dumping is a common cause of post-prandial fullness and requires appropriate dietary manipulation. A rarer cause of fullness in some patients who have had a Roux–en–Y reconstruction is a defect of normal peristalsis in the long limb. This produces hold-up in the propulsion of the meal and results in an unpleasant pain during eating and involuntary, or often voluntary, regurgitation of the meal.[113]

Early dumping syndrome

The rapid filling of the proximal small intestine with hypertonic food leads to rapid movement of fluid into the gut from the extracellular fluid compartment. It also triggers a complex neurohumoral response that in some patients produces a variety of unpleasant gastrointestinal and cardiovascular symptoms. The main importance of the dumping syndrome is that it leads to food avoidance whether because of fullness or other unpleasant symptoms. In severe cases the patient is incapacitated after eating or suffers profuse diarrhoea that prevents normal activities after meals. Quality of life may be very severely restricted and malnutrition can occur rapidly in these patients.

It is perhaps fortunate that patients who have had a total or subtotal gastrectomy have a small reservoir and are usually unable to eat a large hypertonic load. The syndrome is much more common and troublesome in those who have an intact stomach, with the pylorus destroyed or bypassed, or after a partial gastrectomy. Many gastrectomy patients have some dumping symptoms in the first few weeks after surgery, but in most these are relatively mild and improve considerably with simple dietary adjustments that the patients often discover for themselves. During early follow-up it is important to identify significant dumping symptoms. A careful history should be taken and in less clear cases the patient asked to keep a diary recording foods eaten and symptoms experienced. Any patient with post-prandial pain in the first few months after gastrectomy should be suspected of suffering from early dumping as this is much more likely than recurrent disease. It is not that unusual for post-prandial symptoms to be wrongly interpreted as being due to early recurrence and the author has seen patients started on morphine to help control their 'pain'.

Most patients can be treated quite simply by appropriate dietary adaptation. It is important to involve an experienced dietician in the management of patients with dumping.

Reactive hypoglycaemic attacks

This is often incorrectly termed 'late dumping'. In many patients this occurs without early dumping symptoms. Symptoms of hypoglycaemia, including in the most profound cases blackouts and grand mal fits, occur about 2 hours after the last meal. The patient often experiences a craving for sweet food early in the attack.

Dietary assessment is the first step and the patient is then advised to decrease the carbohydrate load in their main meals and to take small amounts of carbohydrate in-between main meals. Careful explanation of the problem is usually sufficient to reassure the patient they do not have a serious disorder. Those with frequent attacks should carry dextrose tablets to eat at the first sign of symptoms.

Diarrhoea

There are several possible causes for diarrhoea after a gastrectomy for cancer:

Truncal vagotomy

This is discussed in Chapter 13.

Early dumping

Diarrhoea not infrequently occurs towards the end or even after a dumping attack and is part of the symptom-complex. Unlike post-vagotomy diarrhoea the attack follows a large hypertonic load and has other associated symptoms.

Bacterial overgrowth

This is relatively common after gastrectomy when there are complex reconstructions or pouches producing a blind limb.[114] Overgrowth in the proximal small intestine may also occur after a Roux-en-Y reconstruction. It is the combination of the loss of gastric acid, which destroys pathogenic ingested bacteria, and the formation of 'blind loops' that allows overgrowth of both aerobic and anaerobic organisms that are usually only present in the large intestine. These faecal bacteria produce toxins that damage the brush border enzymes vital for digestion. They may also utilise important nutrients such as the B vitamins. Pathogenic anaerobes deconjugate and dehydroxylate bile acids that are essential for normal fat absorption in the proximal small intestine.

Faecal fat levels are markedly elevated and in the worst cases the patient has steatorrhoea and loses weight rapidly. The diagnosis can be confirmed by intubation of the proximal jejunum and aspiration of intestinal juice for culture. The best non-invasive test for the detection of overgrowth is the 14C-glycocholate breath test. Proven bacterial overgrowth that causes diarrhoea and malnutrition should be treated with oral antibiotics such as neomycin or metronidazole. Fresh unpasteurised yoghurt or *lactobacillus* preparations should be given with and after a course of antibiotics to inhibit recolonisation by pathogenic bacteria. Only in very resistant cases should further surgery be contemplated.

Steatorrhoea

This may be due to bacterial overgrowth or relative pancreatic insufficiency caused by poor mixing of duodenal contents with food in reconstructions where the duodenum is excluded. Patients with fat malabsorption complain of unpleasant flatus and large bowel colic and pass bulky greasy stools that float and are difficult to flush away. A carefully taken history will identify the problem. If bacterial overgrowth has been excluded or treated then persistent fat malabsorption may respond to pancreatic enzyme supplements taken before or preferably mixed with food.

Bile reflux

Reflux of bile and alkaline juices into the stomach remnant and oesophagus may cause epigastric discomfort, heartburn and vomiting or regurgitation of bile. In the worst cases patients may avoid eating for fear of exacerbating their symptoms. Persistent oesophageal reflux may produce stricturing. The diagnosis is usually made on clinical grounds. Objective evidence can be obtained with a 99m-technetium-HIDA scan.[115] Gastroscopy is important to confirm whether there is mucosal damage and to exclude any other cause for the symptoms.

Treatment is often unsatisfactory and prevention of the problem by a bile-diverting reconstruction in the first place is important. Unremitting symptoms are an indication for further surgery to divert the duodenal contents by changing the reconstruction or lengthening of the Roux limb.

Nutritional problems

These may be divided into general malnutrition, which is reflected by weight loss, and deficits of specific nutrients.

General malnutrition and weight loss

It is important to recognise that malabsorption is a rare cause of malnutrition after a subtotal or total gastrectomy, unless there is bacterial overgrowth.[115] With few exceptions patients who lose weight, or fail to regain their preoperative weight, do so because they fail to ingest sufficient calories. Early satiety and the dumping syndrome are the most common causes and correction of these symptoms is usually sufficient to correct malnutrition.

Patients undergoing a subtotal gastrectomy rarely experience serious problems with weight loss. It is a fallacy that patients who have undergone a total gastrectomy invariably lose weight, although most fail to completely regain their pre-illness weight.[108] Women, and particularly those over 70, do consistently seem to have difficulty maintaining their weight after total gastrectomy. While patients will take sufficient calories under close supervision in hospital, their intake usually decreases on first going home.[116] Nutrition then improves over the first 6 months after surgery, by which time more than half of the patients are taking their recommended calorie intake.[117] It is advised that all patients are kept under close dietary surveillance for at least 12 months after surgery.

Carbohydrate absorption is nearly complete even after total gastrectomy, but the pattern of absorption is abnormal. Protein absorption is decreased, as reflected by an increase in faecal nitrogen, but this is rarely clinically important. Fat malabsorption is the main cause of inadequate calorie absorption. On average post-gastrectomy patients absorb about 80% of ingested fat – easily enough to provide adequate calories provided intake is sufficient. Failure to absorb fat may be caused by bacterial overgrowth or relative pancreatic insufficiency due to poor mixing of food with bile and the duodenal juices.

Specific deficiencies

Vitamin B12

Gastric acid is necessary to release B12 from foodstuffs and, more importantly, gastric parietal cell intrinsic factor is essential for absorption of this vitamin in the terminal ileum. After total gastrectomy patients absorb virtually no vitamin B12 and body stores are gradually depleted, although this may take up to 24 months to become clinically apparent. All patients should receive 1 mg of hydroxycobalamin intramuscularly every 3 months for life.

Other B vitamins

Deficiency only becomes clinically important if there is intestinal bacterial overgrowth. Treatment of the underlying cause of overgrowth is the priority, but oral B complex supplements should be given during treatment and for several weeks afterwards.

Fat-soluble vitamins

Malabsorption is obviously similar to that of fat. Vitamin A deficiency is detectable but remains a subclinical problem even many years after surgery. There is no evidence of vitamin E or K deficiency. Vitamin D malabsorption is of much more importance and particularly in post-menopausal women and long-term survivors. Osteomalacia may develop at an early stage if there is significant fat malabsorption. In those with apparently normal absorption it is recommended that calcium and alkaline phosphatase levels are measured annually.

At 5 years a full assessment for metabolic bone disease should be undertaken in all patients. Post-menopausal women and all patients over 70 should take an oral calcium supplement twice a day for life after a total gastrectomy.

Iron

Absorption is surprisingly normal after total gastrectomy and even if the duodenum has been bypassed. It appears that the jejunum can adapt to absorb iron provided that there are sufficient naturally occurring chelating agents in the food. Iron absorption shows a gradual improvement after gastrectomy and, provided intake is adequate, is near normal 12 months after surgery. An oral iron supplement in combination with vitamin C is given once or twice a day for the first year, but only continued thereafter in those with a poor intake of iron-containing foodstuffs.

Recurrence of cancer

The detection and treatment of recurrent gastric cancer remains a complex issue affected by multiple factors. The mode of recurrence can often be predicted by the stage of the original disease.[118] Cancers that have not penetrated the serosa recur later and usually as liver or distant metastases, whereas those that have invaded through the serosa often recur earlier and within the gastric bed on the peritoneal surfaces.

While radiotherapy or chemotherapy may occasionally be indicated, the majority of patients with clinical recurrence will simply be treated symptomatically. Further surgery for obstructive symptoms is worthwhile, not least because some patients will be found to have another cause for obstruction that is treatable. Malignant obstruction may be relieved by a bypass procedure, but there are often multiple areas of intestinal involvement and the prognosis is generally very poor. The terminal care of patients with recurrent cancer is a subject in itself and does not fall within the scope of this chapter.

References

1. Heberer G, Teichman RK, Kramling H-J et al. Results of gastric resection for carcinoma of the stomach: The European experience. World J Surg 1988; 12:374–81.

2. Hallisey MT, Allum WH, Jewkes AJ et al. Early detection of gastric cancer. Br Med J 1990; 301:513–5.

3. Sue-Ling HM, Martin I, Griffiths J et al. Early gastric cancer; 46 patients treated in one surgical department. Gut 1992; 33:1318–22.

4. Hisamichi S. Screening for gastric cancer. World J Surg 1989; 13:31–7.

5. Maruyama K. Results of surgery correlated with staging. In: Cancer of the Stomach. Preece PE, Cuschieri A, Wellwood JM (eds). London: Grune and Stratton, 1986, pp. 145–63.

6. Fielding JWL. Gastric cancer: Different diseases. Br J Surg 1989; 76:1227.

7. Hundahl SA, Stemmermann GN, Oishi A. Racial factors cannot explain superior Japanese outcomes in stomach cancer. Arch Surg 1996; 131:170–5.

8. Rohde H, Baeuer P, Heitman K. The German Gastric Cancer TNM Study Group. Proximal compared with distal adenocarcinoma of the stomach: differences and consequences. Br J Surg 1991; 78:1242–8.

9. Roder JD, Bonenkamp JJ, Craven J et al. Lymphadenectomy for gastric cancer in clinical trials: update. World J Surg 1995; 19:546–53.

10. Allum WH, Powell DJ, McConkey CC et al. Gastric cancer: a 25-year review. Br J Surg 1989; 76:535–40.

11. MacIntyre IMC, Akoh JA. Improving survival in gastric cancer. Review of operative mortality in English language publications from 1970. Br J Surg 1991; 78:773–8.

12. Sue-Ling HM, Johnston D, Martin I et al. Gastric cancer: a curable disease in Britain. Br Med J 1993; 307:591–6.

13. Bollschweiller E, Boettcher K, Hoelscher AH et al. Is the prognosis for Japanese and German patients with gastric cancer really different? Cancer 1993; 71:2918–25.

14. Schwarz RE, Karpeh MS, Brennan MF. Surgical management of gastric cancer: The Western experience. In: Daly JM, Hennessey TPJ, Reynolds JV (eds.) Management of upper gastrointestinal cancer. London: WB Saunders, 1999.

15. Averbach AM, Jacquet P. Stategies to decrease the incidence of intra-abdominal recurrence in resectable gastric cancer. Br J Surg 1996; 83:726–33.

16. Boku T, Nakane Y, Minoura T et al. Prognostic significance of serosal invasion and free intraperitoneal cancer cells in gastric cancer. Br J Surg 1990; 77:436–9.

17. Iitsuka Y, Kaneshima S, Tanida O et al. Intraperitoneal free cancer cells and their viability in gastric cancer. Cancer 1979; 44:1476–80.

18. Gunderson LL, Sosin H. Adenocarcinoma of the stomach – areas of failure in a reoperation series (second or symptomatic look). Clinicopathological correlation and implications for adjuvant therapy. Int J Radiol Oncol Biol Phys 1982; 8:1–11.

19. Landry J, Tepper JE, Wood WL et al. Patterns of failure following curative resection of gastric cancer. Int J Radiol Oncol Biol Phys 1990; 19:1357–62.

20. Douglass HO, Nava MR. Gastric adenocarcinoma: management of the primary disease. Semin Oncol 1985; 12:32–45.

21. Cunliffe WJ, Sugarbaker PH. Gastrointestinal malignancy: rationale for adjuvant therapy using early postoperative intraperitoneal chemotherapy. Br J Surg 1989; 76:1082–90.

22. Volpe CM, Koo J, Miloro SM. The effect of extended lymphadenectomy on survival in patients with gastric adenocarcinoma. J Am Coll Surg 1995; 181:56–64.

23. Jatsko G, Lisborg PH, Klimpfinger M. Extended radical surgery against gastric cancer: low complication and high survival rates. Jpn J Clin Oncol 1992; 22:102–6.

24. Sasako M, McCulloch P, Kinoshita T *et al.* New method to evaluate the therapeutic value of lymph node dissection for gastric cancer. Br J Surg 1995; 82:346–51.

25. Keller E, Stutzer H, Heitmann K *et al.* Lymph node staging in 872 patients with carcinoma of the stomach and the presumed benefit of lymphadenectomy. German Stomach Cancer TNM Study Group. J Am Coll Surg 1994; 178:38–46.

26. Hamazoe R, Maeta M, Kaibara N. Intraperitoneal thermochemotherapy for prevention of peritoneal recurrence of gastric cancer. Final results of a randomised controlled study. Cancer 1994; 73:2048–52.

27. Yonemura Y, Ninomiya I, Kaji M *et al.* Prophylaxis with intraoperative chemohyperthermia against peritoneal recurrence of serosal-invasion positive gastric cancer. World J Surg 1995; 19:450–55.

28. Sautner T, Hofbauer F, Depisch D *et al.* Adjuvant intraperitoneal cisplatin chemotherapy does not improve long-term survival after surgery for advanced gastric cancer. J Clin Oncol 1994; 12:970–74.

29. Gall FP, Hermanek P. New aspects in the surgical treatment of gastric carcinoma – a comparative study of 1636 patients operated on between 1969 and 1982. Eur J Surg Oncol 1985; 11:219–25.

30. Hornig D, Hermanek P, Gall FP. The significance of the extent of proximal margins on clearance in gastric cancer surgery. Scand J Gastroenterol 1977; 22 (Suppl 133):69–71.

31. Bozzetti F, Bonfanti G, Bufalino R *et al.* Adequacy of margins of resection in gastrectomy for cancer. Ann Surg 1982; 196:682–90.

32. Maehara Y, Okuyama T, Moriguchi S *et al.* Prophylactic lymph node dissection in patients with advanced gastric cancer promotes increased survival time. Cancer 1992; 70:392–5.

33. Hanazaki K, Sodeyama H, Mochizuki Y *et al.* Efficacy of extended lymphadenectomy in the noncurative gastrectomy for advanced gastric cancer. Hepatogastroenterol 1999; 46:2677–82.

34. Japanese Research Society for Gastric Cancer. The general rules for gastric cancer surgery and pathology. Jpn J Surg 1981; 11:127–45.

35. Papachristou DN, Fortner JG. Adenocarcinoma of the gastric cardia. The choice of gastrectomy. Ann Surg 1980; 192:58–64.

36. Harrison LE, Karpeh MS, Brennan MF. Total gastrectomy is not necessary for proximal gastric cancer. Surgery 1998; 123:127–30.

37. Siewert JR, Bottcher K, Stein HJ *et al.* Problem of proximal third gastric carcinoma. World J Surg 1995; 19:523–31.

38. Siewert JR, Stein HJ, Sendler A *et al.* Surgical resection for cancer of the cardia. Semin Surg Oncol 1999; 17:125–31.

39. Wayman J, Dresner SM, Raimes SA *et al.* Transhiatal approach to total gastrectomy for adenocarcinoma of the gastric cardia. Br J Surg 1999; 86:536–40.

40. Aranha GV, Georgen R. Gastric linitis plastica is not a surgical disease. Surgery 1989; 106:758–63.

41. Hallissey MT, Jewkes AJ, Dunn JA *et al.* Resection-line involvement in gastric cancer: a continuing problem. Br J Surg 1993; 80:1418–20.

42. Bozzetti F. Total versus subtotal gastrectomy in cancer of the distal stomach: facts and fantasy. Eur J Surg Oncol 1992; 18:572–9.

43. Bozzetti F, Marubini E, Bonfanti G *et al.* Subtotal versus total gastrectomy for gastric cancer: five-year survival rates in a multicenter randomized Italian trial. Italian Gastrointestinal Tumour Study Group. Ann Surg 1999; 230:170–8.

44. Svedlund J, Sullivan M, Liedman B *et al.* Quality of life after gastrectomy for gastric carcinoma: controlled study of reconstructive procedures. World J Surg 1997; 21:422–33.

45. Davies J, Johnston D, Sue-Ling H *et al.* Total or subtotal gastrectomy for gastric carcinoma? A study of quality of life. World J Surg 1998; 22:1048–55.

46. Skandalakis JE, Gray SW, Rowe SJ. Anatomical complications in general surgery. New York: McGraw Hill, 1983; pp. 63–64.

47. Maruyama K, Gunven P, Okabayashi K *et al.* Lymph node metastases of gastric cancer. General pattern in 1931 patients. Ann Surg 1989; 210:596–602.

48. Maruyama K, Sasako M, Kinoshita T *et al.* Effectiveness of systematic lymph node dissection in gastric cancer surgery. In: Nishi M *et al.* (eds.) Gastric Cancer. Tokyo: Springer Verlag, 1993; pp. 293–305.

49. Kodama Y, Sugimachi K, Soejima K *et al.* Evaluation of extensive lymph node dissection for carcinoma of the stomach. World J Surg 1981; 5:241–8.

50. Noguchi Y, Imada T, Matsumoto A *et al*. Radical surgery for gastric cancer. A review of the Japanese experience. Cancer 1989; 64:2053–62.

51. Soga J, Ohyama S, Miyashita K *et al*. A statistical evaluation of advancement in gastric cancer surgery with special reference to the significance of lymphadenectomy for cure. World J Surg 1988; 12:398–405.

52. Maruyama K, Okabayashi K, Kinoshita T. Progress in gastric cancer surgery in Japan and its limits of radicality. World J Surg 1987; 11:418–25.

53. Nakajima T, Nishi M. Surgery and adjuvant chemotherapy for gastric cancer. Hepatogastroenterology 1989; 36:79–85.

54. Lee JS, Douglass HO. D2 dissection for gastric cancer. Surg Oncol 1997; 6:215–25.

55. Seto Y, Nagawa H, Muto T. Results of extended lymph node dissection for gastric cancer cases with N2 lymph node metastasis. Int Surg 1997; 82:257–61.

56. Roukos DH, Lorenz M, Encke A. Evidence of survival benefit of extended (D2) lymphadenectomy in western patients with gastric cancer based on a new concept: a prospective long-term follow-up study. Surgery 1998; 123:573–8.

57. Hayes N, Ng EK, Raimes SA *et al*. Total gastrectomy with extended lymphadenectomy for 'curable' stomach cancer: experience in a non-Japanese Asian center. J Am Coll Surg 1999; 188:27–32.

58. Maehara Y, Tomoda M, Tomisaki S *et al*. Surgical treatment and outcome for node-negative gastric cancer. Surgery 1997; 121:633–9.

59. Siewert JR, Kestlmeier R, Busch R. Benefits of D2 lymph node dissection for patients with gastric cancer and pN0 pN1 lymph node metastases. Br J Surg 1996; 83:1144–7.

60. Harrison LE, Karpeh MS, Brennan MF. Extended lymphadenectomy is associated with a survival benefit for node-negative gastric cancer. J Gastrointestinal Surg 1998; 2:126–31.

61. Shiu MH, Moore E, Sanders M *et al*. Influence of the extent of resection on survival after curative treatment of gastric carcinoma. Arch Surg 1987; 122:1347–51.

62. Siewert JR, Bottcher K, Roder JD *et al*. Prognostic relevance of systematic lymph node dissection in gastric carcinoma. Br J Surg 1993; 80:1015–18.

63. Siewert JR, Bottcher K, Stein HJ *et al*. Relevant prognostic factors in gastric cancer: ten-year results of the German Gastric Cancer Study. Ann Surg 1998; 228:449–61.

64. Dent DM, Madden MV, Price SK. Randomised comparison of R1 and R2 gastrectomy for gastric cancer. Br J Surg 1988; 75:110–12.

65. Robertson CS, Chung SCS, Woods SDS *et al*. A prospective randomised trial comparing R1 subtotal gastrectomy with R3 total gastrectomy for antral cancer. Ann Surg 1994; 220:176–82.

66. Bonnenkamp JJ, Hermans J, Sasako M *et al*. Extended lymph node dissection for gastric cancer. N Engl J Med 1999; 340:908–14.

 67. Bunt AM, Hermans J, Boon MC *et al*. Evaluation of the extent of lymphadenectomy in a randomised trial of Western- versus Japanese-type surgery in gastric cancer. J Clin Oncol 1994; 12:417–22.

68. Sasako M. Risk factors for surgical treatment in the Dutch Gastric Cancer Trial. Br J Surg 1997; 84:1567–71.

 69. Cuschieri A, Fayers P, Fielding J *et al*. Postoperative morbidity and mortality after D1 and D2 resections for gastric cancer: preliminary results of the MRC randomized controlled surgical trial. Lancet 1996; 347:995–9.

70. Cuschieri A, Weeden S, Fielding J *et al*. Patient survival after D1 and D2 resections for gastric cancer: long-term results of the MRC randomized surgical trial. Br J Cancer 1999; 78:1522–30.

71. Parikh D, Johnson M, Chagla L *et al*. D2 gastrectomy: lessons from a prospective audit of the learning curve. Br J Surg 1996; 83:1595–9.

72. Hayes N, Karat D, Scott DJ *et al*. Radical lymphadenectomy in the management of early gastric cancer. Br J Surg 1996; 83:1421–3.

73. Kampschoer GHM, Maruyama K, van de Velde CJH *et al*. Computer analysis in making preoperative decisions: a rational approach to lymph node dissection in gastric cancer patients. Br J Surg 1989; 76:905–8.

74. Otsuji E, Yamaguchi T, Sawai K *et al*. Total gastrectomy with simultaneous pancreaticosplenectomy or splenectomy in patients with advanced gastric carcinoma. Br J Cancer 1999; 79:1789–93.

75. Griffith JP, Sue-Ling HM, Martin I *et al*. Preservation of the spleen improves survival after radical surgery for gastric cancer. Gut 1995; 36:684–90.

76. Fujita T, Matai K, Kohno S *et al*. Impact of splenectomy on circulating immunoglobulin levels and the development of postoperative infection following total gastrectomy for gastric cancer. Br J Surg 1996; 83:1776–8.

77. Okajima K, Isozaki H. Splenectomy for treatment of gastric cancer: Japanese experience. World J Surg 1995; 19:537–40.

78. Wanabo HJ, Kennedy BJ, Winchester DP *et al*. Role of splenectomy in gastric cancer surgery: adverse effect of elective splenectomy on longterm survival. J Am Coll Surg 1997; 185:177–84.

79. Brady MS, Rogatko A, Dent L *et al*. Effect of splenectomy on morbidity and survival following curative gastrectomy for carcinoma. Arch Surg 1991; 126:359–64.

80. Mishima Y, Hirayama R. The role of lymph node surgery in gastric cancer. World J Surg 1987; 11:406–11.

81. Sugimachi K, Kodama Y, Kuimashiro R *et al.* Critical evaluation of prophylactic splenectomy in total gastrectomy for stomach cancer. Gann 1985; 7:704–9.

82. Kodera Y, Yanamura Y, Shimuzu Y *et al.* Lack of benefit of combined pancreaticosplenectomy in D2 resection for proximal-third gastric carcinoma. World J Surg 1997; 21:622–7.

83. Sasako M. Surgical management of gastric cancer: The Japanese experience In: Daly JM, Hennessey TPJ, Reynolds JV (eds.) Management of upper gastrointestinal cancer. London: WB Saunders, 1999, pp. 107–35.

84. Maruyama K, Sasako M, Kinoshita T *et al.* Pancreas-preserving total gastrectomy for proximal gastric cancer. World J Surg 1995; 19:532–6.

85. Kodama I, Takamiya H, Mizutani K *et al.* Gastrectomy with combined resection of other organs for carcinoma of the stomach with invasion to adjacent organs: clinical efficacy in a retrospective study. J Am Coll Surg 1997; 184:16–22.

86. Kocherling F, Reck T, Gall FP. Extended gastrectomy: who benefits? World J Surg 1995; 19:541–5.

87. Korenaga D, Okamura T, Baba H *et al.* Results of resection of gastric cancer extending to adjacent organs. Br J Surg 1988; 75:12–15.

88. Bozzetti F, Regalia E, Bonfanti G *et al.* Early and late results of extended surgery for cancer of the stomach. Br J Surg 1990; 77:53–6.

89. Iizuka I. Collateral circulation after division of the common hepatic artery – clinical study concerning Appleby's operation. Jpn J Surg 1990; 91:631–8 (English abstract).

90. Sawai K, Takahishi T, Suzuki H. New trends in surgery for gastric cancer in Japan. J Surg Oncol 1994; 56:221–6.

91. Doglietto GB, Pacelli F, Caprino P *et al.* Palliative surgery for far-advanced gastric cancer: a retrospective study of 305 consecutive patients. Am Surg 1999; 65:352–5.

92. Sowa M, Kato Y, Nishimura M *et al.* Surgical approach to early gastric cancer with lymph node metastasis. World J Surg 1989; 13:630–5.

93. Maehara Y, Oshiro T, Endo K *et al.* Clinical significance of occult micrometastases in lymph nodes from patients with early gastric cancer who died of recurrence. Surgery 1996; 119:397–442.

94. Whiting JL, Fielding JW. Radical surgery for early gastric cancer. Eur J Surg Oncol 1998; 24:263–6.

95. Hochwald SN, Brennan MF, Klimstra DS *et al.* Is lymphadenectomy necessary for early gastric cancer? Ann Surg Oncol 1999; 6:664–70.

96. Hiki Y, Shimao H, Mieno H *et al.* Modified treatment of early gastric cancers: evaluation of endoscopic treatment of early gastric cancers with respect to treatment indications. World J Surg 1995; 19:517–22.

97. Kodama M, Koyama K. Indications for pylorus-preserving gastrectomy for early gastric cancer located in the middle third of the stomach. World J Surg 1991; 15:628–34.

98. Goh P, Kum CK. Laparoscopic Billroth II gastrectomy: a review. Surg Oncol 1993; 2 Suppl 1:13–18.

99. Yamashita Y, Kurohiji T, Kakeyama T *et al.* Laparoscopy-guided extracorporeal resection of early gastric carcinoma. Endoscopy 1995; 27:248–52.

100. Sasako M, Kinoshita T, Maruyama K. Prognosis of early gastric cancer. Stomach and intestine 1993; 28:139–46 (in Japanese with English abstract).

101. Namieno T, Koito K, Higashi T *et al.* Tumour recurrence following resection for early gastric carcinoma and its implications for a policy of limited resection. World J Surg 1998; 22:869–73.

102. McCulloch P. Description of the Japanese method of radical gastrectomy. Ann Roy Coll Surg Engl 1994; 76:110–14.

103. Craven JL. Radical surgery for gastric cancer. In: Preece PR, Cuschieri A, Wellwood JM (eds.) Cancer of the stomach. London: Grune and Stratton, 1986; pp. 165–187.

104. Hayes N, Wayman J, Wadhera V *et al.* Peritoneal cytology in the evaluation of gastric carcinoma. Br J Cancer 1999; 79:520–4.

105. Cuschieri A. Reconstruction after gastric resection for cancer. In: Preece P, Cuschieri A, Wellwood JM (Eds) Cancer of the stomach. London: Grune and Stratton, 1986; pp. 209–229.

106. Buhl K, Lehnert T, Schlag P *et al.* Reconstruction after gastrectomy and quality of life. World J Surg 1995; 19:558–64.

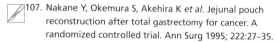

107. Nakane Y, Okemura S, Akehira K *et al.* Jejunal pouch reconstruction after total gastrectomy for cancer. A randomized controlled trial. Ann Surg 1995; 222:27–35.

108. Liedman B, Andersson H, Bossaeus I *et al.* Changes in body composition after gastrectomy: results of a controlled prospective clinical trial. World J Surg 1997; 21:416–21.

109. Fuchs K-H, Thiede A, Engemann R *et al.* Reconstruction of the food passage after total gastrectomy: randomized trial. World J Surg 1995; 19:698–706.

110. Svedlund J, Sullivan M, Liedman B *et al.* Quality of life after gastrectomy for gastric carcinoma: controlled study of reconstructive procedures. World J Surg 1997; 21:422–33.

111. Liedman B, Andersson H, Berglund B *et al.* Food intake after total gastrectomy for gastric cancer: the

role of a gastric reservoir. Br J Surg 1996; 83:1138–43.

112. Ishihara K. Long-term quality of life in patients after total gastrectomy. Cancer Nurs 1999; 22:220–7.

113. Mathias JR, Fernandez A, Sninsky CA *et al.* Nausea, vomiting and abdominal pain after Roux-en-Y anastomosis: motility of the jejunal limb. Gastroenterology 1985; 88:101–7.

114. Troidl H, Kusche J, Vertweber K-H *et al.* Pouch versus oesophagojejunostomy after total gastrectomy: a randomised clinical trial. World J Surg 1987; 11:699–712.

115. Donovan IA, Fielding JWL, Bradby H *et al.* Bile diversion after total gastrectomy. Br J Surg 1982; 69:389–90.

116. Bradley E, Isaacs J, Hersh T *et al.* Nutritional consequences of total gastrectomy. Ann Surg 1975; 182:415–29.

117. Braga M, Zuliani W, Foppa L *et al.* Food intake and nutritional status after total gastrectomy: results of a nutritional follow-up. Br J Surg 1988; 75:477–80.

118. Maehara Y, Emi Y, Babu H *et al.* Recurrences and related characteristics of gastric cancer. Br J Cancer 1996; 74:975–9.

7 Radiotherapy and chemotherapy in the treatment of oesophageal and gastric cancer

Adrian Crellin

INTRODUCTION

The treatment of oesophago-gastric cancer is becoming more complex. The limitations of single modality approaches in producing acceptable long-term survival rates have driven the changing patterns of management of both oesophageal and gastric cancer. Early stage disease can be treated with excellent outcomes. Improvements in staging, imaging and pathology have exposed the fact that the majority of patients present with either locally advanced or metastatic disease. In this context high local recurrence rates and early failure with metastatic disease are easier to understand even in series of patients who in the past would have been accepted as operable and potentially curable.

The changing pattern of disease with rapidly increasing rates of adenocarcinoma of the distal oesophagus and oesophago-gastric junction with reducing numbers of cancers of the body of the stomach may require a different approach to treatment.

Improvements in staging with spiral CT, MRI and endoscopic ultrasound (EUS) now allow patients to be selected for specific approaches to treatment. The early identification of metastases can allow a palliative approach to be followed, thus avoiding the morbidity and mortality associated with resection. Equally, the demonstration of early stage disease can allow the selected use of single modality therapy. There are undoubtedly limitations to the use of imaging, particularly in predicting the response to primary non-surgical treatment, chemotherapy or chemoradiotherapy (CRT), but the addition of new techniques such as positron emission tomography (PET) may offer promise for the future.

An increasingly elderly population with associated comorbid conditions presents particular challenges. It is possible to reduce postoperative mortality by the appropriate selection of patients.[1] Some of these, while not fit for a transthoracic approach to resection, may be appropriate for primary non-surgical treatment such as CRT and so still may be offered a reasonable chance of long-term disease control.

Both oesophageal and gastric cancer show high response rates to chemotherapy. It has been difficult and frustrating, however, to demonstrate the value of chemotherapy in addition to conventional approaches to treatment. This is despite a clearly established role for chemotherapy in the palliative treatment of advanced and metastatic disease.

In oesophageal cancer the changing pattern of squamous and adenocarcinoma has meant some mixed series of cases and variable results. The variable inclusion of lower oesophageal cancer and cancer of the oesophago–gastric junction with gastric adenocarcinoma has also created some difficulty in interpreting the true role of chemotherapy and radiotherapy from the literature.

The identification of improved activity when chemotherapy and radiotherapy are given synchronously has already led to CRT becoming the primary approach in anal cancer with surgery now used for salvage.[2,3] There is good evidence that CRT has a role in oesophageal cancer treatment.

As evidence mounts of the benefit of a multidisciplinary approach to care and assessment and of selected multimodality treatment, it is important that surgeons and oncologists understand more of the strengths and weaknesses of both their own and each other's treatments. Only then can treatment be truly integrated and improved outcomes with minimal morbidity be achieved.

The definition of adjuvant treatment and potentially curative therapy is worth stressing. Adjuvant therapy is usually taken to be additional treatment given after potentially curative therapy, in an attempt to improve the long-term outcome. In this context, surgery can really only be described as potentially curative if the tumour is resected with no residual macroscopic disease and clear histological margins (R0), in the absence of metastatic disease.

The following sections are intended to allow the role of chemotherapy and radiotherapy to be put into context and the strength of evidence assessed. The sections on potentially curative approaches are more detailed. This is the area in which most treatment will be integrated with surgery in current or future approaches.

Potentially curative treatments

Oesophagus

Preoperative radiotherapy

Theoretical advantages of preoperative radiotherapy treatment include: a more easily defined target volume, improved tumour oxygenation at the time of treatment, the potential to improve resectability and reduce the impact of tumour cell spillage at surgery, minimising the impact of microscopic residual disease and reducing local recurrence. This approach has been shown to be of value in rectal cancer.[4]

There have been six randomised trials of preoperative radiotherapy. Three trials were restricted to squamous carcinoma. One of these, by Gignoux et al., reported an improvement in local/regional recurrence[5] (46% versus 67%). Another by Nygaard et al. reports improved survival[6] but this series is complicated by the inclusion of some patients also receiving chemotherapy. One trial included both squamous and adenocarcinoma[7] and two do not specify the histology. Overall it is difficult to draw firm conclusions from these trials.

 A meta-analysis of updated individual patient data from 1147 patients in randomised trials reported a hazard ratio of 0.89 (95% CI 0.78–1.01) with an absolute survival benefit of 4% at 5 years.[8] This result did not reach conventional statistical significance. The benefit therefore seems likely to be small, if any, and there is little evidence of improved resectability.

Postoperative radiotherapy

The main attraction of postoperative radiotherapy is that it can be restricted to selected patients who may have a higher risk of recurrence, in particular of local/regional failure. There are three randomised trials in the literature. The numbers are small (totalling 348 adjuvant patients) and two out of the three include only squamous carcinoma. Teniere et al.[9] showed no survival advantage in 221 patients. There was a small improvement in the failure rate but at the cost of significant side effects. The benefit appears to be limited to node negative patients. Fok et al.[10] included both adenocarcinoma and squamous carcinoma. While both curative and palliative resections were included the patients were separately analysed and received different radiotherapy doses. The results show a significant morbidity (37%) and mortality related to bleeding from the transposed intrathoracic stomach. It should be noted that the dose per fraction of the radiotherapy was high (350 cGy) which may be significant. There was a lower intrathoracic recurrence rate, particularly relating to tracheobronchial disease.

The conclusion is that postoperative radiotherapy may have a limited role in node-negative patients with residual mediastinal disease. Morbidity to the transposed stomach and delayed recovery may be the potential drawbacks. Careful selection of patients and radiotherapy technique seems likely to be important.

Preoperative chemotherapy

The rationale behind preoperative chemotherapy is to improve operability by tumour shrinkage and downstaging and to treat occult metastatic disease as early as possible, thereby trying to reduce late metastatic disease as a cause of failure. A useful additional benefit may be that some patients will improve their swallowing and so gain weight, thus having a better nutritional status in the preoperative phase. Non-responders to chemotherapy will however have surgery delayed and possibly suffer chemotherapy side effects. Preoperative chemotherapy in both squamous and adenocarcinoma appears to consistently achieve good clinical response rates of 47%[11]–61%.[12] Early studies, predominantly in squamous carcinoma, used combinations of cisplatin, vindesine and bleomycin. More recently cisplatin and 5 fluorouracil (5FU) combinations have been used in important randomised trials. New 5HT3 antagonist antiemetic drugs have allowed cisplatin to be used with dramatically reduced toxicity. Protracted venous infusion (PVI) 5FU in combination with cisplatin and epirubicin (the ECF regimen) has produced increased response rates in non-randomised studies. These more modern cisplatin 5FU combinations seem to be active in both squamous[13] and adenocarcinoma.[12]

Randomised trials of preoperative chemotherapy

There are three older randomised trials in the literature. Roth et al.[14] reported the results of 39 patients treated with cisplatin, vindesine and bleomycin. There was no survival advantage between the two arms but responders did seem to have a longer median survival (> 20 months versus overall 9 months versus non-responders 6.2 months). Schlag[11] randomised 75 patients to receiving cisplatin and 5FU. The trial was stopped early due to increased postoperative morbidity and mortality in the chemotherapy treated patients. Nygaard et al.[6]

showed no survival advantage at 3 years. All these trials were small and so were only powered to reliably demonstrate large differences in outcome. A meta-analysis published in 1996[15] did not show a survival benefit for preoperative chemotherapy.

However since then the results from three larger trials have become available and these are influential in suggesting that preoperative chemotherapy does have a role. In a randomised study undertaken by the Rotterdam Esophageal Tumour Study Group,[16] 160 patients with squamous carcinoma were randomised to receive two courses of cisplatin and etoposide or surgery (transhiatal resection) alone. Those patients who demonstrated a good clinical response (69/74) then went on to receive two further courses. Data on 148 patients were analysed with a median follow up of 15 months. There was a significant difference (p = 0.002) in the median survival between the chemotherapy plus surgery and the surgery-alone arm (18.5 months versus 11 months). The conclusion was that neo-adjuvant chemotherapy improves survival. However longer term 2- and 3-year survival figures are not yet available.

The American Intergroup Trial (INT 0113)[17] produced data on 440 ran-domised patients with a median follow up of 46.5 months. Adenocarcinoma (54%) was the predominant histology. The chemotherapy given was three pre-operative courses (cisplatin and 5 days of infusional 5FU) and in stable or responding patients two postoperative courses. Overall 83% of patients received the intended two preoperative cycles of chemotherapy. However only 32% of patients received both postoperative chemotherapy cycles. There was no differ-ence in treatment-related mortality between the two arms (6% surgery (S) versus 7% chemotherapy (CT) plus surgery (S). p = 0.33). On an intent–to–treat basis there was no difference in median survival (16.1 months CT+S versus 14.9 months S), and 1-, 2- and 3-year (23% CT+S versus 26% S) survivals. Disappointingly there was no difference in the pattern of metastatic disease between the two arms. However there was a significantly higher rate of R1 resections in the surgery-alone arm.

Recently the early results of the Medical Research Council (MRC) OEO2 trial have become available.[18] In this trial 802 patients were randomised to receive 2 courses each of cisplatin with a 4-day infusion of 5FU followed by surgery (CS) or immediate surgery alone (S). The majority of patients had ade-nocarcinoma (66%) histology. Although the results are early, there is a significant improvement in median survival as well as 2-year survival (45% CS versus 35% S) with a median time to follow-up of 701 days. There appears to be an improved complete resection rate (84% CS versus 71% S) with no increased postoperative mortality (9% CS versus 10% S).

Thus two out of the three recent trials suggest a survival benefit for preoperative chemotherapy. There are some concerns about the maturity of the data and the quality assurance of both patient staging and surgery.

While the clinical response rates are consistently high, the rate of pathological complete response (pCR) seen in the operative specimens is less impressive.

A new meta-analysis may bring about greater certainty, but it does seem as if pre-operative chemotherapy, as in the OEO2 trial, has become the standard of care against which new treatments must be judged.

Postoperative chemotherapy

There are few useful trials that address the question of adjuvant postoperative chemotherapy. The trials reported by Roth[14] and Kelsen[17] both have an adjuvant component, coupled with preoperative treatment. The failure to complete the postoperative phase in 68% of the Intergroup study[17] underlines a problem with this approach. Patients undergoing major resections for oesophageal carcinoma often have a prolonged postoperative phase. The start of chemotherapy may be delayed due to performance status. Patients may also choose not to continue. A strategy that relies solely on postoperative treatment may have significant problems. Improved patient selection and postoperative supportive care may allow this approach to be practical. The current MRC MAGIC (ST02) Trial now includes tumours of the gastro-oesophageal junction and lower oesophagus and includes three postoperative courses of ECF as well as three given preoperatively in the protocol. There is a current Eastern Cooperative Oncology Group (ECOG) phase II trial (E8296) in the United States giving postoperative cisplatin and paclitaxel, aiming to treat 55 patients. At present, however, postoperative chemotherapy cannot be considered to be the standard of care.

Preoperative chemoradiotherapy

The rationale in using chemotherapy and radiotherapy together is that enhanced tumour-cell kill leads to improved outcomes. Chemotherapy can lead to a decreased ability of tumour cells to repair radiation-induced DNA damage. Many of the commonly used chemotherapy drugs with significant activity in oesophageal and gastric cancer appear to be radiation sensitisers (5FU, cisplatin, mitomycin C, taxanes). There is good evidence that pCR rates are significantly higher than with radiotherapy or chemotherapy given alone. There is the significant attraction of achieving enhanced local therapy coupled with a systemic benefit as desired with preoperative chemotherapy alone. When added to surgery, it is not clear that pCR is necessarily the only useful endpoint. It also has the added advantage in providing direct evidence to guide the process of developing and optimising combination chemotherapy and radiotherapy schedules for use as definitive treatments. This issue will be discussed in the following sections.

Both radiotherapy and chemotherapy rely on achieving an acceptable balance between increased response rates in the tumour on one hand and normal tissue morbidity coupled with patient tolerance on the other. While many of the side effects of chemotherapy are relatively early in presentation e.g. hair loss, emesis and myelosuppression, radiotherapy side effects can present late, after 6 months to years from treatment. If radical surgery is then added the potential for high levels of morbidity become significant.

Non-randomised studies of CRT have appeared in the literature since the late 1980s. The review article by Geh et al. summarises the 46 trials containing 20 patients or more.[19] Pooled data from these studies shows that out of 2704 patients, 79% were operated on with a pCR rate of 24% of those treated and 32% of those resected. The balance of histology in these patients was squamous 68% and adenocarcinoma 32%.

Lessons have been learned as experience with this modality of treatment has grown. Attempts to escalate the dose of radiotherapy can lead to unacceptable rates of morbidity, especially if higher doses per fraction are used.[20,21] Reported CRT-related deaths in the non-randomised series ranged from 0%–15% (mean 3%). Postoperative deaths ranged from 0%–29% (mean 9%). Adult respiratory distress syndrome (ARDS), anastomotic leak and breakdown, pneumonia and sepsis were the commonest causes of death following oesophageal resection. Overall treatment-related deaths ranged from 3% to 25% (mean 9%) of all patients treated. It seems clear that the risk of chemotherapy-related toxicity, particularly myelosuppression, rises with the number of drugs used and the intensity of the CRT regimen.[22,23] An increased risk of tracheobronchial fistula has also been reported.[24]

Consistent reporting of pathology is important and Mandard *et al.* have described a grading of CRT response.[25] Five grades of response ranging from no identifiable tumour to complete absence of regression allow a more objective approach to be adopted. In this paper the significant predictor of disease-free survival after multivariate analysis was the tumour regression grade. There is evidence that pCR confers a survival advantage over those patients not achieving pCR.[26,27,28,29,30] In **Fig. 7.1**, different comparative outcomes such as median survival in months, overall or disease-free survival in years, are plotted together in the series quoting outcomes separately. The importance is in the consistent nature of the difference in outcomes in each series.

There are six reported randomised trials of preoperative CRT compared with surgery alone. In three of these the chemotherapy was given sequentially to the radiotherapy and in three synchronously. Two trials using sequential treatment in squamous carcinoma[6,31] received relatively low doses of radiotherapy and showed no convincing evidence of improved survival with the combined treatment. In a larger European Organisation for Research and Treatment of Cancer (EORTC) trial[21] involving 282 patients the cisplatin chemotherapy was given in close sequence with the radiotherapy. The radiotherapy was given in a split course and at a relatively high dose per fraction (two courses of 18.5 Gy in 5 daily fractions split 2 weeks apart). The CRT patients were more likely to have a curative

Figure 7.1
Relative survival outcomes – pathological complete response to CRT.

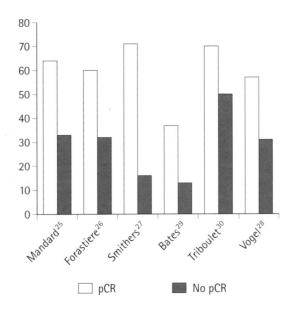

resection. The disease-free survival was significantly longer (3-year CRT+S 40% versus S 28%). There was no difference in the overall survival, largely due to a significantly higher postoperative mortality in the CRT arm (12% versus 4%). Apinop et al.[32] reported a synchronous CRT series of 69 squamous histology patients with no improvement in survival.

There are two larger positive trials of preoperative synchronous CRT.

The Walsh study[33] has been influential in changing practice. In 113 patients with adenocarcinoma, cisplatin and 5FU were given with 40 Gy in 3 weeks of radiotherapy. There was an overall survival benefit in favour of the CRT arm (median 16 months versus 11 months; 3-year 32% versus 6%).

Morbidity in this series was not inconsiderable. The radiotherapy technique and fractionation may explain this. Most open to question however is the noticeably poor survival in the surgery-alone control arm. The basic standards of staging could potentially have led to an imbalance of true staging in the treatment arms. The University of Michigan trial[34] randomised 100 patients with both squamous and adenocarcinoma. The surgery was a transhiatal resection. Patients in the CRT arm received 45 Gy in 30 fractions with cisplatin, 5FU and vinblastine. At first analysis there was no significant difference between the arms but at 3 years a statistically significant benefit emerged with the combined treatment, with an overall survival of 32% versus 15%.

The results of these studies point to a potential for significant improvements in outcome. New trials are necessary that need to be larger. In addition, attention to the quality assurance of all components of treatment and staging is required to ensure that the rather variable results of the past are not replicated.

One such trial has unfortunately closed in the United States (NCCTG-C9781). The results of the Intergroup Study INT-0116 (SWOG9008)[35] were presented at the American Society of Clinical Oncologists (ASCO) 2000 Meeting. While this was predominantly a trial of postoperative CRT in gastric cancer, it included tumours of the gastro-oesophageal junction. It was felt that the positive results of the SWOG 9008 trial would preclude further randomisation to a trial with a surgery-only control arm. In addition recruitment was already poor as a result of preoperative CRT becoming accepted as a standard of care. There are still major questions to be answered, but a surgery-alone arm is not likely to be considered acceptable.

Definitive radiotherapy and chemoradiotherapy

There are no completed randomised trials comparing surgery against primary non-surgical therapy, either radiotherapy alone or chemoradiotherapy. Comparisons of individual series have to be viewed carefully to take selection and staging bias into account. Surgery still remains the gold standard against which new approaches to potentially curative treatment must be compared. However it is clear that there are long-term survivors in series of definitive non-surgical treatment. With an ageing population it must be remembered that 'inoperable' due to the nature of local disease or comorbidity and performance status does not mean treatment is therefore palliative. Indeed in the National

Cancer Institute (NCI) guidelines for treatment, stage by stage, non-surgical treatment is included as an alternative.

Classical quoted figures of the survival from radical radiotherapy come from the paper from Earlam and Cunha-Melo[36] in which mean survival figures of 8489 patients at 1, 2 and 5 years were 18%, 8% and 6% respectively. Approximately 50% of patients were treated with curative intent. Older series tend to be of squamous carcinoma treated with radiotherapy alone. Modern radiotherapy in better selected patients can produce impressive survival results. In a series of 101 patients treated at the Christie Hospital in Manchester[37] between 1985 and 1994, 3- and 5-year survival figures of 27% and 21% respectively were recorded. There was a slightly better survival for adenocarcinoma, but not reaching statistical significance. The majority of tumours (96/101) were 5 cm or less in length. Importantly, the only significant prognostic factor was the use of diagnostic CT, introduced during the latter part of the study. This was used to plan the radiotherapy and led to an increase in field sizes. The conclusion of the paper was that radiotherapy provided an effective alternative to surgery and that modern radiotherapy planning techniques may improve results.

The adoption of combined chemotherapy and radiotherapy (CRT) stems from high response rates and in particular high pCR rates seen in patients going on to resection. Higher morbidity has led to concern about adopting it in all cases. There are four randomised trials comparing radiotherapy alone with CRT. Three of these used low doses or intensity of chemotherapy. A small series of 59 patients from Brazil[38] did not demonstrate a significant survival advantage. The response rates and 5-year survival rates (6% versus 16%) were better in the CRT arm but at a cost of increased acute toxicity. Coia *et al.* report an important non-randomised series[39] in which treatment was with infusional 5FU and mitomycin C with 60 Gy of radiotherapy. Patients with early stage disease are reported separately. The respective 5-year survival and local failure rate, in clinical stages I and II combined, were 30% and 25%. There was no treatment related mortality although there was increased acute toxicity (22% grade III and 6% grade IV).

The biggest series with a major impact on treatment patterns has been the RTOG 85-01 Herskovic study.[40]

A total of 123 patients were randomised to receive either radiotherapy alone to a dose of 64 Gy or two courses of cisplatin and infusional 5FU concurrent with 50 Gy of radiotherapy. Two more courses of chemotherapy were scheduled after the completion of the radiotherapy. A summary of the results of the randomised patients is shown in **Table 7.1**.

In a confirmatory study, 69 non-randomised patients were treated with the CRT protocol and similar results in terms of median survival and with a 3-year survival of 26%. The acute toxicity in the combined treatment arm was significantly higher with notably haematological and renal and mucositis as the major problems. There was no significant difference in the late complication rates. In total 80% of patients in the combined modality arm received the full protocol treatment. The poor overall survival in the radiotherapy-alone control arm remains a question mark against the study.

The high local failure rate of 45% in the Herskovic trial led to the Intergroup study 0122.[41] The dose of radiotherapy was increased to 64.8 Gy and the intensity

	RT	RT–CT	p value
Median survival – months	9.3	14.1	
Overall survival			
1 year	34	52	
2 years	10	36	
5 years	0	30	0.0001
Rate distant metastases	37	21	0.0017
2-year local recurrence rate	59	45	0.0125
Overall disease free	11	36	< 0.001

Table 7.1 *Summary of results: RTOG 85-01. Al-Sarraf et al. 1997[40]*

of the chemotherapy increased in this phase II study of toxicity and survival in 45 patients. The results showed increased toxicity with 11% treatment-related deaths as compared with 2% in the Herskovic study. The protocol was not adopted into a phase III study. Another approach to improved local control was to use brachytherapy to intensify the radiotherapy dose to the tumour. Study RTOG 92-07[42] used the 50 Gy external beam and chemotherapy protocol from the Herskovic protocol and added an intraluminal brachytherapy boost with one of two methods of delivery, high dose rate or low dose rate. Six of the 35 patients developed an oesophageal fistula. This toxicity was deemed unacceptable.

Improvements in CRT seem likely to come from refinements in chemotherapy and radiotherapy technique. Results from preoperative phase II studies suggest a steady improvement in pCR rates with more acceptable toxicity. The rates of pCR range from 24% in 1993[26] to reports of 56%[43] in 1998. Careful staging can ensure that patients with established metastatic disease are appropriately managed. In the preoperative setting new protocols are being assessed for toxicity and response rates[44] before use in a phase III randomised setting. Definitive treatments now report good survival figures[39,40] that, stage for stage, rival those of surgery.[45,46] In squamous carcinoma there seems to be increasing evidence that a policy of primary CRT with surgery as salvage may be the direction for the future.[47] There is a fundamental difficulty in such a policy of primary non-surgical therapy for adenocarcinoma. The stomach and small bowel have more distinct dose-limiting toxicity and extending radiotherapy fields to cover wider areas below the diaphragm seems likely to produce higher levels of morbidity. Areas of potential lymph-node spread may be covered by the extent of surgical resection. Therefore it may be that a more selective approach based on the extent of the primary could allow alternatives of surgery alone, neo-adjuvant chemotherapy/CRT followed by surgery or CRT alone. Tumours primarily of the lower oesophagus or limited to the gastro-oesophageal junction might be candidates for CRT, whereas tumours with significant extension to the cardia or those primarily in the stomach will require surgery.

The ability to predict which patients will respond to chemotherapy or CRT would allow greater certainty in a primary non-surgical approach. Molecular markers hold some promise.[48,49] Conventional reassessment following treatment, with endoscopic biopsy[30] and CT[50] appear unreliable. Reports of the value of endoscopic ultrasound are more variable with some showing a good correlation with final pathological stage[51] and others suggesting it is not reliable.[52] There are reports advocating that this failure to reliably predict pCR necessitates resection.[29] There is as yet no good evidence to show that PET scanning will be useful.

Following successful CRT or radiotherapy alone there is a rate of benign stricture. This ranges from 12%[53] to 25%[37] in more modern studies. However good swallowing function can be maintained in the majority of patients. Even in those with a benign stricture a full or soft diet can be maintained by dilations in 71% of cases.[54] The treatment of post-CRT benign stricture with stents has not been successful in the author's experience and gives rise to mediastinal pain.

The higher pCR rates seen with CRT, the improved local control rates and altered patterns of failure in the literature have all contributed to CRT being largely adopted as a standard of care. There may still be a role for radical radiotherapy alone. This may be for patients with localised disease, particularly squamous carcinoma, who because of age or comorbidity may not tolerate the chemotherapy component of the treatment.

The management of patients with CRT is complex and requires good support from specialist nurses, dieticians and high standards of technical radiotherapy. The risk of morbidity is real but can be overcome. It should be seen as a single integrated modality of therapy rather than two different treatments that happen to be delivered at the same time.

Gastric cancer

Adjuvant chemotherapy

The aim of adjuvant therapy for gastric cancer is to reduce the late patterns of failure following successful surgical resection. The pattern of spread includes nodal and liver metastases. A significant proportion of patients will fail with intrabdominal, peritoneal or omental disease. Extended lymphadenectomy has been advocated as a method to improve the local/regional control rates. Chemotherapy, either systemic or intraperitoneal, has been used to try and reduce the incidence of widespread recurrence. Despite encouraging results of chemotherapy in advanced disease, proof of a benefit for adjuvant chemotherapy has been elusive.

There has been a wide range of randomised adjuvant chemotherapy trials. Regimens with significant activity in the advanced disease setting have been tested since the 1980s. There are variations in the surgery used, the timing of the start of chemotherapy and the toxicity, all of which make interpretation and comparison difficult.

An early trial using 5FU and the nitrosourea compound methyl-CCNU showed promise. In the Gastrointestinal Tumour Study Group[55] trial a significant benefit became apparent 2 years after surgery in 142 randomised patients. The 5-year survival was 50% versus 31% in favour of the chemotherapy arm. These results were not however confirmed in two subsequent studies[56,57] using the same regimen, which together included 314 patients. A regimen using a combination of 5FU, doxorubicin and mitomycin C (FAM) was seen to be active in advanced disease[58] with a good response rate (35%) including 5% complete responses. When used as adjuvant treatment however no survival benefit was seen.[59,60]

A large randomised trial of 2873 patients reported by Hattori *et al.* in 1986, compared 5FU with mitomycin C against mitomycin C alone.[61] Again no difference was seen in overall survival. New orally active pro-drugs of 5FU are now available and have been seen to be active in gastrointestinal cancer. This form of chemotherapy has obvious attractions as an adjuvant therapy in terms of patient acceptability and the scope for longer duration of therapy. The drug tegafur is absorbed orally and is converted to 5FU in the liver. A combination with uracil, acting to potentiate the 5FU, is called UFT.

Recent trials have attempted to make use of these drugs. In a trial reported by Nakajima,[62] 579 patients who had undergone a curative resection with serosa-negative gastric cancer were randomised to have no further treatment or intravenous mitomycin and 5FU immediately after surgery for 3 weeks. Then oral UFT was given for 18 months. There was no difference in survival; the survival of the T1 patients was 92–95% in the two arms. One of the conclusions was that patients with T1 disease can be excluded from future trials as their outlook is already so good. In an attempt to use the same approach in Western patients of AJCCC stage III, Cirera[63] used a large single dose of mitomycin and 3 months of tegafur. The reported improvement in overall 5-year survival of 46% in the control group and 56% in the treated group (p = 0.04) however is open to question by a non-stratified sealed envelope randomisation and an imbalance in node-negative patients between the groups.

Two meta-analyses exist. The first[64] in 1993 excluded trials before 1980 and only included those with a surgery-only control arm. The conclusion was that there was a small benefit, with a common odds ratio of 0.77 (95% CI 0.65–0.88) in favour of adjuvant chemotherapy. The second published in 1999[65] found 13 trials meeting the eligibility criteria. The odds ratio for death in the treated group was 0.80 (95% CI 0.66–0.97). There was thus a small survival benefit of borderline significance, which was more marked in trials with greater than two-thirds of patients having node-positive disease.

Thus there is probably a small benefit to adjuvant chemotherapy for some patients. No regimen seems to be clearly standard. The toxicity of therapy needs to be balanced against this.

The MRC ST02 (MAGIC) trial aims to recruit 500 patients and uses three courses of ECF before and after resection. This regimen is seemingly far more active in the advanced disease setting and it is hoped that this trial will provide more certain evidence of worthwhile benefit. A neoadjuvant approach to treatment seems likely to be the subject of more randomised trials in the future.

Intraperitoneal chemotherapy

The pattern of peritoneal and hepatic recurrence in gastric cancer makes the early use of intraperitoneal chemotherapy attractive. The most positive trial is from Japan[66] using mitomycin C adsorbed onto activated charcoal, acting as a delayed release preparation. Fifty patients with serosal involvement were randomised to immediate treatment or observation. A highly significant difference in survival at

2 years was seen (68.6% versus 26.9%) with the treatment group maintaining an advantage at 3 years. The treatment was reported to be well tolerated.

However, when an attempt was made to repeat these results, in an Austrian multi-centre study,[67] serious toxicity caused the trial to be suspended. A significantly higher postoperative complication rate (35% versus 16%) and 60-day mortality rate (11% versus 2%) were seen in the treatment arm of the study. No benefits were found in overall or recurrence-free survival.

Postoperative chemoradiotherapy

Radiotherapy has not been routinely used in the management of stomach cancer. Local recurrence can, however, be a significant problem. The stomach and nodal areas are close to many critical normal tissues with dose-limiting toxicity, such as kidney, spinal cord and small bowel.

In the British Stomach Cancer Group trial[60] postoperative radiotherapy was one of the arms of the study. The other arms were FAM chemotherapy and a control group with surgery only. There was no difference in survival but the local recurrence rate was significantly better (54% surgery versus 32% with radio-therapy, p < 0.01).

Recently postoperative CRT has been reported to show a significant benefit to survival following gastric resection.[35] The regimen consisted of 5FU/leuco-vorin given in the first and last week of radiotherapy (45 Gy) and two courses of 5-day 5FU/leucovorin given monthly. With a median follow up of 3.3 years both the disease-free survival (49% versus 32%) and overall survival (52% versus 41%) were improved in the CRT arm. There was some significant haematological and gastrointestinal morbidity. However the treatment-related mortality was only 1%. The need for great care in the technical quality and placement of the radio-therapy was stressed. However a significant number of the patients had a D0 resection. It is possible that in this instance the CRT is making up for less than adequate surgery, and may not translate into routine practice where more extens-ive surgery is undertaken. It does open up the question as to whether there is a role for a selected group of patients in whom an R1 resection has occurred with otherwise favourable factors e.g. node-negative, to be given high-quality CRT to reduce the risk of local/regional failure.

Palliative chemotherapy treatment

Squamous carcinoma of the oesophagus

Combination chemotherapy containing cisplatin is the standard for the treatment of advanced and recurrent squamous carcinoma. The indications for use are limited by the relative infrequency of the disease, and in particular the age and performance status of patients requiring palliation. Very often the indications for improvement of symptoms and quality of life are local, and symptomatic therapy with a stent or radiotherapy will be adequate. However good response rates in the order of 35% can be achieved with cisplatin and 4- or 5-day 5FU infusion.[68] Response duration is variable and can range from 3 to 6 months. Consideration should be given to consolidation palliative radiotherapy after successful chemotherapy to improve local control where recurrent growth may produce symptoms for patients with a better performance status and expectation of life. There is some evidence that the improved response rates seen with protracted venous infusion (PVI) 5FU in adenocarcinoma can be achieved in squamous carcinoma.[13] New agents such as paclitaxel have yet to demonstrate their superiority in combination regimens but are clearly active as single agents.

Adenocarcinoma of the oesophagus stomach

While earlier literature tends to report activity in pure gastric cancer, the changing pattern of disease has meant that more recent reports deal with oesophago-gastric cancer.

The single agents most commonly used in the treatment of advanced gastric cancer include 5FU, methotrexate, mitomycin C, the anthracyclines doxorubicin and epirubicin, cisplatin and etoposide. More recently the oral 5FU pro-drugs such as UFT, the taxane drugs, irinotecan and gemcitabine have all featured in new phase II studies.

The FAM regimen (5FU, doxorubicin and mitomycin) initially seemed to have a high response rate of 40%.[69] However in the setting of a randomised trial by the North Central Cancer Treatment Group, seemed to be no better than 5FU alone.[70] In an attempt to modulate the activity of 5FU within the FAM regimen, high-dose methotrexate was given 1 hour before the 5FU in the FAMTX regimen (fluorouracil, doxorubicin and methotrexate). Klein produced impressive results in a study of 100 patients.[71] The response rate was 58% with a complete remission rate of 12%. There were only 3% treatment-related deaths and a long-term survival rate of 6%. The response rate seen in subsequent studies was slightly lower but still confirmed acceptable toxicity. This regimen has now been tested against other combinations.

A randomised EORTC trial[72] with 208 evaluable patients demonstrated its superiority against FAM. Median survival was better (42 weeks versus 29 weeks, p = 0.004) with 41% and 9% of the FAMTX patients alive at 1 and 2 years respectively compared with 22% and 0% for FAM patients.

The EAP regimen (etoposide, doxorubicin, cisplatin) was found to produce similar survival rates and overall response rates, but lower complete remission rates and was significantly more toxic.[73] A recent EORTC trial[74] has compared three regimens: FAMTX, ELF (etoposide, leucovorin and bolus 5FU) and FUP (infusional 5FU and cisplatin) in 399 randomised patients. There was no significant difference in median survival between the regimens. The response rates were lower than in some previous trials (ELF 9%, FUP 20%, FAMTX 12%) but this trial had tight objective response criteria and required measurable disease. The conclusion is that they all produce modest response with comparable survival and toxicity.

The ECF regimen developed at The Royal Marsden Hospital has been shown to have high activity against advanced oesophagogastric cancer,[12] and it has thus become widely used in the United Kingdom. It requires central venous access with a Hickman line; prophylactic warfarin is potentially of value to reduce the thrombotic complication rate. A portable pump delivers the PVI 5FU. The patient requires admission every 3 weeks for epirubicin and cisplatin.

It is well tolerated. Its status as a current gold standard was confirmed in a multi-centre randomised trial of ECF against FAMTX.[75]

A total of 274 patients with adenocarcinoma or undifferentiated carcinoma of the oesophagus, oesophago-gastric junction or stomach were treated. Patients were predominantly of good performance status with a median age of 60 years.

The overall objective response rate was 45% in the ECF arm and 21% in the FAMTX arm (p = 0.0002).

The response of locally advanced disease to ECF has previously been shown to be higher than in metastatic disease.[12] This was confirmed in both arms of the trial (56% ECF versus 23% FAMTX). Of the 121 patients receiving ECF, 10 were able to undergo a resection due to improved status, 6 of whom remain disease free. There were three cases of histological pCR. Only 5% of patients had progression while on either chemotherapy.

The 2-year survival figures and median survival were 14% and 8.7 months for ECF and 5% and 6.1 months for FAMTX respectively (p = 0.03).

The ECF results have opened up a grey area in locally advanced gastric and junctional cancer management. While a patient may not be operable, or it may be deemed inadvisable to operate because of the extent of disease at presentation, it may be possible to consider a potentially curative resection in some cases after chemotherapy. The intent of treatment may therefore need to be revisited by close reassessment after chemotherapy. This emphasises the need for teamwork between the surgeon and oncologist within a multidisciplinary setting. It will take the results of the MAGIC trial to show if it should become standard neo-adjuvant treatment.

In a recent study from Leeds[76] in advanced upper gastrointestinal patients, oral UFT and leucovorin have been substituted for the PVI 5FU in ECF in an attempt to create a more practical, acceptable and cheaper alternative (the ECU regimen) without the need for central lines and pumps. In this dose escalation pilot study 30 patients were treated with acceptable toxicity. Out of 20 assessable patients, 9 out of the 15 with gastro-oesophageal cancer had objective response and 2 of these were complete radiological responses indicating that this deserves further consideration for future randomised studies.

Palliative radiotherapy

External-beam radiotherapy

The literature in the field of radiotherapy in this area is not evidence based in the manner of the preceding sections. The role of radiotherapy in palliation is important however. There are many instances where patients have local symptoms from metastatic disease. As patients receive more chemotherapy, CRT and surgery there is a hope that patients will have longer survivals. With a high proportion of patients presenting with T3N1 disease it is not surprising that many will fail despite more complex and aggressive therapy. The pattern of metastases seems already to be changing in that patients are living to get metastases in brain, bone, skin as well as recurrent nodal masses. These are all amenable to short fractionated radiotherapy treatment and will often see symptom resolution.

The role of external-beam radiotherapy in treating dysphagia has changed with the ready availability of oesophageal stents. Radiotherapy can be very effective in relieving dysphagia but this may take weeks and can even temporarily worsen symptoms with radiation oesophagitis. The role of radiotherapy following successful stent placement is unproven. A UK trial has been proposed, largely to explore the possibility of improvements in survival and symptom-free survival. The attraction is in achieving a measure of local disease control and in treating the mediastinum.

There is a major difference between the fractionation regimens used in the United States and in the UK. 'Palliative' doses of 40–60 Gy in 4–6 weeks are quoted in the US literature. These are in the radical dose range and felt to be inappropriate for UK practice; doses of 20–30 Gy in 1 or 2 weeks are more likely to be used. These can be combined with brachytherapy. Good resolution of tumour and symptom relief in a majority of patients has been reported.[77] Whichever palliative technique is used first, however, other modalities often have a role for patients with longer survival in order to maintain swallowing.

Brachytherapy

Brachytherapy involves the placement of a high–dose rate radioactive source, usually [192]iridium, down the oesophagus in proximity to the tumour. The aim is to get direct tumour-cell kill, thereby relieving dysphagia, or in the case of its use as a boost to external beam radiotherapy, to achieve an increased dose to the tumour with minimal dose to surrounding normal tissues. It does not require a general anaesthetic and can be done as a day-case procedure. Occasionally placement of a nasogastric guide tube is required under endoscopic vision. Pagliero and Rowlands[78] describe a single dose of 15 Gy with a response rate of about 60% measured at 6 weeks from treatment; the dose can be repeated in case of symptomatic relapse.

The optimum dose of brachytherapy has been addressed in a randomised trial using three schedules.[79] Three doses and schedules were tested in 172 patients with advanced oesophageal cancer; these were 12 Gy/2 fractions (A), 16 Gy/2 (B) fractions, and 18 Gy/3 (C) fractions.

Patients were assessed for relief of dysphagia and survival. Dose and tumour length were found to be significant for survival on multivariate analysis. Brachytherapy dose had a significant effect on tumour control. Overall survival for the whole group was 19.4% at 1 year. The survival by group, although not statistically significant, suggests a trend towards better outcomes with the higher dose schedules (at 12 months: A = 9.8%, B = 22.5%, C = 35.3%). There are good published guidelines[80] for the use of brachytherapy that take into account the wide range of possible applications for this technique.

Future directions

In order to achieve the best outcomes for patients, assessment, staging and treatment need to be closely coordinated and integrated in a multidisciplinary setting. Poor outcomes from single modality therapy and increasing evidence of the value of a selective use of multiple modalities will be powerful drivers towards higher quality and more centralised services. Site-specialist clinicians and support services can only meet demands for quality assurance in all possible modalities of treatment with appropriate resources and infrastructure. The essential role of high-quality radiology, including endoscopic ultrasound and expert pathology, cannot be underestimated. Support services such as specialist nursing and dietetic services are particularly important in this area of disease management.

If the lessons from past trials are to be learnt – namely the poor and variable results in control-arm treatments – attention will have to be paid to rigorous quality assurance within each area of defined treatment. This will aid the process of new high-quality research trials aiming to develop new treatment strategies.

There are huge changes in the technology available for radiotherapy treatment. The development of 3D and conformal radiotherapy treatment planning systems directly linked to spiral CT data allows the shape of radiotherapy fields to be individually tailored to an irregularly shaped target volume. In order for this to be successful, however, reliable imaging techniques are essential; by this means a reduction in normal tissue damage and so potentially the toxicity of combining therapy such as CRT and surgery together will be reduced. The ability to define varying dose intensity within a radiotherapy field (intensity modulated radiotherapy treatment – IMRT) may be helpful in being able to grade the dose between a primary tumour and its associated nodal areas.

Improved methods of delivering conventional drugs such as infusional 5FU can give improved response rates with reduced toxicity. New drugs are becoming available, in particular oral 5FU analogues, irinotecan, oxaliplatin and the taxane drugs. These may all have a role in the treatment of oesophago-gastric cancer. Problems in the literature with myelosuppression and in particular toxic deaths may be avoided by the use of growth factors to reduce the incidence of neutropenic sepsis. Many of the problems of severe emesis have already been improved by the use of 5HT3 drugs such as ondansetron and granisetron.

There are important questions to be answered in the method in which different modalities are integrated. The optimum timing of surgery following chemoradiotherapy or chemotherapy has not been defined and may be very important in determining increased morbidity associated with multiple modality therapy. The institution of early nutritional support for patients undergoing prolonged neo-adjuvant therapy will need to be addressed.

As chemoradiotherapy emerges as an alternative to radical surgery, particularly in squamous carcinoma, accurately predicting and defining those patients who will achieve good remission prospectively is important, as is the identification of patients who require salvage surgery. New molecular markers may also be important tools for the future.

The need for quick assessment by site-specialist teams who are able to offer a full range of treatments – from complex combined modality therapy all the way through to quick and efficient palliative care – is only likely to be achieved by teamwork and some degree of reorganisation. Ultimately, an improved understanding of the epidemiology of these diseases will be necessary to allow their identification at a much earlier stage. The current presentation with predominantly nodal and advanced stage disease is likely to limit the improvements that are possible with existing treatments.

The need for continued randomised trials is important. Major centres with high quality assurance and good research support can recruit sufficient patients to answer major questions that are important to improve the outcome for these diseases. The Australasian randomised study of preoperative chemoradiation versus surgery alone is likely to be helpful in answering at least one question. The inclusion in new protocols of a surgery-alone control now seems to be highly unlikely in the United States or United Kingdom settings.

References

1. Bartels HE, Stein HJ, Siewert JR. Preoperative risk analysis and postoperative mortality of oesophagectomy for resectable oesophageal cancer. Br J Surg 1998; 85:840–4.

2. Nigro ND, Seydel HG, Considine B *et al*. Combined preoperative radiation and chemotherapy for squamous cell carcinoma of the anal canal. Cancer 1983; 51:1826–9.

3. Northover JM. Epidermoid cancer of the anus – the surgeon retreats. J R Soc Med 1991; 84:389–90.

4. Swedish Rectal Cancer Trial. Improved survival with preoperative radiotherapy in respectable rectal cancer. N Engl J Med 1997; 336:980–7.

5. Gignoux M, Roussel A, Paillot B *et al*. The value of preoperative radiotherapy in esophageal cancer: results of the EORTC. World J Surg 1987; 11:426–32.

6. Nygaard K, Hagen S, Hansen HS *et al*. Pre-operative radiotherapy prolongs survival in operable esophageal carcinoma: a randomized, multicentre study of pre-operative radiotherapy and chemotherapy. The Second Scandinavian Trial in Esophageal Cancer. World J Surg 1992; 16:1104–10.

7. Arnott SJ, Duncan W, Kerr GR *et al*. Low-dose preoperative radiotherapy for carcinoma of the oesophagus: results of a randomized clinical trial. Radiother Oncol 1992; 24:108–13.

8. Arnott SJ, Duncan W, Gignoux M *et al*. Preoperative radiotherapy in esophageal carcinoma: A meta-analysis using individual patient data (Oesophageal Cancer Collaborative Group). Int J Radiat Oncol Biol Phys 1998; 41:579–83.

9. Teniere P, Hay J, Fingethut A *et al*. Postoperative radiation therapy does not increase survival after curative resection for squamous carcinoma of the middle and lower oesophagus as shown by a multicenter controlled trial. Surg Gynaecol Obstet 1991; 173:123–30.

10. Fok M, Sham JST, Choy D *et al*. Postoperative radiotherapy for carcinoma of the esophagus: A prospective randomized controlled trial. Surgery 1993; 113:138–47.

11. Schlag PM. Randomized trial of preoperative chemotherapy of squamous cell cancer of the esophagus. Arch Surg 1992; 127:1446–50.

12. Bamias A, Hill ME, Cunningham D *et al*. Epirubicin, cisplatin and protracted venous infusion of 5-fluorouracil for esophagogastric adenocarcinoma. Cancer 1996; 77:1978–85.

13. Andreyev HJN, Norman AR, Cunningham D *et al*. Squamous oesophageal cancer can be downstaged using protracted venous infusion of 5-fluorouracil with epirubicin and cisplatin (ECF). Eur J Cancer 1995; 31A:2209–14.

14. Roth JA, Pass HI, Flanagan MM *et al*. Randomized clinical trial of preoperative and postoperative adjuvant chemotherapy with cisplatin, vindesine and bleomycin for carcinoma of the esophagus. J Thorac Cardiovasc Surg 1988; 96:242–8.

15. Bhansali MS, Vaidya JS, Bhatt RG *et al*. Chemotherapy for carcinoma of the oesophagus: a comparison of evidence from meta-analyses of randomized trials and of historical control studies. Ann Oncol 1996; 7:355–9.

16. Kok TC, Lanschot JV, Siersema PD *et al*. for the Rotterdam Esophageal Tumor Study Group. Neoadjuvant chemotherapy in operable esophageal squamous cell cancer: final report of a phase III multicenter randomized controlled trial. Proc Am Soc Clin Oncol 1997; 16:A277.

17. Kelsen DP, Ginsberg R, Pajak TF *et al*. Chemotherapy followed by surgery compared with surgery alone for localized esophageal cancer. N Engl J Med 1998; 339:1979–84.

18. MRC Upper GI Tract Cancer Group. Medical Research Council (MRC) randomised phase III trial of surgery with or without pre-operative chemotherapy in resectable cancer of the oesophagus. Br J Cancer 2000; 83 (Suppl 1):1.

19. Geh IJ, Crellin AM, Glynne-Jones R. A Review of the role of preoperative (neoadjuvant) chemoradiotherapy in oesophageal carcinoma. Br J Surg (in press).

20. Urba SG, Orringer MB, Perez-Tamayo C *et al.* Concurrent preoperative chemotherapy and radiation therapy in localized esophageal adenocarcinoma. Cancer 1992; 69:285–91.

21. Bosset JF, Gignoux M, Triboulet JP *et al.* Chemoradiotherapy followed by surgery compared with surgery alone in squamous-cell cancer of the esophagus. N Engl J Med 1997; 337:161–7.

22. MacKean J, Burmeister BH, Lamb DS *et al.* Concurrent chemoradiation for oesophageal cancer: factors influencing myelotoxicity. Australa Radio 1996; 40:424–9.

23. Minsky BD, Neuberg D, Kelsen DP *et al.* Final report of Intergroup trial 0122 (ECOG PE-289, RTOG 90-12): phase II trial of neoadjuvant chemotherapy plus concurrent chemotherapy and high-dose radiation for squamous cell carcinoma of the esophagus. Int J Radiat Oncol Biol Phys 1999; 43:517–23.

24. Bartels HE, Stein HJ, Siewert JR. Tracheobronchial lesions following oesophagectomy: prevalence, predisposing factors and outcome. Br J Surg 1998; 85:403–6.

25. Mandard AM, Dalibard F, Mandard JC *et al.* Pathologic assessment of tumor regression after preoperative chemoradiotherapy of esophageal carcinoma. Cancer 1994; 73:2680–6.

26. Forastiere AA, Orringer MB, Perez-Tamayo C *et al.* Preoperative chemoradiation followed by transhiatal esophagectomy for carcinoma of the esophagus: final report. J Clin Oncol 1993; 11:1118–23.

27. Smithers BM, Devitt P, Jamieson GG *et al.* A combined modality approach to the management of oesophageal cancer. Eur J Surg Oncol 1997; 23:219–23.

28. Vogel SB, Mendenhall WM, Sombeck MD *et al.* Downstaging of esophageal cancer after preoperative radiation and chemotherapy. Ann Surg 1995; 221:685–95.

29. Bates BA, Detterbeck FC, Bernard SA *et al.* Concurrent radiation therapy and chemotherapy followed by esophagectomy for localized esophageal carcinoma. J Clin Oncol 1996; 14:156–63.

30. Triboulet JP, Amrouni H, Guillem P *et al.* Long-term results of resected esophageal cancer with complete remission to pre-operative chemoradiation. Ann Chir 1998; 52:503–8.

31. Le Prise E, Etienne PL, Meunier B *et al.* A randomized study of chemotherapy, radiation therapy, and surgery versus surgery for localized squamous cell carcinoma of the esophagus. Cancer 1994; 73:1779–84.

32. Apinop C, Puttisak P, Preecha N. A prospective study of combined therapy in esophageal cancer. Hepato-Gastroenterol 1994; 41:391–3.

33. Walsh TN, Noonan N, Hollywood D *et al.* A comparison of multimodal therapy and surgery for esophageal adenocarcinoma. N Engl J Med 1996; 335:462–7.

34. Urba S, Orringer M, Turrisi A *et al.* A randomized trial comparing surgery (S) to preoperative concomitant chemoradiation plus surgery in patients (pts) with resectable esophageal cancer (CA): updated analysis. Proc Am Soc Clin Oncol 1997; 16:277.

35. Macdonald JS, Smalley S, Benedetti J *et al.* Postoperative combined radiation and chemotherapy improves disease-free survival (DFS) and overall survival (OS) in resected adenocarcinoma of the stomach and GE junction. Results of Intergroup Study INT-0116 (SWOG 9008). Proc Am Soc Clin Oncol 2000; 19:A1.

36. Earlam R, Cunha-Melo JR. Oesophageal squamous cell carcinoma: I. A critical review of radiotherapy. Br J Surg 1980; 67:457–61.

37. Sykes AJ, Burt PA, Slevin NJ *et al.* Radical radiotherapy for carcinoma of the oesophagus: an effective alternative to surgery. Radiother Oncol 1998; 48:15–21.

38. Araujo CM, Souhami L, Gil RA *et al.* A randomized trial comparing radiation therapy versus concomitant radiation therapy and chemotherapy in carcinoma of the thoracic esophagus. Cancer 1991; 67 (9):2258–61.

39. Coia LR, Engstrom PF, Paul AR *et al.* Long-term results of infusional 5-FU, mitomycin-C, and radiation as primary management of esophageal cancer. Int J Radiation Oncology Biol Phys 1991; 20:29–36.

40. Al-Sarraf M, Martz K, Herskovic A *et al.* Progress report of combined chemoradiotherapy versus radiotherapy alone in patients with esophageal cancer: an Intergroup study. J Clin Oncol 1997; 15:277–84.

41. Minsky BD, Neuberg D, Kelsen DP *et al.* Neoadjuvant chemotherapy plus high-dose radiation for squamous cell carcinoma of the esophagus: a preliminary analysis of the phase II intergroup trial 0122. J Clin Oncol 1996; 14 (1):149–55.

42. Gaspar LE, Qian C, Kocha WI *et al.* A Phase I/II study of external beam radiation, brachytherapy and concurrent chemotherapy in localized cancer of the esophagus (RTOG 92–07): Preliminary toxicity report. Int J Radiation Oncology Biol Phys 1997; 37 (3):593–99.

43. Raoul JL, Le Prise E, Meunier B *et al.* Neoadjuvant chemotherapy and hyperfractionated radiotherapy with concurrent low-dose chemotherapy for squamous cell esophageal carcinoma. Int J Radiation Biol Phys 1998; 42:29–34.

44. Crellin AM, Sebag-Montefiore D, Martin I *et al.* Preoperative chemotherapy and radiotherapy, plus excision (CARE): A phase II study in esophageal cancer. Proc Am Soc Clin Oncol 2000; 19:A1128.

45. Chan A, Wong A. Is combined chemotherapy and radiation therapy equally effective as surgical resection in localized esophageal carcinoma. Int J Radiation Oncology Biol Phys 1999; 45 (2):265–70.

46. Murakami M, Kuroda Y, Nakajima T *et al.* Comparison between chemoradiation protocol intended for organ preservation and conventional surgery for clinical T1–T2 esophageal carcinoma. Int J Radiation Oncology Biol Phys 1999; 45 (2):277–84.

47. Wilson KS, Lim JT. Primary chemotherapy-radiotherapy and selective oesophagectomy for oesophageal cancer: goal of cure with organ preservation. Radiother Oncol 2000; 54:129–34.

48. Ribiero U, Finklestein SD, Safatle-Ribiero A *et al.* P53 sequence predicts treatment response and outcome of patients with esophageal carcinoma. Cancer 1998; 83:7–18.

49. Yamamoto M, Tsujinaka T, Shiozaki H *et al.* Metallothionein expression correlates with the pathological response of patients with esophageal cancer undergoing preoperative chemoradiation therapy. Oncology 1999; 56:332–7.

50. Jones DR, Parker LA, Detterbeck FC *et al.* Inadequacy of computed tomography in assessing patients with esophageal carcinoma after induction chemoradiotherapy. Cancer 1999; 85:1026–32.

51. Giovannini M, Seitz JF, Thomas P *et al.* Endoscopic ultrasonography for assessment of the response to combined radiation therapy and chemotherapy in patients with esophageal cancer. Endoscopy 1997; 29:4–9.

52. Mallery S, DeCamp M, Bueno R *et al.* Pretreatment staging by endoscopic ultrasonography does not predict complete response to neoadjuvant chemoradiation in patients with esophageal carcinoma. Cancer 1999; 86:764–9.

53. Coia LR, Soffen EM, Schultheiss TE *et al.* Swallowing function in patients with esophageal cancer treated with concurrent radiation and chemotherapy. Cancer 1993; 71:281–6.

54. O'Rourke IC, Tiver K, Bull C *et al.* Swallowing performance after radiation therapy for carcinoma of the esophagus. Cancer 1988; 61:2022–26.

55. Douglass HO, Stabelein DM, Bruckner HM *et al.* Controlled trial of adjuvant chemotherapy following curative resection for gastric cancer. The Gastrointestinal Tumour Study Group. Cancer 1982; 49:1116–22.

56. Engstrom PF, Laqvin PT, Douglass HO *et al.* Postoperative adjuvant 5-fluorouracil and methyl-CCNU therapy for gastric cancer patients. Eastern Cooperative Oncology Group study. Cancer 1985; 55:1868–73.

57. Higgins GA, Amadeo JH, Smith DE *et al.* Efficacy of prolonged intermittent therapy with combined 5-FU and methyl-CCNU following resection for gastric carcinoma. A Veterans Administration Surgical Oncology Group Report. Cancer 1983; 52:1105–12.

58. Cunningham D, Soukop M, McArdle CS *et al.* Advanced gastric cancer: experience in Scotland using FAM. Br J Surg 1984; 71:673–6.

59. Coombes RC, Schein PS, Chilvers CE *et al.* A randomized trial comparing adjuvant 5-fluoro-uracil, doxorubicin and mitomycin C with no treatment in operable gastric cancer. International Collaborative Cancer Group. J Clin Oncol 1990; 8:1362–9.

60. Hallissey MT, Dunn JA, Ward LC *et al.* The second British Stomach Cancer Group trial of adjuvant radiotherapy or chemotherapy in resectable gastric cancer: five-year follow-up. Lancet 1994; 343:1309–12.

61. Hattori T, Inokuchi K, Taguchi T *et al.* Postoperative adjuvant chemotherapy for gastric cancer: the second report. Analysis of data on 2873 patients followed for 5 years. Jpn J Surg 1986; 16:175–80.

62. Nakajima T, Nashimoto A, Kitamura M *et al.* Adjuvant mitomycin and fluorouracil followed by oral uracil plus tegafur in serosa-negative gastric cancer: a randomised trial. Gastric Cancer Surgical Study Group. Lancet 1999; 354 (9175):273–7.

63. Cicera L, Balil A, Batiste-Alentorn *et al.* Randomized clinical trial of adjuvant mitomycin plus tegafur in patients with resected stage III gastric cancer. J Clin Oncol 1999; 17:3810–15.

64. Hermans J, Bonenkamp JJ, Ban MC *et al.* Adjuvant therapy after curative resection for gastric cancer: meta-analysis of randomized trials. J Clin Oncol 1993; 11:1441–7.

65. Earle CC, Maroun JA. Adjuvant chemotherapy after curative resection for gastric cancer in non-Asian patients: revisiting a meta-analysis of randomised trials. Eur J Cancer 1999; 35 (7):1059–64.

66. Hagiwara A, Takahashi T, Kojima O *et al.* Prophylaxis with carbon-adsorbed mitomycin against peritoneal recurrence of gastric cancer. Lancet 1992; 339 (8794):629–31.

67. Rosen HR, Jatzko G, Repse S *et al.* Adjuvant intraperitoneal chemotherapy with carbon-adsorbed mitomycin in patients with gastric cancer: results of a randomized multicenter trial of the Austrian Working Group for Surgical Oncology. J Clin Oncol 1998; 16 (8):2733–8.

68. Bleiberg H, Jacob JH, Bedenne L *et al.* A randomized phase II trial of 5-fluorouracil (5FU) and cisplatin (DDP) versus DDP alone in advanced esophageal cancer. Proc Soc Clin Oncol 1991; 10:A447.

69. Macdonald J, Schein P, Woolley P *et al.* 5-fluorouracil, doxorubicin and mitomycin (FAM) combination chemotherapy for advanced gastric cancer. Ann Intern Med 1980; 93:533–36.

70. Cullinan S, Moertel C, Fleming T *et al.* A comparison of three chemotherapeutic regimens in the treatment of advanced pancreatic and gastric cancer. JAMA 1985; 253:2061–67.

71. Klein HO. Long term results with FAMTX (5-fluorouracil, adriamycin, methotrexate) in advanced gastric cancer. Cancer Res 1989; 9:1025.

72. Wils JA, Klein HO, Wegener DJT *et al*. Sequential high-dose methotrexate and fluorouracil combined with doxorubicin: a step ahead in the treatment of advanced gastric cancer: A trial of the European Organisation for Research and Treatment of Cancer Gastrointestinal Tract Cooperative Group. J Clin Oncol 1991; 9:827.

73. Kelsen D, Atiq O, Saltz L *et al*. FAMTX versus etoposide doxorubicin and cisplatin: a random assignment in gastric cancer. J Clin Oncol 1992; 10:541–48.

74. Vanhoefer U, Rougier P, Wilke H *et al*. Final results of a randomized phase III trial of sequential high-dose methotrexate, fluorouracil, and doxorubicin versus etoposide, leucovorin, and fluorouracil versus infusional fluorouracil and cisplatin in advanced gastric cancer: A trial of the European Organization for Research and Treatment of Cancer Gastrointestinal Tract Cooperative Group. J Clin Oncol 2000; 18:2648–57.

75. Webb A, Cunningham D, Scarffe JH *et al*. Randomized trial comparing epirubicin, cisplatin and fluorouracil versus fluorouracil, doxorubicin, and methotrexate in advanced esophagogastric cancer. J Clin Oncol 1997; 15:261–67.

76. Seymour MT, Dent JT, Papamichael D *et al*. Epirubicin, cisplatin and oral UFT with leucovorin (ECU): a phase I-II study in patients with advanced upper gastrointestinal tract cancer. Annals of Oncology 1999; 10 (11):1329–33.

77. Dawes PJDK, Clague MB, Dean EM. Combined external beam and intracavitary radiotherapy for carcinoma of the oesophagus. Brachytherapy 2 Proceedings of the 5th International Selectron users' meeting 1988. Nucleotron International, 1989; 442–4.

78. Pagliero KM, Rowlands CG. The place of brachytherapy in the treatment of carcinoma of the oesophagus. Brachytherapy HDR and LDR. Proceedings of a brachytherapy meeting: remote afterloading; state of the art. Nucleotron Corporation 1990; 44–51.

79. Sur RK, Donde B, Levin VC *et al*. Fractionated high dose rate brachytherapy in palliation of advanced esophageal cancer. Int J Radiation Oncology Biol Phys 1998; 40 (2):447–53.

80. Gaspar LE, Nag S, Hersokic A *et al*. American Brachytherapy Society (ABS) consensus guidelines for brachytherapy of esophageal cancer. Int J Radiation Oncology Biol Phys 1997; 38 (1):127–32.

8 Palliative treatments of carcinoma of the oesophagus and stomach

Jane M. Blazeby
Derek Alderson

INTRODUCTION

Despite improvements in the detection of oesophageal and gastric cancer the majority of European and American patients still present with advanced disease. Palliative treatments are therefore aimed at lessening the severity of symptoms with minimum morbidity and mortality and maximum quality of life until death occurs. Palliation, despite not having any curative effect on the disease itself, can prolong life especially where relief of dysphagia or gastric outflow obstruction leads to improved nutrition. This chapter concentrates on palliative treatments designed to alleviate symptoms and maintain quality of life in patients with oesophageal and gastric cancer.

Epidemiology and survival

Accurate information about the proportion of patients with oesophageal and gastric cancer who are treated with palliative intent is difficult to obtain. This is because of variations in selection of patients for treatment and because few reported series include consecutive new patients.

Series published from both the East and West show oesophagectomy rates vary between 13 and 85%.[1,2] In 1990 Müller *et al.* published a critical overview of surgery for oesophageal cancer.[3] The outcomes from 1201 papers on the surgical treatment for oesophageal carcinoma were reviewed using a specially designed scoring system. The resectability rate (69 authors) was just 21%. A general statement on resectability could not be made. Variations were thought to reflect situations in particular hospitals, preselection of referrals and surgical attitudes. In any event, most oesophagectomies will prove to be palliative because occult metastatic disease spread was not identifiable at the outset.

Patients with oesophageal cancer selected for palliative treatment have a median survival of 4–6 months and few survive beyond 1 year. Palliative restoration of swallowing is the first priority of treatment to avoid respiratory complications and allow adequate nutrition. This prevents early death, but despite better methods of relieving the obstructed oesophageal lumen, survival advantages have not been proven. Some claim longer survival with combination treatment: external-beam radiotherapy and brachytherapy, chemoradiation, laser and brachytherapy, intubation, chemotherapy or external-beam radiotherapy.[4,5,6,7,8,9,10,11] The addition of external-beam radiotherapy to brachytherapy, laser treatment or intubation has theoretical advantages because deeper tumour penetration may have occurred. Large randomised trials testing this hypothesis have yet to be performed, and small studies (which lack power) have generally failed to support this assumption. A single prospective non-randomised study comparing laser therapy alone to laser therapy with chemotherapy has demonstrated a significant improvement in dysphagia score and survival in the combination group.[8]

The resection rate for patients with gastric cancer is far greater than for oesophageal cancer, because although most patients in the Western hemisphere have widespread disease at presentation, palliative gastrectomy can probably be undertaken with low morbidity and perioperative mortality.[12,13] Rates of total gastrectomy and lymphadenectomy may reflect the proportion of patients treated with curative intent but this is not a standard surgical technique in many centres in the United Kingdom. Most patients are node positive and probably 80% or more of new patients with gastric cancer receive palliative surgery or other palliative treatment.

The median survival for patients with gastric cancer undergoing palliative treatment is poor; 50% of patients die within 6 months of diagnosis and the remainder within 2 years.

There is little evidence to show that surgery or other palliative treatments change the outcome for patients with advanced gastric cancer although increasing interest has centred on the role of chemotherapy.

One small phase III study comparing best supportive care with combination chemotherapy found a significant survival difference between the two groups (3 and 12 months respectively).[14]

The two factors other than disease stage and age which appear to influence survival in patients with oesophageal and gastric cancer are severity of dysphagia and performance status at diagnosis. Derodra et al. showed that patients presenting with dysphagia to solid foods and liquids lived significantly longer than those presenting with complete dysphagia (9 weeks and 3 weeks respectively).[15] This retrospective series only included patients referred to a specialist endoscopy unit and thus patients without dysphagia but with haematogenous disease spread (e.g. liver metastases) were not included in the analysis. Pretreatment performance scores have been shown to predict outcome in patients with advanced oesophageal cancer.[6] This has been clearly demonstrated in other disease groups and performance scores probably reflect disease burden.[16]

Selection of patients for palliative treatment

After establishing a diagnosis, new patients require careful assessment to decide whether treatment is directed towards attempting a cure or if palliation of symptoms is more appropriate. Careful patient selection has been shown to significantly influence results.[1,17] Principal factors are: whether the patient is fit enough to tolerate the procedure; stage and characteristics of the tumour; and consideration of patient preferences.

Fitness for treatment

The place of oesophagectomy in many older patients is often quite easily settled because of general debilitation or multiple coexistent medical problems. Age in itself does not preclude octogenarians from surgery but most series of older patients are carefully selected. In general, patients who are not fit enough for oesophagectomy are also unable to tolerate a radical course of radiotherapy. On the whole, surgery for gastric tumours is tolerated better than oesophageal surgery by the elderly population, but patients still require careful preoperative assessment before undergoing major palliative resections. Anaesthetic assessment for surgery is considered in more detail in Chapter 4.

Staging investigations

Accurate tumour staging plays a critical part in any therapeutic protocol, enabling patients to be assigned appropriately to treatments with either curative or palliative intent. Clear evidence of haematogenous tumour spread (liver, lung or bone metastases) or irresectability (invasion of the aorta, bronchus or pericardium) directs patients with oesophageal cancer to palliative treatment. Despite advances in staging procedures, no single investigation is perfect and a small percentage of patients still require explorative surgery to determine resectability. Palliative resection or bypass surgery to ameliorate bleeding or obstruction may be indicated for patients with gastric cancer despite the presence of haematogenous tumour spread. The decision to proceed with palliative surgery requires careful consideration as many patients rapidly deteriorate in this situation.

Patient preferences

Public demands for new treatments which are based partly upon levels of information in the public domain are beginning to influence the provision of healthcare services in the management of many malignancies. There is increasing awareness of the variable outcome of treatment for cancer and consequently a growing demand to concentrate care in specialist cancer centres. Although little is known at present about the psychology of patients with oesophageal and gastric cancer, all clinicians will be faced with patients who demand every small chance of cure, despite its risks and others who wish to receive minimal dignified intervention. In view of this, clinical decisions should be made with the patient and their family having access to as much information as they require.

Symptoms and signs of advanced oesophageal and gastric cancer

Tumours of the oesophagus and gastric cardia

Proximal gastric tumours are clinically indistinguishable in their presentation from adenocarcinomas of the oesophago-gastric junction or lower oesophagus:

all produce dysphagia, which is the predominant symptom in 90% of patients. The progressive nature of malignant dysphagia is usually readily apparent. Initial difficulties in swallowing solid food may cause bolus obstruction and odynophagia. Solid food intake gradually reduces and patients may present with inability to swallow even saliva. Complete dysphagia may lead to aspiration pneumonia. About 5% develop an oesophago-respiratory fistula. These cause paroxysmal coughing fits, aspiration and, if untreated, eventually death from recurrent chest infections. They occur either because of spontaneous necrosis of the tumour through the oesophageal wall into the bronchial tree or as a sequel of irradiation, laser therapy, surgery or intubation. They are difficult to treat and patients usually die within a month of development.[18] Less commonly oesophageal tumours present with vomiting, haematemesis or with gastro-oesophageal reflux. Often patients have symptoms of metastatic disease including fatigue, anorexia, upper abdominal pain caused by ascites or liver metastases and constipation. Rapid weight loss frequently occurs because of cancer cachexia exacerbated by poor oral intake. Hoarseness because of tumour infiltration of the recurrent laryngeal nerves may be the result of advanced local disease or mediastinal recurrence after oesophagectomy.

Tumours of the body and distal stomach

Gastric cancer commonly has an insidious presentation. Slow blood loss eventually results in symptoms of anaemia. Tumours of the distal stomach can cause outlet obstruction. Patients may complain of epigastric discomfort, early satiety, gastro-oesophageal reflux and effortless vomiting. Occasionally haematemesis is the first presentation. Early tumours produce no physical signs. The presence of an epigastric mass, supraclavicular lymphadenopathy, jaundice, ascites or pleural effusions all reflect advanced disease. Less commonly bony pain and symptoms of increased intracranial pressure are seen. Other troublesome symptoms are iatrogenic, for example the side effects of high-dose opiates, constipation, dry mouth and bloating. Symptoms of oesophageal and gastric cancer are listed in **Table 8.1**.

The provision of rapid relief of dysphagia or gastric obstruction for patients with advanced oesophageal and gastric malignancies is the main priority of palliative treatment. Patients require dietary advice from nutrition teams and palliative care physicians can assist in mobilising multidisciplinary carers.

Palliative treatments for cancer of the oesophagus and gastric cardia

There is a wide variety of approaches available for the palliation of symptoms of advanced tumours of the oesophagus and gastric cardia. Palliative surgery to relieve dysphagia has poor results if macroscopic tumour is left behind. In the pooled patient study published by Müller *et al.*, palliative resection resulted in 3- and 5-year survival rates of 6% and 2% respectively.[3] Hospital mortality rates were around 10% while 46% had significant postoperative complications. The results of bypass surgery are poor, with mortality rates in the range of 20–35%.[19]

Oesophageal cancer	Gastric cancer	Metastatic disease
Dysphagia	Dysphagia	Upper abdominal pain
Odynophagia	Epigastric fullness/discomfort	Epigastric fullness/discomfort
Reflux	Effortless vomiting	Anorexia
Chest pain	Haematemesis	Bone pain
Haematemesis	Nausea	Constipation
Cough	Reflux	Dyspnoea
Dyspnoea	Symptoms of anaemia	Cough
Hoarseness		Weight loss
		Fatigue

Table 8.1 *Symptoms of oesophageal and gastric cancer*

The only notable exception was the series reported by Mannell *et al.*, where the hospital mortality was only 11%, with 82% of patients having complete and lasting relief from dysphagia.[20] Although palliative resection can relieve dysphagia and prevent problems such as haemorrhage, aspiration and the risk of aero-digestive fistulae, all of these can be addressed by other approaches.

The following section will concentrate on non-resectional palliative methods for treating oesophageal cancer. It is divided into four categories:

1. Methods of relieving luminal obstruction
2. Treatment of aero-digestive fistulae
3. Management of recurrent laryngeal nerve palsy
4. Management of chronic bleeding.

Methods of relieving luminal obstruction

Malignant dysphagia may be relieved by repeated dilatations, endoscopic or open insertion of a stent, tumour ablation with laser, diathermy or argon-beam coagulation, or the injection of cytotoxic substances. Many modalities may be viewed as complementary. No one method or combination is greatly superior to the rest and there is a lack of high-quality evidence supporting most interventions. **Table 8.2** summarises the randomised controlled trials of the palliation of dysphagia.

Dilatation

This is essentially of historical interest. Results are short lived and its role is now reduced to that of a temporary measure prior to definitive management of dysphagia. The incidence of perforation after dilatation is 5–10%.[21] Polyvinyl wire-guided bougies and hydrostatic balloons are most commonly used to dilate a stricture. The comparative efficacy of balloons and bougies has not been studied.

Author	n	Group 1	Group 2	Group 3	Dysphagia	Morbidity
Anderson[73]	40	Laser alone	Plastic tube		No difference	No difference
Barr[9]	40	Laser alone	Laser & plastic tube		No difference	Morbidity higher in Group 2
Low[53]	23	Laser alone	Brachytherapy		No difference	Retreatment more frequent in Group 1
Reed[10]	27	Plastic tube	Plastic tube & DXT	Laser and DXT	No difference	In patient stay longer Group 3 than Group 1. Morbidity less Group 3 than Group 1
Angelini[47]	34	Laser alone	Polidocanol		No difference	No difference
Fuchs[74]	40	Laser, DXT and brachy	Plastic tube		No difference	No difference
Sander[6]	39	Laser alone	Laser and brachy		Group 2 squamous cell better	No difference
Carter[40]	40	Laser alone	Plastic tube		Worse in Group 2	No difference
Knyrim[25]	42	Cook plastic tube	Uncovered Wallstent		No difference	Morbidity and in-patient stay worse in Group 1
Lightdale[43]	218	Laser alone	PDT and argon beam		No difference	Morbidity higher in Group 1
Heier[44]	42	Laser alone	PDT		No difference	No difference
De Palma[27]	39	Cook plastic tube	Uncovered Ultraflex stent		No difference	Morbidity worse in Group 1
Adam[41]	60	Covered Wallstent	Uncovered Ultraflex stent	Laser	Worse in Group 3	Stent migration worse in Group 1
Siersema[26]	75	Medoc Celestin tube	Covered Gianturco stent		No difference	Morbidity and in-patient stay worse in Group 1
Roseveare[28]	31	Atkinson tube	Covered Gianturco stent		Worse in Group 1	No difference
Carazzone[49]	47	Laser alone	Ethanol injection		No difference	More pain in Group 2

Note: No differences in 30-day mortality were reported in all of the above trials.

Table 8.2 Prospective randomised controlled trials of the palliation of malignant dysphagia

Intubation

Intubation is probably the most widely used form of palliation at present. Prostheses should be placed endoscopically or radiologically; there is little place for tube insertion by laparotomy, unless a tumour is found to be irresectable.[22] Endoscopic prosthesis insertion is usually possible under intravenous sedation, although some endoscopists continue to use general anaesthesia. Intravenous sedation requires continual attention to the airway. Saliva and regurgitated fluids should be constantly sucked from the patient to prevent aspiration during the procedure.

Prostheses should not be placed less than 2 cm below the upper oesophageal sphincter because of concerns about proximal migration, laryngeal compression, intractable pain and a globus sensation. Modified plastic prostheses have been used in the cervical oesophagus in small studies with reasonable results.[23] There are reports of metal stents being placed near the upper oesophageal sphincter but positioning of the prosthesis is critical and this has not become standard practice.[24] Relative contraindications are more dependent on operator expertise, but these include total luminal obstruction, non-circumferential tumour growth prohibiting proper anchoring of the prosthesis, almost horizontal orientation of the malignant lumen, prior chemoradiation and multiangulated lesions particularly with tumours at the gastro-oesophageal junction. All these situations render endoscopic intubation hazardous. There are two types of stent available: expanding metal prostheses and non-expanding plastic prostheses.

Non-expanding plastic stents

Plastic endoprostheses are still available but their use is diminishing as expanding metal stents are more easily inserted and avoid the need for wide preliminary dilatation, thus minimising the risk of perforation. Prostheses have an internal diameter of 10–12 mm and an outer diameter of 15–18 mm at the mid-position. After insertion patients experience immediate improvement in swallowing although most remain on a semi-solid diet. The most commonly used prostheses are described below.

1. The KeyMed Atkinson prosthesis (KeyMed Ltd., Southend, UK) has a nylon spring incorporated into its rubber wall to prevent kinking. A shoulder is attached to the distal end to prevent migration.
2. The Medoc-Celestin tube (Medoc Ltd., Tetbury, UK) may be inserted either with the traction or pulsion technique. A proximal inkwell funnel is designed to collect food and prevent distal migration.
3. The Wilson-Cook prosthesis (Wilson-Cook Medical, Winston-Salem, NC) is available in a variety of lengths. A model with a modified proximal funnel is available for placement close to the cricopharyngeus.

Method of insertion

There are many methods of endoscopic insertion of a plastic stent; all are based on the same principles. The most important step is dilatation of the stricture before insertion of the stent. Dilatation can be performed gradually a few days before intubation or just prior to intubation. The number of dilators of increasing diameter depends on the length of the stricture, the degree of narrowing and the tortuosity of the lesion.

Figure 8.1
Three of the most frequently used non-expanding plastic oesophageal stents (left to right): Wilson-Cook, Atkinson and Medoc Celestin prostheses.

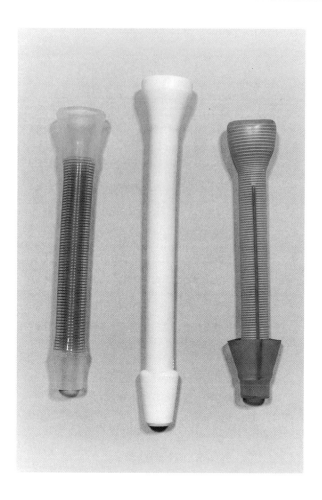

 In all situations, endoscopic guide-wire placement and subsequent dilatation should be performed using fluoroscopy.

A luminal diameter of at least 15 mm is required to accommodate a prosthesis. Some scirrhous malignancies require dilatation to 20 mm. After adequate dilatation the exact measurement of the tumour from the incisors is determined endoscopically and the location point for the proximal funnel edge is marked on the introducer tube. Proximal and distal extents of the tumour may be marked with radio-opaque skin markers or the tumour limitations injected with contrast. The selected tube is then placed on to a supporting device which is passed over the guide-wire to the predetermined position, confirmed by screening. The prosthesis should now be seated properly with its funnel located above the proximal margin of the tumour. With the tube in position, the introducing device is disconnected and withdrawn. The endoscope is then carefully reinserted to check the position of the prosthesis.

Postoperative management

After stent insertion the patient must be instructed to sit upright. Clinical and radiological examination should be performed to exclude perforation before oral fluids are commenced. Patients should receive written dietary information with advice to chew food carefully and drink regularly during and after meals. A daily intake of 10 ml hydrogen peroxide 20 vol. is sometimes recommended.

Complications

Even in experienced hands, intubation with plastic tubes has a complication rate that may be as high as 40%. The procedure-related mortality ranges from 3–16%. Complications are listed in **Table 8.3**.

1. Malposition requires repositioning or removal of the stent.
2. Chest pain may last for several days. It is important to ensure that it does not result from a small perforation.
3. Oesophageal perforation, the most serious complication, is more likely after radiotherapy/chemotherapy or if the tumour is sharply angulated or extensively encases the oesophagus. Rapid development of subcutaneous emphysema, severe pain or radiological evidence of pneumo-mediastinum, air under the diaphragm or a pleural effusion should raise suspicion. Diagnosis is confirmed by contrast radiography. The most appropriate form of therapy depends on the time of detection. If recognised at endoscopy, the insertion of a prosthesis may seal off the perforation and prevent mediastinitis. Alternatively, the procedure may be abandoned and conservative treatment undertaken. This involves administration of broad-spectrum antibiotics, cessation of oral intake and feeding either parenterally or by jejunostomy. An intercostal drain may need to be inserted if there is evidence of pleural contamination. Specific management of this serious complication is covered in detail in Chapter 14.
4. Severe upper gastrointestinal haemorrhage occasionally occurs. This is difficult to treat and supportive measures only may be possible.
5. Early migration occurs in about 1% of patients. Tubes may be left in the stomach although obstruction of the pyloric channel or intestinal perforation necessitates removal at laparotomy.

Early complications	Late complications
Malposition	Migration
Incomplete expansion*	Tumour ingrowth* or overgrowth
Pain	Food bolus obstruction
Perforation	Reflux
Bleeding	Late perforation–fistulation
Migration	Disintegration of prosthesis
Aspiration pneumonia	Stent torsion*
	Bleeding
	Continued eating difficulties

*Specific to metal stents

Table 8.3 *Complications of stent insertion*

Late complications

Late complications occur in at least 20% of patients. They require hospital admission, further endoscopic manoeuvres and occasionally replacement of the prosthesis.

1. Late-distal stent migration has been reported in 7–14%. Patients present with recurrent dysphagia, and a new prosthesis or an alternative method of recanalisation is required.
2. Prostheses may block because of tumour overgrowth at either end of the stent. It may be treated by thermal methods or insertion of another stent within the prosthesis.
3. Food bolus obstruction leads to recurrent dysphagia. Atkinson tubes, which have a narrow diameter, may be more prone to this problem. It is easily dealt with by passage of a paediatric endoscope up and down the tube displacing the impacted food bolus into the stomach. Ogilvie found that food blockage tended to occur more often in tubes over 10 cm in length.[22]
4. Reflux of gastric acid occurs in all patients whenever the tube crosses the gastro-oesophageal junction. It may lead to oesophagitis and occasionally benign stricture formation above the tube. This can be controlled by conservative measures, dilatation and acid suppressive therapy.
5. Pressure necrosis and late oesophageal perforation can occur at the funnel edge of the tube in an area either invaded by tumour or previously irradiated. It is made worse by marked angulation between the oesophagus and prosthesis. This causes pain and may lead to the formation of a mediastinal fistula.
6. Prostheses may deteriorate and disintegrate, although this is rare as most patients do not live long enough. If this occurs the prosthesis needs to be changed to prevent potentially serious complications of disintegration and fracture of the prosthetic tube which in turn may lead to small bowel ulceration and perforation. Endoscopic removal may be achieved by inserting a Wilson-Cook balloon repositioner or a 'through the scope balloon' inside the tube, inflating it and then pulling it out. Other methods have been described, using rat-toothed forceps, polypectomy snares or with the distal end of the scope sharply bent to act as a hook. Operative removal of these tubes is only very occasionally required.
7. Eating difficulties exist due to incomplete relief of dysphagia. Once a prosthesis is in place all food must pass through a rigid tube with a small diameter. Most plastic tubes allow only 10% of patients to eat normally; 50% manage a semi-solid diet while the remainder only drink liquids.[22]

Despite the associated morbidity, the immediate relief of dysphagia in one endoscopy session has made intubation an attractively simple palliative treatment. Expanding metal stents have been introduced to try and overcome the problems associated with dilatation and semi-rigid stent insertion.

Expanding metal stents

Metal stents were first used to palliate malignant dysphagia in 1990. It is claimed that they have numerous advantages compared with plastic tubes although they cost about 10 times more.

The theoretical advantages of metal stents include ease of insertion and a low immediate complication rate because less preinsertion dilatation is required. The stents rapidly relieve dysphagia and have a large internal luminal diameter (16–25 mm compared with 7–12 mm for plastic tubes). There is still a lack of evidence supporting these hypotheses. Four randomised studies comparing metal and plastic stents have been performed.[25,26,27,28] These small studies report a significant reduction in complications and mortality with metal stents. All but one study found that relief of dysphagia is similar with both types of stents. There are an accumulating number of case reports in the literature describing serious complications specific to expanding metal stents.[29,30,31] Confirmation of both clinical and cost-effectiveness is still needed.

Commercially available metal prostheses

At least four systems are available. These are summarised in **Table 8.4**.

1. The Wallstent (Boston Scientific Ltd., Porters Wood, St Albans, Herts) is loaded in a small diameter delivery catheter, constrained in a compressed form by a double plastic membrane. During expansion the stent shrinks by approximately one third. It is partially covered. The conical 'Flamingo' Wallstent is designed to reduce problems with migration.
2. The Ultraflex stent (Boston Scientific Ltd., Porters Wood, St Albans, Herts), made of an alloy of titanium and nickel, has a shape 'memory' as well as super-elastic behaviour. The design incorporates a proximal flare for secure placement. Upon release the stent retracts by approximately 40%.
3. The Gianturco–Rösch covered oesophageal Z stent (Wilson-Cook, Europe, A/S Bjaeverskov, Denmark) is available either fully covered with a polyethylene film and long wire hooks at its mid-portion to facilitate anchoring or a partially coated prosthesis with flange ends to allow greater anchoring. Unlike the Ultraflex and Wallstents it undergoes very little shortening upon release. A patent-pending 'windsock' design to reduce the possibility of gastro-oesophageal reflux is being manufactured.
4. The EsoPhacoil (Instent, Eden Prairie, Minnesota, USA) is a tightly wound coiled spring that shortens and widens on release. The stent is robust and external compression by a tumour is unlikely.

Method of insertion

The principles of metal-stent implantation are similar to those of plastic stent insertion, requiring intravenous sedation and precise radiological measurement. Certain details differ and deployment techniques of the compressed stents vary between commercially available systems. Preinsertion dilatation may be required to a minimum of 10 mm. A guide-wire is passed and the slim delivery device advanced over the guide-wire until the radio-opaque markers of the compressed stent are correctly aligned. Once in position the stent is deployed. It is possible to reposition the Wallstent after partial deployment. Balloon dilatation to improve expansion may be performed up to several days after stent insertion. Clinical care similar to that received by patients with traditional plastic prostheses should be provided after metal stent insertion.

Prosthesis	Description	Advantages	Disadvantages
KeyMed Atkinson	Reinforced silicone	Silicone resists degradation, inexpensive	Requires preliminary dilatation, narrow lumen, semi-rigid
Medoc-Celestin	Reinforced latex rubber	Collapsible distal flange to prevent migration, inexpensive	Requires preliminary dilatation, narrow lumen, semi-rigid
Wilson-Cook	Reinforced silicone	Model available for high tumours, inexpensive	Requires preliminary dilatation, narrow lumen, semi-rigid
Wallstent, Boston Scientific	Partially covered steel wire	Easy delivery, conical design to anchor, good expansion force	Shortens on release, migrates
Gianturco Z stent, Wilson-Cook	Partially covered stainless steel	Non-shortening stent, partially covered, good radiopacity	Migrates
Ultraflex, Boston Scientific	Knitted nitinol mesh	Proximal flare to anchor, covered or uncovered, highly flexible	Tumour ingrowth, shortens on release, poor expansion force
EsoPhacoil Instent	Coiled nitinol spring	Maximum radiopacity, angulation without width loss	Shortens on release, difficult to precisely position, impossible to reposition

Table 8.4 *Properties of plastic and expanding metal stents*

Figure 8.2
Expanding oesophageal metal stents (left to right): Flamingo Wallstent, Ultraflex non-covered stent, Wilson-Cook partially coated Z stent, The EsoPhacoil.

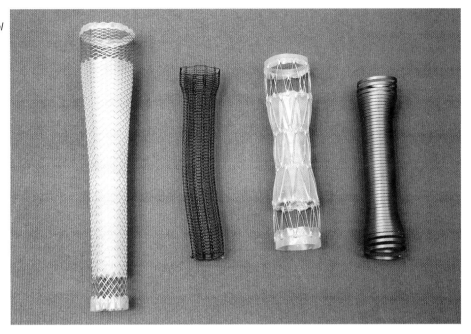

Complications

Expanding metal stents are subject to similar complications associated with plastic tubes as well as problems specific to their design. These are listed in Table 8.3. Combined-case series report a procedure-related mortality of about 2% and early complication rates of between 0 and 40%.[32]

1. Malposition may occur. In this situation a second stent can be inserted to fully cover the tumour.
2. Incomplete stent expansion. This most frequently occurs with the Ultraflex stent. It has been reported in up to 40% of procedures.[33]
3. Chest pain. This seems to be more common with metal stents than plastic prostheses.
4. Oesophageal perforation. This is lower with metal stents than with plastic prostheses.
5. Stent migration. This occurs despite elaborate anchoring devices. Stents crossing the gastro-oesophageal junction are more prone to this complication than those that have both ends anchored within the oesophagus. Endoscopic retrieval has been described but it is not routinely advocated by stent manufacturers. Like their plastic counterparts metal stents may be left in the stomach unless they obstruct the pylorus or cause further complications.

Late complications

Long-term problems with metal stents are similar to those with semi–rigid stents:

1. Stent migration.
2. Tumour ingrowth through the metallic stent latticework or tumour over–growth above or below the ends of the stent. This leads to recurrent

dysphagia and occurs in between 5–30% of patients. It is more frequent if the stent is uncovered.[34] Tumour ingrowth or overgrowth can be managed by a variety of endoscopic methods: balloon trawling, laser treatment, argon-beam coagulation, ethanol injections, intraluminal radiotherapy, dilatation or placement of another stent inside the stent.[35]

3. Food bolus obstruction occurs in metallic stents despite their wide diameter. It is treated in the same way as plastic-stent bolus obstruction.

4. Heartburn and symptoms of gastro-oesophageal reflux. This may be treated with acid suppression therapy or by aiding gastric emptying. It is not yet established if such symptoms are different in patients with metal or plastic prostheses.

5. There are case reports of oesophageal wall necrosis resulting in bleeding related to stent erosion or late perforation.[30,31]

6. Rare complications of stents fracturing or twisting have caused serious morbidity.[29,36]

Trials comparing expanding with non-expanding stents

Three prospective randomised studies have compared metal stents with non-expanding endoprostheses.[25,26,27] Knyrim et al. compared uncovered Wallstents with Wilson-Cook plastic prostheses in 42 patients.[25] Siersema et al. compared a latex prosthesis (Celestin Tube) with the Cook Z stent (Gianturco–Rösch covered design) in 75 patients.[26] De Palma et al. compared the uncovered Ultraflex stent with Wilson-Cook prostheses in 39 patients.[37] Although the strength of evidence is weak from these small studies, it seems that both types of stents were successfully inserted but patients randomised to plastic tubes suffered more immediate complications than those receiving expanding metal stents. Improvement of dysphagia was similar in both groups, and both groups experienced similar amounts of long-term problems with dysphagia. In two of the studies, patients receiving plastic tubes were treated under general anaesthetic whereas those receiving metal stents had only intravenous sedation.[25,26] The third trial does not provide details of the type of anaesthetic used to insert the prosthesis. Despite the higher costs of metal stents, they proved cost effective because of the decreased complication rate and shorter hospital stay. Table 8.2 summarises these trials. The question as to whether ease of placement and versatility offsets the high cost of metal stents remains unanswered. A large detailed UK Health Technology Assessment randomised trial including cost–benefit and quality of life analyses is in progress to provide this answer.[37] Manufacturers are currently developing new designs to decrease the risk of migration, increase the ease of insertion and enable stents to be repositioned or extracted.

Laser treatment

The most widely used laser is based on the solid crystal Neodymium yttrium aluminium garnet (Nd:YAG). This can be used to alleviate obstruction and arrest haemorrhage secondary to metastatic or locally unresectable carcinomas of the oesophagus and stomach. It can also be employed as a temporary measure before definitive operative management of malignant dysphagia. Initial enthusiasm for laser treatment has declined because it takes time and requires repeated hospital visits.

Continued exposure to laser light leads to tissue necrosis with eventual vaporisation. Its effect on the tissue depends on the power output selected, the duration of application, the distance between the fibre tip and target, the aim of the application and the colour of the tissue. When applied to bleeding areas, a black charred appearance develops. Each laser treatment session may recanalise the whole or part of the stricture. Some recommend routine endoscopic review at 48 to 72 hours, when oedema has subsided and accurate assessment of the overall effect can be made. The destroyed tumour may then be evacuated with forceps, polyp graspers, lavage or pushed distally with the endoscope. Others administer treatment as dictated by need.

Endoscopic technique

Laser treatment is usually carried out with intravenous sedation although some centres use a rigid endoscope, general anaesthesia and endotracheal intubation. Those in favour of a rigid scope believe its advantages are that it allows better suction of fluid, smoke and debris, with improved visualisation of the tumour. If a malignant stricture is negotiable, the laser is first applied to the distal end of the tumour. The scope is then withdrawn in a circular fashion into the more proximal tumour. If complete obstruction is encountered, tumours can be vaporised in the antegrade direction or first dilated to allow passage of the endoscope. Antegrade therapy may be more dangerous because information about the luminal axis is lacking, and the areas first treated rapidly become oedematous which impairs access to more distal parts. Pretreatment dilatation also introduces risks.

The most popular type of laser in Britain is the non-contact system. Laser energy is conveyed through a single monofibre which is enclosed in a Teflon sheath. The average power setting of the non-contact Nd:YAG, is 60–120 W. At an irradiation distance of 5–10 mm, multiple pulses for a duration of about 0.5–1 s are given. Coaxial gas (usually CO_2 or NO_2) is administered around the quartz fibre, to cool the probe tip and clear the debris. Gas is removed with the suction channel of the endoscope. A nasogastric tube next to the endoscope can be used to vent the oesophagus. The low-power contact Nd:YAG system uses coaxial water to cool the tip, remove debris and reduce adherence of the contact probe. Essentially the sapphire laser tip acts like a hot knife. Lower power settings theoretically mean that the chances of perforation by excessive laser energy are reduced. Tissue damage only occurs up to 0.5 mm beyond the treatment site. Some find that the tactile feedback of the contact laser probe helps the endoscopist destroy tumour with greater precision and safety.

Complications

The incidence of major complications and mortality (which is in the region of 1–5%) is usually lower for laser destruction than endoscopic intubation (with plastic stents).[38] Early complications are listed in **Table 8.5**.

1. Chest pain may result from extensive mucosal burning. It is common but not severe.
2. Oesophageal perforation is less common following laser recanalisation than intubation. The risk is about 5% and is said to be related to predilatation rather than a direct complication of laser oesophagoscopy.

Early complications	Late complications
Pain	Repeated hospital admissions
Perforation	Tumour recurrence
Pneumatoperitoneum	Benign stictures
Pneumomediastinum	Functional swallowing problems
Gastric distension	
Bleeding	
Aspiration pneumonia	

Table 8.5 *Complications of laser treatment*

3. A benign pneumato-peritoneum or pneumo-mediastinum may be pro-
    duced after laser treatment. This is thought to be related to a jet of coaxial
    gas passing through abnormal, often necrotic, tumour tissue. Patients rarely
    have symptoms. It is detected on routine chest X-ray. Contrast studies do
    not show a leak and patients usually make an uneventful recovery.
4. Gastric distension as a result of carbon dioxide infusion can be quite
    uncomfortable despite using good decompression probes through the
    stenosis. The pain is visceral in nature and may be confused with chest pain
    from excessive mucosal burning.
5. Haemorrhage after laser treatment is rare, occurring in about 1%.

Late complications

Late complications frequently occur following laser destruction and require
repeated endoscopic treatment.

1. The main problem is tumour recurrence. Patients require about monthly
    treatment sessions. It is perceived by the medical profession that this is bur-
    densome and disruptive. There have been few studies, however, objectively
    measuring patients' views about this matter and some may like the contin-
    ued hospital contact.
2. Delayed laser-associated benign strictures can occur in up to 20% of
    patients.[39] They require repeated dilatation and occasionally stent insertion.
3. Swallowing problems. Laser treatment may recanalise 90% of all stenoses
    but the clinical results obtained do not always come up to expectations.
    This appears to be due to a motility disturbance, together with progressive
    cachexia, that may make it impossible for some patients to take solid foods
    again.

In view of these varied responses, means of improving the efficacy of laser treatment by increasing the period between laser therapy and symptomatic relapse
have been explored through combination treatments.

Combination laser treatment

Laser therapy can be combined with external or internal-beam radiotherapy to
prolong the interval between treatments, although the patient must attend for

radiotherapy which does increase hospital attendance. Intraluminal radiotherapy is useful for treating mural invasion following laser debulking of the tumour. Relief of dysphagia may be successfully obtained in 80% of patients.[38] A randomised trial comparing laser treatment alone and laser treatment plus therapy with iridium-192 reported a significantly prolonged first dysphagia-free interval after recanalisation of the stricture in patients with squamous cell tumours receiving combined treatment.[6] Those receiving combined treatment also required significantly more endoscopic procedures.

Laser or stents?

With regard to the incidence of complications and achievement of normal swallowing laser palliation is probably better than intubation with plastic stents.[9,40] One prospective randomised study has compared laser therapy with expanding metal stents and plastic prostheses.[41] This has shown that metal stents are safest and provide the best palliation of dysphagia, although the results of this trial still need confirmation by other groups. Laser treatment may be preferable for non-circumferential, polypoid or exophytic tumours and tubes preferable in sclerotic stenosing tumours.

The main drawback of laser palliation is the need for the patient to attend hospital on a regular basis and the capital cost of the equipment. Laser treatment has nothing to offer patients with an extrinsic lesion causing oesophageal compression, those with a fistula or diffuse subepithelial tumour. If laser is employed as a first-line treatment then salvage intubation can still be used.

Photodynamic therapy

Photodynamic therapy is an investigational treatment which modifies conventional laser treatment. Its role in palliative treatments of upper gastrointestinal malignancies is yet to be determined. It essentially has three elements: light, a photosensitising drug (a haematoporphyrin derivative) and oxygen. The drug acting as a photosensitiser is injected intravenously 3–4 days before irradiation of the tumour. Laser light (administered endoscopically) then activates the drug within the tissue. Once stimulated, the photosensitiser interacts with oxygen to create a high reactive single state. This reacts with cell membranes and organelles and is cytotoxic. Retention of the photosensitiser is longer in dysplastic or frankly neoplastic than normal tissues, at a ratio of about 2:1. Damage to normal tissues heals by regeneration.

Clinical indications

Photodynamic (PDT) therapy may be used to treat patients with small mucosal tumours (uT1, N0) who are unfit or who do not wish to undergo major surgery; it may also be used on larger inoperable lesions. A number of specific complications have been recognised. The activated photosensitiser creates an iatrogenic porphyria which may persist for up to 6 weeks after injection of the drug, leading to skin photosensitivity. Patients are advised to avoid sunlight. Perforation and fistulae may occur, and oesophagitis leading to stricture formation has been reported.[42] Two prospective randomised studies have compared PDT with laser therapy.[43,44] Perforations were more common after laser treatment alone, although relief of dysphagia was similar in both groups. Photodynamic therapy seemed to have a longer duration of response than laser therapy. Until more selective tumour photosensitisers can be developed, it is likely that PDT will remain largely experimental.

Bipolar electrocoagulation

Electrocoagulation, a thermal method of tumour destruction, has always suffered from the problem of adhesion between the tissue and electrode. To overcome this difficulty non-adherent probe tips employing bipolar electrocoagulation energy (BICAP) have been developed. BICAP has the potential advantage of being able to treat a large area, therefore producing rapid relief of dysphagia. It is portable and relatively cheap.[39] Bipolar tumour probes can be used to destroy long tight submucosal tumours, but they must be circumferential. Where there is marked tumour angulation they are less effective, because the probes are rigid and difficult to direct.

Endoscopic technique

BICAP treatment is usually performed under intravenous sedation. The standard kit consists of five probes and a 50 W bipolar generator. Probes are similar to metal olive dilators with bipolar radiant electrode strips in the central portion and must be tested before treatment. Endoscopy is carried out to define the tumour geography and location (dilatation being performed if necessary). Under fluoroscopic control, BICAP probes are inserted over a guide wire to the stricture at the proximal end and five pulses are delivered. The probe is then advanced to the next position and the process repeated. The depth of coagulated tissue depends on forces applied radially by the probe. Usually 2–4 mm of coagulation occurs. Generally one or two treatment sessions are required to treat the entire tumour.

Complications

Like laser treatment, reported technical success is about 90%, but functional relief of dysphagia is only achieved in about 70% of patients. Others have reported about 85% improvement in dysphagia grade, lasting 4–10 weeks.[39] A few small series have reported complications in 10–20% of patients.[34,39] Perforation, fistula formation, strictures and bleeding have occurred.

The BICAP system is portable and costs less than laser equipment. Two prospective non-randomised studies have compared it with laser therapy.[34,39] There were no clear differences in outcome between the two modalities. It was concluded that BICAP should be used to treat long submucosal tumours and laser exophytic tumours. At present more data are needed before firm conclusions can be reached.

Argon-beam coagulation

This is a new technique which ablates tumour tissue. The argon-beam coagulator utilises a jet of ionised argon gas to conduct high frequency electrical energy to the tumour. This is readily applied through an endoscope. This technique allows a no-touch thermal coagulation of the tumour which is more controllable than conventional monopolar electrocautery. Once the surface of the tumour has been coagulated and dried, the electrical current passes through to an adjacent area.

Unlike laser light which is a targeted beam, the argon beam will arc to the nearest point of contact. The depth of extension is minimal (2–3 mm) and thus reduces the risk of perforation. The gas flow is high which means that regular aspiration is required to prevent gastric distension. Several case series have been reported with results that are comparable to other ablative tumour therapies.[45,46]

It is unknown whether argon electrocoagulation has major advantages over other endoscopic treatments for malignant dysphagia. It is not expensive and may be easier to use than the laser. Future trials are needed comparing this method with expanding metal stents.

Chemically induced tumour necrosis

The use of ethanol and polidocanol to induce tumour necrosis in inoperable oesophago-gastric tumours is a cheap and universally applicable method of palliating malignant dysphagia.[47]

Endoscopic technique

Patients require intravenous sedation and flexible endoscopy. Using a sclerotherapy needle, 0.5–1 ml aliquots of chemical are injected into the protuberant part of the tumour. Resistance is felt and blanching and swelling of the tumour observed. In patients with long tumours the injections are started distally so that induced oedema should not impede the passage of the endoscope. There is no limit to the total volume injected in one session (1–36 ml reported). Dilatation is needed if the endoscope is unable to transverse the stricture. Several treatment sessions may be required to improve swallowing.

Complications

An improvement in dysphagia scores is reported in most patients, although it may be made temporarily worse because of tumour oedema and swelling. Retrosternal chest pain and a low-grade pyrexia may occur. Perforation and fistula formation have occurred following injection sclerotherapy.[48]

Injection of chemicals to relieve malignant dysphagia has all the hallmarks of a good technique, being safe, inexpensive and readily available. The technique is less precise than laser treatment because it is difficult to be sure where the alcohol is going once it enters the tissue. A trial comparing injection of 3% polidocanol with laser therapy found both methods to be effective.[47] One prospective trial compared laser treatment with ethanol injections.[49] Significantly more pain was experienced by those being treated by ethanol but dysphagia and other complications were similar in both groups. Despite these reports the use of ethanol has not become widespread and its place may be as an adjunct to more conventional methods for relieving dysphagia. Like thermal methods for recanalisation, it cannot be used for patients with aero-digestive fistula.

Radiotherapy

Radiotherapy aims to recanalise the oesophagus and inhibit local tumour progression. It may be given by external beam or an intraluminal source (brachytherapy). The outcomes of treatment with external beam radiotherapy are difficult to interpret because many series include patients with small (potentially curable) tumours who are not considered for surgery on the basis of their general health. Prior to external-beam therapy a form of endoscopic recanalisation is often recommended because oedema and swelling of the tumour can cause complete dysphagia. Ten or more treatment fractions may be required and the optimum dose is unknown.

Complications

Side effects are common and often serious: pulmonary fibrosis, fistula and benign stricture formation. Acceptable palliation of dysphagia occurs in less than 40% of patients, of whom at least 25% get recurrent dysphagia as a result of cicatricial narrowing of the oesophagus.[50] As a single modality it has been superseded by intracavity irradiation.

Brachytherapy (intracavitary irradiation)

The development of the Selectron (Nucleotron, Zeersum, Holland) remote control after-loading machine has generated considerable interest in recent years. It is a simple and safe procedure, and there is no radiation exposure to staff. The brachytherapy applicator, only 8 mm in diameter, is passed over an endoscopically placed guide-wire and positioned by fluoroscopy in the tumour. This is immobilised at the mouth or nose. The patient is then transferred to a protected treatment room and connected to the Selectron machine. A microprocessor controls the pneumatic transfer of caesium-137 pellets down a flexible tube inserted into the applicator. The optimal dose is unknown and varies between 15 to 20 Gy to a depth of 1 cm in single or multiple fractions. Treatment may be repeated on alternate days leaving the nasogastric tube *in situ* or replacing it as necessary. The great merit of brachytherapy is that the radiation dose is highest to the tumour while adjacent normal tissues are relatively spared. It can be used in combination with laser treatment as discussed above.

Relief of dysphagia

Fast relief of dysphagia is obtained in 70% of patients with squamous cell tumours and 60% of those with adenocarcinoma.[38,51] All patients suffer a varying degree of radiation oesophagitis which leads to painful oesophageal ulceration in up to 30% of patients as well as the development of post-irradiation strictures or tracheo-oesophageal fistula.[52] In a randomised trial, Low and Pagliero compared the efficacy of brachytherapy with laser treatment in 23 patients. No significant differences were found between the two groups but retreatments were three times more common with laser therapy.[53]

Combination treatment

The addition of brachytherapy to external-beam radiotherapy leads to higher doses of radiotherapy to the tumour. Brachytherapy is usually given after the course of external-beam treatment although it may be administered first.[4,54,55] Complications are similar to those experienced with external-beam radiotherapy alone and may occur in up to 50% of patients. The median survival is reported to be better than with other palliative treatments (10 to 13 months), but no randomised comparisons have been performed. The combination of brachy-therapy and laser treatment has been discussed above.

Brachytherapy seems an attractive new development although the cost of an Nd:YAG laser is significantly less than the Selectron unit. It requires an expensive, specially fitted treatment area separate from the endoscopy suite and close liaison with radiotherapy. The endoscopic techniques required for brachytherapy are straightforward. Brachytherapy should be subject to the scrutiny of a large randomised trial to discover whether single or combination treatment provides the best palliation of malignant dysphagia.

Palliative chemotherapy or combination chemoradiotherapy

The role of single agent chemotherapy or combination chemoradiation for patients who are deemed to have inoperable carcinoma of the oesophagus has not yet been defined. The results of phase II studies have generally been modest although enthusiasts continue to report high response rates.[8,56]

There are two small randomised trials which have shown a significant survival benefit of combination chemotherapy when compared with best supportive care on patients with advanced gastric cancer.[14,57] It is not yet known if these results can be extrapolated to patients with advanced oesophageal cancer.

Aero-digestive fistulae

Aero-digestive fistulae cause paroxysmal coughing fits, aspiration and eventually death from recurrent chest infection. They occur in about 5% of patients with oesophageal cancer either because of spontaneous necrosis of the tumour through the oesophageal wall into the bronchial tree or as a sequel of irradiation, laser therapy or intubation. They are difficult to treat and patients often die within 1 month of development.[18] The creation of a cervical oesophagostomy and gastrostomy often seems unnecessary because of the patient's poor prognosis. Palliative bypass surgery with stomach or colon for interposition is highly invasive and the abject general health of the patient produces at least a 50% perioperative morbidity and mortality.[58] Endoscopic insertion of a prosthesis is the treatment of choice although results following the use of rigid prostheses have not been encouraging.[18] Many modifications have been developed. Wilson-Cook produce a fistula prosthesis carrying a circumferential foam-rubber sponge contained in a silicone sheath which expands and closes the fistula once the vacuum is released. A modified Celestin prosthesis is available. An Atkinson tube may be wrapped in a circumferential polyvinyl alcohol (Ivalon) sponge which swells into the fistula and may fill a defect up to 30 mm in diameter. The use of covered metal stents to seal aero-digestive fistulae seems to be a more promising development although no randomised trials have been performed.[59,60,61] Fistulae close to the cricopharyngeus are particularly difficult to manage. In this situation simultaneous tracheal and oesophageal stenting has been described.[62] This is not usually necessary and most fistulae are sealed with an oesophageal stent alone. There is one report of the use of primary chemotherapy in four patients with tracheo-oesophageal fistulae. Two patients healed during treatment.[63] One other report advocates radiation therapy for tracheo-oesophageal fistula, although it had been thought that radiotherapy might enlarge the fistula.[64] At present the role of chemotherapy or radiotherapy in this regard needs further evaluation. The endoscopic placement of fibrin tissue glue may help treat difficult fistulae.

Recurrent laryngeal nerve palsy

Recurrent laryngeal nerve palsy caused by tumour infiltration results in eating difficulties, a weak voice, poor cough and repeated chest infections because of aspiration pneumonia. Patients classically are hoarse, and complain of swallowing difficulties with a choking sensation on consuming solids and liquids. The diagnosis is confirmed by laryngoscopy. Endoscopy may be required to exclude other problems contributing to dysphagia. Characteristically, aspiration is seen during the pharyngeal phase of swallowing on barium studies and endoscopy demonstrates no mechanical obstruction to food passage. The left nerve is more commonly involved because of its largely intrathoracic course, but patients with bilateral palsies may have palpable supraclavicular nodes. Teflon injection to re-establish glottic competence should help swallowing, speech and problems with coughing. In a series of 15 patients all but one improved, who developed stridor and required emergency tracheostomy.[65] Recurrent laryngeal nerve damage at the time of surgery usually causes a temporary paralysis that resolves within 6 weeks.

Bleeding

Bleeding from inoperable oesophageal and cardia tumours causes problems with refractory anaemia and occasionally acute upper gastrointestinal haemorrhage. It is often difficult to completely eradicate because of the advanced nature of the tumour, but symptoms may be controlled by a variety of endoscopic means. Palliative laser therapy can achieve haemostasis by coagulating the exposed bleeding tissues. Injection sclerotherapy (with dilute adrenaline or sclerosant) is effective although it may need to be repeated. Electrocoagulation can control upper gastrointestinal haemorrhage due to controlled tissue heating and argon-beam coagulation may be very useful in this situation. In general this problem may temporarily be relieved but is usually a sign of advanced disease.

Palliative treatments of tumours of the gastric body and antrum

Patients in whom potentially curative radical surgery for gastric cancer is not suitable require adequate palliation of symptoms of pain, vomiting, bleeding and malaise. The treatment of gastric outflow obstruction and chronic bleeding will be discussed separately.

Gastric outlet obstruction

Obstruction associated with cancer of the gastric corpus or antrum is difficult to manage regardless of the therapeutic modality. Such tumours generally involve extensive segments of the stomach and result in interference with both reservoir function and motility patterns. The endoscopic management of malignant gastric outflow obstruction remains controversial.[66,67,68] There is little doubt that whenever possible resection of the primary tumour as a means of providing symptomatic relief provides a better guarantee of success than bypass surgery. Opinions are divided, however, as to the best type of palliative gastrectomy (subtotal or total). Total gastrectomy for advanced gastric cancer may be worthwhile but often at the expense of a higher complication rate. Despite a successful palliative gastrectomy, however, many patients subsequently become anorexic because of the widespread nature of their disease. The role of gastric resection in linitis plastica remains controversial. It probably has little to offer for those patients who additionally have peritoneal or liver metastasis or contiguous organ involvement, where life expectancy is around 4 months. Patients with linitis plastica who have disease limited to the stomach or regional lymph nodes may, however, survive beyond 12 months and thus be appropriately palliated by total gastrectomy.[69,70] Although it is accepted that many operations, undertaken with curative intent, turn out to be entirely palliative procedures, this is becoming less of a problem with modern approaches to preoperative staging.

Patients with non-resectable distal lesions may undergo gastrojejunostomy. The loop of jejunum is anastomosed close to the greater curve of the stomach. There is little consensus regarding anterior or posterior loops. The latter may theoretically be more prone to recurrent obstruction due to proximity to the tumour. The Devine exclusion bypass operation for inoperable antral tumours was thought to increase survival by preventing recurrent tumour obstructing the gastrojejunostomy.[71]

Patients with advanced tumours of the body of the stomach causing problems with bleeding and/or obstruction may undergo palliative total gastrectomy. The morbidity is much higher than partial gastrectomy and opinions remain divided as to its benefits.[70] Total gastrectomy should not be performed if the patient has liver or peritoneal involvement or if the tumour has extension into pancreas or diaphragm. Monson and colleagues concluded that total gastrectomy in selected patients is recommended when technically feasible, but should be performed by an appropriately qualified surgeon.[70]

A variety of approaches are under investigation to expand the role and benefits of palliative surgery. Chemotherapy and radiotherapy are being used by a number of centres. Major drawbacks of chemoradiotherapy for advanced cancer are inevitably toxicity and undesired side effects, which make these treatments unattractive options for many patients if the objective is simply to relieve symptoms. Chemotherapy initially undertaken with palliative intent can, however, render some inoperable patients candidates for gastrectomy. Up to 50% of patients with metastatic and locally advanced gastric adenocarcinomas receiving epirubicin, cisplatin and 5-fluorouracil have been shown to have at least a partial response, without a significant decrease in quality of life.[56] On the whole the regimen was well tolerated. Definitive conclusions are still awaited as these phase II studies have not been confirmed in randomised clinical trials. The recent introduction of chemotherapy administered by protracted venous infusion may be a significant advance. It is generally better tolerated and superior to conventional bolus chemotherapy both in terms of treatment response and side effects.[56]

There are case reports of the placement of self-expanding stents through obstructing antral tumours indicating technical success.[66,67,68] There are no large series to assess the overall effectiveness of this approach. Metal stents may be more successfully placed across recurrent tumours at oesophagojejunal anastomoses and in recurrent peritoneal disease causing high small bowel obstruction following total gastrectomy.[72] Recanalisation of the gastric outlet with laser coagulation has not been used successfully.

The insertion of nasogastric tubes, percutaneous endoscopically placed feeding tubes and jejunostomies enables nutrition to be delivered to patients with inoperable tumours. These manoeuvres alone, however, fail to palliate most of the patient's symptoms. Many believe that such palliation merely perpetuates suffering except in situations where they may be used as an adjunct to recanalisation.

Chronic bleeding

Surgery is again recommended wherever possible to palliate the symptoms of chronic blood loss from gastric tumours. Laser therapy can successfully achieve haemostasis in bleeding gastric malignancies and there are increasing reports of argon-beam coagulation to limit bleeding from gastric tumours.[46] Both methods require repeated hospital admissions.

Summary

The number of therapeutic options available for the palliation of patients with oesophageal and gastric cancer has significantly increased over the past decade. No single treatment completely relieves all symptoms without notable side effects. Common clinical situations such as the management of fistulae, high oesophageal tumours and bleeding inoperable gastric lesions still present formidable problems. The introduction of expanding metal stents, argon-beam coagulation, brachytherapy, infusional chemotherapy and combination treatments offer new hopes, although all require careful evaluation before they become widely available. Referral of suitable patients should be encouraged so that large prospective trials focusing on palliative treatments may be completed expeditiously. The increasing centralisation of cancer services in order to provide high-technology specialised care may improve outcomes but evidence is awaited. There is a need to define outcomes for patients with inoperable malignancies of the upper gastrointestinal tract. Dysphagia scores should be standardised and future palliative trials should include an objective assessment of quality of life of patients as well as cost effectiveness during the follow up period.[75] This ideal approach, however, is not without disadvantages. Severely debilitated patients with a limited life expectancy may be compelled to travel long distances to a centre with specialised endoscopic facilities only to find that treatment has to be performed more than once. Genuine efforts should be made to see if patients with very short survival times (less than 4 weeks) can be identified and perhaps spared unnecessarily aggressive attempts at palliation.

The selection of palliation for patients with advanced disease is difficult. Every patient is unique with regard to tumour histology, stricture location, clinical stage, premorbid state and emotional requirements. Choosing one technique over another must be justifiable on the grounds of treatment efficacy, ease of application, overall adaptability to other therapeutic areas and patient acceptance, while minimising both complications and cost. Skilled clinicians with a thorough understanding of all the available palliative treatments should be aware of the other needs of the patient with advanced malignancy. Close liaison with multi-disciplinary teams including oncologists, dieticians and palliative care services is essential to minimise suffering.

References

1. Hennessy TPJ, O'Connell R. Carcinoma of the hypopharynx, oesophagus and cardia. Surg Gynecol Obstet 1986; 162:243–7.

2. Huang GJ, Wang LJ, Liu JS *et al.* Surgery of oesophageal carcinoma. Semin Surg Oncol 1985; 1:74–83.

3. Müller JM, Erasni H, Stelzner M *et al.* Surgical therapy of oesophageal carcinoma. Br J Surg 1990; 77:845–57.

4. Flores AD, Nelems B, Evans K *et al.* Impact of new radiotherapy modalities on the surgical management of cancer of the oesophagus and cardia. Int J Radiation Oncology Biol Phys 1989; 17:937–44.

5. Coia LR, Engstrom PF, Paul AR *et al.* Long term results of infusional 5-FU, mitomycin-C and radiation as primary management of oesophageal carcinoma. Int J Radiation Oncology Biol Phys 1991; 20:29–36.

6. Sander R, Hagenmueller F, Sander C *et al.* Laser versus laser plus after loading with iridium-192 in the palliative treatment of malignant stenosis of the oesophagus: a prospective, randomised and controlled study. Gastrointest Endosc 1991; 37:433–40.

7. Sargeant IR, Tobias JS, Blackman G *et al.* Radiotherapy enhances laser palliation of malignant dysphagia: a randomised study. Gut 1997; 40:362–9.

8. Highley MS, Parnis FX, Trotter GA *et al.* Combination chemotherapy with epirubicin, cisplatin and 5-fluorouracil for the palliation of advanced gastric and oesophageal adenocarcinoma. Br J Surg 1994; 81:1763–5.

9. Barr H, Krasner N, Raouf A *et al.* Prospective randomised trial of laser therapy only and laser therapy followed by endoscopic intubation for the palliation of malignant dysphagia. Gut 1990; 31:252–8.

10. Reed CE, Marsh WH, Carlson LS *et al.* Prospective, randomised trial of palliative treatment for unresectable cancer of the oesophagus. Ann Thorac Surg 1991; 51:552–6.

11. Schmid EU, Alberts AS, Greeff F *et al.* The value of radiotherapy or chemotherapy after intubation for advanced oesophageal carcinoma – a prospective randomised trial. Radio Oncol 1993; 28:27–30.

12. Brennan MF, Karpen MS. Surgery for gastric cancer: The American view. Sem Oncol 1996; 23:352–9.

13. Irvin TT, Bridger JE. Gastric cancer: an audit of 122 consecutive cases and the results of R1 gastrectomy. Br J Surg 1988; 75:106–9.

14. Pyrhonen S, Kuitunen T, Nyandoto P *et al.* Randomised comparison of fluorouracil, epidoxorubicin and methotrexate (FEMTX) plus supportive care with supportive care alone in patients with non-resectable gastric cancer. Br J Cancer 1995; 71:587–91.

15. Derodra JK, Hale PC, Mason RC. Inoperable oesophageal cancer: factors affecting outcome. Gullet 1992; 2:163–6.

16. Coates AS, Gebski V, Signorini D *et al.* Prognostic value of quality of life scores during chemotherapy for advanced breast cancer. J Clin Oncology 1992; 10: 1833–8.

17. Watson A. A study of the quality and duration of survival following resection, endoscopic intubation and surgical intubation in oesophageal carcinoma. Br J Surg 1982; 69:585–8.

18. Burt M, Diehl W, Martini N *et al.* Malignant oesophago-respiratory fistula: management options and survival. Ann Thorac Surg 1991; 52:1222–8.

19. Abe S, Tachibana M, Shimokawa T *et al.* Surgical treatment of advanced carcinoma of the oesophagus. Surg Gynecol Obstet 1989; 168:115–20.

20. Mannell A, Becker PJ, Nissenbaum M. Bypass surgery for unresectable oesophageal cancer: early and late results in 124 cases. Br J Surg 1988; 75:283–6.

21. Lundell L, Leth R, Lind T *et al.* Palliative dilation in carcinoma of the esophagus and esophagogastric junctions. Acta Chir Scand 1989; 155: 179–84.

22. Ogilvie AL, Dronfield MW, Ferguson R *et al.* Palliative intubation of oesophagogastric neoplasms at fibreoptic endoscopy. Gut 1982; 23:1060–7.

23. Loizou LA, Rampton D, Bown SG. Treatment of malignant strictures of the cervical oesophagus by endoscopic intubation using modified endoprostheses. Gastrointest Endosc 1992; 38: 158–64.

24. Bethge N, Sommer A, Vakil N. A prospective trial of self expanding metal stents in the palliation of malignant oesophageal strictures near the upper oesophageal sphincter. Gastrointest Endosc 1997; 45:300–3.

25. Knyrim K, Wagner HJ, Bethge N *et al.* A controlled trial of an expansile metal stent for palliation of oesophageal obstruction due to inoperable cancer. New Engl J Med 1993; 329:1302–7.

26. Siersema PD, Hop WCJ, Dees J *et al.* Coated self-expanding metal stents versus latex prostheses for esophagogastric cancer with special reference to prior radiation and chemotherapy: a controlled, prospective study. Gastrointest Endosc 1998; 47:113–20.

27. De Palma GD, di Matteo E, Romano G *et al.* Plastic prosthesis versus expandable metal stents for palliation of inoperable esophageal thoracic carcinoma: a controlled prospective study. Gastrointest Endosc 1996; 43:478–82.

28. Roseveare CD, Patel P, Simmonds N *et al.* Metal stents improve dysphagia, nutrition and survival in malignant oesophageal stenosis: a randomised controlled trial comparing modified Gianturco Z-stents with plastic Atkinson tubes. Eur J Gastroenterol Hepatol 1998; 10:653–7.

29. Loser C, Folsch UR. Self-expanding metallic coil stents for palliation of esophageal carcinoma: two cases of decision stent dysfunction. Endoscopy 1996; 28:514–7.

30. Farrugia M, Morgan RA, Latham JA *et al.* Perforation of the oesophagus secondary to insertion of covered Wallstent endoprostheses. Cardiovasc Int Radiol 1997; 20:470–2.

31. Siersema PD, Tan TG, Sutorius FFJM *et al.* Massive hemorrhage caused by a perforating Gainturco-Z stent results in an aortoesophageal fistula. Endoscopy 1997; 29: 416–20.

32. Ell C, May A. Self-expanding metal stents for palliation of stenosing tumours of the esophagus and cardia: A critical review. Endoscopy 1997; 29:392–8.

33. May A, Selmaier M, Hochberger J *et al.* Memory metal stents for palliation of malignant obstruction of the oesophagus and cardia. Gut 1995; 37:309–13.

34. Maunoury V, Brunetaud JM, Cochelard D *et al.* Endoscopic palliation for inoperable malignant dysphagia: long term follow up. Gut 1992; 33:1602–7.

35. Lagattolla NRF, Rowe PH, Anderson H *et al.* Restenting malignant oesophageal strictures. Br J Surg 1998; 85:261–3.

36. Schoefl R, Winkelbauer F, Haefner M *et al.* Two cases of factured esophageal nitinol stents. Endoscopy 1996; 28:518–20.

37. Griffin SM, Bond J *et al.* A pragmatic randomised controlled trial of the cost effectiveness of palliative therapies for patients with oesophageal cancer. NHS Executive Health Technology Assessment 1999.

38. Bader M, Dittler HJ, Ultsch B *et al.* Palliative treatment of malignant stenoses of the upper gastrointestinal tract using a combination of laser and after loading therapy. Endoscopy 1986; 18 (Suppl 1): 27–31.

39. Jensen DM, Machicado G, Randall G *et al.* Comparison of low power YAG laser and BICAP tumour probe for palliation of oesophageal cancer strictures. Gastroent 1988; 94:1263–70.

40. Carter R, Smith JS, Anderson JR. Laser recanalisation versus endoscopic intubation in the palliation of malignant dysphagia: a randomised prospective study. Br J Surg 1992; 79:1167–70.

41. Adam A, Ellul J, Watkinson AF *et al.* Palliation of inoperable oesophageal carcinoma: a prospective randomised trial of laser therapy and stent placement. Radiol 1997; 202:344–8.

42. McCaughan JS, Nims TA, Guy JT *et al.* Photodynamic therapy for oesophageal tumours. Arch Surg 1989; 124:74–80.

43. Lightdale CJ, Heier SK, Marcon NE *et al.* Photodynamic therapy with porfimer sodium versus thermal ablation therapy with Nd:YAG laser for palliation of esophageal cancer: a multicentre randomised trial. Gastrointest Endosc 1995; 42:507–12.

44. Heier SK, Rothman KA, Heier LM *et al.* Photodynamic therapy for obstructing esophageal cancer: light dosimetry and randomised comparison with Nd:YAG laser therapy. Gastroent 1995; 109:63–72.

45. Robertson GSM, Thomas M, Jamieson J *et al.* Palliation of oesophageal carcinoma using the argon beam coagulator. Br J Surg 1996; 83:1769–71.

46. Heindorff H, Wojdemann M, Bisgaard T *et al.* Endoscopic palliation of inoperable cancer of the oesophagus or cardia by argon electrocoagulation. Scand J Gastroent 1998; 33:21–3.

47. Angelini G, Pasini AF, Ederle A *et al.* Nd:YAG laser versus pilodocanol injection for palliation of oesophageal malignancy: a prospective randomised study. Gastrointest Endosc 1991; 37:607–10.

48. Chung SCS, Leong HT, Choi CYC *et al.* Palliation of malignant oesophageal obstruction by endoscopic alcohol injection. Endoscopy 1994; 26:275–7.

49. Carazzone A, Bonavina L, Segalin A *et al.* Endoscopic palliation of oesophageal cancer: results of a

prospective comparison of Nd:YAG laser and ethanol injection. Eur J Surgery 1999; 165:351–6.

50. Earlam R, Cunha-Melo JR. Oesophageal squamous cell carcinoma: II. A critical view of radiotherapy. Br J Surg 1980; 67:457–61.

51. Rowland CG, Pagliero KM. Intracavitary radiation in palliation of carcinoma of oesophagus and cardia. Lancet 1985; ii:981–2.

52. Hishikawa Y, Tanaka S, Miura T. Oesophageal ulceration induced by intracavitary irradiation for oesophageal carcinoma. Am J Radiol 1984; 143:269–73.

53. Low DE, Pagliero KM. Prospective randomised clinical trial comparing brachytherapy and laser photoablation for palliation of oesophageal cancer. J Thorac Cardiovasc Surg 1992; 104: 173–9.

54. Hishikawa Y, Kurisu K, Taniguchi M et al. High-dose-rate intraluminal brachytherapy for oesophageal cancer: 10 years experience in Hyogo College of Medicine. Radio Oncol 1991; 21:107–14.

55. Taal BG, Aleman BMP, Koning CCE et al. High dose rate brachytherapy before external beam irradiation in inoperable oesophageal cancer. Br J Cancer 1996; 74:1452–7.

56. Bamias A, Hill ME, Cunningham D et al. Epirubicin, Cisplatin, and protracted venous infusion of 5-fluorouracil for oesophagogastric adenocarcinoma. Cancer 1996; 77:1978–85.

57. Murad AM, Santiago FF, Petroianu A et al. Modified therapy with 5-fluorouracil, doxorubicin, and methotrexate in advanced gastric cancer. Cancer 1993; 72:37–41.

58. Duranceau A, Jamieson GG. Malignant tracheo-esophageal fistula. Ann Thorac Surg 1984; 37: 346–54.

59. Wu WC, Katon RM, Saxon RR et al. Silicone-covered self-expanding metallic stents for the palliation of malignant oesophageal obstruction and oesophagorespiratory fistulas: experience in 32 patients and a review of the literature. Gastrointest Endosc 1994; 40:22–33.

60. Cook TA, Dehn TCB. Use of covered expandable metal stents in the treatment of oesophageal carcinoma and tracheo-oesophageal fistula. Br J Surg 1996; 83:1417–8.

61. Kozarek RA, Raltz RN, Brugge WR et al. Prospective multicentre trial of oesophageal Z-stent placement for malignant dysphagia and tracheoesophageal fistula. Gastrointest Endosc 1996; 44:562–7.

62. Ellul JPM, Morgan R, Gold D et al. Parallel self-expanding covered metal stents in the trachea and oesophagus for the palliation of complex high tracheo-oesophageal fistula. Br J Surg 1996; 83:1767–8.

63. Malik SM, Krasnow SH, Wadleigh RG. Closure of tracheoesophageal fistulas with primary chemotherapy in patients with oesophageal cancer. Cancer 1994; 73:1321–3.

64. Gschossmann JM, Bonner JA, Foote RL et al. Malignant tracheoesophageal fistula in patients with esophageal cancer. Cancer 1993; 72:1513–21.

65. Griffin SM, Chung SCS, van Hasselt CA et al. Late swallowing and aspiration problems after oesophagectomy for cancer: malignant infiltration of the recurrent laryngeal nerves and its management. Surg 1992; 112:533–5.

66. Lightdale CJ. Self-expanding metal stents for oesophageal and gastric cancer: a new opening. Gastrointest Endosc 1994; 38:86–8.

67. Patton JT, Carter R. Endoscopic stenting for recurrent malignant gastric outlet obstruction. Br J Surg 1997; 84:865–6.

68. Song HY, Yang DH, Kuh JH et al. Obstructing cancer of the gastric antrum: palliative treatment with covered metallic stents. Radiol 1993; 187:357–8.

69. Aranha GV, Georgen R. Gastric linitis plastica is not a surgical disease. Surg 1989; 106:758–63.

70. Monson JRT, Donohue JH, McIlrath DC et al. Total gastrectomy for advanced cancer. A worthwhile palliative procedure. Cancer 1991; 68:1863–8.

71. Kwok SPY, Chung SCS, Griffin SM et al. Devine exclusion for unresectable carcinoma of the stomach. Br J Surg 1991; 78:684–5.

72. Wayman J, Richardson DL, Bliss R et al. Self expanding metal stents in the palliation of small bowel obstruction secondary to recurrent gastric cancer. Gastrointest Endos 1998; 47(3):286–90.

73. Alderson D, Wright PD. Laser recanalisation versus endoscopic intubation in the palliation of malignant dysphagia. Br J Surg 1990; 77:1151–3.

74. Fuchs KH, Freys SM, Schaube H et al. Randomised comparison of endoscopic palliation of malignant oesophageal stenoses. Surg Endos 1991; 5: 63–7.

75. Blazeby JM, Alderson D, Winstone K et al. Development of a EORTC questionnaire module to be used in quality of life assessment for patients with oesophageal cancer. Eur J Cancer 1996; 32:1912–7.

9 Pathophysiology and investigation of GORD and motility disorders

C. Paul Barham
Derek Alderson

INTRODUCTION

Despite being a simple muscular conduit between the mouth and stomach, the oesophagus is the focus of one of the most common health problems afflicting modern Western societies, gastro-oesophageal reflux disease (GORD). Its treatment is the biggest single pharmaceutical expenditure in the NHS, a cost that is rising as the disease becomes more common. GORD is probably responsible for the increasing incidence of oesophageal adenocarcinoma as this cancer arises in a columnar-lined oesophagus, as a consequence of severe reflux disease. Understanding the pathophysiology of GORD and its investigation is becoming increasingly important. Though motility disorders of the oesophagus are much less frequent, they can also cause significant patient morbidity, but remain poorly understood and often inadequately treated.

It is important to have a clear understanding of oesophageal anatomy and physiology to understand the pathophysiology of these disease states.

Adult anatomy

The oesophagus is a muscular tube approximately 25 cm long connecting the pharynx in the neck to the stomach in the abdomen. It is subdivided into three anatomical segments on the basis of position rather than function (cervical, thoracic and abdominal). The cervical oesophagus is a direct continuation of the pharynx, commencing at the cricopharyngeal muscle (the upper oesophageal sphincter) and is about 5 cm in length. The thoracic oesophagus is about 18 cm long, starting at the thoracic inlet at T1 and ending where the oesophagus passes through the hiatal opening of the diaphragm at T10. The abdominal oesophagus is of variable length due to the variable frequency of a hiatus hernia, but is usually only about 1–2 cm in length.

The body of the oesophagus is composed of an outer longitudinal and inner circular layer of muscle, though the longitudinal muscle does spiral slightly down the oesophagus. Though functioning as a single unit, the muscle is unique in being composed of both striated and smooth muscle. At its proximal end (including the cricopharyngeal sphincter) it is entirely striated muscle. Over the next 4–5 cm it is a mixture of both muscle types with smooth muscle becoming more common distally. The middle and lower oesophagus is composed entirely of smooth muscle. This muscular tube is lined by non-keratinised stratified squamous epithelium down to the gastro-oesophageal junction where it abruptly changes to glandular mucosa at the endoscopic Z line. Deep to the mucosa and the muscularis mucosa, but superficial to the circular muscle, lie the connective tissue, blood vessels, nerves and glands that form the submucosa. The blood supply to the upper oesophagus down to the level of the aortic arch is from the inferior thyroid arteries, the middle portion by oesophageal branches from the aorta and the lower part by the oesophageal branches of the left gastric artery. Venous drainage is to the inferior thyroid veins in the neck, into the azygos system in the thorax and most importantly, to the left gastric vein in the abdomen (an important porto-systemic communication). The nerve supply of the oesophagus is predominantly vagal, either from the recurrent laryngeal nerves to the upper oesophagus or the vagus proper to the main bulk of the oesophageal body. Sympathetic supply comes from cell bodies in the middle cervical ganglion supplying the upper part of the oesophagus and from the upper four thoracic ganglia of the sympathetic trunk to the rest of the oesophagus.

The oesophagus lies in the posterior mediastinum in intimate relationship to several important structures for most of its length. In the resting state, therefore, most of the oesophagus lies in the slightly negative pressure environment of the thorax (−5 mmHg compared to atmospheric pressure). This is in contrast to its lower end that, for about 1–2 cm, having passed through the diaphragmatic hiatus, lies in the slightly positive (+5 mmHg) pressure environment of the abdomen. Thus the oesophagus and the stomach are the only part of the gastrointestinal tract where bowel in continuity is contained within cavities of opposing pressure. The pressure gradient across the diaphragm, if unopposed, ought to lead to the free flow of gastric contents into the oesophagus (located in the relative vacuum of the thorax). That this does not usually occur is dependent upon the antireflux barrier at the gastro-oesophageal junction.

Normal oesophageal motility

Normal oesophageal transport occurs through two mechanisms. Primary (or swallow-initiated) peristalsis is centrally mediated, originates in the pharynx and progresses aborally to the stomach (**Fig. 9.1**). If food were to remain in the oesophagus, distending its lumen, then local neural reflexes would induce secondary (or non-swallow initiated) peristaltic activity to clear it.[1] Tertiary contractions (non-peristaltic) are not often seen in normal subjects during short-term radiological or manometric investigations but are more commonly observed during 24-hour manometry investigations. Apart from food and liquid transport, peristalsis also has an important function in clearing refluxed gastric contents, and this occurs by both the primary and secondary mechanisms.

Oesophageal peristalsis depends primarily upon the interaction of myogenic and intrinsic and external neural factors. The electrical activity of the circular muscle appears to be different from the longitudinal muscle as, instead of depolarisation after stimulation, the circular muscle initially hyper-polarises.[2] The resulting time

Figure 9.1
Manometry trace of primary oesophageal peristalsis (P5–P3 are oesophageal body transducers – see Fig. 9.12).

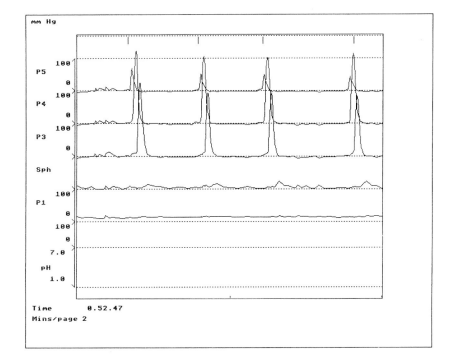

delay allows the longitudinal muscle to contract first, thus providing form and rigidity to the oesophagus during bolus transport. Inherent myogenic properties are necessary for the occurrence of muscle contraction, but central and local neural controls are required for coordination of peristalsis. Peripherally, neural control is mediated via the vagus nerve that links to the intrinsic neurons of the myenteric plexus between the inner and outer muscle layers. Neural mechanisms for afferent input to the central nervous system from the oesophagus are also present. In humans, there is a sensitive system located in the oesophageal body for the detection of volume changes in the oesophageal lumen. There is also evidence that receptors for acidity exist that may produce a centrally mediated peristaltic clearance wave.[3] While the function of afferent nerves from the oesophagus is poorly understood, they probably have an important controlling or modulating effect on normal peristalsis since the vagus is composed largely of sensory fibres. For instance, dry swallows often fail to generate a peristaltic sequence, whereas wet swallows are almost always followed by a propagated contraction of longer duration and greater amplitude.[4,5] The temperature of the swallowed bolus also affects oesophageal peristalsis, with warm substances producing stronger contractions, while the rapid ingestion of ice cream leads to complete absence of distal oesophageal activity.[6]

The antireflux barrier

The upper oesophageal sphincter

This is formed by the lower part of the inferior constrictor of the pharynx, cricopharyngeus and the upper part of the circular muscle of the oesophagus.

This sphincter is closed at rest with a high resting pressure of about 100 mmHg in an anterior posterior direction (less in the lateral direction) protecting the airway from reflux of gastric contents.

Lower oesophageal sphincter

Initially the presence of a lower oesophageal sphincter was doubted because it could not be demonstrated anatomically.[7] Manometric studies however have shown the presence of a high-pressure zone (HPZ) (**Fig. 9.2**) that behaves like a physiological sphincter (relaxing to allow swallowing, belching and vomiting). Subsequent studies showing a statistical correlation between pressures in the distal oesophageal segment and the presence or absence of acid reflux[8] have led to the concept of a physiological sphincter responsible for the control of acid reflux. The finding of a lowered pressure in the HPZ of patients with oesophagitis offered a logical explanation for the development of GORD and explained how some patients with hiatus hernias had no reflux, while others without hiatus hernias could have quite severe oesophagitis.[9] It had previously been held that the presence of a hiatus hernia was an indispensable feature of GORD accounting for its anatomical cause and an explanation for its potential surgical cure.[10]

Basal sphincter tone

Oesophageal manometry has demonstrated the presence of a high-pressure zone extending over the terminal 1–4 cm of the oesophagus with marked axial and radial asymmetry with the highest pressures recorded in the posterior and right

Figure 9.2
Static pull-through manometry with P5 recording LOS pressure (approximately 30 mmHg above gastric pressure) in a patient with achalasia. Note the pH probe (attached at the level of P3) is in the stomach and measuring acid. The marks at the top of the recording indicate each cm withdrawal of the catheter across the LOS.

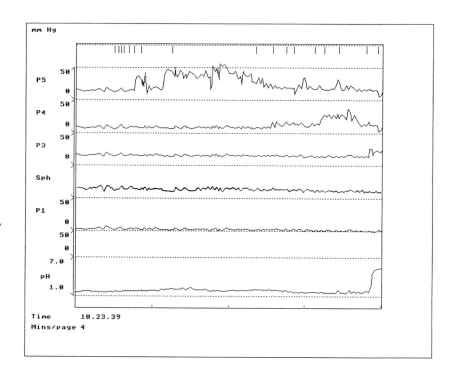

posterior directions.[11,12] The variations in sphincter pressures recorded in the same individual on separate occasions[13] and the findings from prolonged recordings using a perfused sleeve device demonstrate marked diurnal variations in basal LOS pressure in relation to posture,[14] meals[15] and the migrating motor complex.[16]

The regulation of LOS pressure depends on the interplay of myogenic, neural and humoral mediated factors. In humans, resting LOS pressure is reduced by atropine and vagal interruption, suggesting that the neural component is dominant.[17,18] This LOS innervation is by both excitatory and inhibitory autonomic nerves, with the cell bodies of the inhibitory nerves located in the enteric nervous system. Preganglionic vagal fibres originate in the dorsal motor nucleus of the vagus. These vagal fibres synapse on the myenteric ganglionic cell bodies,[19] where the transmitter is acetylcholine. Acetylcholine exerts its effects on the post-ganglionic neurone by both nicotinic and muscarinic receptors, but recent evidence indicates that nitric oxide may be the non-adrenergic, non-cholinergic transmitter between the nerves and the muscle of the LOS.

Adaptive sphincter pressure changes

The pressure gradient across the diaphragm can increase significantly in certain circumstances. These include activities such as abdominal compression, bending, straining and coughing, which produce a rise in intra-abdominal pressure, and sniffing, hiccoughing and deep breathing, which produce a drop in intrathoracic pressure. Several studies have shown an LOS pressure rise in response to these activities. This pressure rise may occur by a reflex-mediated increase in sphincter tone, a change in extrinsic mechanical factors, or perhaps a simple transmission of abdominal pressure to the sphincter.

Sphincter relaxation

The phenomenon of transient lower oesophageal sphincter relaxation (TLOSR) was introduced by Dent following the development of a sleeve device in 1976.[20] This device has a 6-cm unidirectional sensing surface that has been shown to measure the maximum pressure along its length[21] and has been widely used under experimental conditions. It has a major advantage over point sensors as the LOS is known to move up and down by as much as 3 cm during swallowing and breathing[22,23] and so will move up and down relative to a pressure catheter secured to the face. A drop in recorded sphincter pressure from a point sensor may, therefore, be due to either actual sphincter relaxation or to sensor displacement to the stomach or oesophageal body. Results from such sensors must be interpreted with considerable caution.[24,25] The Dent sleeve, by straddling the high-pressure zone, allows some degree of sphincter movement while still maintaining sphincter contact. It has provided an explanation for acid reflux in patients with normal LOS pressure.

Transient lower oesophageal sphincter relaxation can be inappropriate when relaxation occurs spontaneously or after a non-propagated pharyngeal swallow, or appropriate when relaxation follows primary or secondary peristaltic swallows. The relaxations usually occur in less than 5 seconds (from resting pressure to maximal relaxation) and last between 5 and 40 seconds.[26,27]

External mechanical factors

Prior to the identification of a physiological sphincter at the gastro-oesophageal junction in the mid-1950s, mechanical factors were felt to play the main role in preventing GOR. These mechanical factors were the 'flap valve' mechanism and compression of the distal oesophagus by extrinsic forces.

Flap valve mechanism

It is thought that the cardio-oesophageal angle is held in its acute position by contraction of oblique gastric sling fibres in the muscular coat of the stomach and this disappears in cadavers.[28] The oblique angle of entry of the oesophagus into the stomach was said to cause a 'flap-like' mechanism so preventing reflux. However, this angle disappears in a sliding hiatus hernia, yet the presence of a hernia is not always followed by acid reflux. In addition, the gastric sling fibres, which form a cone-like constriction at the cardiac notch, lie at a level below that of a radiologically defined barrier to instilled barium.[29] The role of this mechanism in preventing GOR remains uncertain.

The right pillar of the crus of the diaphragm probably contributes to the measured LOS pressure when there is no sliding hiatus hernia present and may partly explain the marked longitudinal and radial asymmetry of the LOS.[11] Respiratory-induced pressure oscillations are readily seen during manometric measurement of the LOS[22,23] and amplitudes are related to inspiratory depth.[30] Diaphragmatic contractions in man have been shown by one group to augment LOS tone, and this enhancing effect was maximal during deep sustained inspiration when the gastro-oesophageal pressure gradient was greatest.[31] This diaphragmatic pinchcock may work by buttressing the LOS when the greatest gastro-oesophageal pressure gradients occur (deep inspiration, coughing, straining, straight-leg raising and so on).

The mucosal folds (or rosettes) at the junction of the stomach and oesophagus have been proposed as a contributory factor in preventing GOR. These mucosal folds are held in apposition by surface tension and would seem unlikely to offer any sort of barrier to refluxed gastric contents. Indeed, in an animal model, excision of the mucosal rosette or elimination of the acute angle of entry of the oesophagus into the stomach did not result in oesophagitis.[32]

Distal oesophageal compression

Allison was the first to stress the role of the phreno-oesophageal ligament in maintaining competence at the cardia and advised its careful reconstruction during hiatal hernia repair.[10] The phreno-oesophageal ligament is a prolongation of the endo-abdominal fascia from the under-surface of the diaphragm. At the lower margin of the hiatus it decussates into upper and lower leaves. The lower leaf is an ill-defined, loose collection of fibroelastic fibres, which is absent in many cases.[33] The upper layer is a strong, consistent and well-defined membrane that inserts into the oesophagus, and is attached to the submucosa and intramuscular septae of the lower oesophageal wall by fascicles of fibroelastic tissue. This anatomical arrangement anchors the oesophago-gastric junction within the abdomen to prevent herniation through the hiatus, thereby maintaining a portion of the oesophagus within the positive pressure environment of the abdomen.

The height of insertion of the phreno-oesophageal ligament determines the length of the oesophagus that is maintained within the positive pressure environment of the abdomen. This factor would also apply in patients with sliding hiatus hernias who, despite having a portion of the stomach within the anatomical chest, still retain a segment of the oesophagus within an envelope of endo-abdominal fascia. Rises in abdominal pressure will still be transmitted to the lower part of the oesophagus, leaving no net gradient across the gastro-oesophageal junction, thus preventing acid reflux.[34]

The LOS length and the length of the sphincter exposed to intra-abdominal pressure are said by some groups to be important for the prevention of reflux precipitated by increases in intragastric pressure.[35] The overall length is said to be important because a long LOS will exhibit greater resistance to opening by distraction.[36] DeMeester *et al.* have shown in an *in vitro* model system that a short intra-abdominal segment of oesophagus can lead to failure of the sphincter mechanism.[37] They found that in the clinical situation, a low basal LOS pressure (< 5 mmHg) and/or a short intra-abdominal sphincter length (< 1 cm), resulted in a 90% incidence of abnormal GOR.

Clearly, there are mechanical factors that support the LOS in its antireflux function. To what extent these factors contribute to the antireflux barrier, however, remains the subject of considerable debate.

Pathophysiology of GORD

The clinical problem

Symptomatic GOR is one of the most common problems encountered in medical practice. Precise details of its prevalence are, nevertheless, still unknown and figures quoted are often based on guesses rather than facts. Prolonged pH monitoring has shown that even asymptomatic subjects have episodes of GOR which are predominantly shortlived and occur post-prandially.[38,39] Determining the true incidence of symptomatic GOR is made difficult because many people regard heartburn as normal and are content to treat themselves with antacids without seeking medical attention.[40] Furthermore, not all patients with typical reflux symptoms of heartburn and acid regurgitation have oesophagitis. Two studies of patients with reflux symptoms disclosed a normal oesophagus on endoscopy in 32% and 38% of subjects.[41,42] At the other end of the scale oesophagitis is now the commonest finding in upper gastrointestinal endoscopic examinations,[43] yet several studies have shown that up to 20% of patients with endoscopic oesophagitis and its complications never experience heartburn.[44,45]

In view of this difficulty in establishing a diagnosis of GOR disease, a range of diagnostic tests have been developed (**Table 9.1**). From these, 24-hour ambulatory pH monitoring is usually nominated as the gold standard.[46] Even this method can, however, reveal normal pH profiles in symptomatic patients,[47] and in up to 25% of subjects with endoscopic oesophagitis.[48]

Considerable experimental work has been carried out on the pathophysiology of GORD over the last 30 years. This has suggested a multifactorial aetiology, and the various mechanisms thought to be involved are listed in **Table 9.2**.

Endoscopy

Histology

Barium radiology

24-hour pH study

Manometry (standard and prolonged)

Bilitec probe (bile reflux)

Oesophageal scintigraphy

Oesophageal provocation studies
  Acid clearance test
  Standard acid reflux test (SART)
  Bernstein test

Table 9.1 *Diagnostic investigations available for GORD*

1.	Defective lower oesophageal sphincter mechanism
2.	Poor oesophageal body clearance ability
3.	Composition of refluxing fluid
4.	Oesophageal mucosal resistance factors
5.	Delayed gastric emptying

Table 9.2 *Proposed multifactorial pathogenesis of GORD*

Oesophageal motility and GOR disease

Over the years several factors have been thought to be important to prevent the reflux of gastric contents into the oesophagus and these are illustrated in **Table 9.3**, some of which have already been mentioned.

Transient LOS relaxations (TLOSR)

Not only does the sphincter relax to allow the passage of food and liquids, several studies have now confirmed the occurrence of TLSOR (**Figure 9.3**) as a major

1   **Lower oesophageal sphincter**
      Basal tone
      Adaptive pressure changes
      Transient LOS relaxation

2   **External mechanical factors**
      Flap valve mechanism
        Cardio-oesophageal angle
        Diaphragmatic pinchcock
        Mucosal rosette
      Distal oesophageal compression
        Phreno-oesophageal ligament
        Transmitted abdominal pressure

Table 9.3 *Natural barriers to gastro-oesophageal reflux*

Figure 9.3
LOS relaxation (Sph is the sphinctometer transducer in the LOS) allowing acid reflux to occur.

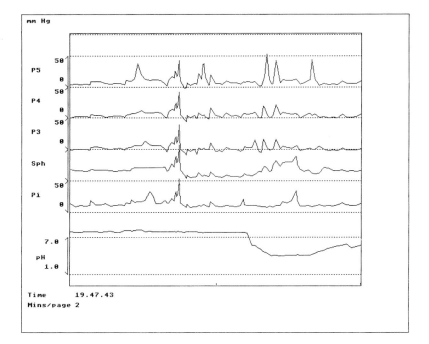

cause of reflux episodes in control subjects.[27,49,50] These studies have shown that the frequency of TLOSRs increases after eating[15,51] and are higher in the sitting position when compared to lying down.[52] The percentage of TLOSRs that led to a reflux episode varied from 34 to 58.[26,53] There are also differences reported in the number of reflux episodes caused by TLOSRs, varying between 30–100%, with the higher figure accepted by most researchers.

TLOSRs have also been shown to be the dominant cause of reflux in symptomatic patients. The proportion of reflux episodes due to TLOSRs varies with the experimental study and the severity of reflux disease. As the disease becomes more severe so a greater proportion of reflux episodes are caused by spontaneous reflux across a low-pressure sphincter. Even in this situation, however, TLOSRs remain the dominant reflux mechanism. The cause of inappropriate TLOSRs has been the subject of much debate. While some have felt that some relaxations were due to failed peristalsis others believe that TLOSRs are a variant of the belch reflex and were primarily a response to gastric distension.[52] Certainly the frequency of TLOSRs increases with gastric distension by gas or by balloons both in controls and reflux patients. Belching occurs through a relaxed sphincter with a manometric pattern very similar to that seen in the TLOSR of a reflux episode. In addition, in ambulant patients, many reflux episodes seem to be precipitated by belching (Fig. 9.4).[54,55] It therefore seems likely that TLOSRs are mediated neurally and are a physiological response to gastric distension. Perhaps the increased rate of TLOSRs in the upright position compared to the supine may be the result of differential gastric distension due to the effects of posture and gravity.

If most reflux episodes in controls and patients are caused by TLOSRs then it is unclear why patients should have more TLOSRs to account for their greater number of reflux episodes. Either they have an abnormality of the reflex (such as undue sensitivity to normal fundal stretch) or the gastric stretch is occurring

Figure 9.4
Manometric pattern of a belch precipitated acid reflux episode (marked by arrow). Pressure rise in stomach (P1) and oesophagus (P5–P3) indicate a common cavity event rather than a simultaneous oesophageal body contraction.

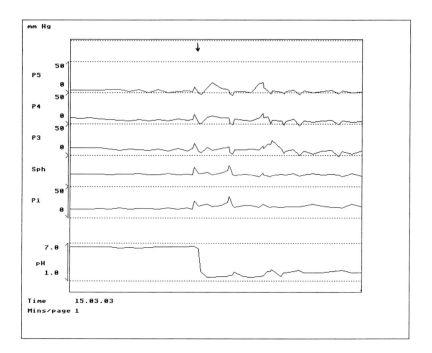

more frequently. As swallowed air is the main source of gastric gas then reflux patients might be swallowing more. Indeed there is some evidence that this occurs as they repeatedly swallow to relieve the discomfort of heartburn.

Sliding hiatus hernia

The presence of a sliding hiatus hernia was originally thought to be characteristic of GORD.[10] Most claimed that the hernia itself was the cause of impaired LOS function, allowing acid reflux to occur. It has also been suggested that GOR and acid-induced damage leads to oesophageal shortening, so pulling the stomach into the chest.[56] The importance placed on the significance of a hiatus hernia in GORD decreased from the time a physiological LOS was identified.[57] When it was found that oesophagitis was associated with deficient sphincter tone, regardless of the presence of a hiatus hernia, sphincter failure took over the aetiological role previously occupied by sliding hiatus hernia.[58,59] Recently there has been a revival of interest in the role of the sliding hiatus hernia. While it is known that the majority of patients with hiatus hernia are asymptomatic, many patients with GORD have a hernia. A previous multicentre study found the endoscopic prevalence of hiatus hernias to be 5.8%, while in patients with oesophagitis this rate rose to 32%.[14] A radiological study of patients with oesophagitis found the incidence to be as high as 90%.[59] There is evidence that GOR is more likely to occur across a deficient LOS in the presence of a hiatus hernia. In addition, oesophageal acid clearance may be impaired in patients with a sliding hiatus hernia.[60] Ambulatory oesophageal pH monitoring has demonstrated both increased frequency of GOR and prolonged acid clearance in patients with hiatus hernia compared to those without.[61] This and other studies have assessed acid clearance indirectly by counting the number of reflux episodes that last longer than five minutes and also measuring the mean acid clearance times over 24 hours (time for the pH to rise above 4 for each reflux episode, divided by the total number of reflux episodes). This indirect assessment does not allow oesophageal peristalsis to be observed and fails to take into account the possibility of repeated reflux episodes occurring during the initial pH fall. If this occurred it would give the appearance of delayed clearance even though oesophageal body peristalsis (i.e. clearance ability) may be normal.

In a study combining oesophageal pH monitoring and observing swallows of radioisotope-labelled hydrochloric acid, Mittal noted that 15 out of 20 patients with hiatus hernia demonstrated retrograde flow of acid from the stomach to the oesophagus. He suggested that a small amount of acid becomes trapped in the hernial sac, which then refluxes into the oesophagus during subsequent swallow-related LOS relaxation.[31] A study combining videofluoroscopy and oesophageal manometry during barium swallows looked at control subjects and patients with small reducing and non-reducing hiatus hernia.[62] Complete oesophageal empty-ing, without retrograde flow of barium, was achieved in 86% of the test swallows in the controls, 66% in the reducing hernia group, and 32% in the non-reducing hernia group. Impaired emptying in the group of patients with a reducing hernia was attributed to late retrograde flow as a small amount of barium flowed into the oesophagus during hernial emptying. In the group with non-reducing hernias, impaired emptying was due to early retrograde flow that occurred immediately after LOS relaxation. The group of patients with non-reducing hernias also demonstrated prolonged acid clearance times compared to control subjects. The authors concluded that the competence of the gastro-oesophageal junction was severely impaired in patients with a non-reducing hiatus hernia and that this would account for its role in the pathogenesis of GORD.

Oesophageal motility and heartburn

Oesophageal body motility in GORD has been the subject of research for many years. Early studies suggested that the symptoms of heartburn were related to various motility patterns. More recent studies[63,64,65] have shown, however, that symptoms of heartburn occur independently of oesophageal body motility changes and are caused instead by a direct action of acid on oesophageal pain receptors. In a small number of patients, motility disorders do coincide with the development of symptoms but few authors have been convinced of a link.[64,66]

Oesophageal acid clearance

Apart from the transport of food and liquid to the stomach, the oesophagus has an important role in the clearance of refluxed gastric contents (**Fig. 9.5**). The concept of oesophageal acid clearance was first proposed by Booth and col-leagues,[67] who introduced the standard acid clearance test. They found that patients with GOR required more swallows to clear the acid than asymptomatic subjects. However, this test is neither specific nor sensitive, as 47% of the patients with GOR had a normal result while subjects with oesophageal motor disorders but no acid reflux had an abnormal result.[68]

Despite the limitations of the above technique, the concept of oesophageal clearance has stimulated considerable research. The first studies of prolonged

Figure 9.5
Refluxed acid is normally cleared by primary peristalsis in a 'stepwise' pattern.

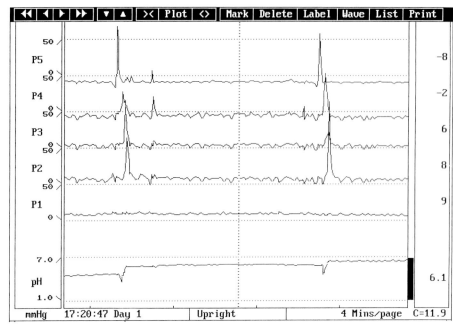

oesophageal pH monitoring[38,69,70] found that normal subjects experienced some episodes of acid reflux, but that this 'physiological' reflux was short lived and occurred mainly after eating, but rarely during sleep. In contrast, GOR patients had a greater number and a greater mean duration of individual reflux episodes. The prolonged mean duration of reflux episodes was taken to reflect a problem with the clearance ability of the oesophagus, as was the finding of the greater number of reflux episodes lasting more than 5 minutes.[71] Recently we described two distinct patterns of apparent acid clearance ability. One group of patients with prolonged acid reflux times had normal motility. In these patients prolonged acid reflux times were due to repeated superimposed acid reflux episodes giving the appearance of poor acid clearance (**Fig. 9.6**). In the other group of patients with poor motility delayed clearance was caused by genuine poor oesophageal body clearance of refluxed acid.[72] In an earlier study DeMeester found different patterns of acid reflux in controls and patients with GOR disease. Patients with oesophagitis were more likely to experience prolonged reflux episodes at night (supine refluxers) compared to shorter daytime episodes (upright refluxers), and he suggested that poor oesophageal clearance during sleep would account for greater oesophageal damage.[39] Further work has reinforced this idea of the importance of delayed acid clearance in recumbent sleeping patients in the development of oesophagitis.[61,73] The supine position is said to be important for two reasons – the effect of gravity and a reduction in oesophageal peristalsis at night. Acid clearance times during a standard acid clearance test are longer when carried out lying down compared to sitting up (and even longer if the head is tilted down).[74] Sleeping with the head of the bed elevated results in improvement in nocturnal acid clearance[75] and healing of microscopic oesophagitis,[68] suggesting that gravity plays an important role in helping to clear acid from the oesophagus. Peristaltic frequency (primary and secondary)

Figure 9.6
A prolonged acid reflux episode may be due to repeated superimposed reflux episodes rather than a single one. Clearance is only partially successful before further reflux occurs.

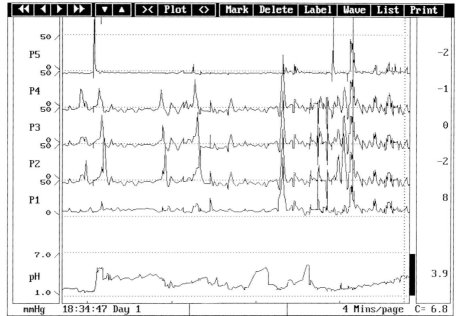

is greatly reduced during sleep[76,77,78] and this by itself is claimed to lead to prolonged acid clearance times in both controls and patients with oesophagitis.[79] Oesophagitis patients therefore have twin risks in that they experience more acid reflux at night when the oesophagus is unprotected by frequent peristalsis[80] and in some there is decreased acid clearance ability.

Several peristaltic abnormalities have been described in patients with GOR. In 1965 Olsen reported a study of oesophageal motility in 50 patients with oesophagitis. Normal peristaltic activity was found in only 28%, 32% had motor incoordination, 37% low amplitude peristalsis and 8% complete motor failure. As the degree of oesophagitis became more severe, so the proportion of patients with motor abnormalities increased.[81] Kahrilas found that patients with GOR had peristaltic dysfunction (failed primary peristalsis or hypotensive peristalsis) that became more prevalent with increasing oesophagitis. Twenty-five per cent of patients with mild oesophagitis had peristaltic dysfunction and this rate increased to 48% in patients with severe oesophagitis.[82] In patients with strictures secondary to GOR, aperistalsis and non-specific motor abnormalities may occur in up to 64% of patients compared to 32% of subjects with GOR but no stricture.[83] Kahrilas has shown the importance of orderly peristalsis in acid clearance by using combined videofluoroscopic and manometric recordings in patients with non-obstructive dysphagia or heartburn. A single normal peristaltic wave resulted in 100% clearance of a barium bolus from the oesophagus. A peristaltic amplitude of greater than 20 mmHg was required to clear barium from the distal oesophagus, though lower pressures were required in the proximal oesophagus.[84]

The fact that a certain percentage of patients with GOR have oesophageal motor abnormalities and that the prevalence increases with the severity of oesophagitis seems to be established.

It is also well known that patients with reflux disease experience intermittent dysphagia in the absence of a mechanical cause. It would seem logical to suppose that a motor abnormality would result in abnormalities of acid clearance and in food bolus transport (causing dysphagia). What is not clear, however, is whether the motor dysfunction is the primary abnormality encouraging the development of oesophagitis or whether it develops secondary to reflux-induced oesophageal inflammation.

Improvements in peristaltic amplitudes and percentage of peristaltic contractions have been found following antireflux surgery, which is said to suggest a secondary effect of acid-induced damage.[25,85] Apart from a report of two patients, however,[86] similar improvements have not been shown to occur following medically induced healing of oesophagitis.[87] Others have found no improvement in oesophageal clearance times or peristaltic behaviour following healing of oesophagitis after medical or surgical treatment.[87,88,89,90] While this could represent a primary motility abnormality, an alternative explanation is that reflux-induced oesophageal myoneuronal damage is irreversible. Against this, Eriksen *et al.*, using 24-hour pH monitoring and solid egg bolus transit times, found no correlation between delayed transit times (found in GOR patients) and severity of oesophagitis. This was taken as evidence of a primary motility problem rather than secondary to oesophageal mucosal damage,[91] a point made earlier by Maddern and Jamieson.[89]

More recently, doubt has been cast on the validity of manometrically determined motor abnormalities in reflux disease. Several studies have shown little correlation between motility and dysphagia after antireflux surgery.[92] Indeed we have shown that while dysphagia and motility abnormalities occur in patients with reflux disease in similar proportions there is no correlation between the two groups – patients with dysphagia are just as likely to have normal or abnormal motility.[93]

Saliva

Oesophageal acid clearance has been shown to depend not only on oesophageal peristalsis, but also on the neutralising ability of saliva. During concurrent radionuclide oesophageal scintigraphy, oesophageal manometry and pH monitoring, Helm found that 95% of an acid bolus was cleared by the first primary or secondary peristaltic wave. Subsequent neutralisation of residual acid occurred in a stepwise fashion with each following swallow-related peristaltic wave.[94] Stimulation of salivation shortened the time required for acid clearance, whereas aspiration of saliva from the mouth abolished acid clearance.[95] The rate of production of saliva is directly related to and determines swallowing frequency[96] which in the resting awake state is about once per minute.[77] Resting salivary flow in normal adults is 0.44 ml/minute with a pH of 7.02 ± 0.05,[97] and is capable of neutralising small amounts of acid over several minutes due mainly to its bicarbonate content. At night, saliva production virtually ceases, as does primary oesophageal peristalsis.[77] Oesophageal submucosal glands can secrete bicarbonate[98] and theoretically, the amount of bicarbonate secreted would be able to neutralise sufficient residual acid from an episode of reflux to raise pH from 2.5 to almost 7. This additional defence mechanism may be important at night when peristalsis and saliva production are greatly reduced.

Gastric abnormalities

As the source of most of the refluxate that produces oesophageal damage, the stomach ought to be a major contributor to the pathophysiology of acid reflux disease either with excessive acid production or with abnormalities of gastric emptying. Conditions that cause mechanical gastric outlet obstruction (benign or malignant causes) can indeed result in quite severe oesophagitis. Delayed gastric emptying (gastroparesis) has also been reported in some patients with GORD[99] and this may be secondary to conditions such as diabetes. In the majority of acid reflux patients, however, no abnormalities in gastric emptying can be determined and the significance of delayed gastric emptying in the pathogenesis of GORD is unclear.

Gastric hypersecretion could also promote oesophageal damage by providing excessive acid volume available for reflux. Acid hypersecretion found in Zollinger–Ellison syndrome is associated with a high rate of oesophagitis.[100] While studies have shown hypersecretion in some patients with GORD[101] as well as differences in basal and peak acid outputs, the majority show little difference in acid secretory levels compared to control subjects.

H. pylori

The available clinical evidence does not support a link between *H. pylori* and acid reflux disease either due to acid hypersecretion or the presence of Barrett's metaplasia.[102]

Duodeno-gastric reflux

There is no doubt that duodenal contents reflux into the stomach as a normal physiological process. From here they can pass into the oesophagus during episodes of gastro-oesophageal reflux. This process has been the subject of much speculation and research over the years in an attempt to determine whether duodenal contents have a role in the oesophageal injury of acid reflux disease, particularly in Barrett's oesophagus where patients appear to have more 'bile' reflux than those with uncomplicated oesophagitis. It was reasonable to suggest that the difference between the development of Barrett's oesophagus and erosive oesophagitis was the influence of duodenal contents. The majority of the studies on this subject have been interpreted as supporting this hypothesis. The problem, in human subjects, is the inability to separate the two components of the refluxate i.e. gastric and duodenal fluid. Many studies, including those aspirating the oesophageal refluxate, have compared Barrett's patients with a group of uncomplicated reflux patients who had lower median 24 hour pH times.[103] In general the greater the duration of acid reflux, the greater the amount of bile reflux[104] but the concentrations of refluxed bile acids are unlikely to be cytotoxic.[105] Acid reflux is clearly the most important factor as reflux symptoms and oesophageal inflammation can be eradicated with potent acid suppressive therapy. While this acid suppression alone will not reverse the metaplastic epithelium, mucosal injury of the Barrett's with laser or argon-gas coagulation returns the epithelium to a squamous phenotype despite continuing 'bile reflux'.[106] At the moment then, the exact role of duodeno-gastric reflux in acid reflux disease is unclear (despite strongly held views to the contrary) and further work is needed.

Oesophageal motor abnormalities

Primary oesophageal motor abnormalities comprise achalasia and diffuse oesophageal spasm. Other abnormalities have been described including nutcracker oesophagus, hypertensive lower oesophageal sphincter and non-specific motor abnormality. These conditions have been largely identified based on variations of the normal manometry pattern on standard motility testing. Their relationship to actual clinical pathology is, however, unknown.

Secondary motility disorders include collagen diseases (e.g. systemic sclerosis and SLE) and pseudoachalasia due to neoplasia and Chagas' disease.

Achalasia

Achalasia is a rare disease with an annual incidence of about 1 in 100 000. Males and females are equally affected. It can occur at any age but usually presents after the age of 30. Loss of ganglion cells in the oesophagus results in an inability to produce coordinated peristaltic contractions down the oesophageal body and a failure of appropriate lower oesophageal sphincter relaxation. The cause of this destruction is unknown but histological examination of muscle taken at the time of cardiomyotomy or oesophageal resection[107] often shows inflammatory cells around the ganglion cells. Nerve destruction is not always confined to the oesophageal body alone as some studies have suggested that abnormalities may extend to the vagus nerve itself and its dorsal motor nucleus.[108] Whatever the cause of the nerve destruction, the loss of coordinated function results in the diagnostic features of the disease of a hypertensive, non-relaxing LOS with simultaneous oesophageal body contractions. Early in the condition, before oesophageal dilatation occurs the simultaneous contractions can be quite power-ful and (in addition to the non-relaxing lower oesophageal sphincter) may contribute to the dysphagia. Once the oesophagus has dilated excessively the oesophageal body muscle is unable to contract to oppose its wall. This produces the manometric pattern of low amplitude, simultaneous pressure rises due to the swallowed material raising the pressure in the dilated cavity (**Fig. 9.7**).

The clinical features of the disease are of dysphagia, regurgitation and pain. Traditionally the dysphagia is for both liquids and solids, though the majority of patients have dysphagia for solids alone. Large quantities of food and liquid in a dilated oesophagus can lead to regurgitation and to aspiration during sleep.

In classical achalasia with a dilated oesophagus the diagnosis is readily made by barium radiology. This shows a dilated oesophagus with a 'bird beak' appearance to the lower oesophageal sphincter (**Fig. 9.8**). The peristaltic stripping wave is absent. The manometric features are of a hypertensive sphincter on pull-through (in about 50% of the patients) and the complete absence of peristaltic contrac-tions in the oesophageal body. As mentioned in the section on reflux disease, any degree of sphincter relaxation using point transducers (so casting doubt on a diagnosis of achalasia) should be considered with great caution. In early achala-sia, before the classical radiological features have developed, manometry is the

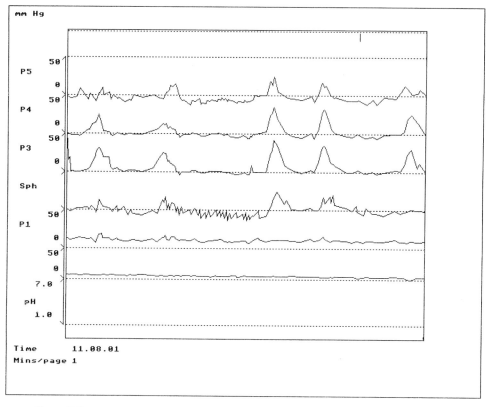

Figure 9.7
Manometric pattern of achalasia. Low amplitude simultaneous oesophageal body contractions.

Figure 9.8
Classical radiological appearance of achalasia. Dilated oesophagus tapering to a 'bird's-beak' LOS.

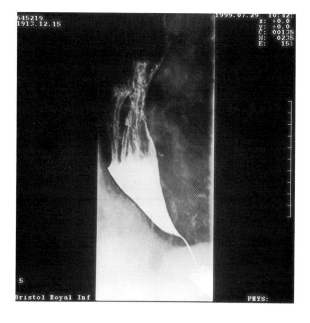

investigation of choice, as all patients will demonstrate the complete absence of peristalsis. All contractions (if visible) are simultaneous.

Treatment for the majority of patients aims to destroy the resistance of the lower oesophageal sphincter so improving dysphagia. This can be achieved by overstretching and tearing the muscle with a wide diameter (35 or 40 mm) balloon at endoscopy – this is presently the first-line treatment. The injection of botulinum toxin (blocking the presynaptic release of acetylcholine at the neuromuscular junction) has been used in recent years as a less invasive treatment, but only has a temporary effect and thus poor long-term results. Open or laparoscopic surgical myotomy, with or without an antireflux procedure, is the treatment of choice after failed balloon dilatation. The exact indications for an antireflux procedure and the best type of procedure have yet to be ascertained.

A few patients continue to experience dysphagia after ablation of their LOS (confirmed by radiology and conventional manometry) and in these a 24-hour study combined with a pH catheter may reveal the cause (such as intermittent powerful oesophageal body contractions (Fig. 9.3) or acid reflux (Fig. 9.4).

Diffuse oesophageal spasm

Diffuse oesophageal spasm is a rare disorder characterised by retrosternal chest pain and/or dysphagia and radiological and manometric abnormalities interspersed with normal peristalsis.[109] The presence of peristalsis differentiates this condition from achalasia, where peristalsis is always absent. In addition, a few patients who have had myotomies for intractable pain or as part of treatment for an associated pulsion diverticulum, muscle biopsies have revealed no histological abnormalities in the myenteric plexus (unpublished observations). Although some authors have implied that achalasia and diffuse oesophageal spasm may represent ends of a spectrum of primary motor abnormality,[110,111] it seems unlikely that there is a common aetiology.

The typical manometric features in this abnormality are high amplitude (> 180 mmHg), prolonged (> 6 seconds), multipeaked and simultaneous contractions down the oesophageal body (**Fig. 9.9**). Interspersed with these contractions are peristaltic waves that are usually of high amplitude. While not all abnormal contractions produce symptoms, those that do should have a temporal relationship with the abnormal manometry.[112] Because of the frequency of simultaneous contractions interspersed with peristaltic contractions, the diagnosis of DOS has increasingly been made by the finding on standard manometry of two or more simultaneous contractions (of the 10 wet swallows) with at least some peristalsis.[113] This has almost certainly over-diagnosed the condition and at the same time has missed some patients with quite severe but intermittent symptoms. We have shown that some patients with the typical symptoms (chest pain and dysphagia) and typical 'spasm' contractions on prolonged manometric recordings can have entirely normal standard manometry. This is perhaps not surprising in a condition that is intermittent in nature. Another feature of the disease, revealed by 24-hour manometry, is the very frequent occurrence of nocturnal 'spasm' waves that if severe can wake the patient from sleep. The radiological feature of DOS is the classical corkscrew oesophagus, but is only seen if the abnormal contractions occur during the investigation (**Fig. 9.10**). Food

Figure 9.9
Classical manometric contraction of DOS, high amplitude, multi-peaked and prolonged contractions of the oesophageal body.

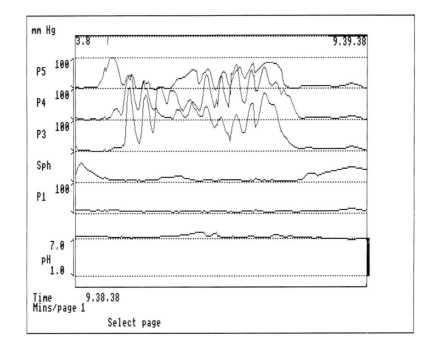

Figure 9.10
Classical radiological appearance of DOS or 'corkscrew oesophagus'.

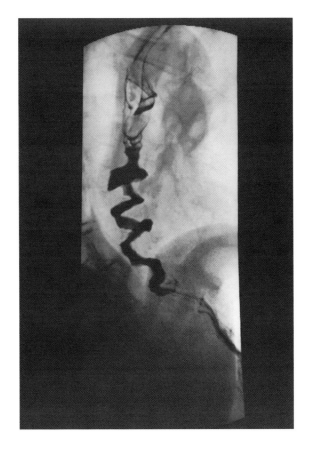

retention and oesophageal dilatation are not features of this disease but the powerful simultaneous contractions can predispose to the formation of oesophageal diverticulum.

Nutcracker oesophagus

The finding of high amplitude peristaltic contractions (greater than two standard deviations of that for normal subjects) of otherwise normal-looking waves in patients with angina-like chest pain led to the coining of the term 'nutcracker' oesophagus. Many studies have been carried out to determine its pathophysiology. There is often poor correlation between contractions and symptoms; hypertensive contractions can be found in patients investigated for reflux disease (without symptoms of chest pain or dysphagia) and in over 1000 24-hour manometric studies we have rarely been able to make this diagnosis. In contrast other groups have suggested that it is the most common of the primary oesophageal motor abnormalities (on the basis of standard manometry).[114] It seems likely that patients with chest pain and dysphagia who are found to have high amplitude contractions during standard manometry (yet without symptoms during that study) may well have DOS, but did not experience their intermittent abnormal simultaneous contractions during a short-term study. Further work is needed to determine if this diagnosis is a separate entity from diffuse oesophageal spasm or if they are both part of a spectrum of abnormal symptomatic oesophageal contraction.

Hypertensive lower oesophageal sphincter

Short-term manometric studies have also described a hypertensive LOS.[115] Usually this is found in patients with DOS if the diagnosis has been possible during the standard study but it has also been reported as an isolated abnormality. Again whether this is a true abnormality or part of the spectrum of intermittent manometric abnormalities found in DOS is unclear. The diagnosis rests on a pull-through pressure greater than 2 SD of normal subjects (40 mmHg in our laboratory). Its finding should be recorded but, in our view, usually ignored when found in isolation.

Non-specific oesophageal motor abnormality

While nutcracker oesophagus and hypertensive LOS may or may not be separate entities, this is certainly a catch-all diagnosis! It appears to be a diagnosis of anything that doesn't fit the above manometric categories but falls outside the normal pattern of standard motility testing. This would include abnormalities such as intermittent failure of peristalsis, occasional absent peristalsis to a wet swallow and low-amplitude contractions. These findings are common, particularly in reflux patients. 24-hour studies almost always show improvements in peristaltic behaviour and abnormalities rarely correlate with patient symptoms.

Secondary oesophageal motor abnormalities

There are a variety of secondary oesophageal motility problems that can occur in certain systemic conditions (**Table 9.4**). Most produce non-specific motility

Collagen-vascular diseases
   Systemic sclerosis
   Mixed connective tissue disease
   Polymyositis and dermatomyositis
   Systemic lupus erythematosis

Endocrine and metabolic disorders
   Diabetes
   Amyloidosis

Neuromuscular diseases
   Myotonic dystrophy
   Myasthenia gravis
   Multiple sclerosis
   Cerebrovascular diseases

Chronic idiopathic intestinal pseudo-obstruction

Chagas' disease

Ageing

Table 9.4 *Conditions associated with secondary oesophageal motor dysfunction*

abnormalities such as low-amplitude contractions or failure of peristaltic propagation and their rarity leaves them outside the scope of this publication. Some however produce more specific oesophageal abnormalities.

Scleroderma

Scleroderma or systemic sclerosis is a disease characterised by fibrosis and degenerative changes in the skin, synovium and parenchyma of certain organs, notably the heart, kidneys, lungs and intestines. The oesophagus is involved in approximately 75–85% of patients by either manometric or radiological criteria. Histological studies of the oesophagus show that the smooth muscle layers are atrophied with some fibrous replacement, whereas the striated portion remains essentially normal. Involvement of the lower oesophagus initially results in a patulous lower oesophageal sphincter with negligible pressure. Acid reflux is common, leading to oesophagitis which is compounded by the poor clearance ability of the oesophageal body involved. Patients complain of a variety of symptoms including dysphagia (related to the motor abnormality), regurgitation, aspiration and heartburn (related to acid reflux). The diagnosis of oesophageal involvement is readily made with standard manometry which reveals a low lower-oesophageal sphincter pressure on pull-through and feeble or non-existent peristalsis in the mid and lower oesophageal body. In contrast, pressure waves are normal in the striated portion of the upper oesophageal body. Treatment of the oesophageal involvement centres on the control of acid reflux, usually with a proton pump inhibitor and dilatation of any peptic stricture. Antireflux surgery should only be considered as a last resort due to the poor oesophageal body motility and should be as non-obstructing as possible (partial fundoplication).

Mixed connective tissue disease

This disorder demonstrates clinical features found in systemic sclerosis, polymyositis and systemic lupus erythematosis (SLE). More than 60% of patients have oesophageal involvement and the manometric findings are very similar to systemic sclerosis.

Polymyositis and dermatomyositis

Polymyositis (dermatomyositis if accompanied by the classical skin eruption) is a diffuse inflammatory disease of striated muscle. The proximal striated portion of the oesophagus is involved in about 60–70% of cases and produces symptoms of aspiration, nasopharyngeal regurgitation and oropharyngeal dysphagia. These features are more readily observed by radiology than by manometry.

Chronic idiopathic intestinal pseudo-obstruction

Chronic idiopathic intestinal pseudo-obstruction produces intermittent symptoms and signs of intestinal obstruction in the absence of a mechanical blockage. Motility abnormalities can occur throughout the intestine and the oesophagus is frequently involved, even if asymptomatic. Most patients demonstrate a lack of peristalsis (either simultaneous waves or none at all) with varying degrees of failure of lower oesophageal relaxation. Indeed the manometric picture can be very similar to achalasia, even when patients do not complain of dysphagia.

Chagas' disease

Chagas' disease is produced by the protozoan *T. cruzi* and is confined to the South American continent. Typically it affects the heart, producing cardiomyopathy and the oesophagus resulting in a megaoesophagus. Oesophageal involvement results in symptoms very similar to severe achalasia with intermittent dysphagia that worsens as oesophageal dilatation progresses. As in achalasia there is destruction of the myenteric nerve plexus. The diagnosis is made by barium radiology in combination with the appropriate immunological investigations. Treatment in the early stage (before significant oesophageal dilatation) is the same as in achalasia, namely dilatation of the oesophageal sphincter. Later, with increasing dilatation of the oesophagus, oesophagectomy may be required.

Achalasia in neoplasia

The association of achalasia with oesophageal and proximal gastric cancer has been known about for some time. In these cases it is presumed that the achalasia develops as a consequence of a paraneoplastic process affecting the myenteric nerves or by direct malignant invasion of the plexus. It has also been described as occurring in malignancy away from the oesophagus itself such as bronchial carcinoma. This pseudoachalasia can be indistinguishable from primary achalasia on manometry and often on radiology. Features that would be more in keeping with pseudoachalasia would be sudden onset of progressive symptoms with excessive weight loss. It is important to realise that malignant pseudoachalasia is distinct from squamous carcinoma of the oesophagus developing in longstanding achalasia that is presumed to be a result of chronic stasis and mucosal irritation.

Ageing (Presbyoesophagus)

Based on early radiological and manometric studies it was initially felt that ageing produced certain patterns of oesophageal dysfunction such as increased tertiary contractions, abnormal contractions (multipeaked waves) and greater failure of peristaltic propagation. This has been confirmed in recent studies showing reduced LOS pressure and peristaltic amplitudes as well as greater failure of peristaltic contractions.[116,117] If patients with diseases that are known to affect the oesophagus are excluded, then ageing produces motility changes that are of only minor functional significance.

Methods of investigation

The oesophagus is the easiest part of the GI tract to investigate because of its accessibility. Consequently many techniques have been developed over the years to study structure and function. Some tests are widely used in clinical practice (barium radiology and flexible endoscopy) while others are predominantly research tools (oesophageal aspiration studies). Some of the techniques used to investigate the oesophagus are described below but a detailed description of individual methodologies is beyond the scope of this chapter.

Endoscopy

Flexible endoscopy is often the first line of investigation in patients with symptoms that may involve the oesophagus. In addition to visual examination of the mucosa, histological and cytological specimens can be obtained and therapeutic procedures such as stricture dilatation, oesophageal stent insertion and arresting haemorrhage can be performed. Not only can endoscopy detect mucosal abnormalities, but it may also give a clue to the presence of an oesophageal motility abnormality. A dilated oesophagus containing food debris with a tight but passable lower oesophageal sphincter may suggest achalasia. An oesophageal diverticulum might suggest a motility abnormality. For the most part, however, the endoscope is a poor method of investigating motility problems as it detects mucosal structural problems rather than muscular functional abnormalities.

Radiology

Contrast radiology plays an important part in the investigation of oesophageal problems, detecting anatomical, mucosal and functional abnormalities. It can be used for both acid reflux disease and certain motility problems.

A simple chest X-ray may show lung changes that would support a history of aspiration or reveal the presence of a large hiatus hernia.

A double contrast barium study can reveal the mucosal abnormalities of oesophageal inflammation and strictures. It will demonstrate the presence of webs, rings, diverticulae and hiatus hernias, along with the presence or absence of normal propagating contractions. As such it may reveal the classical motility abnormalities of achalasia or diffuse oesophageal spasm ('corkscrew' appearance). The diagnosis, however, in early achalasia and DOS patients is often missed. While endoscopy has overtaken radiology in the investigation of reflux disease, radiology still retains an important role in the investigation of patients with motility abnormalities. Techniques such as videofluoroscopy combined with solid and liquid bolus swallows can help in the diagnosis of pharyngeal and upper oesophageal motility disorders.

pH studies

The development of miniaturised pH catheters, digital recording devices and computer analysis software has allowed prolonged (24-hour) ambulatory pH recordings to become widely available in clinical practice. Not only does the equipment record acid reflux episodes as they occur, it also allows a correlation between patient symptoms and those episodes to be made using an event marker (**Figure 9.11**). Computerised software then analyses the recording to produce tables of standard variables that can be compared to known control values. With prolonged recordings of frequent reflux episodes several measures have become standard. These include the total number of reflux episodes, the number lasting more than 5 minutes and the total acid reflux time (as a percentage of the total recording time). The latter is probably the single most useful measurement and, in most centres, an oesophageal pH of <4, recorded 5 cm above a manometrically defined LOS, should be present for less than 4% of a 24-hour period in normal individuals. If the recording is further divided into daytime, night-time and post-prandial periods a large number of values are possible. As there is a wide spectrum of severity of acid reflux disease, with day-to-day variation, the recorded variables have to be referenced to known

Figure 9.11
24 hour pH study showing excessive acid reflux in a patient with Barrett's oesophagus. Note correlation of patient's pain with acid in the oesophagus.

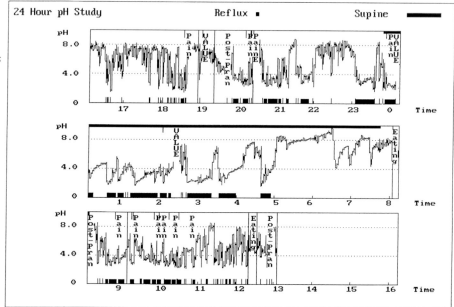

control values. One such system that is widely used is the revised Johnson/ DeMeester score that tries to produce a score based on the above variables (from control subjects) above which acid reflux is likely (**Table 9.5**). While this may be helpful, an abnormal score should not be used in isolation to other clinical information. In addition, consideration has to be given to the symptom (event) marker so that the patient's typical symptoms can be correlated with what is happening in the oesophagus at the moment of the symptoms. For example a patient may still be considered to suffer from acid reflux disease if every typical symptom is correlated in time with acid in the oesophagus despite an overall oesophageal pH time within the normal range. At the other extreme a patient with no correlation of their symptoms with acid in the oesophagus and with pH study variables above the normal range does not necessarily have acid reflux disease. The result of a pH study should be taken into consideration with the clinical history, endoscopy and radiology findings and response to acid suppression with a proton pump inhibitor. Furthermore, most patients with reflux disease do not need a pH study. A typical history, endoscopic evidence of oesophagitis and a good response to acid suppression are enough for a diagnosis without the need for a pH study. A pH study should be used for atypical symptoms, incomplete or poor response to acid suppression or before contemplating antireflux surgery.

pH	Total	Upright	Supine	Eating	Post-prandial	Fasting
Duration (hrs)	20:48	12:50	7:58	0:55	2:30	0:00
No. of reflux episodes	123	106	17	1	19	–
Time below pH 4.0	426:34	228:19	198:15	0:03	53:17	–
% Time below pH 4.0	34.1	29.6	41.4	0.1	35.5	–
No. of episodes > 5 min	24	15	9	0	4	–
Longest reflux (mins)	42:27	27:15	42:27	0:03	12:16	–

Scores according to Johnson and DeMeester for pH < 4

Component	Patient value	95% values	Score
% Total time	34.1	4.45	24.96
% Upright time	29.6	8.42	12.64
% Supine time	41.4	3.45	41.77
No. of episodes	123	46.90	9.08
No. > 5 min	24	3.45	20.62
Longest episode	42:27	19.80	5.54
Composite score			**114.61**

95 percentile score at pH < 4 for normals is 14.72

Table 9.5 *pH values and Johnson and DeMeester score for patient illustrated in Fig. 9.11*

While the precise details of the technique of pH studies are beyond the scope of this chapter, a few important points are worth mentioning. In order to produce standardised and reproducible results most studies are carried out in an agreed way. An acid reflux episode, as recorded by a pH probe, starts when the oesophageal pH drops below 4 and ends when it rises above 5 (or 4 in some laboratories). The pH probe is positioned so that it lies 5 cm above the top of the lower oesophageal sphincter. If the probe is positioned too low it will slip into the stomach on the upward movement of the lower oesophagus and will then result in excessive acid reflux times. Conversely if the probe is too high then acid reflux times will be underestimated. As different subjects have different distances from the tip of the nose (where the probe is secured) to the LOS, a guess of the distance cannot be used. *The only reliable way of accurate pH probe placement is to determine the position of the LOS by manometry.* Using the number of reflux episodes that last more than 5 minutes to imply poor clearance and hence poor motility is inaccurate. Long-lasting reflux episodes on a pH study are just as likely to be due to multiple superimposed reflux episodes than to poor clearance of a single reflux event.[72] Assuming pH rises above 7.5 are due to alkaline reflux is also inaccurate.[105] Completion of a diary sheet to record symptoms, activities and ingested food types is also important. Several foods and drinks are acidic and may be inaccurately recorded as a reflux episode if not eliminated from the analysis. The alternative is to restrict the patient to particular neutral foodstuffs, but this then becomes increasingly less of a physiological outpatient ambulatory study. Patients should eat and drink the 'normal' foods that would result in a typical day of reflux symptoms. At the completion of the study the quantity and type of symptoms experienced should also be recorded to help in the analysis of the data. Instruction to the patient on the use of the event marker and to document in a diary what symptom was being recorded is also important, particularly if the event marker can be pressed accidentally.

Manometry

As the main function of the oesophagus is the transport of food and drink into the stomach manometry ought to be a useful technique for studying disorders of this organ. Its usefulness, however, has probably been overstated. Two methods of manometric recording are available – the standard static study and ambulatory study.

Standard manometry

Manometry recordings can be obtained from catheters containing solid-state pressure transducers or water-perfused channels. The manometry catheter is passed into the stomach and then slowly withdrawn 1 cm at a time so that the pressure ports pass through the lower oesophageal sphincter. This allows the base-line sphincter pressure (above resting gastric pressure) to be measured along with estimations of sphincter length. The values of several pressure ports can be averaged out to give a mean sphincter pressure and sphincter length. Next the pressure ports are positioned in the oesophageal body, usually three, placed 5 cm apart. Motility is assessed by the use of the standard 10 wet swallow test. Like the pH study, control data are used to compare the findings from patients including such parameters as the number of peristaltic contractions that occur in response to the wet swallows, the amplitude and velocity of the contractions and the occurrence of abnormal contractions such as simultaneous or non-propagated waves. A further procedure that can be added to the standard study using a water-perfused catheter assembly is measurement of LOS relaxation. This has to be performed with a sleeve device that straddles the LOS, allowing up and down movement of the LOS relative to the catheter. As the catheter needed is water-perfused these studies have to be performed with patients immobile in the laboratory. While LOS function is of prime importance in the pathogenesis of acid reflux disease, its clinical measurement is of limited value (outside of research studies) as detection of GORD is by other methods and treatment ignores LOS behaviour.

The standard motility study is extensively used in physiology laboratories but could be criticised as being un-physiological. In a 24-hour period there are between 1000–2000 peristaltic swallows along with many other contraction types. Several meals and drinks are consumed and many pressure events occur. If motility abnormalities occur, particularly if they are intermittent, they may be missed on a study measuring just 10 water swallows.

Ambulatory pH and manometry

The development of solid-state pressure transducers, miniaturised digital recording devices and modern computer technologies have allowed the introduction of prolonged manometric studies in ambulatory patients (**Fig. 9.12**). Several studies have described their use in intermittent problems such as non-cardiac chest pain and obscure motility abnormalities.[118] It may be that some of the primary oesophageal motility abnormalities need to be reclassified on the basis of a prolonged study e.g. diffuse oesophageal spasm, particularly if symptoms and abnormal motor events occur intermittently or at night.

One of the advantages of some of the modern systems is the ability to combine simultaneous pH and motility recordings (and even ECG) to further help in the diagnosis of obscure chest pain. Further work is needed in defining the role of these types of recording systems.

Measurement of duodeno-gastric oesophageal reflux

While many believe that duodeno-gastric oesophageal reflux may contribute to the pathophysiology of reflux disease, the paucity of convincing clinical evidence and the lack of effective treatment (excluding surgery) in combination with the eradication of inflammation and symptoms with acid suppression alone makes the routine investigation of bile reflux unnecessary. In the past a rise in oesophageal pH above 8 and aspiration studies were the only methods available for detecting duodeno-gastric reflux. However, pH rises above 8 have been shown to be too unreliable to detect alkaline reflux[105] and aspiration studies too cumbersome and uncomfortable to be clinically useful.[103] The development of the 'Bilitec' (Synectics) recorder uses the spectrophotometric detection of bilirubin as an indirect measure of bile salt reflux and the studies can be performed in much the same way as ambulatory pH recordings. Its clinical role has still to be determined.

Figure 9.12
Combined pH and manometry catheters for ambulatory recordings. The pH probe is positioned 5 cm above the top of the LOS.

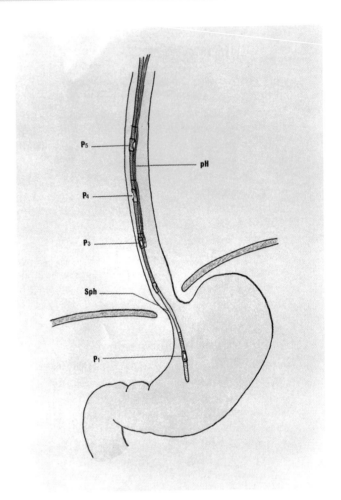

Provocation studies

In the past a variety of provocation tests were developed to try to help in the diagnosis of oesophageal disease (particularly GORD). With the widespread use of prolonged pH monitoring and oesophageal manometry these have largely disappeared from clinical use.

Oesophageal scintigraphy

Oesophageal scintigraphy has been adapted to investigate the oesophagus as an alternative to radiological investigation. The reported advantage over conventional radiology is the production of dynamic data with objective measurements of oesophageal transit. Solid or liquid boluses can be labelled with Technetium 99 m and the transport of the boluses measured with a gamma camera and graphs produced. Except for enthusiasts or researchers, the data generated by this technique have little discriminatory advantage over conventional methods of studying the oesophagus.

References

1. Castell DO. Anatomy and physiology of the esophagus and its sphincters. In: Esophageal Motility Testing. Castell DO, Richter JE, Dalton CB (eds.). New York: Elsevier Science, 1987, pp. 13–27.

2. Sugarbaker DJ, Rattan S, Goyal RJ. Mechanical and electrical activity of esophageal smooth muscle during peristalsis. Am J Physiol 1984; 246:G145–50.

3. Madsen T, Wallin L, Larsen VH. Oesophageal peristalsis in normal subjects: influence of pH and volume during imitated gastro-oesophageal reflux. Scand J Gastroenterol 1983; 18:513–18.

4. Dodds WJ, Hogan WJ, Reid DP et al. A comparison between primary esophageal peristalsis following wet and dry swallows. J Appl Physiol 1973; 35:851–7.

5. Hollis JB, Castell DO. Effect of dry swallows and wet swallows of different volumes on esophageal peristalsis. J Appl Physiol 1975; 38:1161–1164.

6. Winship DH, Viegas DE, Andrade SR et al. Influence of bolus temperature on human esophageal motor function. J Clin Invest 1970; 49:243–50.

7. Higgs B, Shorter RG, Ellis FH. A study of the anatomy of the human esophagus with special reference to the gastroesophageal sphincter. J Surg Res 1965; 5:503–7.

8. Skinner DB, Booth DJ. Assessment of distal esophageal function in patients with hiatal hernia and/or gastroesophageal reflux. Ann Surg 1970; 172:627–37.

9. Cohen S, Harris LD. Does hiatus hernia affect competence of the gastroesophageal sphincter? N Engl J Med 1971; 289:1053–6.

10. Allison PR. Reflux esophagitis, sliding hiatal hernia, and the anatomy of repair. Surg Gynecol Obstet 1951; 92:419–31.

11. Kaye MD, Showater JP. Manometric configuration of the lower esophageal sphincter in normal human subjects. Gastroenterology 1971; 61:213–23.

12. Bemelman WA, Van Der Hulst VPM, Dijkhuis T et al. The lower esophageal sphincter shown by a computerized representation. Scand J Gastroenterol 1990; 25:601–8.

13. Goodall RJR, Hay DJ, Temple JG. Assessment of the rapid pull through technique in oesophageal manometry. Gut 1980; 21:169–73.

14. Baldi F, Ferrarini F, Labate AMM et al. Prevalence of esophagitis in patients undergoing routine upper endoscopy: A multicenter survey in Italy. In: Esophageal Disorders: Pathophysiology and therapy. DeMeester TR, Skinner DB (eds.). New York: Raven Press, 1985; pp. 213–19.

15. Dent J, Dodds WJ, Friedman RH et al. Mechanism of gastroesophageal reflux in recumbent asymptomatic human subjects. J Clin Invest 1980; 65:256–67.

16. Dent J, Dodds WJ, Sekiguchi T et al. Interdigestive phasic contractions of the human lower esophageal sphincter. Gastroenterology 1983; 84:453–60.

17. Dodds WJ, Dent J, Hogan WJ et al. Effect of atropine on esophageal motor function in humans. Am J Physiol 1981; 240:G290–96.

18. Rattan S, Goyal RK. Neural control of the lower esophageal sphincter. Influence of the vagus nerves. J Clin Invest 1974; 54:899–906.

19. Gonella J, Niel JP, Roman C. Vagal control of lower oesophageal sphincter motility in the cat. J Physiol 1977; 273:647–64.

20. Dent J. A new technique for continuous sphincter pressure measurement. Gastroenterology 1976; 71:263–67.

21. Linehan JH, Dent J, Dodds WJ et al. Sleeve device functions as a Starling resistor to record sphincter pressure. Am J Physiol 1985; 248:G251–G255.

22. Dodds WJ, Stewart ET, Hogan WJ et al. Effect of esophageal movement on intraluminal esophageal pressure recording. Gastroenterology 1974; 67:592–600.

23. Winans CS. Alteration of lower esophageal sphincter characteristics with respiration and proximal esophageal balloon distension. Gastroenterology 1972; 62:380–88.

24. Corazziari E, Bontempo I, Anzini F et al. Motor activity of the distal oesophagus and gastro-oesophageal reflux. Gut 1984; 25:7–13.

25. Gill RC, Bowes KL, Murphy PD et al. Esophageal motor abnormalities in gastroesophageal reflux and the effects of fundoplication. Gastroenterology 1986; 91:364–69.

26. Dodds WJ, Dent J, Hogan WJ et al. Mechanisms of gastroesophageal reflux in patients with reflux esophagitis. N Engl J Med 1982; 307:1547–52.

27. Mittal RK, McCallum RW. Characteristics of transient lower esophageal sphincter relaxations in humans. Am J Physiol 1987; 252:G636–G641.

28. Atkinson M, Summerling MD. The competence of the cardia after cardiomyotomy. Gastroenterologia 1954; 92:123–34.

29. Clark MD, Rinaldo JA, Eyler WR. Correlation of manometric and radiological data from the esophagogastric area. Radiology 1970; 94:261–70.

30. Welch RW, Gray JE. Influence of respiration on recordings of lower esophageal sphincter pressure in humans. Gastroenterology 1982; 83:590–94.

31. Mittal RK, Rochester DF, McCallum RW. Effect of diaphragmatic contraction on lower oesophageal sphincter pressure in man. Gut 1987; 28:1564–8.

32. Meiss JH, Grindlay JH, Ellis FH. The gastroesophageal sphincter mechanism. J Thorac Surg 1958; 36:156–65.

33. Bombeck CT, Dillard DH, Nyhus LM. Muscular anatomy of the gastroesophageal junction and role of the phrenoesophageal ligament. An autopsy study of the sphincter mechanism. Ann Surg 1966; 164:643–52.

34. De Caestecker JS, Heading RC. The pathophysiology of reflux. In: Reflux oesophagitis. Hennessy TPJ, Cuschieri A, Bennett JR (eds.). London: Butterworth, 1989, pp. 1–36.

35. Joelsson BE, DeMeester TR, Skinner DB et al. The role of the esophageal body in the antireflux mechanism. Surgery 1982; 92:417–23.

36. Pettersson GB, Bombeck CT, Nyhus LM. The lower esophageal sphincter: mechanisms of opening and closure. Surgery 1980; 80:307–14.

37. DeMeester TR, Wernly JA, Bryant GH et al. Clinical and in vitro analysis of determinants of gastroesophageal competence: a study of the principal of antireflux surgery. Am J Surg 1979; 137:39–45.

38. Johnson LF, DeMeester TR. Twenty-four hour pH monitoring of the distal oesophagus: a quantative measure of gastroesophageal reflux. Am J Gastroenterol 1974; 62:325–32.

39. DeMeester TR, Johnson LF, Joseph GJ et al. Patterns of gastroesophageal reflux in health and disease. Ann Surg 1976; 184:259–70.

40. Graham DY, Smith JL, Patterson DJ. Why do apparently healthy people use antacid tablets? Am J Gastroenterol 1983; 78:257–60.

41. Johansson KE, Ask P, Boeryd B et al. Oesophagitis, signs of reflux, and gastric acid secretion in patients with symptoms of gastro-oesophageal reflux disease. Scand J Gastroenterol 1986; 21:837–47.

42. Fuchs KH, DeMeester TR, Albertucci M. Specificity and sensitivity of objective diagnosis of gastroesophageal reflux disease. Surgery 1987; 102:575–80.

43. Stoker DL, Williams JG, Leicester RG et al. Oesophagitis – a five year review. Gut 1988; 29:A1450.

44. Palmer ED. The hiatus hernia – esophagitis – esophageal stricture complex. Am J Med 1968; 44:566–79.

45. Patterson DJ, Graham DY, Smith JL et al. Natural history of benign esophageal stricture treated by dilatation. Gastroenterology 1983; 85:346–50.

46. Gotley DC, Cooper MJ. The investigation of gastro-oesophageal reflux. Surg Res Comm 1987; 2:1–17.

47. Johnsson F, Joelsson BO. Reproducibility of ambulatory oesophageal pH monitoring. Gut 1988; 29:886–9.

48. Johnsson F, Joelsson B, Gudmundsson K et al. Symptoms and endoscopic findings in the diagnosis of gastroesophageal reflux disease. Scand J Gastroenterol 1987; 22:714–18.

49. Baldi F, Ferrarini F, Balestra R et al. Oesophageal motor events at the occurrence of acid reflux and during endogenous acid exposure in healthy subjects and in patients with oesophagitis. Gut 1985; 26:336–41.

50. Smout AJPM, Akkermans LMA, Bogaard JW et al. 'Inappropriate' lower esophageal sphincter relaxations in normal subjects (Abstract). Dig Dis Sci 1985; 30:795.

51. Freidin N, Mittal RK, McCallum RW. Does body posture affect the incidence and mechanism of gastro-oesophageal reflux? Gut 1991; 32:133–6.

52. Wyman JB, Dent J, Dodds WJ et al. Control of belching by the lower oesophageal sphincter. Gut 1990; 31:639–46.

53. Dent J, Holloway RH, Toouli J et al. Mechanisms of lower oesophageal sphincter incompetence in patients with symptomatic gastro-oesophageal reflux. Gut 1988; 29:1020–8.

54. Barham CP, Gotley DC, Miller R et al. Pressure events surrounding acid reflux episodes and acid clearance in ambulant healthy control subjects. Gut 1993; 34:444–9.

55. Barham CP, Gotley DC, Mills A et al. Precipitating causes of acid reflux episodes in ambulant patients with gastro-oesophageal reflux disease. Gut 1995; 36:505–10.

56. Orringer MB, Stirling MB. Short esophagus and peptic stricture. In: Surgery of the chest, 5th edn, vol. 1. Sabiston DC and Spencer FC (eds). Philadelphia: WB Saunders, 1990, pp. 930–50.

57. Fyke FE, Code CF, Schlegel JF. The gastroesophageal sphincter in healthy human beings. Gastroenterologia 1956; 86:135–50.

58. Atkinson M, Edwards DAW, Honour AJ et al. The oesophagogastric sphincter in hiatus hernia. Lancet 1957; ii:1138–42.

59. Ott DJ, Wu WC, Gelfand DW. Reflux esophagitis revisited: prospective analysis of radiological accuracy. Gastrointest Radiol 1981; 6:1–7.

60. DeMeester TR, Lafontaine E, Joelsson BE et al. Relationship of a hiatus hernia to the function of the body of the esophagus and the gastroesophageal junction. J Thorac Cardiovasc Surg 1981; 82:547–58.

61. Johnson LF, DeMeester TR, Haggitt RC. Esophageal epithelial response to gastroesophageal reflux, a quantitive study. Dig Dis Sci 1978; 23:498–509.

62. Sloan S, Kahrilas PJ. Impairment of esophageal emptying with hiatal hernia. Gastroenterology 1991; 100:596–605.

63. Atkinson M, Bennett JR. Relationship between motor changes and pain during esophageal acid perfusion. Am J Dig Dis 1968; 13:346–50.

64. Richter JE, Johns DN, Wu WC et al. Are esophageal motility abnormalities produced during the intraesophageal acid perfusion test? J Am Med Assoc 1985; 253:1914–17.

65. Burns TW, Venturatos SG. Esophageal motor function and response to acid perfusion in patients with symptomatic reflux esophagitis. Dig Dis Sci 1985; 30:529–35.

66. Kjellen G, Tibbling L. Oesophageal motility during acid provoked heartburn and chest pain. Scand J Gastroenterol 1985; 20:937–40.

67. Booth DJ, Kemmerer WT, Skinner DB. Acid clearing from the distal esophagus. Arch Surg 1968; 96:731–34.

68. Stanciu C, Bennett JR. Oesophageal acid clearing: one factor in the production of reflux oesophagitis. Gut 1974; 15:852–7.

69. Spencer J. The use of prolonged pH recording in the diagnosis of gastro-oesophageal reflux. Br J Surg 1969; 56:912–14.

70. Pattrick FG. Investigation of gastroesophageal reflux in various positions with a two-lumen pH electrode. Gut 1970; 11:659–67.

71. DeMeester TR, Wang CI, Wernly JA et al. Technique, indications and clinical use of 24 hour esophageal pH monitoring. J Thorac Cardiovasc Surg 1980; 79:656–70.

72. Barham CP, Gotley DC, Mills A, Alderson D. Oesophageal acid clearance in patients with severe oesophagitis. Br J Surg 1995; 82:333–37.

73. Little AG, DeMeester TR, Kirchner PT et al. Pathogenesis of esophagitis in patients with gastroesophageal reflux. Surgery 1980; 88:101–07.

74. Kjellen G, Tibbling L. Influence of body position, dry and wet swallows, smoking and alcohol on oesophageal acid clearing. Scand J Gastroenterol 1978; 13:283–8.

75. Johnson LF, DeMeester TR. Evaluation of elevation of the head of the bed, bethanechol and antacid foam tablets on gastroesophageal reflux. Dig Dis Sci 1981; 26:673–80.

76. Wallin L, Madsen T. 12-hour simultaneous registration of acid reflux and peristaltic activity in the oesophagus. A study in normal subjects. Scand J Gastroenterol 1979; 14:561–66.

77. Lichter I, Muir RC. The pattern of swallowing during sleep. Electroencephalogr Clin Neurophysiol 1975; 38:427–32.

78. Lear CSC, Flanagan JB, Moorrees CFA. The frequency of deglutition in man. Arch Oral Biol 1965; 10:83–96.

79. Orr WC, Robinson MG, Johnson LF. Acid clearance during sleep in the pathogenesis of reflux esophagitis. Dig Dis Sci 1981; 26:423–27.

80. Kruse-Anderson S, Wallin L, Madsen T. Acid gastro-oesophageal reflux and oesophageal pressure activity during postprandial and nocturnal periods. Scand J Gastroenterol 1987; 22:926–30.

81. Olsen AM, Schlegel JF. Motility disturbances caused by oesophagitis. J Thorac Cardiovasc Surg 1965; 50:607–12.

82. Kahrilas PJ, Dodds WJ, Hogan WJ et al. Esophageal peristaltic dysfunction in peptic esophagitis. Gastroenterology 1986; 91:897–904.

83. Ahtaridis G, Snape WJ, Cohen S. Clinical and manometric findings in benign peptic strictures of the esophagus. Dig Dis Sci 1979; 24:858–61.

84. Kahrilas PJ, Dodds WJ, Hogan WJ. Effect of peristaltic dysfunction on esophageal volume clearance. Gastroenterology 1988; 94:73–80.

85. Escandell AO, De Haro LFM, Paricio PP et al. Surgery improves defective oesophageal peristalsis in patients with gastro-oesophageal reflux. Br J Surg 1991; 78:1095–7.

86. Marshall JB, Gerhardt DC. Improvement in esophageal motor dysfunction with treatment of reflux esophagitis: a report of 2 cases. Am J Gastroenterol 1982; 77:351–4.

87. Eckardt VF. Does healing of esophagitis improve esophageal motor function? Dig Dis Sci 1988; 33:161–5.

88. Russell COH, Pope CE, Gannan RM et al. Does surgery correct esophageal motor dysfunction in gastroesophageal reflux? Ann Surg 1981; 194:290–95.

89. Maddern GJ, Jamieson GG. Oesophageal emptying in patients with gastro-oesophageal reflux. Br J Surg 1986; 73:615–17.

90. Baldi F, Ferrarini F, Longanesi A et al. Oesophageal function before, during and after healing of erosive oesophagitis. Gut 1988; 29:157–60.

91. Eriksen CA, Sadek SA, Cranford C et al. Reflux oesophagitis and oesophageal transit: evidence for a primary oesophageal motor disorder. Gut 1988; 29:448–52.

92. Baigrie RJ, Watson DI, Myers JC et al. Outcome of laparoscopic Nissen fundoplication in patients with disordered preoperative peristalsis. Gut 1997; 40:381–85.

93. Anthony A, Barham CP, Mills A et al. Non-obstructive dysphagia in patients with gastro-oesophageal reflux disease – is manometry helpful?

Accepted for presentation to the Association of Surgeons, 2000.

94. Helm JF, Dodds WJ, Riedel DR *et al*. Determinants of esophageal acid clearance in normal subjects. Gastroenterology 1983; 85:607–12.

95. Helm JF, Dodds WJ, Pele LR *et al*. Effect of esophageal emptying and saliva on clearance of acid from the esophagus. N Engl J Med 1984; 310:284–288.

96. Kapila YV, Dodds WJ, Helm JF *et al*. Relationship between swallow rate and salivary flow. Dig Dis Sci 1984; 29:528–33.

97. Helm JF, Dodds WJ, Hogan WJ *et al*. Acid neutralising capicity of human saliva. Gastroenterology 1982; 83:69–74.

98. Meyers RL, Orlando RC. *In vivo* bicarbonate secretion by human esophagus. Gastroenterology 1992; 103:1174–8.

99. Dubois A. Pathophysiology of gastroesophageal reflux disease: role of gastric factors. In: Castell DO (ed) The esophagus. Boston, MA: Little, Brown, 1992, pp. 479–92.

100. Miller LS, Vinayek R, Frucht H *et al*. Reflux esophagitis in patients with Zollinger-Ellison syndrome. Gastroenterology 1990; 98:341–6.

101. Barlow AP, DeMeester TR, Ball CS *et al*. The significance of the gastric secretory state in gastroesophageal reflux disease. Arch Surg 1989; 124:937–40.

102. Oberg S, Peters JH, Nigro JJ *et al*. *Helicobacter pylori* is not associated with the manifestations of gastro-oesophageal reflux disease. Arch Surg 1999; 134:722–726.

103. Nehra D, Howell P, Williams CP *et al*. Toxic bile acids in gastro-oesophageal reflux disease: Influence of gastric acidity. Gut 1999; 44:598–602.

104. Marshall REK, Anggiansah A, Owen WA *et al*. The temporal relationship between oesophageal bile reflux and pH in gastro-oesophageal reflux disease. Euro J Gastroenterol Hepatol 1998; 10:385–92.

105. Gotley DC. Bile acids and trypsin are unimportant in alkaline oesophageal reflux. J Clin Gastroenterol 1992; 14:2–7.

106. Barham CP, Jones R, Hardwick R *et al*. Photothermal ablation of Barrett's oesophagus: endoscopic and histological evidence of squamous re-epithelialisation. Gut 1997; 41:281–84.

107. Goldblum JR, Whyte RI, Orringer MB *et al*. Achalasia. A morphological study of 42 resected specimens. Am J Surg Pathol 1994; 18:327–37.

108. Cassella RR, Brown AL, Sayre GP *et al*. Achalasia of the esophagus: pathologic and etiologic considerations. Ann Surg 1964; 160:474–86.

109. Fleshler B. Diffuse esophageal spasm. Gastroenterology 1967; 52:559–64.

110. Kramer P, Harris LD, Donaldson RM. Transition from symptomatic diffuse spasm to cardiospasm. Gut 1967; 8:115–19.

111. Vantrappen G, Janssens J, Hellemans J *et al*. Achalasia, diffuse esophageal spasm and related motility disorders. Gastroenterology 1979; 76:450–7.

112. Barham CP, Gotley DC, Fowler AL *et al*. Diffuse oesophageal spasm: The diagnosis is made by ambulatory 24-hour manometry. Gut 1997; 41:151–5.

113. Dalton CB, Castell DO, Henson EG *et al*. Diffuse esophageal spasm: A rare motility disorder not characterised by high amplitude contractions. Dig Dis Sci 1991; 36:1025–8.

114. Stuart RC, Hennessy TPJ. Primary disorders of oesophageal motility. Br J Surg 1989; 76:1111–20.

115. Traube M, Lagarde S, McCallum RW. Isolated hypertensive lower esophageal sphincter: treatment of a resistant case by pneumatic dilatation. J Clin Gastroenterol 1984; 6:139–42.

116. Ferriolli E, Dantas RO, Oliveira RB *et al*. The influence of ageing on oesophageal motility after ingestion of liquids with different viscosities. Eur J Gastroenterol Hepatol 1996; 8:793–8.

117. Grande L, Lacima G, Ros E *et al*. Deterioration of esophageal motility with age: a manometric study of 79 healthy subjects. Am J Gastroenterol 1999; 94:1795–1801.

118. Peters L, Maas L, Petty D *et al*. Spontaneous non-cardiac chest pain. Evaluation by 24-hour ambulatory esophageal motility and pH monitoring. Gastroenterology 1988; 94:878–86.

10 Treatment of gastro-oesophageal reflux disease

David I. Watson
Glyn G. Jamieson

INTRODUCTION

Gastro-oesophageal reflux is a common problem throughout the developed world, affecting between 10 and 40% of the population of most Western countries.[1,2] Whether its incidence is increasing is a moot point. What is certainly increasing is the treatment of the condition and this has led to a dramatic rise in the overall cost of medical therapy in many countries over recent years. In addition there is now good evidence that distal oesophageal adenocarcinoma is increasing,[3] and this provides circumstantial evidence that complications of gastro-oesophageal reflux (e.g. the development of Barrett's oesophagus) are also increasing.

Gastro-oesophageal reflux disease is caused by excessive reflux of gastric contents, which contain acid and sometimes bile and pancreatic secretions, into the oesophageal lumen. While a certain amount of reflux occurs physiologically in everyone, pathological reflux leads to symptoms such as heartburn, upper abdominal pain and the regurgitation of gastric contents into the oropharynx. Gastro-oesophageal reflux is associated with a range of contributing factors, and a multifactorial aetiology is likely. First is hiatus herniation, which is found in approximately half of the patients who undergo surgical treatment.[4,5] This results in widening of the angle of His, effacement of the lower oesophageal sphincter, and loss of the assistance of positive intra-abdominal pressure acting on the lower oesophagus. Second is the reduced lower oesophageal sphincter pressure which is often found, although in many patients with reflux the resting lower oesophageal sphincter pressure is normal. Reflux in these patients results from an excessive number of transient lower oesophageal sphincter relaxation events.[6] Other factors which might contribute to the genesis of reflux include abnormal oesophageal peristalsis (which causes poor clearance of refluxed fluid) and delayed gastric emptying.

The treatment of reflux is usually incremental, commencing with various levels of medical measures, surgery being reserved for patients with more severe disease, who either fail to respond adequately to medical treatment, or who do not wish to take medication life long. Non-operative therapy treats the effects of reflux, as the underlying reflux problem is not corrected, and therapy for most patients must be continued indefinitely.[7] Surgical procedures are, however, curative, preventing reflux by reconstructing an antireflux valve at the gastro-oesophageal junction.[6,8] In the past, surgery has tended to be reserved for patients with complicated reflux disease or those with very severe symptoms. Recently the role of surgery has changed and there is an increasing tendency to utilise surgery at earlier stages in the course of reflux disease. This is probably because of the introduction of laparoscopic surgical approaches.[9]

Medical treatment

Simple measures

A variety of simple measures can be helpful for the management of patients who experience mild symptoms. Many of these options are initiated by patients themselves or in consultation with their general practitioner. Such measures include antacids together with the avoidance of precipitating factors such as spicy foods and alcohol. Additional measures include weight loss (when appropriate), avoiding cigarette smoking, modification of the timing and quantity of meals (e.g. avoiding going to bed with a full stomach) and raising the bed head. Unfortunately, while these measures are appealing in their simplicity, they are rarely effective for patients with moderate to severe disease, and most patients who present for surgery cannot be adequately treated with these measures. Furthermore, while obesity seems to be an important factor in reflux, it is unusual for patients to achieve sustained weight loss sufficient to eliminate the need for other treatment options.

H2-receptor antagonists

The first effective non-operative treatment for reflux was the development of medications which reduced the production of stomach acid. The histamine type 2 (H2) receptor antagonists (cimetidine, ranitidine, famotidine and nizatidine) sometimes relieve mild to moderate reflux symptoms if given in an adequate dose. When first used in the 1970s they revolutionised the medical approach to duodenal ulcer disease; they were, however, much less effective for reflux disease and few patients achieve complete relief of reflux symptoms with these medications.[10] Even so, in milder forms of the disease they can reduce symptoms. When medications are ceased, however, symptoms usually return, and treatment has to be recommenced. Many patients comment on the diminishing effectiveness of these medications, necessitating progression to more active therapy.

Proton pump inhibitors

Proton pump inhibitors (omeprazole, lanzoprazole, raseprozole and pantoprazole) were introduced into clinical practice in the late 1980s.[7] They are much more effective for the relief of symptoms, and achieve better healing of oesophagitis than H2 receptor antagonists. However, patients with worse oesophagitis such as Savary Miller grade 2 or 3, have a higher failure rate with these medications,[11] and in addition many patients who initially achieve good symptom control, go on to develop 'break through' symptoms at a later date, usually requiring an increased dose of medication to maintain symptom control. It is presumed that failure is the result of inadequate acid suppression although in some cases the presence of bile or duodenal fluid in the refluxate may play a role. In patients who respond well to proton pump inhibitors, symptoms usually recur rapidly (sometimes in less than 24 hours) following cessation of medication, and for this reason medical treatment is likely to be required lifelong, unless surgery is performed.[7] The long-term use of proton pump inhibitors has not been shown to cause any clear adverse outcome to date, and in particular there has been no direct evidence of carcinogenic effects from long-term use. A recent study has shown, however, that long-term use may be associated with the development of atrophic gastritis with intestinal metaplasia in patients with concurrent *Helicobacter pylori* infection.[12] Long-term use can also be associated with parietal cell hyperplasia.[13] This latter phenomenon may be the reason why symptoms recur so rapidly in some patients on cessation of therapy.

Prokinetic agents

Cisapride is the only prokinetic agent which has been shown to be better than placebo for the treatment of reflux disease.[14] It acts by accelerating oesophageal and gastric emptying, thereby improving acid clearance from the distal oesophagus, and emptying gastric contents more quickly, leaving less gastric content available to be refluxed. Its therapeutic benefit is similar to that of the H2 receptor antagonists, and it is also synergistic when combined with H2 antagonist acid suppression. Studies have not shown an objective benefit of combining the proton pump inhibitors with cisapride. Cisapride also increases lower oesophageal sphincter resting pressure.[15] Its clinical role has been limited since proton pump inhibitors became widely available. At present however cisapride has been withdrawn from the UK and European markets pending further investigation of its effects on cardiac function.

Surgical treatment

The principle underlying the surgical management of gastro-oesophageal reflux disease is the creation of a mechanical antireflux barrier between the oesophagus and stomach. This works independently of the composition of the refluxate, and its success is not influenced by the specific aetiology of the reflux problem. While medical therapy is effective in relieving symptoms for many patients with acid reflux, only surgery achieves effective control of duodenogastro-oesophageal reflux.

Selection criteria for surgery

As a general rule, all patients who undergo antireflux surgery should have objective evidence of reflux. This may be the demonstration of erosive oesophagitis on endoscopy or an abnormal amount of acid reflux demonstrated by 24-hour pH monitoring. Neither of these tests are sufficiently reliable to base all preoperative decisions on their outcome,[16] as a number of patients with troublesome reflux will have either a normal 24-hour pH study or no evidence of oesophagitis at endoscopy (and very occasionally, both). For this reason the tests have to be interpreted in the light of the patient's clinical presentation, and a final recommendation for surgery must be based on all available clinical and objective information.[16]

Patients selected for surgery fall into two general groups:

1. Patients who have failed to respond (or have responded only partially) to medical therapy;
2. Patients whose symptoms are fully controlled by medications, but who do not wish to continue lifelong with medication. The latter group are more likely to be younger patients who face decades of acid suppression to alleviate their symptoms. In the first group, the response to surgery is usually more certain if the patient has had a good response to acid suppression in the past, or at least has had some symptom relief from medication. In patients who have had no response to proton pump inhibitors, their symptoms are often due to something other than reflux, despite concurrent objective evidence of reflux (which can be asymptomatic). Such patients will not benefit from antireflux surgery, at least in a symptomatic sense.

Failure of medical treatment can be defined as continuing symptoms of reflux while on an adequate dose of acid suppression. In most countries this means at least a standard dose of a proton pump inhibitor for a minimum period of 3 months. In some countries such as Australia and Belgium, where government imposed prescribing restrictions limit the availability of proton pump inhibitors to less than the full range of reflux patients, some patients will be selected for surgery who have only been treated with H2 receptor antagonists. Cost has become a significant issue in some countries, and in Australia despite prescribing restrictions, medication for reflux consumes more than 10% of national expenditure on prescription drugs. Proton pump inhibitors are more effective in controlling the symptom of heartburn rather than volume regurgitation, and it is this latter symptom which is often the dominant problem in patients who have failed on medical therapy.

A further classification of patients who undergo surgery for gastro-oesophageal reflux disease can be made as follows:

1. Patients who have complicated reflux disease; and
2. Patients who have straightforward disease without complications.

Patients with complicated reflux disease

Reflux with stricture formation

The treatment of peptic oesophageal strictures has been greatly altered since proton pump inhibitors became available, and this is one area where the role of surgery seems to have lessened.[17] In the past, surgery was the only effective treatment for strictures, and when the stricture was densely fibrotic this even meant resection of the oesophagus. Fortunately it is now unusual to see patients with such advanced disease. Strictures in young and fit patients are usually best treated by antireflux surgery and dilatation. However, many patients who develop strictures are elderly or infirm and the use of proton pump inhibitors with dilatation is usually effective in this group.

Reflux with respiratory complications

When gastro-oesophageal regurgitation spills over into the respiratory tree, this can cause chronic respiratory illness, such as recurrent pneumonia or asthma. This is a firm indication for antireflux surgery, as proton pump inhibitors' predominant action is to block acid secretion, and the volume of reflux is not greatly altered. Such problems as halitosis, chronic cough, chronic laryngitis, chronic pharyngitis, chronic sinusitis and loss of tooth enamel are sometimes attributed to gastro–oesophageal reflux. While there is little doubt that on occasions such problems do arise in refluxing patients, these problems in isolation are not reliable indications for surgery. As acid is usually the damaging agent, antireflux surgery is probably not advisable unless proton pump inhibition unequivocally reverses the problem.

Columnar-lined (Barrett's) oesophagus

At present it remains an open question whether Barrett's oesophagus alone is an indication for antireflux surgery. There is little argument that patients with Barrett's oesophagus who have reflux symptoms should be selected for surgery on the basis of their symptoms and their response to medication, and not simply because they have a columnar-lined oesophagus.[18] There is some experimental evidence to suggest that continuing reflux may be deleterious with regard to malignant change in oesophageal mucosa[19] and one prospective randomised trial has suggested that antireflux surgery gives superior results to drug therapy in this patient group.[19] However, proton pump inhibitors were only introduced into the medical arm of that trial in its later years.

There is emerging evidence that abolition of symptoms with proton pump inhibition does not equate to 'normalising' the pH profile in a patient's oesophagus.[20] Since antireflux surgery does usually abolish acid reflux, this may become a further reason to recommend surgery in patients with Barrett's oesophagus. There is no evidence to support the contention that either surgical or medical treatment of reflux in patients with Barrett's oesophagus consistently leads to regression of the columnar lining,[21] although in the future it is possible that a combination of medical or surgical therapy with ablation of the columnar lining might offer a better long-term outcome for this group of patients.

Patients with uncomplicated reflux disease

Medical therapy in the form of proton pump inhibitors is so effective today that only a small minority of patients do not get substantial or complete relief of their symptoms using these agents. Despite this, patients continue to present for antireflux surgery in large numbers for reasons already discussed. An additional factor which has emerged in recent years is the rising incidence of adenocarcinoma of the cardia associated with gastro–oesophageal reflux disease.[3] Whether antireflux surgery is more effective than long-term proton pump inhibition at preventing the development of columnar-lined oesophagus and subsequently carcinoma of the cardia is controversial. If duodenal fluid has a role in the pathogenesis of adenocarcinoma of the oesophagus, then antireflux surgery would be preferable to acid suppression alone in patients with Barrett's oesophagus, and of course it may also prevent the development of Barrett's oesophagus in the first place. However, this hypothesis has yet to be adequately tested, and at present there is insufficient evidence to support a position that antireflux surgery should be performed to prevent subsequent malignant transformation.

Medical versus surgery therapy

The issue of the most appropriate treatment for gastro-oesophageal reflux disease has been the subject of disagreement between surgeons and gastro-enterologists. Whilst most would agree that a single management strategy is unlikely to be appropriate for all patients, there is a need for better comparative data for medical versus surgical therapy. Three randomised trials have been reported which have investigated this issue, although all were performed before the availability of either laparoscopic antireflux surgery, or proton pump inhibitor medication, and hence there is scope for more work in this area. Behar et al.[22] reported in 1975 a small trial of 31 patients randomised to undergo either the Belsey Mark IV procedure or medical therapy at the time. Surgery achieved good to excellent results in 73% versus 19% for the medical group.

The next study was reported by Spechler et al.[23] in 1992. In this study, 247 patients (predominantly men) were randomised to either continuous medical therapy with a H2 blocker, medical therapy for symptoms only, or an open Nissen fundoplication. Seven patients' symptoms persisted on medical therapy to the extent that they were reallocated to a surgical procedure. Overall patient satisfaction was highest in the surgical group at both the 1- and 2-year follow-up intervals. However, neither the surgical approach, nor the medical treatment investigated in this study, would now be regarded as optimal.

Ortiz et al.[19] more recently reported a study which randomised 59 patients at the more severe end of the reflux spectrum with Barrett's oesophagus. Twenty-seven patients had the best medical treatment available and 32 patients underwent a short Nissen fundoplication. Satisfactory symptomatic control was achieved in 24 and 29 patients respectively. However, there was significantly better control of oesophageal inflammation and stenosis in the surgical group. Since proton pump inhibitors were only used in the last few years of the study, this trial also becomes of historical rather than present relevance.

It is clear from the reported studies that surgery produced better results in the era before the introduction of proton pump inhibitors. The early results of a large randomised Swedish study comparing surgery with omeprazole are yet to be published. However, early reports (personal communication) suggest that the gap between medical and surgical therapy has been reduced by the introduction of better medical therapy.

What are the advantages and disadvantages of antireflux surgery?

The advantages of surgery are fairly clear. Operation is the only treatment which actually cures the problem, i.e. it stops gastric contents from refluxing into the oesophagus. Hence patients treated by surgery can usually eat whatever foods they choose, they can lie down flat and bend over without reflux occurring and, importantly, they do not need to take any medication.

The first disadvantage is the morbidity associated with the operation (see discussion of complications). While laparoscopic surgery has meant that the pain of an open operation has been greatly reduced, most patients have some difficulty in swallowing in the immediate postoperative period, although in the great majority this is only temporary.[24] However, the time taken to get better is quite variable, and several months are often required.[5] Furthermore, the great majority of patients feel full quickly after eating even small meals, and this often leads to some postoperative weight loss.[5] In patients who are overweight at the time of surgery (the majority!) this is sometimes seen as an advantage rather than a disadvantage. This restriction on meal size also usually disappears over a few months.

Because fundoplication produces a one-way valve, swallowed air which has passed into the stomach usually cannot pass back through the valve. Thus, patients have to be forewarned that they will not be able to belch effectively after the operation and so should be cautious about drinking gassy drinks.[25] This applies particularly to patients who undergo a Nissen (total) fundoplication. For similar reasons, patients will usually be unable to vomit after the procedure, and should be informed of this. As swallowed gas cannot be belched effectively, the great majority of patients are aware of increased flatulence with increased borborygmi and increased passage of wind after the procedure.[26] Although patients who undergo a partial fundoplication (particularly anterior) have a lower incidence of these problems,[27] difficulties can still occur. Despite these possible disadvantages, the overwhelming majority of patients claim that the disadvantages are far outweighed by the advantages of the operation.[24,27,28] To date it has not been possible to predict preoperatively those patients who will develop problems following surgery.

Preoperative investigations

Apart from the assessment of each patient's general suitability for surgery by determining comorbidities, some specific investigations should be performed before undertaking antireflux surgery.

Endoscopy

Endoscopy is a prerequisite. It enables oesophagitis to be documented (confirming reflux disease), strictures to be dilated, oesophageal tumours to be excluded, and other gastro-oesophageal pathology to be documented and treated. The position of the squamo-columnar junction and the presence and size of any hiatus hernia is also assessed. The presence of a large hiatus hernia is not a contraindication to a laparoscopic approach, although the surgery is technically more difficult, and conversion to an open procedure is more likely.[29,30] An inexperienced surgeon is well advised to seek the assistance of a more experienced colleague in this situation.

Manometry

Manometry is used to exclude primary motility disorders such as achalasia. It is also able to document the adequacy of oesophageal peristalsis.[16] The presence of weak peristaltic amplitudes or poor propagation of peristalsis is not a contraindication to antireflux surgery. Although many surgeons recommend a tailored approach to patient selection by choosing a partial fundoplication in patients with poor peristalsis[31,32] there is no strong evidence to support this.[33,34]

Evidence from one randomised trial[35] and two uncontrolled case series[33,34] has shown good results following the Nissen procedure in patients with very poor peristalsis.

Nevertheless, common sense suggests that a partial fundoplication procedure is likely to be safer in patients with a true adynamic oesophagus. Manometry also assists in the precise placement of a pH probe if pH monitoring is required.

Oesophageal pH monitoring

While most surgeons advocate the routine assessment of patients with 24-hour ambulatory pH monitoring before antireflux surgery, the authors use a selective approach. This test is not sufficiently accurate to be regarded as the 'gold standard' for the investigation of reflux, and if an abnormal pH profile is used to select patients for surgery, up to 20% of patients who have oesophagitis and typical reflux symptoms will be excluded unnecessarily from antireflux surgery. Hence, we apply this investigation in patients with endoscopy negative reflux disease, and in patients with atypical symptoms.[16] The test's ability to clarify whether symptoms are associated with reflux events is useful for the assessment of these patients. Nevertheless the use of preoperative pH monitoring does allow comparison to be made made with the postoperative situation.

The role of bile reflux (Bilitec) monitoring has yet to be defined in gastro-oesophageal reflux disease, although in the future the measurement of bile reflux may be helpful in patients who fail to respond to acid suppression.

Operations available

To the non-surgeon, it might seem that there is a bewildering array of operations available for the treatment of reflux. In fact, the fundoplication introduced by Rudolf Nissen in 1956, or some variant of it, is overwhelmingly the most popular antireflux operation in the world today. Total fundoplications, such as the Nissen, or partial fundoplications, whether anterior or posterior, probably all work in a similar fashion,[8,36] and that fashion may be as much mechanical as physiological, as it has been demonstrated that these procedures are effective, not only when placed in the chest *in vivo*[37] but also on the bench top, i.e. *ex vivo*.[8] The principles of fundoplication are to mobilise the lower oesophagus and to wrap the fundus of the stomach, either partially or totally, around the oesophagus. When the oesophageal hiatus is enlarged, it is narrowed by sutures to prevent para-oesophageal herniation postoperatively, and also to prevent the wrap being pulled up into the chest (although the fundoplication will work in the chest, other complications such as gastric ulceration and gastric obstruction sometimes occur in this situation). Complications of reflux such as fibrotic stricturing with shortened oesophagus, are seen much less frequently today than in the past. In this circumstance, in order to provide a long enough oesophagus to reach the abdomen, an oesophageal lengthening (Collis') procedure is often undertaken. The upper lesser curvature of the stomach is used to produce the new oesophagus and the stomach is then wrapped around this.

Mechanism of action of antireflux operations

Exactly how various procedures work is often debated, and the range of possible mechanisms of action indicate the lack of consensus on the mode of action of an antireflux operation. Some of the proposed mechanisms include:

1. The creation of a floppy valve by maintaining close apposition between the abdominal oesophagus and the gastric fundus. As intragastric pressure rises the intra-abdominal oesophagus is compressed by the adjacent fundus.
2. Exaggeration of the flap valve at the angle of His.
3. Increase in the basal pressure generated by the lower oesophageal sphincter.
4. Reduction in the triggering of transient lower oesophageal sphincter relaxations.
5. Reduction in the capacity of the gastric fundus, thereby speeding proximal and total gastric emptying.
6. Prevention of effacement of the lower oesophagus (which effectively weakens the lower sphincter).

Since the procedures seem to work, even *ex vivo*,[8] it seems likely that the first two mechanisms account for the efficacy of the majority of antireflux procedures. The increase in lower oesophageal sphincter pressure following surgery is not important, and in some partial fundoplication procedures, there is very little increase in pressure, yet reflux is well controlled.[27,38] The trend towards increasingly looser and shorter total fundoplications or greater use of partial fundoplication procedures suggests that there is no such thing as a fundoplication which is 'too loose'.

Techniques of antireflux surgery

A range of different antireflux operations are currently performed and all have their advocates. No one procedure currently yields perfect results, that is, 100% cure of reflux without side effects. Despite this, published reports can be found which support every known procedure, and it is probably better to consider results from randomised trials when assessing the merits of these procedural variants (see below), rather than relying on uncontrolled outcomes reported by advocates of a single procedure. It should also be recognised that the experience of the operating surgeon is of great importance for achieving a good postoperative outcome.[39] Variability can be reduced, but not eliminated, by detailed technical descriptions and effective surgical training. The arrival of laparoscopic antireflux surgery has also changed the way in which the vast majority of antireflux surgery is now performed. Over the last decade this approach has become standard for primary antireflux surgery, making operation more acceptable to patients and their physicians.

Nissen fundoplication (**Fig. 10.1**)

This is probably the most commonly performed antireflux operation worldwide. Nissen originally described a procedure which entailed mobilisation of the oesophagus from the diaphragmatic hiatus, reduction of any hiatus hernia into the abdominal cavity, preservation of the vagus nerves and mobilisation of the posterior gastric fundus around behind the oesophagus, without dividing the short gastric vessels, and suturing of the posterior fundus to the anterior wall of the fundus using non-absorbable sutures, thereby achieving a complete wrap of stomach around the intra-abdominal oesophagus.[40] The original fundoplication was 5 cm in length and an oesophageal bougie was not used to calibrate the wrap.

Because this procedure was associated with an incidence of persistent postoperative dysphagia, gas bloat syndrome and an inability to belch, the procedure has been progressively modified in an attempt to improve long-term outcome. Most

Figure 10.1
Nissen fundoplication.

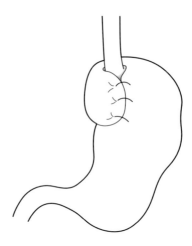

surgeons now agree that calibration of the wrap with a large (52 Fr or bigger) intraoesophageal bougie, and shortening the fundoplication to 1 to 2 cm in length achieve a better outcome.[41,42] Furthermore, while the need for routine hiatal repair was uncertain in the era of open surgery, most surgeons routinely include this step during laparoscopic antireflux surgery. Omission of this step is associated with a higher incidence of postoperative hiatal herniation.[43] The hepatic branch of the vagus nerve is usually preserved during this procedure.

However, controversy exists about the need to divide the short gastric vessels to achieve full fundal mobilisation. The so-called floppy Nissen procedure described by Donahue,[44] relies on extensive fundal mobilisation. On the other hand the modification of the Nissen fundoplication using the anterior fundal wall alone, also first described by Nissen and Rossetti,[40,45] does not require short gastric vessel division to construct the fundoplication. This simplifies the dissection, although more judgement and experience may be required to select the correct piece of stomach to use for the construction of a sufficiently loose fundoplication. Both procedures have their advocates, and good results (90% good or excellent long-term outcome) have been reported for both variants.[41,45] Nevertheless, strong opinions are held about whether the short gastric vessels should be divided or not, and this controversy has been heightened by the introduction of laparoscopic fundoplication.

Posterior partial fundoplication (**Fig. 10.2**)

A variety of fundoplication operations have been described in which the fundus is wrapped partially round the back of the oesophagus, with the aim of reducing the possible side effects of total fundoplication due to overcompetence of the cardia, such as dysphagia and gas-related problems. Toupet described a posterior partial fundoplication in which the fundus is passed behind the oesophagus and sutured to the left lateral and right lateral walls of the oesophagus, as well as to the right diaphragmatic pillar, creating a 270° posterior fundoplication.[46] A very similar procedure was described by Lind.[47] This entails a 300° posterior fundoplication, which is constructed by suturing the fundus to the oesophagus at the left and right lateral positions, and additionally anteriorly on the left, leaving a 60° arc of oesophageal wall uncovered anteriorly. The hiatus is repaired if necessary.

Figure 10.2
Posterior partial fundoplication.

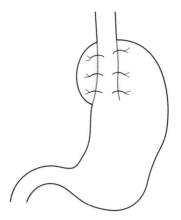

Anterior partial fundoplication

Several anterior fundoplication procedures have been described, and all purport to reduce the incidence of dysphagia and other side effects. The Belsey Mark IV procedure entails a 240° anterior partial fundoplication which is usually performed through a left thoracotomy approach.[48] The distal oesophagus is mobilised, sutured to the gastric fundus and sutured to the diaphragm. Any hiatus hernia is repaired, and the anterior two-thirds of the abdominal oesophagus covered by the fundoplication. This procedure has been common in cardiothoracic surgical practice in the past, although the open thoracic access is associated with significant morbidity, and for this reason it has fallen from favour since the arrival of laparoscopic antireflux surgery. A minimally invasive thoracoscopic approach has been recently described, although clinical outcomes remain unreported.[49]

The Dor procedure is an anterior hemifundoplication which involves suturing of the fundus to the left and right sides of the oesophagus.[50] This procedure is commonly used in combination with an abdominal cardiomyotomy for achalasia as it is unlikely to cause dysphagia, and it may reduce the risk of gastro-oesophageal reflux following cardiomyotomy.

A 120° anterior fundoplication has also been described.[38] This entails reduction of any hiatus hernia, posterior hiatal repair, suture of the posterior oesophagus to the hiatal pillars posteriorly, suture of the fundus to the diaphragm to accentuate the angle of His, and creation of an anterior partial fundoplication by suturing the fundus to the oesophagus on the right anterolateral aspect. Satisfactory medium-term reflux control following open surgery has been reported for this procedure, and a low incidence of gas-related problems. Published laparoscopic experience is however limited,[51] and its application has been limited to a few centres only.

The present authors recently reported the results of a prospective randomised trial of a laparoscopic 180° anterior partial fundoplication (**Fig. 10.3**) versus a Nissen procedure[27] (see below). This procedure entails hiatal repair, suture of the distal oesophagus to the hiatus posteriorly and construction of an anterior fundoplication which is sutured to the oesophagus and the hiatal rim on the right and anteriorly. This variant of anterior fundoplication shows promise, but until longer term outcomes are available it should remain under evaluation.

Figure 10.3
180° anterior partial fundoplication performed by the transabdominal route.

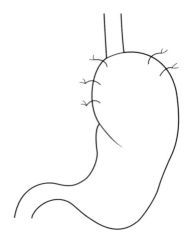

Other antireflux procedures

Hill's procedure Hill described a procedure which is often regarded as a gastropexy rather than a fundoplication.[52] However, it also plicates the cardia, and when examined endoscopically the intragastric appearances are similar to a fundoplication. The procedure entails suturing the anterior and posterior phreno-oesophageal bundles to the preaortic fascia and the median arcuate ligament. While excellent results have been reported by Hill,[52,53] it has not been widely applied because most surgeons have difficulty understanding the anatomical principles; in particular, the so-called phreno-oesophageal bundles are not clear structures. Hill also emphasises the need for intraoperative manometry. This is not widely available, limiting the dissemination of his technique.

Collis' procedure (**Fig. 10.4**) This is useful for patients whose oesophago-gastric junction cannot be reduced below the diaphragm.[54] However, this situation has become uncommon in recent years, possibly due to the reduced incidence of stricture formation which has accompanied the introduction of effective medical therapy for reflux. The Collis procedure involves the construction of a tube of gastric lesser curve to recreate an abdominal length of oesophagus, around which

Figure 10.4
Collis gastroplasty with subsequent Nissen fundoplication.

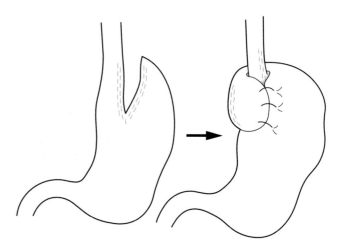

a fundoplication can then be constructed. This is a useful procedure for patients with true oesophageal shortening, where the gastro-oesophageal junction cannot be reduced satisfactorily into the abdomen. It is often constructed by using a circular end-to-end stapler to create a transgastric window, and a linear cutting stapler is used from this hole up to the angle of His to construct the neo-oesophagus. Laparoscopic and thoracoscopic techniques for this procedure have been described, although longer term outcomes are not available.[55,56,57] A disadvantage of this procedure is that the gastric tube does not have peristaltic activity, and furthermore it can secrete acid. This leads to a poorer overall success rate for this procedure, although some of this could be due to the end stage nature of the reflux disease which led to the choice of this procedure in the first place.

Anatomical repair Earlier in the twentieth century it was believed that gastro-oesophageal reflux was associated with an anatomical derangement at the oesophageal hiatus of the diaphragm due to the development of a hiatus hernia, and this provided the basis for the first surgical treatment for reflux. This was popularised by Allison who advocated 'anatomical' repair of hiatus hernia. Using an open transthoracic approach, this procedure involved the reduction of the hiatus hernia, narrowing of the hiatal ring and accentuation of the angle of His. This successfully corrected pathological reflux, and early follow-up reported excellent results in 91% of cases. At 20-year follow-up, however, this figure had dropped to 66% in Allison's hands,[58] and partly as a result of this the operation fell into disfavour, despite the fact that excellent long-term outcomes had been reported by some other surgeons. However, Allison's repair demonstrated that restoration of normal hiatal anatomy, without a fundoplication, resulted in control of gastro-oesophageal reflux symptoms, without the side effects typically associated with total fundoplication.

Angelchik prosthesis Perhaps the most interesting thing about this prosthesis is that it actually controlled reflux and induced a rethink about the pathophysiology of reflux. It may work by preventing proximal gastric distension, which in turn mitigates against transient lower oesophageal sphincter relaxation, or effacement and weakening of the lower oesophageal sphincter, or both mechanisms.[59] The procedure involves the placement of a gel-filled silastic prosthesis around the gastro-oesophageal junction. It has largely been consigned to surgical history, as long-term follow-up revealed an unacceptably high rate of surgical revision, particularly for troublesome dysphagia as well as migration of the prosthesis into the mediastinum and even into the lumen of the gastrointestinal tract.[60,61]

Complete or partial fundoplication?

Because fundoplication is associated with an incidence of postoperative dysphagia, gas bloat and other gas-related symptoms such as increased flatulence, the relative merits of the Nissen fundoplication procedure versus various partial fundoplication variants have been debated for many years. The introduction of laparoscopic approaches has only served to heighten this controversy. On the one hand the Nissen procedure produces an overcompetent gastro-oesophageal junction, which is the cause of some of the problems with dysphagia and gas bloat. On the other hand, it has been suggested that partial fundoplication reduces the risk of overcompetence, although perhaps at the expense of a less durable anti-reflux repair.

Several prospective randomised trials of Nissen versus a partial fundoplication have been performed. However, all but two of these have enrolled only small numbers of patients, and they therefore lack the statistical power necessary for firm conclusions to be drawn. Furthermore most investigated a posterior partial fundoplication, and data are more limited for the other procedures. DeMeester et al.[62] had the distinction of reporting the first randomised study in the field of surgery for reflux disease in 1974. Their trial randomised 45 patients to undergo either a Nissen, Hill, or a Belsey procedure, and followed their patients for 6 months following surgery. The dysphagia rate was similar for all three procedures and reflux recurred early in one patient following the Hill procedure, in two following a Belsey procedure, but in no patients in the Nissen group. Those surgeons who think that early dysphagia is commoner with laparoscopic than open surgery should take note of this paper, since early dysphagia was recorded in 13/15, 13/15, and 6/15 respectively for the Nissen, Hill and Belsey procedures.

Nissen versus posterior fundoplication

Thor and Silander[63] reported the next small trial in 1989, with follow-up for 5 years. They randomised 31 patients to undergo either a Nissen or a Toupet fundoplication. The Nissen wrap was 4 cm in length, and it was calibrated over a 40 Fr bougie, the oesophageal hiatus was not repaired, the hepatic branch of the vagus nerve was divided routinely and the short gastric vessels were not divided. A good or excellent outcome was achieved in 8/12 of the Nissen group and 18/19 of the Toupet group. However, because of the small number of patients enrolled, this difference was not significant. Three of the patients who underwent Nissen fundoplication underwent further surgery for dysphagia. In each instance this was for the development of a 'slipped Nissen'. No reoperations were required in the Toupet group. The incidence of reoperation for the 'slipped Nissen' phenomenon, however, is far in excess of the low rates reported in other more recent studies.[41,64,65,66]

Walker et al.[64] reported the results of their randomised trial in 1992. This study compared a Nissen fundoplication (3 cm long, with selective division of the short gastric vessels, and calibrated over a 40 Fr bougie), with a 300° posterior partial fundoplication (Lind). As only 26 patients were enrolled in each group, lack of statistical power again applies to this study. New dysphagia was seen equally in both groups at early (6 weeks) and late follow-up, and the incidence of gas-bloat problems was also identical.

Lundell et al. have reported in several publications the outcome of a trial of Nissen fundoplication without dividing the short gastric vessels versus Toupet partial fundoplications into which 137 patients were entered. Early outcomes at 6-months' follow-up were similar.[67] Interestingly at the 5-year follow-up[65] there was a trend towards more dysphagia following partial than with a Nissen wrap, although in all instances the symptom was reported to be mild. On the other hand, flatulence was commoner after Nissen fundoplication at 2 and 3 years but not at other earlier or later time intervals. Long-term reflux control was similar for the two procedures at 5 years (6% following Toupet, 5% after Nissen). Reoperation was more common following Nissen fundoplication, with one patient in the Toupet group undergoing further surgery for severe gas-bloat symptoms, and 5 of the Nissen group undergoing reoperation for postoperative paraoesophageal herniation. Hiatal repair was performed infrequently in this trial, and in only one of the five patients who developed a postoperative hernia.

A further recent reanalysis of the data from this trial[35] sought to answer the question of whether a tailored approach to antireflux surgery should be applied. There were no demonstrable disadvantages for the Nissen procedure in those patients who had manometrically abnormal peristalsis before surgery.

Following the introduction of laparoscopic techniques, Laws *et al.*[68] recently reported a small trial in which 39 patients were randomised to undergo either a laparoscopic Nissen or Toupet fundoplication. Again, no significant short-term outcome differences were demonstrated between the two procedures.

If one combines all the data of the Nissen versus posterior fundoplication trials together, the available evidence appears to support the view that the only differences in outcome between the total fundoplication and the posterior fundoplication, is in the wind-related problems. Certainly, the hypothesis that dysphagia is less of a problem following a posterior partial fundoplication has not been substantiated by these trials.

Although these pooled data are essentially short-term follow-up (because most trials have not reported longer term outcomes), the longer term data of Lundell *et al.*[65] suggest these results may be representative of the longer term also.

Nissen versus anterior fundoplication

In 1999 the present authors reported the first prospective randomised trial to compare a Nissen fundoplication with an anterior partial fundoplication techniques.[27] Both procedures were performed laparoscopically. This study enrolled 107 patients to undergo either a Nissen or anterior partial fundoplication. The partial fundoplication variant entailed a 180° fundoplication which was anchored to the right hiatal pillar and the oesophageal wall.

While no overall outcome differences between the two procedures were demonstrated at 1 and 3 months follow-up, at 6 months patients who underwent an anterior fundoplication were less likely to experience dysphagia for solid food, less likely to be troubled by excessive passage of flatus, more likely to be able to belch normally, and the overall outcome was better.

These differences have continued to be evident 2 years following surgery, and control of reflux has been similar following partial fundoplication (unpublished data). Despite this data, this trial has not resolved which procedure will be the most appropriate in the long term. However, if its durability is as good as the Nissen fundoplication, then the results of this study are likely to support the argument for routine application of an anterior (but not posterior) partial fundoplication procedure. This is yet to be proven, however, and therefore long-term follow-up is needed to clarify this issue.

The controversy of division/no division of short gastric vessels

Until recently, the issue of division versus non-division of the short gastric vessels was rarely discussed. However, following anecdotal reports of increased problems with postoperative dysphagia following laparoscopic Nissen fundoplication without division of the short gastric vessels,[69,70] this aspect of surgical technique has become a much debated topic. Routine division of the short gastric vessels during fundoplication, to achieve full fundal mobilisation and thereby ensure a loose fundoplication, is thought by some to be an essential step during laparoscopic (and open) Nissen fundoplication.[41,42] This opinion has been popularised by the publication of studies that have compared experience with division of the short gastric vessels with historical experience of a Nissen fundoplication performed without dividing these vessels.[45,44] Other uncontrolled studies of Nissen fundoplication either with or without division of the short gastric vessels confuse the issue further, as good results have been reported whether these vessels were divided or not.[43,56]

Two randomised trials have been reported which investigate this aspect of technique. Luostarinen et al.[66,71,72] reported the outcome of a small trial of division versus no division of the short gastric vessels during open total fundoplication. Fifty patients were entered into this trial, and the most recent report[72] described outcomes following a median 3-year follow-up period. Both procedures effectively corrected endoscopic oesophagitis. However, there was a trend towards a higher incidence of disruption of the fundoplication (5 versus 2), and reflux symptoms (6 versus 1) in patients whose short gastric vessels were divided, and furthermore 9 out of 26 patients who underwent vessel division developed a postoperative sliding hiatus hernia, compared to only 1 out of 24 patients whose vessels were kept intact. The likelihood of long-term dysphagia or gas-related symptoms was not influenced by mobilising the gastric fundus in this trial.

In 1997, we reported a randomised trial which enrolled 102 patients undergoing a laparoscopic Nissen fundoplication, to have a procedure either with or without division of the short gastric blood vessels.[5] No difference in overall outcome was demonstrated at short-term follow-up of 6 months, with the exception of increased operating time if the vessels were divided. In particular, this trial failed to show that dividing the short gastric vessels during laparoscopic Nissen fundoplication reduced the incidence or severity of dysphagia following surgery, nor was there any significant difference in lower oesophageal sphincter pressure, oesophageal emptying time or barium meal X-ray appearances. Longer term follow-up, however, is needed to assess the durability of each operative variant.

 Nevertheless, the currently available evidence from both published trials does not support the proposition that the short gastric vessels should be divided routinely during either laparoscopic or open Nissen fundoplication.

Laparoscopic antireflux surgery

Initial results and complications following laparoscopic fundoplication

Laparoscopic fundoplication was first reported in 1991[73,74] and it has rapidly established itself as the procedure of choice for reflux disease, with the vast majority of antireflux procedures now being performed this way (**Fig. 10.5 and 10.6**). The results of several large prospectively followed series have been published, with short and medium term (up to 3 years) outcomes available.[26,28,75] Overall results from these studies suggest that laparoscopic antireflux surgery is

Figure 10.5
Laparoscopic view of completed Nissen fundoplication.

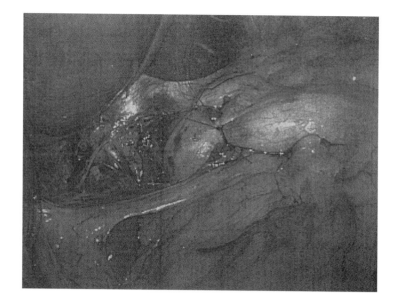

Figure 10.6
Laparoscopic view of completed anterior partial fundoplication. This particular fundoplication was fashioned as a 90° wrap, leaving an area of exposed oesophagus on the right side.

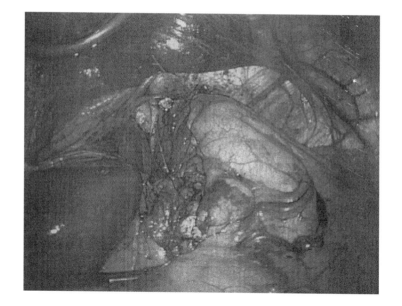

effective, and that it results in an overall reduction in the short-term morbidity associated with surgery for reflux. However, several complications unique to the laparoscopic approach have also been described (**Table 10.1**).[9] Long-term results remain unknown, although it is probably reasonable to extrapolate outcomes from open surgery if the same principles have been adhered to. In terms of curing reflux, the laparoscopic Nissen procedure has been successful, with only a 2% incidence of recurrence of reflux at 2 to 3 years follow-up. It is likely that this procedure will be as durable as open fundoplication, where a 70–80% success rate can be expected up to 25 years follow-up.[76] It has been suggested that dysphagia could be more common following laparoscopic fundoplication, although

Pneumothorax[94,105,106,107,108]

Pneumomediastinum[109,110]

Pulmonary embolism[93,111,112]

Injury to major vessels[95]

Paraoesophageal hiatus hernia[43,85,112]

Hiatal stenosis[89]

Mesenteric thrombosis[100,113]

Bilobed stomach[93]

Oesophageal perforation[112,114,115,116,117]

Gastric perforation[93,112,114]

Duodenal perforation[99]

Bowel perforation[117]

Cardiac laceration and tamponade[97,98]

Pleuropericarditis[118]

Necrotising fasciitis[86]

Table 10.1 *Unique or common complications following laparoscopic antireflux surgery*

this impression could also be erroneous due to the more intense nature of the prospective follow-up applied in many centres. Furthermore, in our experience dysphagia has been less of a problem following fundoplication than it was prior to surgery, with a reduction in the incidence from approximately 30% before surgery to less than 10% at 12 months following it,[4,5] and for the majority of these patients dysphagia has not been troublesome in the long term. The overall satisfaction rate is quite high, with about 90% of patients stating that given the same choice they would have the operation again.

Nevertheless, up to 10% of patients are dissatisfied. Some of this is because of a complication of the original surgery, in the authors' experience this has usually been either the development of a paraoesophageal hernia (which accounts for about half of all reoperations), or because of continuing troublesome dysphagia (with either the wrap or the hiatus being too tight). Some patients are dissatisfied, however, even though their reflux has been cured and they have not had any complications.[77] This is usually because they do not like the flatulence which can follow the procedure. It is also important to recognise that there is a learning curve associated with this form of surgery, and we have demonstrated that the first 20 patients in an individual surgeon's experience are associated with a higher complication rate, and as experience increases the reoperation rates fall to below 5% and probably to below 2%.[39] There are no specific contraindications to the laparoscopic approach, and the repair of giant hiatal hernias and reoperative antireflux surgery are both feasible (although technically more demanding).

There are some differences between the management of patients during and after laparoscopic and open fundoplication procedures. Laparoscopic surgery may increase the risk of thromboembolic complications (see below) and therefore prophylaxis for deep vein thrombosis is mandatory. Other differences are primarily due to the accelerated recovery following laparoscopic surgery. The authors' practice is to avoid the use of a nasogastric tube, commence oral intake within 24 hours of surgery and to arrange a barium meal X-ray within 2 days to check the postoperative anatomy at a time when problems are easily corrected. Since implementing this approach, a similar strategy has been applied to patients undergoing open surgery (usually revision procedures) and this has facilitated a quicker recovery in some of these patients too.

Laparoscopic versus open antireflux surgery

Non-randomised comparisons between open and laparoscopic fundoplication have generally shown that laparoscopic surgery requires more operating time than the equivalent open surgical procedure,[78,79] that the incidence of postoperative complications is reduced, the length of postoperative hospital stay is shortened by 3 to 7 days, patients return to full physical function between 6 and 27 days earlier, and overall hospital costs are reduced following laparoscopic antireflux surgery. The efficacy of reflux control appears to be similar between the two approaches.

Five randomised controlled trials have been reported which compare a laparoscopic Nissen fundoplication with its open surgical equivalent.[80,81,82,83,84] However, all describe early results only, and two of the studies have been reported as published abstracts only. Nevertheless, the results of all these trials confirm advantages for the laparoscopic approach, albeit less dramatic than the advantages expected from the results of non-randomised studies.

The trials of laparoscopic versus open Nissen fundoplication reported by Watson *et al.*,[81] Franzen *et al.*[82] and Perttila *et al.*[84] which enrolled 42, 36 and 20 patients respectively, demonstrated equivalent short-term clinical outcomes, shortening of the postoperative stay by about 1 day (3 versus 4 median), longer operating times (extended by approximately 30 minutes) and an overall reduction in the incidence of complications following laparoscopic fundoplication. The reduction in the length of the postoperative hospital stay by only 1 day was unexpected. This was achieved entirely by a shorter hospital stay following open fundoplication, suggesting that at least some of the apparent benefits of the laparoscopic approach could be due to a general change in management policy, and if any surgeon uses an open approach then there are probably significant gains to be made by encouraging earlier oral intake, avoiding nasogastric tubes and encouraging earlier discharge from hospital.

Heikkinen *et al.*[83] reported a trial of 42 patients who underwent either an open or a laparoscopic Nissen fundoplication. However, the operation performed laparoscopically was usually different from that performed in the open surgical group, as the short gastric vessels were rarely divided at laparoscopic fundoplication, but almost always at open surgery, and the oesophageal hiatus was repaired in all patients at laparoscopic fundoplication, but selectively at open surgery. Laine *et al.*[80] recently reported the outcome of a larger trial of 110 patients randomised to undergo laparoscopic or open Nissen fundoplication. In this study hospital stay was halved from 6.4 to 3.2 days, patients returned to work quicker (37 versus 15 days), but operating time was also prolonged by 31 minutes.

Unfortunately none of the currently reported trials report postoperative outcomes beyond 12 months. Nevertheless, the overall results of all 5 trials confirm that laparoscopic antireflux surgery has short-term advantages over the open approach, and short-term (3–12 months) control of reflux is similar to that following open surgery.

Complications of laparoscopic antireflux surgery

As experience with laparoscopic approaches for antireflux surgery has grown, complications unique to the laparoscopic approach have emerged (Table 10.1). These include postoperative paraoesophageal hiatus hernia, reoperation for dysphagia and gastrointestinal perforation. Nevertheless, the risk of complications should be balanced against the advantages of the laparoscopic approach, as it is likely that the overall complication rate is reduced following laparoscopic surgery.[9] The likelihood of complications can be influenced by a number of factors including; surgeon experience and expertise, operative technique and perioperative care. Furthermore the final outcome of some complications can be moderated significantly by applying appropriate early management strategies.

Complications which are more common following laparoscopic antireflux surgery are described below.

Paraoesophageal hiatus hernia

Paraoesophageal hiatus herniation has been thought to be an uncommon finding following open fundoplication, presenting usually in the late follow-up period, although its frequency could have been underestimated in the past. Most large series of laparoscopic procedures report the occurrence of paraoesophageal herniation following surgery (**Figure 10.7**), particularly in the immediate postoperative period.[43,85,86] The incidence of this complication ranges up to 7% in

Figure 10.7
Barium meal X-ray demonstrating a large paraoesophageal hiatus hernia 3 months after laparoscopic fundoplication.

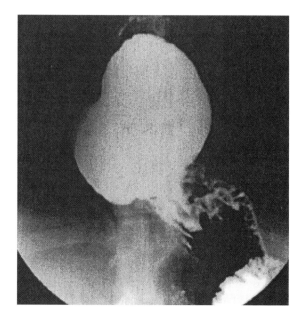

published reports,[9,43] and it seems that this is exacerbated by some factors inherent in the laparoscopic approach. These include a tendency to extend laparoscopic oesophageal dissection further into the thorax than during open surgery, an increased risk of breaching the left pleural membrane,[87] and the effect of reduced postoperative pain. Loss of the left pleural barrier can allow the stomach to slide more easily into the left hemithorax, and less pain permits more abdominal force to be transmitted to the hiatal area during coughing, vomiting or other forms of exertion in the initial postoperative period, pushing the stomach into the thorax, as the normal anatomical barriers have been disrupted by surgical dissection. Early resumption of heavy physical work also has been associated with acute herniation. Strategies are available which can reduce the likelihood of herniation. Routine hiatal repair has been shown to reduce the incidence by approximately 80%.[43] In addition, excessive strain on the hiatal repair during the early postoperative period should be avoided by the routine use of antiemetics, and advising patients to avoid excessive lifting or straining for about 1 month following surgery.

Dysphagia

The debate in the laparoscopic era is whether or not dysphagia is more likely to occur following laparoscopic antireflux surgery. Nearly all patients, including those who undergo a partial fundoplication, experience dysphagia requiring dietary modification in the first weeks to months following laparoscopic surgery. However, it is dysphagia which is severe enough to need further surgery which is of most concern. Early severe dysphagia requiring surgical revision has been reported in a number of series.[88,89,90] Conversion of a Nissen fundoplication to a partial fundoplication has been performed for troublesome dysphagia for both open and laparoscopic techniques, usually with success.[90,91,92]

More common with the laparoscopic approach, however, is the problem of a tight oesophageal diaphragmatic hiatus causing dysphagia (**Figs. 10.8** and **10.9**).[89,91] Two factors may cause this problem; over-tightening of the hiatus during hiatal repair, and excessive perihiatal scar tissue formation. Most surgeons use an intraoesophageal bougie to distend the oesophagus and to assist with calibration of the hiatal closure. However, this will not always prevent over-tightening; if a problem does arise in the immediate postoperative period, it can usually be corrected by early laparoscopic reintervention with release of one or more hiatal sutures. Later narrowing of the oesophageal hiatus due to postoperative scar tissue formation in the second and third postoperative weeks, even in patients not undergoing initial hiatal repair, has also been described. In the authors' experience, endoscopic dilatation has usually only provided temporary relief of symptoms, rather than a long-term solution. Correction of this problem requires widening of the diaphragmatic hiatus. This can be achieved by a laparoscopic approach, with anterolateral division of the hiatal ring and adjacent diaphragm until the hiatus is sufficiently loose.

Pulmonary embolism

Pulmonary embolism has been more common in some of the early reports of laparoscopic Nissen fundoplication,[93] and in particular following conversion of cases to open surgery, suggesting that prolonged operating times might be an important aetiological factor. In addition, several mechanical factors inherent in

Figure 10.8
Barium meal X-ray demonstrating usual appearance following laparoscopic Nissen fundoplication.

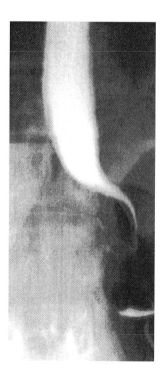

Figure 10.9
Day 2 postoperative barium meal in a patient with total dysphagia following Nissen fundoplication due to a tight oesophageal hiatus. The problem was corrected by widening the hiatus and removing the hiatal repair sutures.

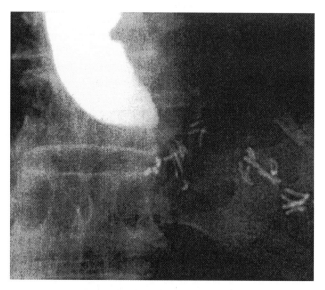

the laparoscopic antireflux surgery environment, create a scenario in which venous thrombosis is more likely. The combination of head-up tilt of the operating table, intra-abdominal insufflation of gas under pressure and elevation of the legs in stirrups, greatly reduces venous flow in the leg veins, potentially predisposing to deep venous thrombosis. This problem may be minimised by the routine use of vigorous antithromboembolism prophylaxis, including low-dose heparin, antiembolism stockings and mechanical compression of the calves.

Complications unique to laparoscopic antireflux surgery

Bilobed stomach

A technical error which has been described during early experiences with laparoscopic Nissen fundoplication is the 'bilobed stomach'.[93] This problem occurs using too distal a piece of stomach to form a Nissen fundoplication, usually the gastric body rather than the fundus, resulting in a bilobular shaped stomach (**Fig. 10.10**). This may not be recognised at the time because of the different angle of view provided by the laparoscope. While most patients are asymptomatic, in extreme cases it is possible for the upper part of the stomach to become obstructed at the point of constriction in the gastric body resulting in post-prandial abdominal pain, which requires surgical revision (**Fig. 10.11**). Ensuring that the correct piece of stomach (the fundus) is used for construction of the fundoplication prevents this problem from arising.

Pneumothorax

Intraoperative pneumothorax occurs in up to 2% of patients due to injury to the left pleural membrane during retro-oesophageal dissection, particularly if dissection is directed too high within the mediastinum.[94] Careful dissection behind the oesophagus, ensuring that the tips of instruments passed from right to left behind the oesophagus do not pass above the level of the diaphragm, and experience with laparoscopic dissection at the hiatus, reduce its likelihood. The occurrence of a pneumothorax does not usually require the placement of a chest drain, as

Figure 10.10
Barium meal image of a 'bilobed' stomach. This patient continues to have an excellent clinical result at 7 years follow-up.

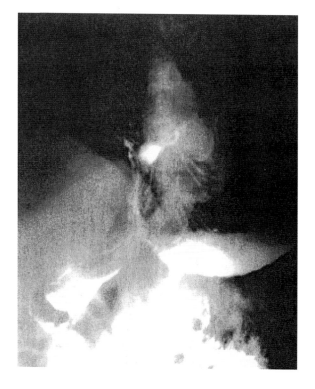

Figure 10.11
Barium meal image of a more severe 'bilobed' stomach. This patient developed gastric obstruction and required surgical revision.

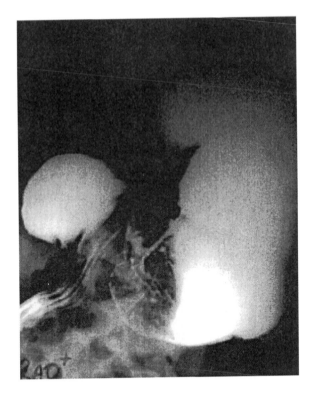

CO_2 gas in the pleural cavity is rapidly reabsorbed at the completion of the procedure, allowing the lung to re-expand rapidly.

Vascular injury

Vascular injury to the inferior vena cava, the left hepatic vein and the abdominal aorta have all been reported.[95,96] This problem may be associated with aberrant anatomy, inexperience, the excessive use of monopolar diathermy cautery dissection, or a combination of all of these. Intraoperative bleeding more commonly follows inadvertent laceration of the left lobe of the liver by a laparoscopic liver retractor or other instrument, and haemorrhage from poorly secured short gastric vessels during fundal mobilisation. A rare complication is cardiac tamponade. This has been reported twice,[97,98] once as a result of laceration of the right ventricle by a liver retractor, and once due to an injury of the cardiac wall from a suture needle. Certainly the proximity of the heart, inferior vena cava and aorta to the distal oesophagus, render potentially life-threatening injuries a distinct possibility if surgeons are unfamiliar with the hiatal anatomy as seen via the laparoscope. Nevertheless, the overall risk of perioperative haemorrhage during and after antireflux surgery is probably reduced by the laparoscopic approach, and the likelihood of splenectomy is significantly reduced by the laparoscopic approach.

Perforation of the upper gastrointestinal tract

Oesophageal and gastric perforation are specific risks, with an incidence of approximately 1% reported in most series.[9,26,99] Gastric perforation is usually an avulsion injury of the gastric cardia due to excessive traction by the surgical assistant. Perforation of the back wall of the oesophagus usually occurs during dissection of the posterior oesophagus. The anterior oesophageal wall is probably at greatest risk when a bougie is passed to calibrate the tightness of a Nissen fundoplication or the oesophageal hiatus. All these injuries can be repaired by sutures, placed either laparoscopically or by an open technique. Awareness that injury can occur enables surgeons to institute strategies which reduce the likelihood of their occurrence. Furthermore, injury is less likely with greater experience.

Mortality

Three deaths have been reported following laparoscopic antireflux procedures: one caused by peritonitis secondary to duodenal perforation,[99] one arising from thrombosis of the superior mesenteric artery and the coeliac axis,[100] and one following infarction of the liver.[101] No other deaths have been reported, suggesting that the overall mortality of laparoscopic antireflux surgery is very low, and that the laparoscopic approach is safe compared with open surgical approaches.

Avoiding complications following laparoscopic antireflux surgery and minimising their impact

To avoid or minimise complications following a laparoscopic antireflux procedure, a range of strategies should be considered and applied whenever possible. Surgeons should apply a surgical technique which will reduce the likelihood of an adverse outcome arising. Most agree that the oesophageal hiatus should be narrowed or reinforced with sutures, irrespective of whether a hiatus hernia is present or not.[43] However, as complications will occur in a small number of patients following any surgical procedure, a strategy should be sought which will minimise the impact of problems when they arise. One such strategy is to perform a barium swallow examination on the first or second postoperative day to confirm that the fundoplication is in the correct position and that the stomach is entirely intra-abdominal. If there is any uncertainty endoscopic examination may clarify the situation. If the appearances are not acceptable, or if other problems such as severe dysphagia or excessive pain occur, then laparoscopic re-exploration should be performed. Early laparoscopic reintervention is associated with minimal morbidity, and usually delays the patient's recovery by only a few days. Most complications requiring reintervention can be readily dealt with laparoscopically within a week of the original procedure.[24] Beyond this time, however, laparoscopic reoperation becomes difficult, and for this reason we have a relatively low threshold for laparoscopic re-exploration in the first postoperative week if early problems arise.

If complications become apparent at a later stage, laparoscopic reoperation is often still feasible if an experienced surgeon is available.[91] However, the likelihood of success is reduced in the intermediate period following the original procedure. Waiting, if possible, until scar tissue has matured (i.e. at least 3 to 6 months), simplifies subsequent laparoscopic dissection, and increases the likelihood of completing the procedure laparoscopically.

Other randomised trials

The Angelchik prosthesis

Three small trials have compared the Nissen fundoplication with the Angelchik antireflux prosthesis. Hill *et al.*[60] randomised 61 patients to undergo either a Nissen fundoplication or the placement of an Angelchik antireflux prosthesis. Follow-up was over a 7-year period, with good long-term results obtained in 17/22 from the Angelchik group and 20/25 of the Nissen group. Two of the Angelchik prostheses were removed for persistent dysphagia and one more because of postoperative infection. Five patients also had persistent dysphagia following prosthesis placement. No Nissen procedures required surgical revision. Long-term outcomes were similar. Kmiot *et al.*[61] randomised 50 patients to a similar trial. The incidence of persistent dysphagia was greater following placement of the Angelchik prosthesis (20% versus 0%) and 3 patients required removal of the prosthesis for this problem. The authors chose to stop this trial early because of this problem. Eyre-Brook *et al.*[102] reported a trial of 48 patients with similar outcomes following the Angelchik prosthesis.

 The overall results of the 3 trials suggest a higher dysphagia rate and reoperation rate following placement of the Angelchik prosthesis and for these reasons this operation is now rarely performed.

The Ligamentum Teres cardiopexy

Janssen *et al.*[103] enrolled 20 patients in a randomised study of Nissen fundoplication versus Ligamentum Teres cardiopexy. Although both procedures effectively corrected reflux for the first 3 months following surgery, by 12 months, 6 of the 10 patients who underwent the Ligamentum Teres repair required further surgery for recurrent reflux.

 Despite the small number of patients entered, the results of the Ligamentum Teres repair were so poor that continued use of this procedure can no longer be justified.

Antrectomy with Roux-en-Y duodenal diversion

Washer *et al.*[104] randomised 42 patients with 'severe reflux oesophagitis' (most with reflux strictures) to receive either a total fundoplication or an antrectomy with Roux-en-Y duodenal diversion. At an average of 5 years follow-up good to excellent results were achieved in 20 of 22 patients having an antrectomy and Roux-en-Y anastomosis, compared with 13 of 20 patients having a fundoplication. The study was originally reported in 1984 and since the advent of more effective medical treatment, the type of patients enrolled in this study is now rarely seen. Furthermore, most surgeons think that gastrectomies add a disease dimension in their own right and so remain unconvinced of the utility of this approach, at least for first-time operations for reflux.

Summary of the results from prospective randomised trials

The results of randomised trials can be assessed together to facilitate the development of guidelines for antireflux surgery (**Table 10.2**). Some of these will meet with wide acceptance as they support the current body of thought of the international surgical community. However, others are controversial, as they do not support the opinions of the majority of experts in the field. Nevertheless, in the hierarchy of evidence, the results of prospective randomised trials should take precedence over the opinion of experts. It should be remembered that well-regarded expert opinions from the past have sometimes been shown to be wrong as more evidence becomes available.

Few surgeons will disagree with the conclusion that the Nissen fundoplication outperforms the Angelchik prosthesis and the Ligamentum Teres cardiopexy and that the latter procedures should no longer be undertaken. Furthermore most surgeons performing surgery for reflux agree that the laparoscopic approach has been a major advance in surgical technique for this condition and that this has led to surgery becoming a more attractive management option. Controversy, however, will be raised by conclusions drawn about division of the short gastric blood vessels and the place of partial fundoplications in the surgeon's armamentarium. The only published trials which have investigated division of the short gastric vessels support the position that this manoeuvre is not necessary for the creation of a satisfactory Nissen fundoplication. Further trials are, however, required to confirm this conclusion.

It is perhaps surprising that the four studies of posterior versus Nissen fundoplication have demonstrated no real advantages for the posterior partial fundoplication technique (with the exception of gas-related problems), particularly as the data from these trials are often used to support the positions of either selective or routine use of the posterior fundoplication technique. Nevertheless, the combined

---

- Laparoscopic Nissen fundoplication is associated with fewer complications overall and a shorter convalescence than open Nissen fundoplication*

- The Nissen fundoplication has a lower complication and reoperation rate than the Angelchik prosthesis*

- The Nissen fundoplication controls reflux better than the Ligamentum Teres cardiopexy

- Whether both vagus nerves are included or excluded from the wrap makes no difference

- Division of the short gastric blood vessels does not improve the outcome following Nissen fundoplication*

- Dysphagia and recurrent reflux following posterior partial fundoplication and Nissen fundoplication are similar
    in unselected patients*
    in patients with poor oesophageal motility

- The incidence of dysphagia and 'gas-related' complications is reduced following anterior partial fundoplication

- Partial fundoplications are associated with less wind-related problems than total fundoplication*

---

* = statement is supported by evidence from more than one randomised trial

Table 10.2 *Evidence from prospective randomised trials for antireflux surgery*

data of the reported trials do not support the proponents of the posterior partial fundoplication; anterior partial fundoplication could on the other hand be a better alternative, although with only one trial reported so far, more studies are needed.

The large caseload of many surgical units performing laparoscopic surgery for gastro-oesophageal reflux is now providing opportunities to conduct further trials of antireflux surgery techniques, and this should contribute to a rapid expansion of the evidence base from which future conclusions can be drawn.

References

1. Nebel OT, Fornes MF, Castell DO. Symptomatic gastroesophageal reflux: incidence and precipitating factors. Am J Dig 1976; 21:953–56.

2. Thompson WE, Heaton KW. Heartburn and globus in apparently healthy people. Can Med Assoc J 1982; 126:46–8.

3. Lord RVN, Law MG, Ward RL et al. Rising incidence of oesophageal adenocarcinoma in men in Australia. J Gastroenterol Hepatol 1998; 13:356–62.

4. Watson DI, Jamieson GG, Pike GK et al. Laparoscopic vs anterior fundoplication; a randomised double blind controlled trial. Aust NZ J Surg 1999; 69 (Suppl):A57 (Abstract).

5. Watson DI, Pike GK, Baigrie RJ et al. Prospective double blind randomised trial of laparoscopic Nissen fundoplication with division and without division of short gastric vessels. Ann Surg 1997; 226:642–52. *A randomised trial of 102 patients who underwent a total fundoplication with versus without division of the short gastric vessels. No clinical outcome differences were seen, and in particular dysphagia rates were identical. However, reported follow-up remains short.*

6. Ireland AC, Holloway RH, Toouli J et al. Mechanisms underlying the antireflux action of fundoplication. Gut 1993; 34:303–8.

7. Dent J. Australian clinical trials of omeprazole in the management of reflux oesophagitis. Digestion 1990; 47:69–71.

8. Watson DI, Mathew G, Pike GK et al. Comparison of anterior, posterior and total fundoplication using a viscera model. Dis Esoph 1997; 10:110–14.

9. Watson DI, Jamieson GG. Antireflux surgery in the laparoscopic era (Review). Br J Surg 1998; 85:1173–84.

10. Bate CM, Keeling PW, O'Morain C et al. Comparison of omeprazole and cimetidine in reflux oesophagitis: symptomatic, endoscopic, and histological evaluations. Gut 1990; 31:968–72.

11. Hetzel DJ, Dent J, Reed WD et al. Healing and relapse of severe peptic esophagitis after treatment with omeprazole. Gastroenterol 1998; 95:903–13.

12. Kuipers EJ, Lundell L, Klinkenberg-Knol EC et al. Atrophic gastritis and *Helicobacter pylori* infection in patients with reflux esophagitis treated with omeprazole or fundoplication. New Engl J Med 1996; 334:1018–22.

13. Driman DK, Wright C, Tougas G et al. Omeprazole produces parietal cell hypertrophy and hyperplasia in humans. Dig Dis Sci 1996; 41:2039–47.

14. Verlinden M. Review article: A role for gastrointestinal prokinetic agents in the treatment of reflux oesophagitis? Aliment Pharmacol Therap 1989; 3:113–31.

15. Watson DI, Jamieson GG, Myers JC et al. The effect of 12 weeks of Cisapride on oesophageal and gastric function in patients with gastro-oesophageal reflux disease. Dis Esoph 1996; 9:48–52.

16. Waring JP, Hunter JG, Oddsdottir M et al. The preoperative evaluation of patients considered for laparoscopic antireflux surgery. Am J Gastroenterol 1995; 90:35–8.

17. Bischof G, Feil W, Riegler M et al. Peptic esophageal stricture: is surgery still necessary? Wei Klin Wochenschr 1996; 108:267–71.

18. Farrell TM, Smith CD, Metreveli RE et al. Fundoplication provides effective and durable symptom relief in patients with Barrett's esophagus. Am J Surg 1999; 178:18–21.

19. Ortiz EA, Martinez de Haro LF, Parrilla P et al. Conservative treatment versus antireflux surgery in Barrett's oesophagus: long-term results of a prospective study. Br J Surg 1996; 83:274–8.

20. Ortiz A, De Maro LT, Parrilla P et al. 24-h pH monitoring is necessary to assess acid reflux suppression in patients with Barrett's oesophagus undergoing treatment with proton pump inhibitors. Br J Surg 1999; 86:1472–4.

21. Sagar PM, Ackroyd R, Hosie KB et al. Regression and progression of Barrett's oesophagus after antireflux surgery. Br J Surg 1995; 82:806–10.

22. Behar J, Sheahan DG, Biancani P. Medical and surgical management of reflux oesophagitis, a

38-month report on a prospective clinical trial. New Engl J Med 1975; 293:263–8.

23. Spechler SJ. Comparison of medical and surgical therapy for complicated gastroesophageal reflux disease in veterans. New Engl J Med 1992; 326:786–92.

    The only large prospective randomised trial to compare medical with surgical therapy for gastro-oesophageal reflux. This study demonstrated superior outcomes following an open Nissen fundoplication procedure compared to the use of H2 receptor antagonists.

24. Watson DI, Jamieson GG, Baigrie RJ et al. Laparoscopic surgery for gastro-oesophageal reflux: beyond the learning curve. Br J Surg 1996; 83:1284–7.

25. Ackroyd R, Watson DI, Game PA. Fizzy drinks following laparoscopic Nissen fundoplication: a cautionary tale of explosive consequences. Aust NZ J Surg 1999; 69:887–8.

26. Gotley DC, Smithers BM, Rhodes M et al. Laparoscopic Nissen fundoplication – 200 consecutive cases. Gut 1996; 38:487–91.

27. Watson DI, Jamieson GG, Pike GK et al. A prospective randomised double blind trial between laparoscopic Nissen fundoplication and anterior partial fundoplication. Br J Surg 1999; 86:123–30.

    The only randomised trial to compare an anterior partial fundoplication with the Nissen procedure. Short term (6 months) follow-up of 107 patients demonstrated a reduction in the incidence of dysphagia and gas related side effects following anterior partial fundoplication. Longer term follow-up, however, is yet to be reported, and for this reason long term reflux control remains unknown.

28. Trus TL, Laycock WS, Branum G et al. Intermediate follow-up of laparoscopic antireflux surgery. Am J Surg 1996; 171:32–5.

29. Oddsdottir M, Franco AL, Laycock WS et al. Laparoscopic repair of paraesophageal hernia. New access, old technique. Surg Endosc 1995; 9:164–8.

30. Watson DI, Devitt PG, Jamieson GG. Importance of dissection of the hernial sac in laparoscopic surgery for very large hiatus hernias. Arch Surg 1999; 134:1069–73.

31. Kauer WKH, Peters JH, DeMeester TR et al. A tailored approach to antireflux surgery. J Thorac Cardiovasc Surg 1995; 110:141–7.

32. Little AG. Gastro-oesophageal reflux and oesophageal motility diseases; Who should perform antireflux surgery? Ann Chir Gynaecol 1995; 84:103–5.

33. Beckingham IJ, Cariem AK, Bornman PC et al. Oesophageal dysmotility is not associated with poor outcome after laparoscopic Nissen fundoplication. Br J Surg 1998; 85:1290–3.

34. Baigrie RJ, Watson DI, Myers JC et al. The outcome of laparoscopic Nissen fundoplication in patients with disordered pre-operative peristalsis. Gut 1997; 40:381–5.

35. Rydberg L, Ruth M, Abrahamsson H et al. Tailoring antireflux surgery: A randomized clinical trial. World J Surg 1999; 23:612–18.

36. Watson DI, Mathew G, Pike GK et al. Efficacy of anterior, posterior and total fundoplication in an experimental model. Br J Surg 1998; 85:1006–9.

37. Collard JM, De Koninck XJ, Otte JB et al. Intrathoracic Nissen fundoplication: long-term clinical and pH-monitoring evaluation. Ann Thorac Surg 1991; 51:34–8.

38. Watson A, Jenkinson LR, Ball CS et al. A more physiological alternative to total fundoplication for the surgical correction of resistant gastro-oesophageal reflux. Br J Surg 1991; 78:1088–94.

39. Watson DI, Baigrie RJ, Jamieson GG. A learning curve for laparoscopic fundoplication. Definable, avoidable, or a waste of time? Ann Surg 1996; 224:198–203.

40. Nissen R. Eine einfache operation zur beeinflussung der refluxoesophagitis. Schweiz Med Wochenschr 1956; 86:590–2.

41. DeMeester TR, Bonavina L, Albertucci M. Nissen fundoplication for gastroesophageal reflux disease. Evaluation of primary repair in 100 consecutive patients. Ann Surg 1986; 204:9–20.

42. DeMeester TR, Stein HJ. Minimizing the side effects of antireflux surgery. World J Surg 1992; 16:335–6.

43. Watson DI, Jamieson GG, Devitt PG et al. Paraoesophageal hiatus hernia: an important complication of laparoscopic Nissen fundoplication. Br J Surg 1995; 82:521–3.

44. Donahue PE, Bombeck CT. The modified Nissen fundoplication – reflux prevention without gas bloat. Chir Gastroent 1977; 11:15–27.

45. Rossetti M, Hell K. Fundoplication for the treatment of gastroesophageal reflux in hiatal hernia. World J Surg 1977; 1:439–44.

46. Toupet A. Technique d'oesophago-gastroplastie avec phrenogastropexie appliquee dans la cure radicale des hernies hiatales et comme complement de l'operation d'heller dans les cardiospasmes. Med Acad Chir 1963; 89:394.

47. Lind JF, Burns CM, MacDougal JT. 'Physiological' repair for hiatus hernia – manometric study. Arch Surg 1965; 91:233–7.

48. Belsey R. Mark IV repair of hiatal hernia by the transthoracic approach. World J Surg 1977; 1:475–81.

49. Nguyen NT, Schauer PR, Hutson W et al. Preliminary results of thoracoscopic Belsey Mark

IV antireflux procedure. Surg Lapar Endosc 1998; 8:185–8.

50. Dor J, Himbert P, Paoli JM *et al.* Treatment of reflux by the so-called modified Heller–Nissen technic. Presse Med 1967; 75:2563–9.

51. Watson A, Spychal RT, Brown MG *et al.* Laparoscopic 'physiological' antireflux procedure: preliminary results of a prospective symptomatic and objective study. Br J Surg 1995; 82:651–6.

52. Hill LD. An effective operation for hiatal hernia: an eight year appraisal. Ann Surg 1967; 166:681–92.

53. Aye RW, Hill LD, Kraemer SJM *et al.* Early results with the laparoscopic Hill repair. Am J Surg 1994; 167:542–6.

54. Jobe BA, Horvath KD, Swanstrom LL. Postoperative function following laparoscopic Collis gastroplasty for shortened esophagus. Arch Surg 1998; 133:867–74.

55. Swanstrom LL, Marcus DR, Galloway GQ. Laparoscopic Collis gastroplasty is the treatment of choice for the shortened esophagus. Am J Surg 1996; 171:477–81.

56. Johnson AB, Oddsdottir M, Hunter JG. Laparoscopic Collis gastroplasty and Nissen fundoplication. A new technique for the management of esophageal foreshortening. Surg Endosc 1998; 12:1055–60.

57. Falk GL, Harrison RI. Laparoscopic cut Collis gastroplasty: a novel technique. Dis Esoph 1998; 11:260–2.

58. Allison PR. Hiatus hernia: a 20-year retrospective survey. Ann Surg 1973; 178:273–6.

59. Maddern GJ, Myers JC, McIntosh N *et al.* The effect of the Angelchik prosthesis on esophageal and gastric function. Arch Surg 1991; 126:1418–22.

60. Hill ADK, Walsh TN, Bolger CM *et al.* Randomized controlled trial comparing Nissen fundoplication and the Angelchik prosthesis. Br J Surg 1994; 81:72–4.

61. Kmiot WA, Kirby RM, Akinola D *et al.* Prospective randomized trial of Nissen fundoplication and the Angelchik prosthesis. Br J Surg 1991; 78:1181–4.

62. DeMeester TR, Johnson LF, Kent AH. Evaluation of current operations for the prevention of gastroesophageal reflux. Ann Surg 1974; 180:511–25.

63. Thor KBA, Silander T. A long-term randomized prospective trial of the Nissen procedure versus a modified Toupet technique. Ann Surg 1989; 210:719–24.

64. Walker SJ, Holt S, Sanderson CJ *et al.* Comparison of Nissen total and Lind partial transabdominal fundoplication in the treatment of gastro-oesophageal reflux. Br J Surg 1992; 79:410–14.

65. Lundell L, Abrahamsson H, Ruth M *et al.* Long-term results of a prospective randomized comparison of total fundic wrap (Nissen-Rossetti) or semifundoplication (Toupet) for gastro-oesophageal reflux. Br J Surg 1996; 83:830–35.
The only randomised trial of total versus posterior partial fundoplication to enrol a large cohort of patients, and to report long-term follow-up. No advantages for the partial fundoplication technique were seen, except for a reduction in gas-related side effects at 2 and 3 years following surgery. In particular dysphagia rates and reflux control were similar for the two procedures.

66. Luostarinen M, Koskinen M, Reinikainen P. *et al.* Two antireflux operations: Floppy versus standard Nissen fundoplication. Ann Med 1995; 27:199–205.

67. Lundell L, Abrahamsson H, Ruth M *et al.* Lower esophageal sphincter characteristics and esophageal acid exposure following partial or 360° fundoplication: Results of a prospective, randomized clinical study. World J Surg 1991; 15:115–21.

68. Laws HL, Clements RH, Swillies CM. A randomized, prospective comparison of the Nissen versus the Toupet fundoplication for gastroesophageal reflux disease. Ann Surg 1997; 225:647–54.

69. Hunter JG, Swanstrom L, Waring JP. Dysphagia after laparoscopic antireflux surgery. The impact of operative technique. Ann Surg 1996; 224:51–7.

70. Dallemagne B, Weerts JM, Jehaes C *et al.* Causes of failures of laparoscopic antireflux operations. Surg Endosc 1996; 10:305–10.

71. Luostarinen MES, Koskinen MO, Isolauri JO. Effect of fundal mobilisation in Nissen-Rossetti fundoplication on oesophageal transit and dysphagia. Eur J Surg 1996; 162:37–42.

72. Luostarinen ME, Isolauri JO. Randomized trial to study the effect of fundic mobilization on long-term results of Nissen fundoplication. Br J Surg 1999; 86:614–18.

73. Geagea T. Laparoscopic Nissen's fundoplication: preliminary report on ten cases. Surg Endosc 1991; 5:170–73.

74. Dallemagne B, Weerts JM, Jehaes C *et al.* Laparoscopic Nissen fundoplication: Preliminary report. Surg Lapar Endosc 1991; 1:138–43.

75. Anvari M, Allen C. Laparoscopic Nissen fundoplication. Two-year comprehensive follow-up of a technique of minimal paraesophageal dissection. Ann Surg 1998; 227:25–32.

76. Luostarinen M, Isolauri J, Laitinen J *et al.* Fate of Nissen fundoplication after 20 years. A clinical, endoscopical, and functional analysis. Gut 1993; 34:1015–20.

77. Watson DI, Chan ASL, Myers JC *et al.* Illness behaviour influences the outcome of laparoscopic antireflux surgery. J Am Coll Surg 1997; 184:44–8.

78. Rattner DW, Brooks DC. Patient satisfaction following laparoscopic and open antireflux surgery. Arch Surg 1995; 130:289–94.

79. Peters JH, Heimbucher J, Kauer WKH *et al.* Clinical and physiological comparison of laparoscopic and open Nissen fundoplication. J Am Coll Surg 1995; 180:385–93.

 80. Laine S, Rantala A, Gullichsen R *et al.* Laparoscopic vs conventional Nissen fundoplication. A prospective randomized study. Surg Endosc 1997; 11:441–4.

81. Watson DI, Gourlay R, Globe J *et al.* Prospective randomised trial of laparoscopic versus open Nissen fundoplication. Gut 1994; 35 (Suppl 2):S15 (Abstract).

 82. Franzen T, Anderberg B, Tibbling L *et al.* A report from a randomized study of open and laparoscopic 360° fundoplication. Surg Endosc 1996; 10:582 (Abstract). *A randomised trial of laparoscopic versus open total fundoplication that enrolled 110 patients. Short-term outcomes were improved following laparoscopic Nissen fundoplication, including a quicker recovery and reduced overall complication rate. At short-term follow-up, the clinical outcomes of control of reflux and various side effects have been similar.*

83. Heikkinen T-J, Haukipuro K, Koivukangas P *et al.* Comparison of costs between laparoscopic and open Nissen fundoplication: a prospective randomized study with a 3-month followup. J Am Coll Surg 1999; 188:368–76.

84. Perttila J, Salo M, Ovaska J *et al.* Immune response after laparoscopic and conventional Nissen fundoplication. Eur J Surg 1999; 165:21–28.

85. Johansson B, Glise H, Hallerback B. Thoracic herniation and intrathoracic gastric perforation after laparoscopic fundoplication. Surg Endosc 1995; 9:917–18.

86. Viste A, Vindenes H, Gjerde S. Herniation of the stomach and necrotizing chest wall infection following laparoscopic Nissen fundoplication. Surg Endosc 1997; 11:1029–31.

87. Watson DI, Jamieson GG, Britten-Jones R *et al.* Pneumothorax during laparoscopic dissection of the diaphragmatic hiatus. Br J Surg 1993; 80:1353–4.

88. Wetscher GJ, Glaser K, Wieschemeyer T *et al.* Tailored antireflux surgery for gastroesophageal reflux disease: Effectiveness and risk of post-operative dysphagia. World J Surg 1997; 21:605–10.

89. Watson DI, Jamieson GG, Mitchell PC *et al.* Stenosis of the esophageal hiatus following laparoscopic fundoplication. Arch Surg 1995; 130:1014–16.

90. Collard JM, Romagnoli R, Kestens PJ. Reoperation for unsatisfactory outcome after laparoscopic antireflux surgery. Dis Esoph 1996; 9:56–62.

91. Watson DI, Jamieson GG, Game PA *et al.* Laparoscopic reoperation following failed antireflux surgery. Br J Surg 1999; 86:98–101.

92. Vertruyen M, Cadiere GB, Himpens J *et al.* Reoperation for total and irreversible food intolerance after laparoscopic adjustable silicone gastroplasty banding (LASGB). Surg Endosc 1996; 10:570 (Abstract).

93. Jamieson GG, Watson DI, Britten-Jones R *et al.* Laparoscopic Nissen fundoplication. Ann Surg 1994; 220:137–45.

94. Watson DI, Mitchell PC, Game PA *et al.* Pneumothorax during laparoscopic dissection of the oesophageal hiatus. Aust NZ J Surg 1996; 66:711–12.

95. Baigrie RJ, Watson DI, Game PA *et al.* Vascular perils during laparoscopic dissection of the oesophageal hiatus. Br J Surg 1997; 84:556–7.

96. McKenzie T, Esmore D, Tulloh B. Haemorrhage from aortic wall granuloma following laparoscopic Nissen fundoplication. Aust NZ J Surg 1997; 67:815–16.

97. Firoozmand E, Ritter M, Cohen R *et al.* Ventricular laceration and cardiac tamponade during laparoscopic Nissen fundoplication. Surg Lapar Endosc 1996; 6:394–7.

98. Farlo J, Thawgathurai D, Mikhail M *et al.* Cardiac tamponade during laparoscopic Nissen fundoplication. Eur J Anaesthesiol 1998; 15:246–7.

99. Hinder RA, Filipi CJ, Wetscher G *et al.* Laparoscopic Nissen fundoplication is an effective treatment for gastroesophageal reflux disease. Ann Surg 1994; 220:472–83.

100. Mitchell PC, Jamieson GG. Coeliac axis and mesenteric arterial thrombosis following laparoscopic Nissen fundoplication. Aust NZ J Surg 1994; 64:728–30.

101. Schorr RT. Laparoscopic upper abdominal operations and mesenteric infarction. J Laparoendosc Surg 1995; 5:389–91.

102. Eyre-Brook IA, Codling BW, Gear MWL. Results of a prospective randomized trial of the Angelchik prosthesis and a consecutive series of 119 patients. Br J Surg 1993; 80:602–4.

103. Janssen IM, Gouma DJ, Klementschitsch P *et al.* Prospective randomised comparison of teres cardiopexy and Nissen fundoplication in the surgical therapy of gastro-oesophageal reflux disease. Br J Surg 1993; 80:875–8.

104. Washer GF, Gear MWL, Dowling BL *et al.* Randomized prospective trial of Roux-en-Y duodenal diversion versus fundoplication for severe reflux oesophagitis. Br J Surg 1984; 71:181–4.

105. Reid DB, Winning T, Bell G. Pneumothorax during laparoscopic dissection of the diaphragmatic hiatus. Br J Surg 1993; 80:670.

106. Joris JL, Chiche J-D, Lamy ML. Pneumothorax during laparoscopic fundoplication: Diagnosis and treatment with positive end-expiratory pressure. Anesth Analg 1995; 81:993–1000.

107. Matkinen M-T, Yli-Hankala A, Kansanaho M. Early detection of CO_2 pneumothorax with continuous spirometry during laparoscopic fundoplication. Acta Anaesthesiol Scand 1995; 39:411–13.

108. Biswas TK, Smith JA. Laparoscopic total fundoplication: Anaesthesia and complications. Anaesth Intensive Care 1993; 21:127–8.

109. Stallard N. Pneumomediastinum during laparoscopic Nissen fundoplication. Anaesthesia 1995; 50:667–8.

110. Overdijk LE, Rademaker BM, Ringers J et al. Laparoscopic fundoplication: A new technique with new complications? J Clin Anesth 1994; 6:321–23.

111. Pike GK, Bessell JR, Mathew G et al. Changes in fibrinogen levels in patients undergoing open and laparoscopic Nissen fundoplication. Aust NZ J Surg 1996; 66:94–6.

112. Munro W, Brancatisano R, Adams IP et al. Complications of laparoscopic fundoplication: The first 100 patients. Surg Lapar Endosc 1996; 6:421–3.

113. Medina LT, Vientimilla R, Williams MD et al. Laparoscopic fundoplication. J Laparoendosc Surg 1996; 6:219–26.

114. Schauer PR, Meyers WC, Eubanks S et al. Mechanisms of gastric and esophageal perforations during laparoscopic Nissen fundoplication. Ann Surg 1996; 223:43–52.

115. Lowham AS, Filipi CJ, Hinder RA et al. Mechanisms of avoidance of esophageal perforation by anesthesia personnel during laparoscopic foregut surgery. Surg Endosc 1996; 10:979–82.

116. Swanstrom LL, Pennings JL. Safe laparoscopic dissection of the gastroesophageal junction. Am J Surg 1995; 169:507–11.

117. Collet D, Cadiere GB. Conversions and complications of laparoscopic treatment of gastroesophageal reflux disease. Am J Surg 1995; 169:622–6.

118. Viste A, Horn A, Lund-Tonnessen S. Reactive pleuropericarditis following laparoscopic fundoplication. Surg Lapar Endosc 1997; 7:206–8.

11 Barrett's oesophagus, dysplasia and the complications of gastro-oesophageal reflux disease

Hugh Barr

Barrett's oesophagus

Barrett's oesophagus is a most intriguing pathological condition of the oesophagus. It is assumed that the squamous epithelium is injured by chronic gastro-oesophageal reflux and repair is effected in this abnormal environment by columnar, instead of squamous, cells. Three distinct types of this columnar metaplasia have been identified. The most common is intestinal, and this is the most likely to undergo malignant transformation. The other two types, cardiac and fundic, are difficult to distinguish from gastric mucosa at these sites.

Adenocarcinoma of the gastro-oesophageal junction is at present reaching epidemic proportions, and is strongly associated with Barrett's oesophagus. Currently adenocarcinoma in Barrett's oesophagus has an incidence of 800 per 100 000. This can be compared with lung cancer in men over 65, where the incidence is 500 per 100 000. Cancer incidence may be expressed as a percentage of a particular population developing cancer per year. For adults with Barrett's oesophagus the annual rate is 0.8%.[1] The significance of the problem is emphasised by the current rate of rise in the incidence of oesophageal adenocarcinoma that is outstripping any other cancer including melanoma, lymphoma and small cell lung cancer.[2,3]

Intestinal metaplasia (**Fig. 11.1**) in the columnar-lined segment and at the gastro-oesophageal junction has been identified as the precursor lesion. It is usually heterogeneous and can only be detected by careful biopsy, and it can be present in mucosa of macroscopically normal appearance.[4] The significance of this change and the relationship of this condition to the rising incidence of gastric cancer at the gastro-oesophageal junction is hotly debated.[5]

Historical considerations

Norman Rupert Barrett first described this condition of columnar-lined oesophagus in combination with oesophagitis and an ulcer, in 1950.[6] He defined the oesophagus as being lined by squamous epithelium and observed that in some

Figure 11.1
Histological slide of specialised intestinal metaplasia with goblet cell formation.

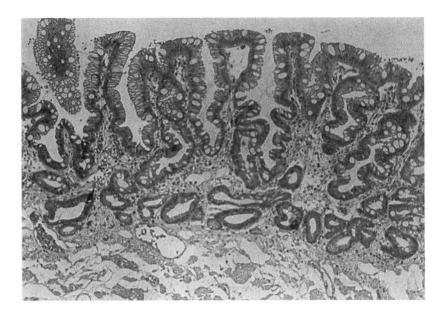

patients the distal oesophagus was lined by gastric-like columnar epithelium. He misinterpreted his findings as a congenitally short oesophagus with a tubular intrathoracic stomach. It was Allison and Johnstone[7] who demonstrated that the columnar epithelium was proximal to the lower oesophageal sphincter and established that the condition was clearly an oesophageal problem. Confirmation was secured by Lortat-Jakob, who described 'endobrachyoesophagus' with shortening of the oesophageal mucosa but not the muscular tube.[8] The argument over whether this was an acquired or congenital condition continued until Bremner in 1970 demonstrated columnar cell regeneration in the distal oesophagus in an experimental model of chronic gastro-oesophageal reflux.[9] Although columnar-lined oesophagus is called Barrett's oesophagus, the first description was by Tileston in 1906.[15]

Definitions

The precise definition of a condition would usually be a prerequisite to full understanding. The commonly used definition of Barrett's oesophagus is described as the 'condition in which the distal oesophagus is lined by a variable length of columnar epithelium'. This statement may be regarded as too simplistic; the term Barrett's oesophagus is imprecise as the eponym acknowledges only a historical description. And although it would seem self-evident that the oesophagus can be accurately defined, this is not the case; unfortunately at endoscopic examination its precise boundaries can be mistaken. The problem occurs because Barrett's oesophagus occurs at the junction of the oesophagus and the gastric cardia. Some consideration must be given to an accurate assessment of the anatomy and hence the pathology.

Anatomical and endoscopic considerations

The main problem is that the anatomy and position of the gastro-oesophageal junction are difficult to define. There is a lack of universally accepted and reproducible set of criteria to identify the cardia of the stomach from the distal oesophagus. The manometrically defined lower oesophageal sphincter can be identified. The assumption that the oesophagus is normally lined by squamous mucosa above this has not been rigorously tested.[10] During endoscopy it is important to identify certain important landmarks in order to allow some delineation of abnormal columnar-lined oesophagus (Barrett's oesophagus). The squamo-columnar junction is usually visible as the pale squamous epithelium merges into redder columnar mucosa. The gastro-oesophageal junction is imaginary but at present is defined endoscopically as the level of the most proximal gastric fold. Some patients with a hiatus hernia have defective and weak lower oesophageal sphincters, and there is therefore no clear-cut flare as one enters the stomach with the endoscope. The proximal margin of the gastric folds must be determined when the distal oesophagus is minimally inflated. Over-inflation will flatten and obscure all the gastric folds. If the squamo-columnar and gastro-oesophageal junction coincide, the entire oesophagus is lined with squamous mucosa. When the squamo-columnar junction is proximal to the gastro-oesophageal junction, there is a columnar-lined segment or Barrett's oesophagus (**Fig. 11.2**).

Pathological considerations

The hope that pathology would be less subjective is not securely founded. Oesophageal squamous mucosa is easily identified. Standard teaching is that the gastric cardia is lined by columnar cardiac or junctional epithelium, but pathologists are not uniform in their definitions. This epithelium can extend into the oesophagus, but it is unclear as to whether this is normal or a variant of Barrett's oesophagus. Some would contend that up to 2 cm of this epithelium in the distal oesophagus is normal.[5,11]

An important alternative pathological classification has been proposed based on the importance of the presence of specialised intestinal metaplasia (Fig. 11.1). Yet it would be wrong to define Barrett's oesophagus solely on the criteria of finding specialised intestinal metaplasia, since biopsies of the cardia and stomach may contain metaplastic changes that are indistinguishable from those obtained

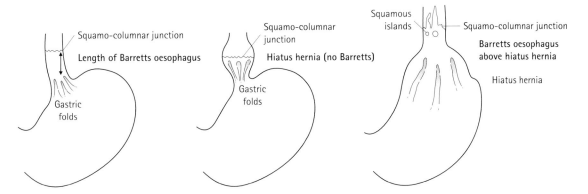

Figure 11.2
Endoscopic difficulties and landmarks allowing an accurate diagnosis of Barrett's oesophagus.

from the columnar-lined oesophagus. Spechler and Goyal suggest that whenever endoscopically visible columnar-lined oesophagus is seen then the condition is called columnar-lined oesophagus. Biopsies are then taken from this area to look for specialised intestinal metaplasia (SIM). The condition is then classified as columnar-lined oesophagus with or without specialised intestinal metaplasia. If the biopsy comes from the squamo-columnar junction at the gastro-oesophageal junction then the condition is known as specialised intestinal metaplasia at the gastro-oesophageal junction.[12,13]

Although this can all appear confusing to the clinical surgeon, we must ask if there are any definite markers in a biopsy that may identify its origin from the stomach or the oesophagus. The answer is affirmative but these signs are only rarely evident. A clear indication of oesophageal origin is the presence of an oesophageal gland or more usually (in a biopsy sample) a duct from these glands (**Fig. 11.3**). The depth of biopsy makes these findings unusual.

At present it is still clinically useful to measure the length of Barrett's oesophagus. Long-segment Barrett's oesophagus exceeds 3 cm of the lower oesophagus, short segment is less than 3 cm and intestinal metaplasia at the gastro-oesophageal junction is called oesophago-gastric junction with specialised intestinal metaplasia.[14] The endoscopic feature most strongly associated with a finding of specialised intestinal metaplasia on biopsy is the length of the Barrett's segment. The likelihood of finding histological evidence for patients with long-segment Barrett's oesophagus (> 3 cm) being 90%. Other features that increase the possibility of finding SIM are a jagged squamo-columnar junction with tongues extending upwards in the oesophagus (**Fig. 11.2**) and discrete patches of metaplasia.

Figure 11.3
Histological slide to show intestinal metaplasia with a deep oesophageal gland (lower right) and the squamous lined duct.

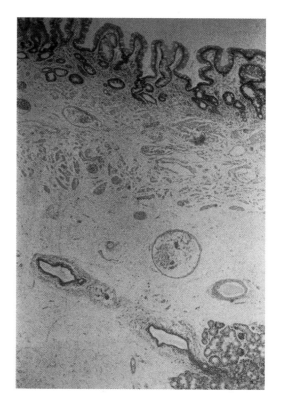

Pathophysiology of Barrett's oesophagus (**Fig. 11.4**)

The precise pathogenesis and derivation of columnar metaplasia in the lower oesophagus is still uncertain. Although not proven, our current understanding is based on the concept of a mucosal 'adaptive' response to the increased cell loss as a result of chronic inflammation, secondary to gastro-oesophageal reflux disease. Barrett's oesophagus is found in patients undergoing endoscopy for reflux disease, and they have been shown to have an increased exposure of their lower oesophagus to acid and the components of the refluxate.[16] Oesophageal squamous epithelium is highly sensitive to acid, alkaline and biliary reflux and it becomes inflamed, with cell loss, necrosis and ulceration. This results in an increase in the proliferative zone height and length to maintain epithelial thickness. The oesophageal stem cells located at the tip of the papillae are thus susceptible to damage, being more superficial than their daughter cells. Paradoxically, the more severe the reflux the more superficial and at risk the all-important functional stem cell becomes. The only cells that can survive in this milieu are the acid or bile-resistant lineages.[17] Subsequently, increased apoptosis in the basal compartments purifies these metaplastic cell lineages. There is a significant increase in apoptotic activity in intestinal-type Barrett's compared to gastric type. As progress occurs in the neoplastic sequence apoptosis is seen to be less in dysplastic and carcinomatous epithelium with a significant increase in proliferation.[18] Effective intraoesophageal acid suppression has been shown to favour differentiation and decrease proliferation, raising, the possibility that acid suppression may slow or even prevent malignant degeneration.[19]

The symptoms of gastro-oesophageal reflux are an extremely common problem with up to 9% of adults having heartburn daily and about 20% weekly.[20] There is a strong and quite possibly a causal relationship between symptomatic gastro-oesophageal reflux disease and oesophageal adenocarcinoma.

This has been clearly demonstrated in a Swedish case–control study. Patients with recurrent reflux symptoms when compared with asymptomatic patients had an odds ratio of 7.7 for oesophageal adenocarcinoma and 2 for adenocarcinoma of the gastric cardia. Patients with severe symptoms of long standing had an odds ratio of 43.5 and 4.4 for oesophageal and cardia adenocarcinoma respectively. The main conclusion is that symptomatic reflux is a risk for oesophageal adenocarcinoma regardless of the presence of Barrett's oesophagus, which was not specifically identified in this nationwide population-based study.[21]

Prevalence of Barrett's oesophagus and oesophageal cancer

The precise prevalence of Barrett's oesophagus is yet to be determined. Autopsy data suggest that 1 in 20 may have the disease.[22] Approximately 1% of unselected patients undergoing endoscopy for dyspepsia are found to have Barrett's oesophagus.[23] It is certainly very much more common in patients undergoing endoscopy for gastro-oesophageal reflux disease, being found in 12%.[24] The prevalence increases with age. It is predominantly a disease of Caucasians with a male to female ratio of 2:1.[25] The problem of prevalence estimation is compounded since the metaplastic columnar epithelium may not cause any symptoms and indeed

Definition of Barrett's oesophagus	Patients	Follow-up (mean years)	Incidence (patient years)	Reference
> 3 cm or SIM	50	5.2	1/52	26
> 3 cm or SIM	166	2.9	1/59 male 1/167 female	27
SIM	177	4.8	1/208	28
> 5 cm	56	2.9	1/55	29
> 2 cm with SIM	29	1.8	1/52	30
> 3 cm	81	3.6	1/96	31
> 5 cm	102	4.2	1/115	32
SIM	71	3	1/55	33

* (Specialised intestinal metaplasia SIM)

Table 11.1 *Prospective series that estimate the risk of developing an oesophageal adenocarcinoma in patients with Barrett's oesophagus or SIM**

the pain of gastro-oesophageal reflux may improve in patients when this reflux-resistant epithelium develops.

The risk of adenocarcinoma has been estimated following several prospective (**Table 11.1**) and retrospective series. Overall the estimated incidence of carcinoma in patients with Barrett's oesophagus is of the order of 1 in 150 patient years, with a 30–50 fold increase of cancer over the general population.[34] Intriguingly, this figure tallies quite nicely with the odds ratio of approximately 45 for patients with severe reflux oesophagitis.[21] Certain features are associated with an increased risk of dysplasia and cancer. These include the length of the Barrett's segment,[14,32] smoking,[35] obesity and a lack of raw fruit, vegetable and fibre in the diet.[36] Patients with benign metaplastic columnar-lined oesophagus who are smokers have a 2.3-fold risk of developing a carcinoma, and a doubling of the length of the metaplastic segment results in a 1.7 times increased risk.[46]

Dysplasia

Carcinogenesis in Barrett's oesophagus is thought to follow a sequence from intestinal metaplasia through low- and high-grade dysplasia and finally to invasive cancer (**Fig. 11.4**). The presence of dysplasia is regarded as the best marker for malignant transformation in the epithelium. Dysplasia is classified histologically into low and high grade, with 'indefinite' used when dysplasia cannot be clearly differentiated from the reactive or regenerative changes associated with inflammation. This classification is a modification of histopathological classifications used in the rest of the gastrointestinal tract, most notably for colonic dysplasia associated with inflammatory bowel disease.[37] High-grade dysplasia is diagnosed when there are distinct cytological changes; in particular the nuclei vary markedly in size, shape and there is a loss of polarity. There is also loss of crypt architecture with gross distortions occurring (**Figs. 11.5** and **11.6**). Low-grade

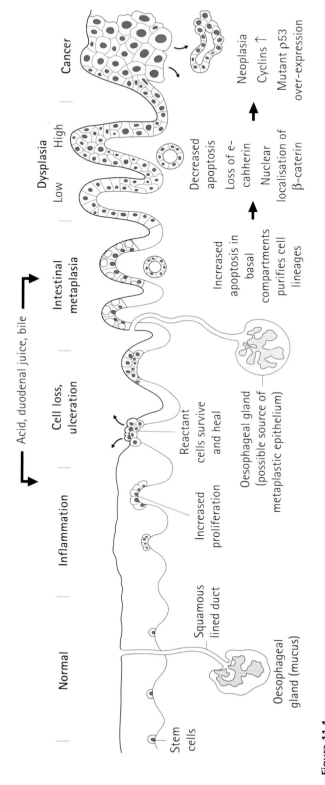

Figure 11.4
Neoplastic progression from squamous mucosa to adenocarcinoma.

Figure 11.5
Histological section of low-grade dysplasia. Note loss of goblet cells and cytological abnormalities.

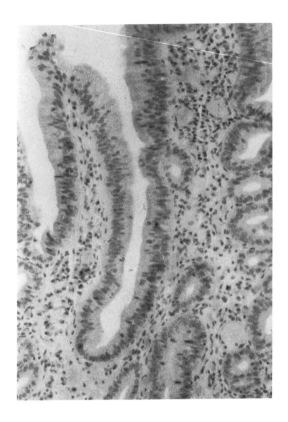

Figure 11.6
Histological section to show high-grade dysplasia with very bizarre cytological changes.

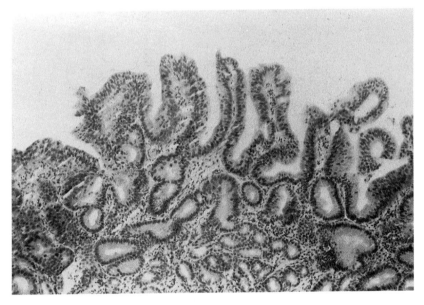

dysplasia is harder to classify but occurs with loss of cellular differentiation with loss of goblet cells. The crypt and cytological changes are milder changes than with high-grade dysplasia. Intramucosal cancer is said to have occurred when there is invasion through the basement membrane into the lamina propria. The term carcinoma *in situ* has been abandoned because of the confusion it caused. There is considerable inter- and intraobserver variation among experienced pathologists in the histological diagnosis of dysplastic Barrett's oesophagus.[38]

The molecular events associated with transformation from metaplasia to dysplasia are very important and quite distinct. It is important to note that most Barrett's epithelium is stable and will not undergo malignant transformation. However, some cells, usually of the intestinal type, develop increased proliferative indices[18,19] and transform to express an oncogenic phenotype. They are visibly different and express oncogenes such as c-erbB2.[39] Cell-cycle abnormalities may well occur during the early malignant transformation. Cells are mobilised from the G0 to G1 phase, there is loss of the G1–S transition and there are more cells in the G2 phase.[40] Cyclins as regulators of the cell cycle are in particular over-expressed in oesophageal adenocarcinomas.[41] Cell-cycle regulation is also a function of p53 as the 'guardian of the genome'. Any DNA damage upregulates p53 which then stops the cell cycle at the G1–S checkpoint and stimulates repair of the nucleic acids. Mutant p53s are inactive and their accumulation is the basis for the detection of the protein by immunohistochemical methods. The detection of p53 protein in Barrett's oesophagus and cancer is now well documented. It is not present in non-dysplastic epithelium, but is seen in 9% of specimens indefinite for or with low-grade dysplasia, 55% of those with high-grade dysplasia, and 87% of carcinomas.[42] It appears that p53 may be a useful prognostic marker. Patients with low-grade dysplasia who express p53 are likely to progress to high-grade or indeed carcinoma. Those that show no expression are less likely to undergo further malignant degeneration.[43] Thus the subgroup of patients with low or indefinite dysplasia and p53 expression should be followed with a more rigorous surveillance regimen. It must be emphasised that not all oesophageal adenocarcinomas express p53, and patients without expression have progressed to cancer.[42]

Other molecular and histological markers are being sought to identify patients at high risk of malignant transformation. Analysis of the DNA content using flow cytometry has shown that aneuploidy or increase in the G2/tetraploidy fraction is an increased risk factor for malignant progression.[44] Another critical event in the neoplastic progression is loss of cell adhesion with aberrant expression of adhesion molecules. Most notably there is reduced expression of e-cadherin with localisation of catenins, to the nucleus as the mucosa becomes more malignant.[45]

Dysplasia: the natural history

The natural history of the malignant progression of Barrett's oesophagus is a crucial but as yet unanswered question. There are several questions that must be addressed. First, we must ask how many patients who have a preoperative histological diagnosis of high-grade dysplasia are found to have invasive cancer after surgery. This group is selected because is does exclude patients unfit for the extensive surgery required to surgically remove the oesophagus (Table 11.2). In some series up to 50% of patients with a preoperative diagnosis of high-grade dysplasia are found to have a carcinoma. This confirms the importance of precise histological assessment and the use of rigorous biopsy protocols. Patients with dysplasia must be biopsied according to protocol. Large 9 mm open-span biopsy forceps (Olympus FB13K) must be used with the suck and twist technique

Patients High-grade dysplasia	Invasive cancer postoperative histology	Reference
8	4	47
18	9	48
16	6	49
9	2	50
7	0	51
9	5	52
11	8	53
12	4	54
30	13	55
15	8	56
19	2	57
15	5	58*

All series are compiled after 1990- *indicates a review of the pre-1990 experience

Table 11.2 *Carcinoma identified in patients having a resection for high-grade dysplasia*

(turn-and-suction) to maximise the mucosal biopsy size. It is therefore necessary to use a large channel endoscope. After detailed identification of all landmarks, the Barrett's segment is biopsied from its lowermost to above the squamo-columnar junction. Samples must be taken from all areas of mucosal abnormality and any areas where high-grade dysplasia had been identified previously. All four quadrants of the oesophagus are also biopsied at 2 cm intervals.

The number of samples removed may be, and often should be, greater than 50. Patients who have this aggressive surveillance regimen[51] can have their cancers detected very early, and proceed to appropriate oesophagectomy. If high-grade dysplasia is the indication for oesophagectomy then there is a valid concern that some with only a small area of dysplasia may have a prophylactic oesophagectomy. Unfortunately, some of these patients have died of the postoperative complications.[57] In one series the operative mortality of patients operated on for high-grade dysplasia was 14% with no mortality from a missed cancer.[51] There can be no doubt that patients who undergo surveillance and have a surveillance-detected cancer will survive longer following surgery than patients who develop symptomatic cancers.[52] Therefore the debate remains as to whether the endpoint of surveillance is the initial diagnosis of high-grade dysplasia, the persistence of high-grade dysplasia or the definitive diagnosis of invasive cancer.

Although difficult and confounding to analysis, some attempt must be made to examine whether high-grade dysplasia always progresses to cancer in the lifetime of the patient. **Tables 11.3** and **11.4** are an attempt to examine in longitudinal series the time for low-grade and high-grade dysplasia to progress to cancer. The data are few and insubstantial. The most important and informative single study was of 58 patients with high-grade dysplasia.[51] These patients were extremely closely examined with a rigorous biopsy protocol. Seven progressed

Low grade → High grade → Cancer			Number of patients	Reference
	13		2	29
32		6	5 and 5	26
	43		2	31
22		14	1 and 5	68
	29		1	48
	38		7	51
24		15	1 and 3	

Low Grade → Cancer	Number of patients	Reference
52	1	31
56	1	64
42	1	Barr 1999 (personal series)

(Time of progression is in months. The data is extracted from figures and is therefore approximate)

Table 11.3 *Summary of the longitudinal studies of patients with dysplasia that progresses to cancer*

High grade → High grade	Patients	Reference
32	21	51
48	1	26
Low grade → Low grade		
6–84	13	31
69	2	26
Low grade → Metaplasia		
6–60	3	31

(Time span is in months of follow-up)

Table 11.4 *The natural history of dysplasia*

to intramucosal cancer over a mean period of 38 months, and 21 remained with stable high-grade dysplasia over a 32-month follow-up. We cannot assume that all patients will progress fromhigh-grade dysplasia. The situation of patients with low-grade dysplasia is even more confusing; some will progress to carcinoma without high-grade dysplasia being detected and some will regress to metaplastic epithelium. An important question remains as to whether high-grade dysplasia may regress. Unfortunately the data are unclear. Some series have documented that high-grade dysplasia has appeared to resolve.[19] We must remain cautious, since there are problems of sampling error and longer-term follow-up is required.

Management of Barrett's oesophagus

It is now clear that heartburn due to gastro-oesophageal reflux disease is a serious symptom that now must be appropriately addressed, since it may be the precursor of malignant degeneration at the gastro-oesophageal junction.[20,21] Although symptoms of chronic reflux precede the development of Barrett's oesophagus,[59] it is a resistant epithelium. Barrett's columnar-lined mucosa is an adaptive response to injury and is therefore resistant to further injury and is less sensitive, and more likely to be asymptomatic. Indeed, patients may find their symptoms improving as the metaplasia develops. There is evidence that they are less aware of acid reflux than those patients with uncomplicated reflux and symptom relief is an unreliable measure of control of acid reflux.[60] If the endpoint of treatment of patients with Barrett's oesophagus is the relief of heartburn then it is unlikely that the acid control is adequate.[61] Since patients with symptomatic heartburn may or may not have Barrett's oesophagus an initial endoscopy is essential. If columnar-lined metaplasia is present then proper biopsy is necessary.

In view of the epidemiological Swedish data that symptomatic heartburn is associated with an increased risk of adenocarcinoma, the issue of therapy must be addressed.[21] Most patients self treat or are treated empirically with antacid medication. Some will be treated aggressively with proton pump inhibitors or indeed surgically. More often such treatment is reserved for those with erosive oesophagitis. Treatment regimens are intermittent and dependent on the patient's response. Thus it is likely that the patient will receive short-term treatment allowing frequent relapse of symptoms and further erosive changes and damage to the lower oesophagus.[20] Reflux oesophagitis is a chronic condition that calls for long-term maintenance therapy,[62] after proper endoscopic diagnosis. There is no doubt that proton pump inhibitor therapy and/or surgery can be very effective in healing oesophagitis and improving symptoms.[62] The crucial question is whether it can have an effect on Barrett's oesophagus and malignant degeneration. The molecular evidence is that effective acid suppression favours differentiation and decreases proliferation.[19] There is also clinical evidence that with prolonged continuous treatment with omeprazole, certain histological parameters of Barrett's oesophagus are improved. There is a decrease in the length of the Barrett's segment with an increase in the number of squamous islands. There is also a reduction in the proportion of sulphomucin-rich intestinal metaplasia.[63]

A randomised double blind study has confirmed that profound acid suppression with a proton pump inhibitor, leading to elimination of acid reflux, induces a partial regression of the columnar-lined segment.[64]

Controversy also remains as to whether surgery is effective in causing regression of Barrett's oesophagus or halting progression. One study of 56 patients has demonstrated that the mean length of affected oesophagus was reduced from 8 cm to 4 cm after fundoplication in 24 patients; 9 patients showed progression of disease; 23 patients showed no change; and 1 patient developed an invasive carcinoma.[65] Overall there appears to be no clear evidence of regression or reduction of neoplastic transformation after antireflux surgery, although the rate of progression may be reduced.[66] Patients with reflux oesophagitis and Barrett's oesophagus require full medical antireflux therapy. Those with intestinal metaplasia should have regular surveillance endoscopy and biopsy, and a 2-yearly interval is recommended by the author. There are many unresolved issues regarding treatment and surveillance. Some guidance can be obtained from previous reports[67] but these reports must be modified in the light of our increasing knowledge; they appear somewhat dated and must urgently be updated.

Barrett's oesophagus with indefinite or low-grade dysplasia

Intensive medical therapy with a proton pump inhibitor is recommended for a period of 8–12 weeks. If there is histological improvement then 6-monthly surveillance with repeat biopsy is necessary until at least two consecutive examinations reveal no dysplastic change. Surveillance can then be decreased to 2-yearly intervals. The patient should remain on a proton pump inhibitor. If the dysplasia persists then continued intensive control of reflux is necessary and should be confirmed with appropriate investigation. The surveillance should continue at 6-monthly intervals. The development of endoscopic mucosal ablation techniques means that consideration must be given to this form of therapy if low-grade dysplasia persists.

Barrett's oesophagus with high-grade dysplasia

The diagnosis of high-grade dysplasia must be confirmed by at least one further expert pathologist. It is recommended that these patients be subject to a surgical and pathological meeting. If any doubt remains then the endoscopy is repeated immediately and the biopsy protocol must be rigorous[51] and adequate time given to obtaining large and multiple specimens. Some would recommend that the detection of high-grade dysplasia is an indication to end surveillance and proceed to surgery if the patient is well enough for surgical excision. Others have clearly demonstrated that surveillance with biopsy protocols strictly adhered to can differentiate dysplasia from intramucosal cancer.[51] Patients considered to be too great an operative risk should be considered for endoscopic mucosal resection or endoscopic mucosal ablation. These techniques must also be considered for patients with persistent high-grade dysplasia as an alternative to surgical resection and continued surveillance. The operative mortality for oesophagectomy is between 3–10% with a morbidity of 30%. There is therefore a clear need for a minimal targeted therapy for mucosal destruction.

Endoscopic treatments for dysplasia in Barrett's oesophagus

Endoscopic mucosal ablation

Endoscopic mucosal resection has the advantage of removing the mucosa for histological staging. Two techniques are possible: either the lift and cut technique following submucosal injection of saline under the lesion, or the suck and cut method. Both involve diathermy-snare removal after the production of an artificial polyp. The first method involves direct injection in order that a cushion of saline may allow safe snare removal. The latter requires aspiration of the mucosa into a variceal bander and ligation with a band or tie and subsequent snare removal.[69]

Thermal ablation

Endoscopic destruction of the superficial mucosa in a non-selective fashion is possible using the laser, multipolar electrocoagulation or argon-beam plasma coagulation. Barrett's columnar metaplastic tissue is slightly thicker than normal squamous mucosa at 0.5 mm.[70] This does not imply that this is the depth to which treatment should be limited, since consideration must be given as to how the tissue will heal. However, the amount of tissue that needs to be ablated is very small and superficial measuring between 1–2 mm. Full thickness or deep damage risks immediate or delayed perforation with the consequences of mediastinitis, peritonitis and death. Damage that does not penetrate to the external surface, yet reaches the muscle causing damage could result in healing by fibrosis and stricture formation. Limitation of the depth of thermal destruction may be important to allow regeneration with squamous rather than columnar cells. The type of epithelium that regrows is in part determined by the depth of injury. For squamous regeneration it is probable that some of the superficial squamous-lined ducts of the oesophageal mucus glands must survive. The choice of laser or thermal device to destroy the tissue is therefore critical.

Three lasers, Nd:YAG (1064 nm), KTP (532 nm), the Diode (805 nm) and the argon-beam coagulator have been compared for the thermal destruction of superficial areas of mucosa in the oesophagus. A thermal imaging system was used to measure the depth of penetration and the thermal profile in tissue produced using each device at various powers and energy. The purpose was to find parameters of between 60–100°C (coagulative necrosis + vaporisation) on the luminal (mucosal) surface with less than 37°C (no risk of full thickness necrosis) on the external surface.[71,74] Irradiation with the KTP laser, power 15–20 W for 1 second, produced surface temperatures of greater than 65°C with external temperature of 21°C. It was extremely difficult to generate high temperatures on the external surface of the oesophagus using this laser. The diode laser (25 W for 5 seconds) could produce surface temperatures of 90°C but with external temperature of 38°C. The Nd:YAG laser tended to produce worrying temperatures through to the external surface at energy levels that were sufficient to produce thermal destruction on the mucosa. The argon plasma coagulator generated very intense superficial temperatures with little transmission to the external surface of the oesophagus. Both the KTP laser and the argon-beam coagulator have proved to be very effective in treatment and eradication of high- and low-grade dysplastic epithelium and metaplastic mucosa when combined with control of gastro-oesophageal reflux with proton pump inhibitor therapy.[71,72] Unfortunately argon-beam coagulation has been associated with two perforations, one of which resulted in the patient's death.[72] Neo-squamous epithelium was restored in 70% of patients with eradication of dysplasia and intestinal metaplasia; in 30% however, the neo-squamous epithelium covered metaplastic glands.[72,73]

Photodynamic therapy

Photodynamic therapy (PDT) is an interesting technique with the potential for selective destruction of cancers. It is based on the systemic administration of certain photosensitising agents that are retained with some selectively in malignant tissue. When exposed to appropriate wavelength laser light a cytotoxic reaction occurs causing cellular destruction. In extracranial tissues the maximum tumour:normal ratio that can be obtained with a variety of photosensitising agents is 2–3:1. Investigation of photodynamic therapy in experimental gastrointestinal neoplasms has demonstrated important biological advantages. Full thickness intestinal damage produced by photodynamic therapy, unlike thermal damage, does not reduce the mechanical strength of the bowel wall or cause perforation because the submucosal collagen is preserved. In addition, selective necrosis of small areas (less than 2 mm) is possible, with preservation of adjacent non-malignant structures. It is clear that this process is limited to small areas of tissue.

The problem of targeting the photosensitiser to the dysplastic mucosa, and avoiding systemic photosensitisation may be overcome by using endogeneous photosensitisation. Following an excess administration of 5-aminolaevulinic acid (5-ALA), a precursor of haem, an intracellular accumulation of the photosensitiser protoporphyrin IX (PpIX), is induced. The synthesis of 5-ALA from glycine and succinyl-CoA is the first step in porphyrin biosynthesis and ultimately haem. This pathway is tightly regulated by end-product inhibition. If excess endogeneous 5-ALA is administered then this regulation is bypassed and an intracellular accumulation of the photosensitiser protoporphyrin IX (PpIX) is induced. The level of photosensitisation is kept to a few hours and the photosensitiser can be administered orally. The photosensitiser is activated in tissue using 630 nm laser light from a KTP pumped dye laser.

Ten patients with biopsy proven high-grade dysplasia in Barrett's oesophagus were given 60 mg kg^{-1} of 5 amino-laevulinic acid orally, dissolved in fruit juice. After 4 hours treatment was performed at endoscopy under intravenous sedation with 4–10 mg midazolam. The patients were kept in subdued lighting for 24 hours only. All patients were treated using 630 nm light from a dye laser (Laserscope Dye Module 2000, San Jose, California) delivered via a 3 cm cylindrical diffusing fibre, placed in a purpose-made 10–14 mm perspex dilator to provide even light distribution. An energy fluence of 90–150 Jcm^{-2} was delivered to all areas of Barrett's oesophagus by repositioning the diffusing fibre. Acid reflux was suppressed using 40 mg omeprazole daily. Follow-up endoscopy and multiple biopsies at 2-monthly intervals for 8–30 months demonstrated squamous regeneration in the dysplastic columnar-lined oesophagus in four patients with regeneration over metaplastic tissue in two patients.[75] Subsequent studies have confirmed that this method is particularly effective for the eradication of high-grade dysplasia and tumours less than 2 cm.[76] KTP laser destruction was also equally effective in this group of patients.[77] Often a combination of methods is necessary to fully eradicate areas of dysplasia and neoplasia. Photodynamic therapy with an exogeneous, parenterally administered photosensitiser can produce deeper damage to the oesophageal wall. This has the advantage that there may well be a more effective control of occult cancer.[78] This more radical therapy is associated with an oesophageal stricture rate of 34%, a consequence of deep damage to the muscular wall of the oesophagus.

The crucial concept that must be grasped is that mucosal ablation with either endoscopic mucosal resection, thermal or photodynamic ablation is not the end-point of surveillance. The squamous re-epithelialisation that occurs is with neo-squamous mucosa, the destruction is often incomplete[73] and the oncogenic potential of the mucosa is reduced but not abolished. It is essential to continue surveillance. It may be necessary to repeat ablation at intervals. The treatment should be regarded as 'mowing the lawn rather paving the garden'.

Complications of reflux oesophagitis

Severe reflux disease can be complicated by peptic ulceration and stricture formation. An ulcer in the oesophagus is a serious event and is characterised by the complications of ulceration in other parts of the upper gastrointestinal tract. Reflux or peptic strictures occur just above the squamo-columnar junction and may arise in 10% of patients with severe reflux symptoms. As well as heralding a metaplastic change, the spontaneous resolution of symptoms may signify the development of a stricture. Patients with scleroderma may develop particularly intractable strictures. The fibrous replacement of oesophageal smooth muscle results in poor oesophageal peristalsis and decreased lower oesophageal sphincter pressure. The Schatzki–Inglefinger ring is a complication of reflux disease.[80] A well-defined fibrous narrowing occurs in the distal oesophagus at the squamo-columnar junction and consists of fibrosis in the mucosa and the submucosa. These strictures are particularly well treated by oesophageal dilatation.

Most peptic reflux strictures can be managed by oesophageal dilatation and aggressive proton pump inhibitor therapy. These strictures must be dilated progressively rather than abruptly.[79] In resistant cases repeated dilatations may be necessary to achieve an adequate lumen. Benign strictures that persist despite dilatation and full medical treatment must be investigated carefully to ensure that there is not an underlying carcinoma or an extrinsic lesion. A CT scan or preferably endoscopic ultrasound is indicated for resistant strictures.

A small group of patients with resistant strictures or who have recurrence despite appropriate medical therapy may require antireflux surgery. Rarely, a Roux-en-Y biliary diversion with antrectomy may be required for patients with intractable problems. It is important that the duodeno-jejunal anastomosis is at least 45 cm distal to the gastro-jejunostomy to ensure that bile is completely diverted from the remaining stomach and subsequently the oesophagus.

References

1. Spechler SJ. Barrett's esophagus. Sem Oncol 1994; 21:431–7.

2. Blot WJ, Devesa SS, Kneller RW et al. Rising incidence of adenocarcinoma of the esophagus and gastric cardia. JAMA 1991; 265:1287–9.

3. Blot WJ, Devesa SS, Fraumeni JF Jr. Continuing climb in rates of esophageal adenocarcinoma: an update. JAMA 1993; 270:1320.

4. Spechler SJ, Zeroogian JM, Antonioli DA et al. Prevalence of metaplasia at the gastroesophageal junction. Lancet 1994; 344:1533–6.

5. Spechler SJ. The role of gastric carditis in metaplasia and neoplasia at the gastroesophageal junction. Gastroenterology 1999; 117:218–28.

6. Barrett NR. Chronic peptic ulcer of the oesophagus and 'oesophagitis'. Br J Surg 1950; 38:175–82.

7. Allison PR, Johnstone AS. The oesophagus lined with gastric mucous membrane. Thorax 1953; 8:87–110.

8. Lortat-Jakob JL. L' endobrachy-oesophage. Ann Chir 1957; 11:1247–52.

9. Bremner CG, Lynch VP, Ellis FH. Barrett's esophagus: congenital or acquired? An experimental study of esophageal mucosal regeneration in the dog. Surgery 1978; 68:209–16.

10. Kim SL, Waring JP, Spechler SJ et al. Diagnostic inconsistencies in Barrett's esophagus. Gastroenterology 1994; 107:945–9.

11. Hayward J. The lower end of the oesophagus. Thorax 1961; 16:36–41.

12. Spechler SJ, Goyal RK. The columnar-lined esophagus, intestinal metaplasia, and Norman Barrett. Gastroenterology 1996; 110:614–21.

13. Spechler SJ. Esophageal columnar metaplasia (Barrett's esophagus). Gastrointest Endosc Clin N Am 1997; 7:1–18.

14. Hirota WK, Loughney TM, Lazas DJ et al. Specialized intestinal metaplasia, dysplasia, and cancer of the esophagus and esophagogastric junction: prevalence and clinical data. Gastroenterology 1999; 116:277–85.

15. Tileston W. Peptic ulcer of the oesophagus. Am J Sci 1906; 132:240–2.

16. Vaezi MF, Singh S, Richter JE. Role of acid and duodenogastric reflux in esophageal mucosal injury: a review of animal and human studies. Gastroenterology 1995; 108:1897–1907.

17. Jankowski J. Molecular events in Barrett's metaplasia. Gastroenterology 1993; 104:1235.

18. Whittles CE, Biddlestone LR, Burton A *et al.* Apoptotic and proliferative activity in the neoplastic progression in Barrett's oesophagus: a comparative study. J Pathol 1999; 187:535–40.

19. Ouata-Lascar R, Fitzgerald RC, Triadafilopoulos G. Differentiation and proliferation in Barrett's esophagus and the effects of acid suppression. Gastroenterology 1999; 117:327–35.

20. Cohen S, Parkman HP. Heartburn – a serious symptom. N Engl J Med 1999; 340:878–9.

21. Lagergren J, Bergstrom R, Lindren A *et al.* Symptomatic gastroesophageal reflux as a risk factor for esophageal adenocarcinoma. N Engl J Med 199; 340:825–31.
Important confirmation in a case-controlled study that symptomatic reflux oesophagitis leads to adenocarcinoma of the oesophagus.

22. Cameron AJ, Zinsmeister AR, Ballard DJ *et al.* Prevalence of columnar-lined Barrett's esophagus. Comparison of population-based clinical and autopsy findings. Gastroenterology 1990; 99:918–22.

23. Cameron AJ, Lomboy CT. Barrett's esophagus: age, prevalence and extent of columnar epithelium. Gastroenterology 1992; 103:1241–5.

24. Winters C Jr, Spuring TJ, Chobanian SJ *et al.* Barrett's esophagus: a prevalent, occult complication of gastroesophageal reflux disease. Gastroenterology 1987; 92:118–24.

25. Caygill CPJ, Reed PI, McIntyre A *et al.* The UK national Barrett's oesophagus registry: a study of two centres. Eur J Cancer Prevention 1998; 7:161–3.

26. Hameeteman W, Tytgat GN, Houthoff HF *et al.* Barrett's oesophagus: development and adenocarcinoma. Gastroenterology 1989; 96:1249–56.

27. Wright TA, Gray MR, Morris AI *et al.* Cost effectiveness of detection Barrett's cancer. Gut 1996; 39:574–9.

28. Drewitz DJ, Sampliner RE, Garewal HS. The incidence of adenocarcinoma in Barrett's esophagus: a prospective study of 170 patients followed for 4.8 years. Am J Gastroenterol 1997; 92:212–15.

29. Robertson CS, Mayberry JF, Nicholson DA. Value of endoscopic surveillance in the detection of neoplastic change in Barrett's oesophagus. Br J Surg 1988; 75:760–3.

30. Weston AP, Kirmpotich PT, Cherian R *et al.* Prospective long-term endoscopic and histological follow-up of short segment Barrett's esophagus: comparison with traditional long segment Barrett's esophagus. Am J Gastroenterol 1997; 92:407–13.

31. Miros M, Kerlin P, Walker N. Only patients with dysplasia progress to adenocarcinoma in Barrett's oesophagus. Gut 1991; 32:1441–6.

32. Iftikar SY, James PD, Steele R. Length of Barrett's oesophagus: an important factor in the development of dysplasia and adenocarcinoma. Gut 1992; 33:1155–8.

33. Bonelli L. Barrett's esophagus: results of a multicentre survey. Endoscopy 1993; 25:652–4.

34. Van den Boogert J, Van Hillegersberg R, De Bruin RWF *et al.* Barrett's oesophagus: pathophysiology, diagnosis, and management. Scand J Gastroenterol 1998; 33:449–53.

35. Gammon MD, Schoenberg JB, Ahsan H *et al.* Tobacco, alcohol and socioeconomic status and adenocarcinoma of the oesophagus and gastric cardia. J Natl Cancer Inst 1997; 89:1277–84.

36. Brown LM, Swanson CA, Gridley G *et al.* Adenocarcinoma of the esophagus: role of obesity and diet. J Natl Cancer Inst 1995; 87:104–9.

37. Haggitt RC. Barrett's esophagus, dysplasia, and adenocarcinoma. Hum Pathol 1988; 25:982–93.

38. Reid BJ, Haggitt RC, Rubin CE *et al.* Observer variation in the diagnosis of dysplasia in Barrett's oesophagus. Hum Pathol 1988; 19:166–78.

39. Jankowski J, Coghill G, Hopwood D *et al.* Oncogenes and the p53 oncosuppressor gene in adenocarcinoma of the oesophagus. Gut 1992; 33:1033–8.

40. Reid BJ, Sanchez CA, Blount PL *et al.* Cell cycle abnormalities in advancing stages of neoplastic progression. Gastroenterology 1993; 105:119–29.

41. Jiang W, Zhang YJ, Kahn SM *et al.* Altered expression of cyclin D1 and human retinoblastoma genes in human oesophageal cancer. Proc Natl Acad Sci 1993; 90:9026–30.

42. Younes M, Lebovitz RM, Lechago LV *et al.* p53 protein accumulation in Barrett's metaplasia, dysplasia and carcinoma follow-up study. Gastroenterology 1993; 105:1637–42.

43. Younes M, Ertan A, Lechago LV *et al.* p53 protein accumulation is a specific marker of malignant potential in Barrett's metaplasia. Dig Dis Sci 1997; 42:697–701.

44. Menke-Pluymers MBE, Mulder AH, Hop WC *et al.* Dysplasia and aneuploidy as markers of malignant degeneration in Barrett's oesophagus. The Rotterdam Oesophageal Tumour Study Group. Gut 1994; 35:1348–51.

45. Bailey T, Biddlestone L, Shepherd N *et al.* Altered cadherin and catenin complexes in the Barrett's esophagus-dysplasia-adenocarcinoma sequence. Correlation with disease progression and dedifferentiation. Am J Pathol 1998; 152:1–10.

46. Menke-Pluymers MBE, Hop WCJ, Dees J *et al.* Risk factors for development of an adencarcinoma in columnar-lined (Barrett) esophagus. Gastroenterology 1993; 72:1155–8.

47. Altorki NK, Sunagawa M, Little AG *et al.* High-grade dysplasia in the columnar-lined esophagus. Am J Surg 1991; 161:97–9.

48. Pera M, Trastek VF, Carpenter HA *et al.* Barrett's esophagus with high-grade dysplasia: an indication for esophagectomy? Ann Thorac Surg 1992; 54:199–204.

49. Rice TW, Falk GW, Achkar E. Surgical management of high-grade dysplasia in Barrett's esophagus. Am J Surg 1997; 174:1832–6.

50. Steitz JM Jr, Andrews CW Jr, Ellis FH Jr. Endoscopic surveillance of Barrett's oesophagus. Does it help? J Thorac Cardiovasc Surg 1993; 105:383–8.

51. Levine DS, Haggitt RC, Blount PL *et al.* An endoscopic biopsy protocol can differentiate high-grade dysplasia from early adenocarcinoma in Barrett's esophagus. Gastroenterology 1993; 105:40–50.

52. Peters JH, Clark GW, Ireland AP *et al.* Outcome of adenocarcinoma in Barrett's esophagus in endoscopically surveyed and non-surveyed patients. J Thorac Cardiovasc Surg 1994; 108:813–21.

53. Edwards MJ, Gable DR, Lentsch AB *et al.* The rationale for esophagectomy as the optimal therapy for Barrett's esophagus with high-grade dysplasia. Ann Surg 1996; 223:585–9.

54. Collard JM, Romagnoli R, Hermans BP *et al.* Radical esophageal resection for adenocarcinoma arising in Barrett's esophagus. Am J Surg 1997; 174:307–11.

55. Heitmeller RF, Redmond M, Hamilton SR. Barrett's esophagus with high-grade dysplasia. An indication for prophylactic esophagectomy. Ann Surg 1996; 224:66–71.

56. Ferguson MK, Naunheim KS. Resection for Barrett's mucosa with high-grade dysplasia: implications for prophylactic photodynamic therapy. J Thorac Cardiovasc Surg 1997; 114:824–9.

57. Cameron AJ, Carpenter HA. Barrett's esophagus, high-grade dysplasia, and early adenocarcinoma: a pathological study. Am J Gastroenterol 1997; 92:586–91.

58. Palley SL, Sampliner RE, Garewal HS. High-grade dysplasia in Barrett's oesophagus. J Clin Gastroenterol 1989; 11:369–72.

59. Spechler SJ, Goyal RK. Barrett's esophagus. N Engl J Med 1986; 315:362–71.

60. Trimble KC, Pryde A, Heading RC. Lowered oesophageal sensory thresholds in patients with symptomatic but not excessive gastro-oesophageal reflux: evidence for a spectrum of visceral sensitivity in GERD. Gut 1995; 37:7–12.

61. Ouatu-Lascar R, Triadafilopoulos G. Complete elimination of reflux symptoms does not guarantee normalization of acid reflux in patients with Barrett's esophagus Am J Gastroenterol 1998; 93:711–16.

62. Vigneri S, Termini R, Leandro G *et al.* A comparison of five maintenance therapies for reflux esophagitis. N Engl J Med 1995; 333:1106–10.

63. Gore S, Healey CJ, Sutton R *et al.* Regression of columnar lined (Barrett's) oesophagus with continuous omeprazole therapy. Aliment Pharmacol Ther 1993; 7:623–8.

64. **Peters FTM, Ganesh S, Kuipers EJ *et al.* Endoscopic regression of Barrett's oesophagus during omeprazole treatment; a randomised double blind study. Gut 1994; 45:489–94.**
    A blinded randomised trial showing that acid suppression can result in alterations in Barrett's metaplasia.

65. Sagar PM, Ackroyd R, Hosie KB *et al.* Regression and progression of Barrett's oesophagus after antireflux surgery. Brit J Surg 1995; 82:806–10.

66. Ortiz A, Martinez de Haro LF, Parrilla P *et al.* Conservative treatment versus antireflux surgery in Barrett's oesophagus: long-term results of a prospective study. Br J Surg 1996; 83:274–8.

67. Dent J, Bremmer CG, Collen MJ *et al.* Working party report to World Congress of Gastroenterology, Sydney 1990: Barrett's oesophagus. J Gastroenterol Hepatol 1991; 6:1–22.

68. Reid BJ, Blount PL, Rubin CE *et al.* Flow-cytometric and histological progression to malignancy in Barrett's esophagus: prospective endoscopic surveillance of a cohort. Gastroenterology 1992; 102:1212–19.

69. Soehendra H, Binmoeller KF, Bohnacker S *et al.* Endoscopic snare mucosectomy in the esophagus without any additional equipment: A simple technique for resection of flat early cancer. Endoscopy 1997; 29:380–3.

70. Ackroyd R, Brown NJ, Stephenson TJ *et al.* Ablation treatment for Barrett oesophagus: what depth of tissue destruction is needed? J Clin Pathol 1999; 52:509–12.

71. Barham CP, Jones RL, Biddlestone LR *et al.* Photothermal laser ablation of Barrett's oesophagus: endoscopic and histological evidence of squamous re-epithelialisation. Gut 1997; 41:281–384.

72. Byrne JP, Armstrong GR, Attwood SEA. Restoration of the normal squamous lining in Barrett's esophagus by argon beam plasma coagulation. Am J Gastroenterol 1998; 93:1810–15.

73. Biddlestone LR, Barham CP, Wilkinson SP *et al.* The histopathology of treated Barrett's esophagus. Am J Surg Pathol 1998; 22:239–45.

74. Dix T, Barr H. Photothermal ablation of metaplastic columnar-lined (Barrett's) oesophagus, experimental studies for safe endoscopic laser therapy. Progress in Biomedical Optics 1996; 2922:275–80.

75. Barr H, Shepherd NA, Dix A *et al.* Eradication of high grade dysplasia in columnar-lined (Barrett's) oesophagus using photodynamic therapy with endogenously generated protoporphyrin IX. Lancet 1996; 348:584–5.

76. Gossner L, Stolte M, Stroka R *et al.* Photodynamic ablation of high-grade dysplasia and early cancer in Barrett's esophagus by means of 5-aminolaevulinic acid. Gastroenterology 1998; 114:448–55.

77. Gossner L, May A, Stolte M *et al.* KTP laser destruction of dysplasia and early cancer in columnar-lined Barrett's esophagus. Gastrointest Endosc 1999; 49:8–12.

78. Overholt BF, Panjepour M, Haydek JM. Photodynamic therapy for Barrett's esophagus: follow-up in 100 patients. Gastrointest Endosc 1999; 49:1–7.

79. Spechler SJ. American Gastroenterological Association Medical position statement on treatment of patients with dysphagia caused by benign disorders of the distal esophagus. Gastroenterology 1999; 117:229–32.

80. Spechler SJ. AGA technical review on treatment of patients with dysphagia caused by benign disorders of distal esophagus. Gastroenterology 1999; 117:233–54.

12 Benign ulceration of the stomach and duodenum

John Wayman
Simon A. Raimes

INTRODUCTION

Few areas of surgery can have seen such dramatic changes in practice in the last few years as surgery for peptic ulcer disease. With the advent of modern medical treatments the need for elective surgery in cases of peptic ulcer disease has become extremely rare. Operations that were once the 'bread and butter' of both general surgeons and their trainees have virtually disappeared from all but specialist practice. Current strategies for both elective and, more importantly, emergency treatment of peptic ulcers have to take account of modern medical treatment and also decreasing surgical experience.

The need for hospital admission of patients with peptic ulceration has fallen markedly in the last 50 years along with the need for elective surgery. This is due to a decrease in incidence that is quite separate from the advances in treatment. Nevertheless, the incidence of complications of peptic ulceration, such as perforation and haemorrhage, has remained constant and mortality has risen in the last decade. The role of surgery in peptic ulceration has become the surgery of resistant ulcers, of ulcer complications and surgery for the sequelae of previous ulcer operations.

Epidemiology

Study of the epidemiology of peptic ulceration is frequently flawed. Since the introduction of H2 antagonists (H2RA), proton pump inhibitors (PPIs), and eradication therapy for *Helicobacter pylori* (HP), most cases of peptic ulcer disease have been treated in the community.[1] A decline in incidence of peptic ulcer disease based on hospital admission statistics owes more to these changes in treatment than true change in the incidence of disease. Hospital admission data are more accurately applied in situations where hospital admission has remained mandatory; the incidence of perforation has shown little change with time.[2] This still does not take account of changes in iatrogenic aetiological factors, such as the increasing use of non-steroidal inflammatory drugs (NSAIDs).

Mortality from peptic ulcer disease accounted for less than 1% of deaths in England and Wales in 1990.[3] Mortality statistics suggest that death from the complications of peptic ulcer disease is much more common in the elderly and especially females. In the UK, there has been a small increase in the rate of peptic ulcer perforation in elderly women since 1960.[4] In contrast the incidence of perforation in males and younger female patients has fallen.[5] This difference may be largely due to the increased prescription of NSAIDs.

Factors that affect the incidence of peptic ulcer

The incidence and prevalence of peptic ulcer disease varies with time, sex, geography and socioeconomic development.

Temporal factors Both duodenal and gastric ulceration appear to be contemporary diseases, although their incidence has fluctuated. It has been suggested that this is due to a cohort phenomenon secondary to antecedent fluctuating economic prosperity and recession.[6] Since 1960, a period of relative prosperity in the West, the incidence of peptic ulcer disease has fallen, while it has remained high in the underdeveloped world.

Geographical factors Study of geographical variation is confounded by inconsistency of data collection and diagnostic criteria. Such studies have illustrated regional variation in the relative frequencies of duodenal and gastric ulceration and their complications.[7] Even within the UK regional variation has been observed with an increasing incidence of perforated duodenal ulcer south to north.[5]

Socioeconomic variation Closely allied to temporal and geographical variation is socioeconomic variation. Contrary to the 'traditional' characterisation of the patient with duodenal ulceration as affluent and the patient with gastric ulceration as poor, both are more common in the poorer classes.[8] The observation that incidence varies according to occupation and educational attainment is similarly closely related to socioeconomic disparity.[9]

Aetiology

Helicobacter pylori overshadows all other factors implicated in the pathogenesis of peptic ulcer disease. Most peptic ulcers treated in modern practice are caused by *Helicobacter* infection or NSAID ingestion. Other factors, particularly smoking, may facilitate ulcerogenesis in the presence of one or other of the former causative factors. There remains a small group of patients with idiopathic ulceration in whom there are several possible aetiological factors.

Diet

There is no strong evidence for the role of diet in the aetiology of either duodenal or gastric ulceration. Cohort studies in the US have shown an association between caffeine consumption at a young age and a propensity to peptic ulceration later in life.[10] In the same study milk was shown to be protective, while alcohol had no effect.

Acid and pepsin

Reports conflict with respect to the relative roles of acid and pepsin in the aetiology of duodenal and gastric ulcers.

Duodenal ulcers Patients with duodenal ulceration have been shown in several studies to have increased gastric acid production at night and have greater peak secretion levels. This may be due to a larger parietal cell mass, increased sensitivity of parietal cells to gastrin or an increased production of gastrin from the gastric antrum. It is postulated that increased acid production together with the increased gastric emptying recognised in some patients with duodenal ulceration leads to an increased exposure of the duodenum to gastric acid and pepsin.[11]

Gastric ulcers There appear to be several different types of gastric ulcer. Each has a different pathogenesis:

Type 1 – Lesser curve ulcers which are preceded by chronic atrophic gastritis. These ulcers are generally associated with low basal and peak acid output. Interestingly, they appear to develop at the junction between the antral gastrin-secreting mucosa and the parietal cells of the body.

Type 2 – Associated with duodenal ulcer disease. They are usually HP-positive and produce normal or increased amounts of gastric acid.

Type 3 – Prepyloric ulcers within 2 cm of the pyloric ring. They are associated with a diffuse antral gastritis and increased acid production.

Type 4 – Proximal gastric ulcers in the parietal cell mucosa of the body or fundus. They are usually close to the oesophago-gastric junction and are associated with chronic atrophic gastritis.

Smoking

Patients who smoke are more prone to peptic ulceration and are more likely to die from the complications of ulceration than non-smokers.[12] Smoking appears to have no consistent effect on acid secretion; it does, however, impair the therapeutic effects of antisecretories, it may stimulate pepsin secretion and promote reflux of duodenal contents into the stomach. Smoking increases the harmful effects of HP, and increases production of free radicals, endothelin and platelet-activating factor. Smoking also affects the mucosal protective mechanisms. It decreases gastric mucosal bloodflow and inhibits gastric mucous secretion, gastric prostaglandin generation, salivary epidermal growth factor secretion, duodenal mucosal bicarbonate secretion and pancreatic bicarbonate secretion. The adverse effects of smoking on aggressive and protective factors qualify it as an important contributor to the pathogenesis of peptic ulcer disease and indicate that smoking plays a significant facilitative role in the development and maintenance of peptic ulcer disease.[13] Medical and surgical ulcer treatments are more likely to fail with those who smoke. Current smoking increases the risk for ulcer perforation 10-fold.[14]

Associated disease

Diseases associated with peptic ulceration are chronic liver disease, hyperparathyroidism and chronic renal failure, particularly during dialysis and after successful transplantation. Other disease associations have been observed, but are probably biased by the fact that patients under close medical supervision and regular attenders are more likely to have investigations performed and the diagnosis made than infrequent attenders of medical care.

Non-steroidal anti-inflammatory drugs and aspirin

The association between NSAIDs and gastritis and gastroduodenal ulceration has been known for some time. Use of NSAIDs is associated with an increase in the prevalence of gastric and duodenal ulceration, particularly in complicated cases and especially in elderly people where the risk of bleeding is increased between 2- and 4-fold compared with non-NSAID users.[15] It should be appreciated that perhaps one-third of patients who develop ulcers while on NSAIDs have had underlying ulcer disease.[16] A useful source of information for the role of aspirin in peptic ulceration comes from controlled trials of therapy for thromboembolic disease. These consistently indicate a 2-fold increase in the risk of upper gastro-intestinal bleed for patients given aspirin-containing regimens compared with controls.[17] The mechanism of injury appears to be through the disturbance of prostaglandin synthesis caused by inhibition of the cyclo-oxgenase enzyme, specifically the COX-1 isoform. Newly developed drugs selectively block the action of COX-2 isoform, thereby avoiding the COX-1 related gastro-duodenal ulcer complications. In a combined analysis of 8 trials of patients with osteoarthritis, treatment with the newer COX-2 selective inhibitor NSAID was associated with a significantly lower incidence of peptic ulcer disease and complications than treatment with existing NSAIDs.[18]

Helicobacter pylori

This is a spiral-shaped gram-negative microaerophilic bacterium that colonises gastric epithelium and mucus. Humans are its principal host. The discovery of *H. pylori*, formerly *Camplyobacter*, has revolutionised our understanding of the pathogenesis of peptic ulceration.[19] *Helicobacter* organisms have been isolated from areas of antral gastritis seen in association with duodenal ulceration, areas of gastric metaplasia adjacent to areas of duodenal ulceration and also areas of chronic active gastritis, the precursor of gastric ulceration.[20]

Epidemiology of infection

There are several putative modes of transmission and acquisition of HP infection. Transmission from animals or foods seems unlikely.[21] Transmission through water supply seems more likely in certain situations: South American studies have shown that differences in water supply predict infection rate and that PCR products can be demonstrated in the water supplied to families of high infection rate.[22] The greatest evidence supports direct contact, person-to-person transmission of infection; areas where people live in close proximity – such as the Third World and institutionalised patients in the West – show a high prevalence of infection.[23] The clustering of infection within families with identical strains of organisms also supports this theory.[24] Accidental and experimental ingestion of the organism leads to infection.[25,26] Whether transmission is oral–oral or faecal–oral is not clear since organisms have been isolated from both the faeces and saliva of infected patients. Acquisition of infection appears to be in childhood with an annual acquisition rate in Western adults of around 3%. In recent years, there has been a decline in the incidence of HP infection. This may be because of improved hygiene, improved nutrition during childhood, smaller family size, greater interval between children and increased consumption of antimicrobials.[27] Many of the previously observed socioeconomic, geographical and temporal trends in the prevalence of peptic ulcer are more likely to be a reflection of prevalence of *H. pylori* infection. Hence the prevalence of infection is higher in developing countries (70% by the age of 20) compared with Western countries (60% by the age of 65).[28] *H. pylori* is present with a presumed causative role in 95–99% of cases of non-NSAID-induced duodenal ulceration.[29] It has, however, been estimated that only 10% of patients infected with HP will in fact go on to develop an ulcer in the future. Future epidemiological studies will need to concentrate not simply on infection rates and sero-positivity but deal separately with individual strains with their evident different outcomes.

The clinical outcome of H. pylori *infection*
The clinical outcome of infection seems to be related to interplay of organism and host factors.

Bacterial factors
Recent studies have demonstrated that *H. pylori* isolates possess substantial phenotypic and genotypic diversity that may engender differential host inflammatory responses that influence clinical outcome.[30] Genetic studies of *H. pylori* suggest that there are strains that share similarities and are each associated with a particular disease; one subgroup associated with gastritis alone, one with gastritis and ulceration, and another with complicated ulcer disease.[31] The analysis of strains of bacteria isolated from ulcer and non-ulcer patients reveals that certain factors, particularly the ability of bacteria to adhere to epithelial cells and release toxins, may facilitate infection and ulcerogenesis.[32,33] *In vitro* studies show that certain strains of *H. pylori* exert a characteristic cytopathic effect on mammalian cells in culture with the formation of intracytoplasmic vacuoles.[34] Between 50–60% of strains can be induced to release this vacuolation cytotoxin *in vitro*, although all strains possess the vacA gene that encodes it. Strains producing vacuolating cytotoxin activity are more commonly isolated from people with peptic ulcers than without. The vacA genotype influences cytotoxin activity and signal sequence type correlates closely with peptic ulceration. Another marker of virulence is the protein product of the cytotoxin associated gene A (cagA). The function of the high molecular weight (128 kDa) cagA gene product is unknown, but expression strongly correlates with severity of gastritis and development of peptic ulceration. Infection with strains possessing cagA (cytotoxin associated gene A) is more common among people with peptic ulceration than without. CagA is a marker for the cag pathogenicity island, which includes genes necessary for the enhanced inflammation induced by pathogenic strains. The cagA-linked gene picB (Permits Induction of Cytokines) is necessary for enhanced interleukin-8 release from cultured cells.[35] This may be one factor responsible for the increased mucosal inflammation seen in association with cagA-positive strains. Other virulence factors have been proposed such as HP neutrophil-activating protein (HP NAP); further evidence is needed before any can be considered of importance.[30]

Despite rapid advances in the understanding and characterisation of *H. pylori* virulence factors, there is currently little practical clinical application. Identification of strains for clinical practice remains problematic; functional tests of vacuolating cytotoxin activity require culture of gastric biopsies in cell lines. The interpretation of serological tests of VacA by ELISA technique remains uncertain because of the differing response of different genotypes within the strain. CagA serology is more easily and reliably measured by ELISA. For practical purposes, *H. pylori* in association with peptic ulcer disease must be eradicated regardless of the supposed 'virulence' of the organism.

Patient factors

The host epithelium not only provides a protective barrier, but also initiates immune inflammatory responses to infections that may be deleterious to the host. *H. pylori* binds preferentially to Lewis antigens on the surface of gastric epithelial cells.[36] Lewis antigens form part of the complex that determines blood group, particularly blood group O. This may be the explanation for the long-observed tendency for duodenal ulceration to occur in patients of this blood group. The age at which infection was acquired may have some bearing on the clinical outcome; childhood infection is associated with a pangastritis similar to that found in gastric ulceration and gastric cancer, but different from that observed in cases of duodenal ulceration.[37]

Proposed mechanism of mucosal injury

Direct injury

The precise mechanism by which *H. pylori* exerts its ulcerogenic effects is not established. The observation that ulceration occurs in the duodenum only in areas of gastric metaplasia colonised by *H. pylori* suggests that direct local damage to the epithelium plays at least some part. It is probable that release of cytokines from the organism itself, or by the patient's cellular response to infection, is relevant to this process.[38] Cytotoxic substances released from the bacterium itself include membrane lipopolysaccharide, urease (which acts as a chemotaxin for monocytes and neutrophils *in vitro*), the vacuolating cytotoxin and heat shock proteins. These have a deleterious effect on the mucus layer and mucosal protection allowing acid to permeate directly to the epithelial cells thereby causing cellular injury. This in turn excites chemotaxis of leukocytes to the scene, with release of further cytokines such as IL8 and production of damaging oxygen free radicals which exacerbate and perpetuate this mucosal insult.[39] There is also direct activation of neutrophils by *H. pylori* in part at least through a recently isolated HP neutrophil activating protein (HP NAP) has been identified and its encoding gene (nap A) sequenced.[40]

Increased gastric acid production

H. pylori causes antral gastritis and increased gastrin and pepsinogen release (Hyperpepsinogenaemia I). Acid production in the more proximal stomach inhibits the colonisation by bacteria and inhibition of gastric acid secretion by antisecretory drugs facilitates the proximal migration of organisms. This relative sparing of the body of the stomach facilitates normal and in many cases, increased gastrin-induced acid production. Gastrin release may be exaggerated as a result of the local action of cytokines from the inflammatory cells on the albeit reduced G-cell mass.[41] The function of the G-cells is further augmented by the reduced capacity of adjacent D-cells to secrete the acid inhibitory peptide, somatostatin.[42] Eradication of *H. pylori* lowers gastrin levels and hence acid secretion by approximately two-thirds.[43]

Interaction with NSAIDs

While the mechanisms of injury of NSAID-induced ulceration and *H. pylori* are separate and distinct, there is some suggestion that there is also an interaction of *H. pylori* in NSAID-induced gastropathy. Unfortunately NSAID ingestion and *H. pylori* infection are both common in the aged population and hence studies are frequently confounded. NSAID ingestion does not increase susceptibility to *H. pylori* infection; there is some evidence that NSAID ingestion is toxic to the organism. Nor is there any convincing evidence that *H. pylori* exacerbates NSAID-associated mucosal injury.[44] Nevertheless, there have been two small recent studies which demonstrate that HP eradication prior to NSAID ingestion reduces the incidence of ulceration.[45,46]

Management strategies for peptic ulceration

Endoscopic confirmation

Patients with dyspeptic symptoms should undergo endoscopic examination to confirm the presence of an ulcer and exclude other potentially serious pathology. Gastric ulcers must be carefully biopsied as there is a risk that an apparently benign gastric ulcer is in fact an early malignancy.[47] Direct endoscopic inspection, adequate tissue biopsy and expert histological interpretation are essential in order to identify dysplasia and neoplasia. Repeat endoscopy to confirm healing and rebiopsy is essential for all gastric ulcers.

Diagnosis of helicobacter infection

Multiple diagnostic tests are available for determining the presence of *H. pylori* infection. Some tests rely on endoscopy while others are non-invasive. The accuracy of a test depends on the clinical situation in which it is used. Most tests have been evaluated in untreated individuals, while few studies have investigated their performance post-treatment when bacterial counts might be low. HP infection can be determined non-invasively by carbon isotope (13C or 14C)-urea breath test, serologically by ELISA, or using endoscopic biopsy material by functional assay of urease activity and histological analysis. Which test should be regarded as the 'gold standard' is uncertain. A commercially available CLO (Campylobacter-like organisms) urease test involves a small well containing urea agar with a phenol red buffer. The test has around 90% sensitivity and > 95% specificity in untreated patients. Several drugs including proton pump inhibitors, bismuth and antibiotics temporarily suppress HP and render functional assays falsely negative. The sensitivity may be less following treatment although using more than one biopsy may improve sensitivity.[48] Histological diagnosis is most sensitive with the Warthin-Starry stain and the modified Giemsa stain, the latter being the simpler and cheaper and hence the most commonly used. Although frequently used as the reference method for other studies this method is prone to inter-observer variability. False negative diagnosis occurs in about 5–15% of cases depending on the laboratory experience. Since the inoculum in the post-treatment case may be low and there may be proximal migration of the infection, diagnosis in this circumstance can be enhanced by analysis of biopsies from both the antrum and body of the stomach.[49] Immunohistochemistry using polyclonal antisera to HP can improve sensitivity and reduce inter-observer variation.[50] Use of the polymerase chain reaction (PCR) allows detection of the presence of HP DNA in the absence of viable bacteria. Although this test may have the highest sensitivity, there are frequent false positive results and the test adds little to existing diagnostic techniques.[51] The ^{13}C (non-radioactive) and ^{14}C (radioactive) breath tests rely on the urease activity of HP. Carbon-labelled urea is fed to the patients; only those with urea-producing HP will hydrolyse the urea to ammonia and CO_2 which is exhaled and $^{13}CO_2$ or $^{14}CO_2$. Detection of $^{13}CO_2$ is by gas isotope ratio–mass spectrometer (expensive) or more recently infrared spectroscopy (NDIRS) and Laser-assisted ratio analysis (LARA); detection of $^{14}CO_2$ is by scintillation beta-counter (available in most medical physics departments). The test has over 90% sensitivity and specificity, although the sensitivity is dramatically reduced by concurrent use of PPIs. The urea breath test is particularly well suited to assessing HP status post-treatment.[52]

Although serological detection of IgA, IgM and IgG response are all feasible, IgG response measured by ELISA or latex agglutination has been proven the most useful marker of infection. Laboratory-based kits have 90% sensitivity and specificity, but the tests are not useful as measures of treatment success as titres take a variable time to return to normal; matched pre- and 6/12 post-treatment serum assays may improve accuracy but this is logistically difficult in clinical practice. The latest promising test is the faecal antigen detection kit. This is quick, technically simple, non-invasive and early reports suggest high degree of accuracy and good prediction of successful eradication.[53]

In the absence of NSAID ingestion HP infection is so likely in cases of duodenal ulceration that a negative test result should be viewed with some scepticism. Further testing by an alternative method, particularly serologically, or even empirical treatment with subsequent re-evaluation may be justified.[54]

Determination of NSAID or aspirin ingestion

Careful inquiry is needed to elucidate whether NSAIDs or aspirin are being taken regularly. Ingestion is especially common among elderly people, but patients may fail to declare such information unless specific inquiry is made.

Treatment of peptic ulcers

NSAID-induced ulceration

H. pylori should be tested for and eradicated even in patients taking NSAIDs. Half of patients on NSAIDs with peptic ulceration have HP infection contributing to ulceration.[55] NSAIDs should be stopped or their dose reduced if cessation is absolutely contraindicated. If continued NSAID use is deemed necessary, most ulcers will heal with H2 receptor antagonist therapy or, more quickly, with proton pump inhibitors. Maintenance therapy is likely to be required in some form. The newer COX-2 selective inhibitors are likely to have fewer complications.[18]

Eradication of Helicobacter pylori

There is no consensus on the optimum treatment for *H. pylori*. However, once eradication has been achieved, reinfection rates are less than 0.5% in developed countries.[56] Ulcer recurrence in the absence of *H. pylori* infection is rare according to long-term follow-up studies.[57]

Antimicrobial drugs

Successful eradication of *H. pylori* is inhibited by the inaccessibility of the habitat between the adherent mucus gel and the epithelial cell surface in which it exists and antimicrobial resistance, especially to metronidazole and clarithromycin of some strains. In order to overcome these factors prolonged therapy with complex multiple drug regimens has been suggested and proven nearly completely (98–100%) effective. However, poor compliance and cost suggests that such aggressive therapy should be reserved for resistant infection.

The choice of antibiotic regimen should take account of previous antibiotic exposure and local prevalence of antibiotic resistance. Classical triple therapy consists of colloidal bismuth, metronidazole and tetracycline or amoxicillin. Bismuth-based triple therapies are more effective than dual therapies in eradicating *H. pylori* infections. However, poor compliance and frequent adverse effects have made these combinations less favourable in clinical practice. Proton pump inhibitor-based triple therapies have shown more consistent and higher eradication rates with a short duration of treatment, good patient compliance, fewer side effects, prompt symptom relief and fast ulcer healing. Results from PPI-based quadruple therapies are promising; however, large multicentre clinical trials are needed to confirm the effect and the complex regimen may again compromise compliance outside the clinical trial setting.[58] The most recent evidence suggests that a 1 week 'triple therapy' course of a proton pump inhibitor, with clarithromycin and either metronidazole or amoxycillin will cure HP infection in 90% of cases.[59]

 Currently UK and European guidelines suggest a 1-week long, twice daily dose of a proton pump inhibitor and two of clarithromycin, metronidazole or amoxicillin. This regimen has an acceptable balance of efficacy in association with good compliance, effectiveness against metronidazole-resistant strains of *H. pylori* and acceptable cost.[60]

Failure to eradicate HP by one regimen should prompt the prescription of a second course of treatment after consideration of previous antibiotic exposure and sensitivities. A quadruple regimen (a proton pump inhibitor with 'classical' triple therapy) is justified in these circumstances. Inevitably more studies are being carried out to devise better strategies and further guidelines will be issued. As with other infectious diseases, consultation with microbiologists and development of local antibiotic policies should be considered with resistant *H. pylori* infection.

Antisecretory drugs

Conventional antiulcer therapy is also necessary in addition to *H. pylori* eradication to facilitate mucosal healing and symptom relief.

H2 receptor antagonists selectively and competitively block the Class 2 histamine receptors of parietal cells to reduce secretion of gastric acid and pepsin. *Misoprostol*, an analogue of prostaglandin E1, inhibits the secretion of acid and proteolytic enzymes at the same time as increasing bicarbonate and mucus secretion. *Pirenzepine* is a specific antagonist for muscarinic M2 receptors, which reduce gastric acid secretion by a pharmacological interruption of the vagus.

Proton pump inhibitors inhibit the Na^+/K^+ ATPase which is the final common pathway through which histamine, vagal acetylcholine and gastrin stimulate gastric acid production. This class of drugs induces virtual achlorhydria. The long-term effects and risks of this remain unknown.

The choice of therapy is largely an economic one. H2RAs and proton pump inhibitors are both effective ulcer-healing agents. Proton pump inhibitors are more effective in cases of gastric ulcer, while the differences between the two in cases of duodenal ulceration is less marked.[61]

Investigation of ulcers which fail to heal

The natural history of peptic ulceration has been transformed by pharmacological and bacteriological developments. The stage at which one defines failure of medical treatment is open to conjecture. Duodenal ulcers are generally considered refractory if healing is not evident by 8 weeks and gastric ulcers if healing is not at least progressing by 12 weeks.[54]

Persistent symptoms without refractory ulcer

Endoscopic re-evaluation of duodenal ulcers should differentiate between a refractory ulcer and persistence of symptoms despite ulcer healing. If satisfactory ulcer healing and *H. pylori* eradication are demonstrated, alternative diagnoses should be considered.

Persistent *Helicobacter* infection

The first step in the evaluation of refractory ulcers should be to confirm successful eradication of *H. pylori*. Biopsies should be repeated at the same time as the endoscopy when failure of healing is confirmed. A higher than usual rate of false-negative results should be anticipated with carbon isotope breath tests within the first 3 weeks following therapy due to suppression of bacterial function, but not necessarily eradication. Serum antibody titres can be expected to fall after successful eradication but this is slow (up to 6 months) and variable. Possible causes of failure of HP eradication are antibiotic resistance (most commonly to metronidazole or clarythomicin) or if the patient has not complied with the prescribed regimen. The former may be overcome by appropriate modification of the eradication regimen with directed treatment based on bacteriological culture.

Failure of ulcer healing if *H. pylori* negative

Ingestion of NSAIDs should be re-evaluated. Surreptitious aspirin ingestion has been observed and if suspected may be established by assay of plasma salicylate levels. Any other factor that may be facilitating ulceration, such as smoking or intercurrent disease, should be sought and eliminated where possible. Smoking in particular is associated with failure of medical treatment of peptic ulcer disease.

The truly resistant ulcer

Resistant ulcers are of two types:

1. *Refractory resistant ulcer* fails to heal despite the exclusion of *Helicobacter pylori* infection and ingestion of ulcerogenic drugs.
2. *Relapsing resistant ulcer* heals initially but recurs in the absence of *Helicobacter pylori* or ingestion of ulcerogenic drugs.

Refractory or relapsing ulceration should prompt multiple biopsies of the ulcer margin and base to identify the several neoplastic, infectious and inflammatory conditions that can mimic peptic ulcer (see **Fig. 12.1**). Gastric ulceration should be viewed with caution and biopsied from the outset. A diagnosis of Zollinger–Ellison should be suspected in cases of *Helicobacter*-negative, non-NSAID-induced refractory ulceration and especially where there is ulceration of the second part

Figure 12.1
Proposed management protocol for resistent ulcers

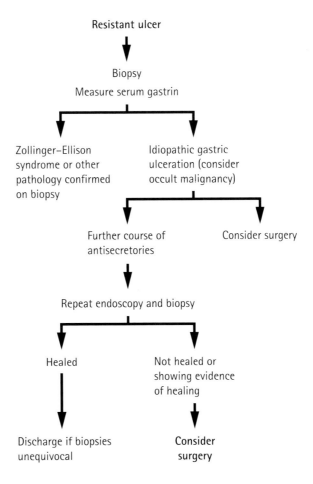

of the duodenum or large confluent ulcers in the duodenum. Hypergastrinaemia should be excluded prior to a decision to treat a refractory ulcer.

Treatment of idiopathic refractory ulceration

Where no cause for persistent ulceration can be found it may be necessary for the patient to take long-term antisecretory drugs. Alternatively, elective surgery may be considered in this highly selected group of patients. Inherent in this decision is a careful calculation of the relative risks and benefits of surgery (see below) against the potential risks and costs of continued medical treatment. The risks of complication of persistent ulcer disease, the degree of disability experienced by patients and their fitness for surgery should all be considered in the decision of whether or not to operate. In the case of refractory gastric ulcers there is the concern of unidentified malignancy.

Zollinger–Ellison syndrome

In 1955 Zollinger and Ellison described a condition of a non-insulin-secreting tumour of the pancreas associated with gastric hypersecretion and fulminant peptic ulceration.[62]

Clinical features

The syndrome typically presents with epigastric pain, although 40% of patients complain of diarrhoea and weight loss and a third present with oesophagitis only.[63] The disease may present with perforation, haemorrhage, oesophageal stricture, jejunal ulceration or anastomotic breakdown. The condition should also be suspected when a duodenal ulcer coexists with primary hyperparathyroidism or metastatic carcinoma of unknown origin.

Historically this syndrome was only recognised after a protracted course of ulcer disease leading to a delay in diagnosis of between 3 and 9 years.[64] The diagnosis should now be considered in the small group of patients who fail to respond to medical treatment.

Pathology

Although originally described as a pancreatic endocrine tumour, the definition has also come to include extrapancreatic gastrin-secreting tumours. Where the condition is due to a pancreatic tumour, in two-thirds of cases the tumour will be multifocal within the pancreas.[65] At least two-thirds will be histologically malignant.[66] One third will already have demonstrable metastases by the time of diagnosis.[67] The most common extrapancreatic site is in the wall of the duodenum. Less frequently (6–11% of cases) ectopic gastrinoma tissue has been identified in the liver, common bile duct, jejunum, omentum, pylorus, ovary and heart.[68,69] These extrapancreatic tumours rarely metastasise to the liver and, even though they do metastasise just as frequently to regional lymph nodes, they tend to have a better prognosis than primary pancreatic tumours.[70]

Multiple endocrine neoplasia

One-quarter of patients with ZE have other endocrine tumours as part of a familial Multiple Endocrine Neoplasia (MEN I) syndrome and particularly hyperparathyroidism.[67] This group of patients has a much worse prognosis than sporadic ZE syndrome, in part due to the multifocal nature of the tumour within the pancreas. Cure is rarely possible and treatment is conservative with attempted surgical resection being contraindicated.

Sporadic gastrinomas

The majority of cases of ZE syndrome arise sporadically. Such tumours are more likely to occur in extrapancreatic sites than familial types. Prognosis is better in this group of patients.

Diagnosis

The diagnosis of ZE syndrome can be established by radioimmunoassay of serum gastrin levels and measurement of gastric acid hypersecretion. Diagnosis may be confirmed by the finding of fasting hypergastrinaemia. False-positive results may occur in cases of achlorhydria or hypochlorhydria, such as ingestion of anti-secretory drugs, post-vagotomy, pernicious anaemia and atrophic gastritis. Hypergastrinaemia may also be detected in conditions that increase antral G-cell gastrin production, such as gastric outlet obstruction and antral G-cell hyperplasia. It also occurs in conditions that impair the elimination of gastrin from the body, such as renal failure. If there is diagnostic uncertainty or the basal serum gastrin level is marginally elevated, dynamic assay of serum gastrin following secretin (or alternatively calcium or glucagon) provocation may be required. Gastrin response to a standard meal helps to differentiate between hypergastri-naemia due to antral G-cell hyperplasia, which will result in an increase in serum gastrin levels, while no response would be expected in cases of gastrinoma.

Treatment

There are two main aims of treatment in patients with ZE syndrome. The first is control of gastric acid hypersecretion and the second is treatment of the tumour itself.

Treatment of gastric hypersecretion

Before the introduction of histamine H2 receptor antagonists in the mid-1970s a total gastrectomy was often necessary to control the gastric hypersecretion and prevent recurrent and life-threatening complications. Lesser acid-reducing operations were associated with a very high recurrence rate. Complete resolution of symptoms only follows adequate acid suppression, although very large doses of H2RAs were often needed. Since parietal cell vagotomy has been shown to reduce the need for H2RAs by 75%, this procedure has been advocated at the time of exploratory laparotomy.[71] The introduction of the more potent proton pump inhibitors has led to a more acceptable twice-daily dosing. The consensus of opinion has moved to a general acceptance of proton pump inhibition as the preferred therapy with parietal cell vagotomy becoming infrequently used.[72]

However, long-term follow-up reveals that even in patients cured surgically, 40–70% require continued acid suppression leading many to advocate parietal cell vagotomy at the time of exploratory laparotomy. This is especially appropriate for women of childbearing age for whom the teratogenic risk of proton pump inhibitors remains unknown. Patients in whom exploratory laparotomy is not indicated due to obvious dissemination should not be considered for surgery and are treated with a dose of PPI 'titrated' against endoscopic and symptomatic response. Patients in whom metastases are only discovered at the time of laparotomy should also be treated with PPIs.

Treatment of tumour

Preoperative localisation

A tumour of the pancreas should be sought and localised by computerised tomography. Percutaneous ultrasound is of little benefit, but endoscopic and intraoperative ultrasound have proved useful. EUS is highly accurate in the localisation of pancreatic tumours and gastrinomas as small as 4 mm in the duodenal wall. Use of EUS early in the preoperative localisation strategy leads to a reduction in the number of other investigations that need to be performed.[73] More elaborate diagnostic tools including selective angiography and splenic venous catheter sampling of blood gastrin levels may improve the detection of both solitary gastrinomas and metastases. These techniques are more sensitive than CT or even intraoperative ultrasound by 16 and 28% respectively.[74]

 Somatostatin receptor scintigraphy with [111In-DTPA-DPhe1] octreotide (SRS) is emerging as the most sensitive of all techniques for detecting gastrinomas; detecting 30% of gastrinomas greater or equal to 1.1 cm, 64% of those 1.1–2 cm, and 96% of those > 2 cm.[75]

The test involves whole-body imaging which is advantageous for the detection of extrapancreatic sites. Liver metastases can frequently be detected by conventional imaging but SRS has proved a more sensitive investigation that may prevent unnecessary surgical exploration. SRS is superior to any other single modality including ultrasonography, computerised tomography, magnetic resonance image, angiography and bone scan.[76] SRS has been shown to alter management in about half of cases assessed by these more traditional modalities primarily by improved tumour localisation and clarification of equivocal localisation results.[77]

Surgical excision of primary gastrinoma

How aggressively surgery should be pursued in cases of gastrinoma is controversial. A prospective audit of outcome of cases treated surgically between 1981 and 1998 has been reported. Surgical exploration and resection resulted in excellent long-term results with 10-year survival of 94%.[68] Some argue that exploration should only be undertaken if a definite lesion has been identified preoperatively. If resectable solitary or multiple gastrinomas can be identified, surgical management should be considered in view of the high risk of malignancy. Patients with MEN1 and those with diffuse liver metastases should not be treated surgically. Surgical resection of localised liver gastrinoma provides a cure rate similar to that of extrahepatic gastrinoma and an excellent long-term survival.[78]

Surgical strategy

Exploration of the pancreas despite failure of preoperative investigations to localise a tumour is controversial. A surgical procedure will detect a third more gastrinomas than even SRS.[75] If surgical exploration is performed then the pancreas must be mobilised along its entire length, inspected, palpated and if the facilities are available rescanned intraoperatively by endoluminal or laparoscopic ultrasound. If a tumour cannot be localised by these means, the next step in the search should be directed toward the duodenum. Palpation of the duodenal wall will only identify 61% of duodenal gastrinomas. Duodenal transillumination by endoscopy will improve detection to 84%, and duodenotomy usually identifies the remaining cases.[79] If no gastrinoma is found in the usual locations, other ectopic sites should be examined carefully (*vide supra*).[68,69] Resection of these primary ectopic tumours can lead to durable biochemical cures.[69] Gastrinomas may be identified in 96% of surgical explorations if these approaches are adopted.[68] If no tumour is identified then at most an acid-reducing operation should be performed, but there is no place for blind pancreatic resection. Further non-operative localisation tests should be repeated 6–12 months later, but further surgery only contemplated if a tumour is definitely detected.

Elective surgery for peptic ulceration

In developed Western countries very few patients will now even be considered for an elective ulcer procedure. There will still be rare patients with ulcers resistant to treatment in whom all the common aetiological factors have been excluded. Throughout the second half of the twentieth century elective surgical treatment was reserved for those with non-healing or rapidly recurring symptomatic ulcers and for those who did not comply with their treatment. On the basis of the concept that peptic ulcer disease is a spectrum of a disease rather than a single entity, those undergoing surgery were generally at the worse end of this spectrum. With the development of increasingly strong antisecretory drugs the indications have narrowed even further and by the late 1980s very few elective ulcer operations were required and only those at the very far end of the severity spectrum. The discovery of the importance of eradication of *Helicobacter pylori* in the healing and maintenance of ulcer healing has narrowed the indications even further. Even the so-called 'giant peptic ulcer' which has hitherto been considered an indication for surgical rather than medical treatment can be safely managed with current medical therapy. Intractability and complications should be considered the only indications for peptic ulceration in the modern era.[80]

Duodenal ulcer surgery

Definitive surgery for duodenal ulcer evolved around the concept of acid reduction, either by resection of most of the parietal cell mass, vagal denervation of the parietal cells or resection of the antral gastrin-producing cells. The balance lay in minimising the chance of ulcer recurrence while at the same time trying to avoid the symptomatic side effects and metabolic sequelae of the procedure that would affect the patient for the rest of their life.

The trend by the mid-1970s was towards highly selective or proximal gastric vagotomy (HSV or PGV) which denervated the parietal cell mass, but left the antrum and pylorus innervated and so allowed a gastric emptying pattern that while not completely normal, did not require a drainage procedure.[81] This was the first ulcer procedure that did not involve bypass, destruction or removal of the pylorus and as a result has significantly fewer side effects than other ulcer operations.

HSV in most series has a mortality of well under 1%.[82] The incidence of side effects such as early dumping, diarrhoea and bile reflux is also very low.[83] The main concern with this operation, whether for duodenal or gastric ulcer, has been the recurrence rate. In the best hands recurrence rates of 5–10% have been achieved.[84,85] Many others were not able to produce this level of excellence and even at the time of the introduction of H2RAs the truncal versus highly selective vagotomy debate continued. Once cimetidine was available, recurrent ulceration became a less significant problem as patients who had undergone an unsuccessful vagotomy could be treated with H2 receptor antagonists and actually appeared to be more sensitive than patients who had not had their parietal cells denervated.[86] Improvement in the intraoperative testing of completeness of vagotomy and particularly the use of the endoscopic congo red test have also improved the performance of HSV and lessened the risk of ulcer recurrence.[87,88]

Anterior seromyotomy with posterior truncal vagotomy probably denervates the proximal stomach more consistently.[89] This later operation has never been compared with HSV in a large trial and so its place in ulcer surgery remains uncertain. It has proved that the posterior vagal trunk can be divided and the patient not experience significant diarrhoea, provided the pylorus is intact and innervated. There is really now no place for truncal vagotomy with destruction, bypass or excision of the pylorus because of the lifelong risk of diarrhoea, which in a significant proportion of patients is socially disabling.[90]

Some surgeons, particularly in the USA, have advocated the use of truncal vagotomy and antrectomy, suggesting that this operation is the most effective for reducing acid secretion and has a very low recurrence rate of about 1%. The procedure was subsequently modified to a selective vagotomy and antrectomy, leaving the hepatic and coeliac fibres of the vagi intact. This did reduce the incidence of side effects, especially diarrhoea, though dumping was still a problem. Bile gastritis and oesophagitis were also troublesome side effects unless a Roux-en-Y reconstruction was used, though recurrent stomal ulceration was then more frequent unless a more extensive gastric resection was performed (*vide infra*). The perfect ulcer operation has remained elusive and indeed there is none that has no side effects or risks.

By the early 1980s it was becoming apparent that the introduction of H2 antagonists had significantly narrowed the indications for elective ulcer surgery and that recurrent ulceration rates after HSV were rising. There were several studies that attempted to address this concern by comparing HSV with selective vagotomy and antrectomy. Overall the balance of opinion considered that the higher rate of ulcer recurrence but better side effect profile of HSV were preferable as it was easier to treat recurrent ulcers than other more debilitating side effects which the patient would suffer for the rest of his or her life.[84,91,92]

The last paper of importance about HSV was a report from Johnston's group in Leeds in 1988. This confirmed that as the group of ulcer patients undergoing elective surgery became more selected the recurrence rate after HSV was increasing.[93] Looking at the group of duodenal ulcer patients who were refractory to healing with a 3-month course of full dose H2RAs (1 g cimetidine or 300 mg ranitidine a day) they found an 18% recurrent ulcer rate at 2 years rising to 34% at 5 years. In comparison the respective figures for those who had healed on H2RAs, but did not wish to take long-term maintenance therapy, were 1.5% and 3%. In the past the single most important factor in determining ulcer recurrence after HSV was the surgeon who had performed the operation.[86] However in the H2RAs-resistant group even the best surgeon had a 3-year recurrence rate of over 20%. There are presently no figures available for those patients who are *Helicobacter* negative and are refractory to healing with proton pump inhibitors, but the recurrence rate would be predicted to be very much higher. It has to be concluded that HSV almost certainly does not have a place in the treatment of refractory duodenal ulcers in the twenty-first century. Since the operation is so operator-dependent few trainee surgeons will have the opportunity to learn the correct technique, and indeed those who have already done so will have scant opportunity to maintain their experience. Surgery for benign ulcers will have to be centralised to a few specialised units.

Recommended operations for refractory duodenal ulcers

The plain fact is that at the time of writing no one knows what operation should be recommended for refractory duodenal ulcer. After eradication of *Helicobacter* and exclusion of other causes of persistent ulceration we are left with a very small number of patients with aggressive ulcer disease who are often female and smokers. If they are under 60 and otherwise healthy then surgery should be considered. In view of the predicted poor results of HSV in this group of patients it is likely that resection of the antral gastrin-producing mucosa and either resection or vagal denervation of the parietal cell mass is necessary.

Selective vagotomy and antrectomy Selective denervation is preferred because of a lower incidence of side effects. It is not an easy procedure; the dissection around the lower oesophagus and cardia has in particular to be done very carefully. The vagotomy should be performed before the resection and tested intraoperatively. The reconstruction should either be a gastroduodenal (Billroth I) anastomosis or a Roux-en-Y gastro-jejunostomy. The latter is associated with less bile reflux into the gastric remnant and oesophagus, but carries a higher risk of stomal ulceration and so at least a two-thirds gastrectomy is advised.

Subtotal gastrectomy Removal of a large part of the parietal cell mass is sound in theory and indeed ulcer recurrence after this operation is unusual. However, there is a high incidence of post-prandial symptoms and in particular epigastric discomfort and fullness that significantly limits calorie intake. Importantly there is a high incidence of long-term nutritional and metabolic sequelae that require lifelong surveillance and can be difficult to prevent, particularly in women.

Pylorus-preserving gastrectomy There is interesting work from China on a form of highly selective vagotomy with resection of about 50% of the parietal cell mass and the antral mucosa, but preserving the pyloric mechanism and the vagus nerves to the distal antrum and pylorus.[94] This operation is physiologically sound and may prove to be nearer to the ideal operation for refractory ulcers in the

West. Limited, non-randomised data suggest that this may be a superior technique with fewer sequelae compared with the traditional approach.[95]

Surgery for gastric ulcer

Surgical treatment for benign gastric ulcer is now very rarely required as failure to heal after exclusion of aetiological factors and up to 6 months treatment with a PPI is extremely uncommon. Type 2 and 3 ulcers should be treated in the same way as duodenal ulcers – it is important to realise that HSV is not recommended for prepyloric ulcers. The choice of operation for a Type 1 ulcer is between excision of the ulcer with HSV or Billroth 1 partial gastrectomy. The recurrence rate is higher after HSV/excision, but the operative mortality is lower and side effects fewer after this procedure. There are no reliable data on which to base a recommendation for surgical treatment of refractory gastric ulcers at the present time.

Laparoscopic peptic ulcer surgery

Interest in minimally invasive procedures has led to many publications proving the feasibility of laparoscopic definitive ulcer operations. The simple fact is that the issue is not whether the operation can be done, but whether it needs to be done. The indications for laparoscopic surgery are exactly the same as for open procedures.

Surgery for the complications of peptic ulcers

Although the number of patients requiring elective surgery has declined, the number who require surgery for the complications of peptic ulcer disease has remained constant.[96,97]

Perforation

With the changing emphasis towards medical treatment of peptic ulcers, surgery is now mainly performed in the emergency situation. Those requiring emergency surgery are a selected group of high-risk patients with higher mortality. A number of factors associated with poor outcome in perforated peptic ulcer have been identified; delay in diagnosis, coexistent medical illness, shock on admission, leukocytosis and age over 75.[98] A delay in treatment of greater than 24 hours is associated with a 7-fold increase in mortality, 3-fold risk of morbidity and a 2-fold increase in hospital stay;[99] the elderly are particularly vulnerable and often more difficult to diagnose because of poorly localised symptoms and signs and fewer preceding symptoms.[100] There is a range of treatment options for peptic ulcer perforation. At one extreme is conservative non-surgical treatment and at the other early operation involving definitive antiulcer procedures at the same time.

Conservative management

Study of the natural history of perforated peptic ulcers suggests that they frequently sealed spontaneously by omentum or adjacent organs. Since 1951 the argument for conservative management has been advocated, but never gained widespread acceptance. Taylor showed that the mortality in his series of patients with peptic ulcer disease was half that of the contemporary reported mortality for perforation treated surgically.[101] In a recent small series, mortality by the conservative approach was 3% with conversion to operation in 6/34 because of progressive deterioration; 5 for unsealed gastric or duodenal ulceration and one for gangrenous cholecystitis.[102] A small, randomised controlled trial comparing conservative treatment with surgical treatment showed no difference in morbidity or mortality.[103] Eleven of 40 patients treated conservatively, ultimately required surgical treatment; these cases were more often over 70 years of age. Hence some authors advocate an initial, closely monitored trial of conservative therapy of parenteral broad-spectrum antibiotics, intravenous acid antisecretories, intravenous fluid resuscitation and nasogastric aspiration in patients under the age of 70. Another adjunct suggested by some is a gastrograffin swallow; if the perforation is sealed, the patient can be treated non-surgically.[104] Such a policy requires careful interval assessment by an experienced surgeon with a low threshold for performing laparotomy if clinical improvement is not apparent both to confirm the diagnosis and oversew an unsealed perforation.

Open surgery

In most centres the treatment of choice for patients with perforation of the duodenum is still laparotomy, peritoneal lavage and simple closure of perforation usually by omental patch repair. The routine use of drains is unnecessary and may in fact increase morbidity.[105] Additional biopsy of perforated gastric ulcers is mandatory. This simple treatment is safe and effective in the long term, when combined with pharmacological acid suppression.[106] Since 90% of perforations are associated with *H. pylori* infection,[107] it is not surprising that *H. pylori* eradication further significantly reduces the ulcer recurrence.[108]

Traditionally there has been a school of thought that at the time of emergency laparotomy, definitive ulcer surgery should be performed. In particular, HSV has been strongly advocated to reduce the risk of recurrent ulceration and its complications. The advances in understanding of the treatment of ulcers together with the decrease in experience of elective antiulcer surgery have made this argument no longer tenable. The indications for emergency definitive surgery are exactly the same as the criteria for elective surgery and should now be extremely rare in the patient presenting with an acute perforation.

Laparoscopic surgery

Over recent years there has been a movement towards minimally invasive surgery in the acute situation. Laparoscopic treatment of peptic ulcer perforation was first reported in 1990.[109] Subsequent modifications have been described. In the combined laparoscopic/endoscopic approach the omental plug is drawn into the lumen endoscopically in the hope of reducing postoperative leakage.[110] In the laparoscopy-assisted approach simple closure of perforated peptic ulcers is performed though a small right upper-quadrant incision using conventional instruments and techniques and abdominal wall lifting laparoscopy.[111] Tissue-adhesive glue and repair of perforation by falciform ligament patch repair have had some success.[112,113] The limited series reported suggest that laparosopically performed omental patching is feasible, safe and has comparable results to open surgery with the established advantages of laparoscopic surgery, such as less postoperative discomfort, less wound infection and less risk of incisional herniation (**Table 12.1**).[114] There may be a tendency in such series for fitter patients to undergo laparoscopic repair by experienced enthusiasts, during office hours, thus spuriously improving the outcome for this approach in comparison to the open approach. There does not appear to be a clinically significant improvement in speed of restoration of gastrointestinal function or discharge from hospital. By contrast the operations take significantly longer and there is a significant need for reoperation for persistent leakage. Inexperience with the technique can lead to significant intraoperative complications such as gall bladder perforation.[115] The physiological affects of laparoscopy such as changes in pulmonary and cardiovascular function and reduction in renal and hepatic blood flow may contribute to morbidity in the sick patient. It may be that only selective patients should be considered: shocked patients and patients operated on after 24 hours tend to fair worse with laparoscopy.[116]

Before this technique becomes more widely adopted larger, randomised studies are required and such surgery should probably only be conducted within such trials.

Though technically feasible, laparoscopic definitive surgery has no place in the emergency treatment of peptic ulcer disease for exactly the same reasons described above.

Bleeding

Management of acute haemorrhage from peptic ulceration of the stomach and duodenum has been revolutionised by rapidly developing endoscopic technology and expertise. The traditional teaching of immediate surgery for all actively bleeding ulceration needs to be tempered by the availability of such endoscopic developments. Successful management is by meticulous resuscitation, accurate diagnosis and the timely application of appropriate therapy (see also vol. 1).

Medical therapy

In laboratory and animal studies, both platelet aggregation and gastric mucosal bleeding time were shown to be extremely sensitive to different pH levels. High intragastric pH facilitates platelet aggregation, deceases bleeding time and prevents lysis of clots.[123] The largest randomised trial to date demonstrated no benefit of cimetidine in stopping active bleeding or preventing rebleeding.[124] A review of smaller trials, on subgroup analysis demonstrated a slightly better outcome for patients taking H2RAs with gastric ulcers.[125] Varying outcome measures, lack of specificity of source of bleed and differences in study design prevent any firm conclusions being drawn. A large (n = 1147) double blind placebo-controlled trial has demonstrated no benefit in acute bleeding even for the more potent acid suppression of proton pump inhibitors.[126] Nevertheless, this study was unselective and looked at all types of non-variceal bleeding and all degrees of severity; patients without stigmata of recent haemorrhage have a low risk of rebleed anyway and inclusion of these in the study was likely to dilute the beneficial effects of proton pump inhibitors. A smaller randomised double-blind (n = 220) study from India found that omeprazole 40 mg/day significantly reduced the risk of rebleeding in patients with stigmata of recent haemorrhage such as an adherent clot who did not

Study		No cases	Design	Average operation time (min)	Time to oral diet (days)	Hospital stay (days)	Surgical complications/ reoperation	Mortality
Robertson et al. 2000 (116)	Open	16	Retrospective	72	5	7	–	6%
	Laparoscopic	20		77	4	5	GB perforation × 2 Reoperation × 1	10%
Khoursheed et al. 2000 (118)	–	–	Consecutive series	–	–	–	–	–
	Laparoscopic	21		71.6	3	5.2	Reoperation × 1	0
Naesgaard et al. 1999 (119)	Open	49	Retrospective	100	–	8	Reoperation × 1	12%
	Laparoscopic	25		50	–	8	Reoperation × 2	20%
Bergamaschi et al. 1999 (123)	Open	62	Retrospective	65	5	9	Reoperation × 1	19%
	Laparoscopic	17		92	4	7	–	12%
KatKhouda et al. 1999 (117)	Open	16	Prospective (non-randomised)	63	3	8	Reoperation × 1	6%
	Laparoscopic	30		106	5	3	Reoperation × 1	3%
Druart et al. 1997 (120)	–	–	Prospective multicentre trial	–	–	–	–	–
	Laparoscopic	100		80	4	9	Reoperation × 3	5%
Miserez et al. 1996 (115)	Open	18	Retrospective	75	–	11	–	13%
	Laparoscopic	16		90	–	10	Reoperation × 2	5.5%
Johansson et al. 1996 (121)	Open	17	Prospective (non-randomised)	30	–	7	Reoperation × 1	12%
	Laparoscopic	10		60	–	6	Reoperation × 1	10%
So et al. 1996 (122)	Open	38	Retrospective	65	–	9	Incisional hernia	10%
	Laparoscopic	15		80	–	5	–	0%

Table 12.1 Studies of laparoscopic repair of perforated peptic ulcer

undergo endoscopic therapy.[127] A randomised prospective study (n = 100) from Taiwan has demonstrated that omeprazole therapy is better than cimetidine in reducing the risk of rebleed where a visible vessel has been injected.[128]

The most recent evidence comes from a randomised controlled study (n = 240) from Hong Kong. This study has demonstrated a significant reduction in rebleeding following endoscopic treatment with a protocol of intravenous omeprazole (omeprazole 80 mg i.v. bolus followed by 8 mg/hr infusion for 72 hours).[129]

Tranexamic acid can inhibit the dissolution of fibrin clot through inhibition of plasminogen and the fibrinolytic effect of pepsin. Meta-analysis of randomised, double blinded trials reveal no significant difference in the incidence of rebleeding, but an increase in complications related to therapy such as stroke, MI, DVT and PE.[130]

Somatostatin decreases gastric acid and pepsin secretion. However there is no proven benefit for somatostatin or its analogue (octreotide) in the management of active non-variceal upper gastrointestinal bleeding.[131] Prostaglandin E2 and its analogue (misoprostol) inhibit gastric acid production, stimulate mucosal perfusion and promote bicarbonate and mucus secretion. Small studies to date have demonstrated no benefit in stopping acute bleeding or preventing rebleeding.

Endoscopic therapy

The various techniques of endoscopic haemostasis have dramatically reduced the need for emergency surgery for bleeding due to peptic ulceration.

Meta-analysis suggests that endoscopic therapy reduces the mortality of acute upper gastrointestinal bleed in patients with active bleeding or non-bleeding visible vessel by avoiding the often-considerable morbidity or mortality of emergency surgery.[132]

Currently available techniques are laser photocoagulation, bipolar diathermy, heater probe, injection sclerotherapy and adrenaline injection. Which technique is to be employed depends on local availability and expertise; there is little evidence on which to rate one technique above another. Over 90% of bleeding ulcers can be initially controlled by endoscopic techniques.[133]

Operative therapy

Indications for surgery

Operative intervention is mandatory if initial control of bleeding is not possible endoscopically. Surgery is also indicated if rebleeding occurs following successful endoscopic treatment. Rebleeding may be observed directly by endoscopy or indirectly by continuing visible blood loss or need for transfusion. If there is doubt as to whether rebleeding has occurred, check endoscopy should be performed before subjecting a patient to surgery. Some recommend a second attempt at endoscopic treatment for rebleeding before considering surgery. A recent prospective randomised study from the Prince of Wales Hospital (Chinese University of Hong Kong) looking at 92 patients who rebled found that retreatment with adrenaline injection and heater probe led to a 73% control.[134] Overall, morbidity and mortality were greater in the group randomised to surgery; the complications of those re-endoscoped related to those of salvage surgery. Of those patients who failed to respond to second injection therapy, hypotension at randomisation and ulcer size

Characteristic	Risk of rebleeding
Clean base	<5%
Flat red or black spot	10%
Adherent clot	22%
Visible vessel	43%
Active, non-pulsatile bleeding ('oozing')	30–50%
Active arterial bleeding	55%

Table 12.2 *Stigmata of recent haemorrhage and risk of rebleed*

greater than 2 cm were significant risk factors. Although this is a thorough, well-conducted randomised trial, it should be remembered that the Chinese University of Hong Kong is an internationally renowned centre for endoscopic treatment whose results are invariably superior to others reported. Whether such a policy of retreatment can work outside this centre requires further evaluation. Even at this centre the mortality of 'salvage' surgery is high. Since the need for salvage surgery is likely to be greater in less specialised centres, a policy of early operation in the presence of rebleed is likely to be the safer option until further studies are complete.

Surgical intervention should be anticipated where there is a significant risk of rebleeding. Several criteria can be used to assess the risk of rebleeding including stigmata of recent haemorrhage (**Table 12.2**). In addition, the proximity of the ulcer to major vessels such as the gastro-duodenal ulcer on the posterior inferior wall of the duodenal bulb and the left gastric artery high on the lesser curve of the stomach suggests a high risk of massive bleeding. Other risk factors of poor outcome, which should prompt the need for surgical intervention, include age over 60 and shock or anaemia on admission.

Surgical technique

There is little evidence upon which to base the decision of surgical technique. Many studies of treatment of bleeding peptic ulceration have considered the need for surgery as an unfavourable outcome measure rather than a treatment option and few randomised trials of surgical therapy have been reported.

Bleeding duodenal ulcer

The first step is to make a longitudinal duodenotomy immediately distal to the pyloric ring. Haemostasis can be initially achieved by digital pressure. While it may be necessary to extend the duodenotomy through the pyloric ring, unless vagotomy is planned, the pylorus should be preserved if at all possible. Older texts frequently assume that vagotomy is an integral part of ulcer surgery and recommend larger pyloro-duodenotomy. The stomach and duodenum should be cleared of blood and clots using suction to obtain optimal view of the bleeding site. If access is still difficult, kocherisation of the duodenum may help along with drawing up of the posterior duodenal mucosa using tissue forceps.

The actively bleeding or exposed vessel should be secured. Points of note in securing the vessel are the limited access, the proximity to underlying structures such as the common bile duct and the tough fibrous nature of the base of a chronic ulcer. In view of these problems, a small, heavy, round-bodied or taper-cut semicircular needle with 0 or No. 1 suture material should be used. The argument of absorbable versus non-absorbable suture is irrelevant as the sutures inevitably slough off as the ulcer heals. If feasible the ulcer base should be excluded from the lumen by apposing the mucosa over the ulcer with a transverse row of interrupted sutures of an absorbable material.

The duodenotomy may be closed transversely if it is not too long and the duodenum has been fully kocherised. If vagotomy has been performed the pyloric ring should be divided and the duodenotomy closed transversely to create a Heinke–Mickulicz pyloroplasty (**Fig. 12.2**). If transverse closure is difficult because of the length of the duodenotomy, longitudinal closure may be performed and a gastro-jejunostomy fashioned. Alternatively, a Finney pyloroplasty (or gastro-duodenostomy) may be fashioned (**Fig. 12.2b**).

In a giant ulcer the first part of the duodenum may be virtually destroyed and, once opened, impossible to close. In this situation it is necessary to proceed to partial gastrectomy. The right gastric and right gastroepiploic arteries are divided. The stomach is disconnected from the duodenum by a combination of blunt and sharp dissection. Antrectomy is performed and continuity restored by gastro-jejunostomy with Roux-en-Y. The duodenal stump can then be closed. Although this can be achieved by pinching the second part of the duodenum away from the ulcer to allow conventional closure, this is probably more safely achieved by the technique of Nissen (**Fig. 12.3**). If closure is difficult then the duodenal stump may be drained by a tube or Foley catheter either through the duodenal suture-line or more securely though the healthy side wall of the second part of the duodenum (**Fig. 12.4**).

With the advent of proton pump inhibitors, vagotomy is not an essential part of surgery for bleeding duodenal ulceration and particularly if the patient is *helicobacter*-positive or has been ingesting aspirin or NSAIDs. The present advice is that definitive ulcer surgery is not indicated in the acute situation and that the ulcer disease should be treated postoperatively in the same way as uncomplicated ulcer disease. Long-term acid suppression may be required postoperatively if no precipitating factors for ulceration can be identified.

Bleeding gastric ulcer

The precise site of bleeding should already have been identified endoscopically. If not then intra-operative endoscopy and careful palpation of the stomach for induration should identify the site of bleeding ulcer. If there is still doubt a generous incision should be made across the pylorus and duodenum followed by a more proximal gastrotomy if the source of bleeding is still not clear. Most chronic gastric ulcers are in the antrum or at the incisura. The traditional treatment for such ulcers that fail endoscopic therapy is partial gastrectomy. Some groups have advocated simple underrunning of bleeding gastric ulcers.[135] While this may be appropriate in selected cases with small bleeding gastric ulcers such as the Dieulafoy lesion, the only randomised trial to date (n = 129) suggests that this 'conservative' approach has a higher mortality and is more likely to result in rebleeding if used unselectively.[136] If the ulcer is not removed then mucosal apposition over the ulcer base is advisable to lessen the risk of rebleeding. Where

Figure 12.2
*(a) Heinecke–
Mickulicz
pyloroplasty;
(b) Finney
pyloroplasty.*

A   Heinecke–Microlicz
pyloroplasty

Ulcer under-run

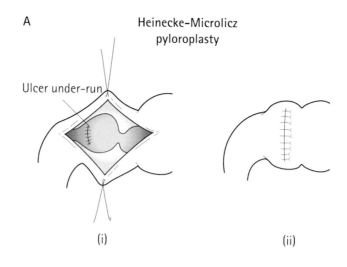

(i)   (ii)

B   Finney pyloroplasty

Ulcer under-run

Long
gastroduodenotomy

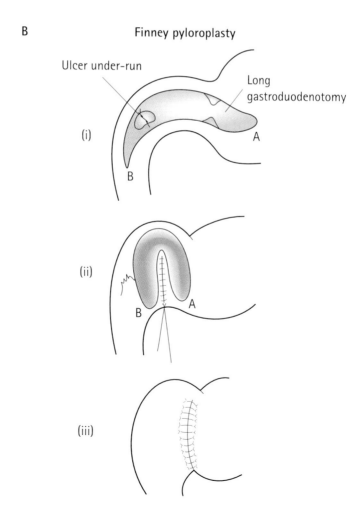

(i)

A

B

(ii)

B   A

(iii)

Figure 12.3
Nissen technique.

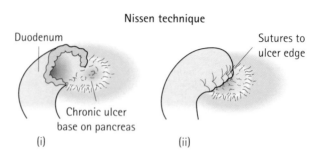

Nissen technique

Duodenum

Sutures to
ulcer edge

Chronic ulcer
base on pancreas

(i)   (ii)

Figure 12.4
*Duodenal drainage
following partial
gastrectomy for
duodenal ulcer.*

Tube drainage

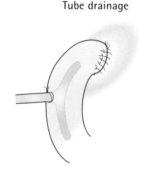

technically feasible the safest approach is to excise the ulcer and close the defect transversely.

For proximal gastric ulcers, typically those high on the lesser curve eroding through into the left gastric artery, the choice of operation lies between total gastrectomy or local excision of the lesser curve (Pauchet's manoeuvre). Limited surgery is recommended, as the mortality is much lower than a major gastric resection. This can be combined with ligation of the feeding left gastric artery to reduce the risk of rebleeding.

Pyloric stenosis

Gastric outlet obstruction can result from peptic ulcer disease of the duodenum or prepyloric region. It is a condition usually associated with chronic relapsing ulceration and is now fairly uncommon in the Western world.

Resuscitation and medical therapy

Initial management should consist of active parenteral fluid and biochemical restoration with nutritional and vitamin supplementation as necessary. Nasogastric incubation with a wide-bore tube allows gastric wash out of undigested food and so reduces antral stimulation. High-dose parenteral antisecretory therapy is given and *Helicobacter* eradication achieved, if appropriate. In cases where the obstruction has been caused by oedema and spasm, the situation may be expected to resolve once medical treatment has healed the ulcer.[138] In cases where the obstruction results from fibrosis and cicatrisation of a pyloric ulcer, some form of intervention will be necessary.

Endoscopic treatment

The group of patients who develop gastric outflow obstruction are generally elderly people, often with intercurrent disease, who tolerate major surgery poorly. Minimally invasive approaches are often appropriate in the first instance. Initial reports of successful resolution of pyloric stenosis following endoscopic balloon dilatation were challenged because of the relatively high number of cases that ultimately required open surgery (50% within 2 years).[139,140] Nevertheless this remains a useful first-line endoscopic procedure which can be repeated on several occasions with good long-term results in up to 80% of patients.[141] The main risk of endoscopic dilatation is perforation and the procedure should only be performed on patients who have been appropriately worked up for surgical intervention if needed. Only if a combination of intensive medical treatment and dilatation fails to reopen the gastric outlet is surgery indicated.

Surgery

The most appropriate operation to perform in cases of gastric outlet obstruction must take into account all those factors outlined for elective surgery of gastric and duodenal ulceration. The procedure must also restore drainage of the stomach. There are no published series that prove which procedure best achieves these aims. Initial fears about the capacity of a large atonic stomach to resume function have not realised. The operation with least complications is simple pyloroplasty (or gastroenterostomy where the inflammation around the pylorus is particularly intense), with highly selective vagotomy. Antrectomy and selective vagotomy or subtotal gastrectomy are more aggressive alternatives less likely to result in restenosis, but with a higher mortality and incidence of both short- and long-term side effects.

Laparoscopic surgery

In keeping with the trends for minimally invasive surgery, laparoscopic highly selective vagotomy with balloon dilatation has been attempted with some success in cases of pyloric stenosis.[141] This has not been proven to be superior to dilatation and long-term acid suppression. More recently laparoscopic truncal vagotomy and gastroenterostomy has proven a technically feasible solution with good symptomatic response at 6 months follow-up.[141] This operation cannot be recommended as a definitive ulcer procedure; laparoscopic techniques may have a role in the future for patients who have failed endoscopic balloon dilatation therapy, but are not a first-line intervention for pyloric stenosis.

References

1. Kurata JH, Honda GD, Frankl H. Hospitalisation and mortality rates for peptic ulcers: a comparison of a large health maintenance organisation and US data. Gastroenterology 1982; 83:1008–16.

2. Coggon D, Lambert P, Langman MJS. Twenty years of hospital admission for peptic ulcer in England and Wales. Lancet 1981; i:302–4.

3. Mortality statistics, cause. England and Wales 1990. Office of Population, Censuses and Surveys: HMSO, 1991.

4. Walt R, Katschinski B, Logan R et al. Rising frequency of ulcer perforation in elderly people in the United Kingdom. Lancet 1986; i:489–92.

5. Brown RC, Langman MJS, Lambert PM. Hospital admission for peptic ulcer during 1968–1972. BMJ 1976; 1:35–7.

6. Susser S, Stein Z. Civilisation and peptic ulcer. Lancet 1962; i:115–8.

7. Langman MJS. The Epidemiology of Chronic Digestive Disease. London: Edward Arnold, 1979.

8. Mendelhoff AI. What has been happening to duodenal ulcer? Gastroenterology 1974; 67:1020–2.

9. Friedman GD, Siegelaub AB, Seltzer CC. Cigarettes, alcohol, coffee and peptic ulcer. New Engl J Med 1974; 290:469–73.

10. Paffenberger PS, Wing PL, Hyde RT. Chronic disease in former college students. XIII. Early precursors of peptic ulcer. Am J Epidemiol 1974; 100:307–15.

11. Maddern GH, Horowitz M, Hetzel DJ et al. Altered solid and liquid gastric emptying in patients with duodenal ulcer disease. Gut 1985; 26:689–93.

12. McCarthy DM. Smoking and ulcers – time to quit. New Engl J Med 1984; 311:726–8.

13. Eastwood GL. Is smoking still important in the pathogenesis of peptic ulcer disease? J Clin Gastroenterol 1997; 25 (Suppl 1):S1–7.

14. Svanes C, Soreide JA, Skarstein A et al. Smoking and ulcer perforation. Gut 1997; 41 (2):177–80.

15. Faulkner G, Prichard P, Sommerville K et al. Asprin and bleeding peptic ulcers in the elderly. BMJ 1988; 297:1311–13.

16. Griffin MR, Piper JM, Daugherty JR et al. Non-steroidal anti-inflammatory drug use and increased risk for peptic ulcer disease in elderly persons. Ann Int Med 1991; 114:735–40.

17. Group AR. A randomised controlled trial of asprin in persons recovered from myocardial infarction. JAMA 1980; 243:661–9.

18. Langman MJ, Jensen DM, Watson DJ et al. Adverse upper gastrointestinal effects of rofecoxib compared with NSAIDs. JAMA 1999; 282 (20):1929–33.

19. Warren RJ, Marshall BJ. Unidentified curved bacilli on gastric epithelium in active chronic gastritis. Lancet 1983; i:1273–5.

20. Dixon MF. Helicobacter pylori and peptic ulceration: histopathological aspects. Gastroenterol Hepatol 1991; 6:125–30.

21. Feldman RA, Eccersley AJ, Hardie JM. Epidemiology of Helicobacter pylori: acquisition, transmission, population prevalence and disease-to-infection ratio. British Medical Bulletin 1998; 54 (1):39–53.

22. Hulten K, Han SW, Enroth H et al. Helicobacter pylori in the drinking water in Peru. Gastro 1996; 110:1031–5.

23. Berkowicz J, Lee A. Person to person transmission of Compylobacter pylori (letter). Lancet 1987; ii:681–2.

24. Drumm B, Perez-Perez G, Blazer M et al. Intrafamilial clustering of Campylobacter pylori infection. New Engl J Med 1990; 312:359–63.

25. Morris A, Nicholson G. Ingestion of Campylobacter pyloridis causes gastritis and raised fasting gastric acid. Am J Gastroenterol 1987; 82:192–9.

26. Langenberg W, Rauws EAJ, Oudbier JH et al. Patient to patient transmission of Helicobacter pyloris infection by fibreoptic gastroduodenoscopy and biopsy. J Infect Dis 1991; 61:307–11.

27. Tytgat GNJ. HP – reflections for the next millenium. Gut 1999; 45 (Suppl 1):145–7.

28. Pounder RE, Ng D. The prevalence of Helicobacter pylori infection in different countries. Ali Pharmacol Therap 1995; 9 (Suppl 2):33–9.

29. NIH consensus conference. Helicobacter pylori in peptic ulcer disease. JAMA 1994; 272:65–9.

30. Atherton JC. H. pylori virulence factors. British Medical Bulletin 1998; 54 (1):105–20.

31. Go MF, Tran L, Chan KY et al. REP-PCR finger print analysis reveals gastro–duodenal disease specific clusters of Helicobacter pylori strains. Am J Gastroenterol 1993; 88:1591–4.

32. Hessey ST, Spenger J, Wyatt JI. Bacterial adhesion and disease activity in Helicobacter-associated chronic gastritis. Gut 1990; 31:134–8.

33. Tee W, Lambert JR, Pegorer M et al. Cytotoxin production by Helicobacter pylori more common in peptic ulcer disease. Gastroenterology 1993; 104:A789.

34. Leunk RD. Production of a cytotoxin by Helicobacter pylori. Rev Infect Dis 1991; 13:S686–9.

35. Tummuru MKR, Sharma SA, Blaser MJ. Helicobacter pylori picB, a homolog of the Bordetella pertussis toxin secretion protein, is required for induction of IL-8 in

gastric epithelial cells. Mol Microbiol 1995; 18:867–76.

36. Boren T, Falk P, Roth KA *et al.* Attachment of *Helicobacter pylori* to human gastric epithelium mediated by blood group antigens. Science 1993; 262:1892–5.

37. The Eurogast Study Group. An international association between *Helicobacter pylori* infection and gastric cancer. Lancet 1993; 391:1359–62.

38. Playford R. Cytokines and *Helicobacter pylori* – a growth area. Gut 1996; 39:881–2.

39. Dunn B. Pathogenic mechanisms of *Helicobacter pylori*. Gastroenterol Clin North Am 1993; 22:43–57.

40. Peek RM Jr, Blaser MJ. Pathophysiology of *Helicobacter pylori*-induced gastritis and peptic ulcer disease. Am J Med 1997; 102 (2):200–7.

41. Graham DY, Go MF, Lew GM *et al. Helicobacter pylori* infection and exaggerated gastrin release. Effects of inflammation on progastrin processing. Scand J Gastroenterol 1993; 28:690–4.

42. Graham DY, Lechago J. Antral G-cell and D-cell numbers in *Helicobacter pylori* infection; effect of *Helicobacter pylori* eradication. Gastroenterology 1993; 104:1655–60.

43. El-Omar E, Panman I, Dorrain CA *et al.* Eradicating *Helicobacter pylori* infection lowers gastrin mediated acid secretion by two thirds in patients with duodenal ulcer. Gut 1993; 34:1060–65.

44. Barkin J. The relation between HP and NSAIDs. Am J Med 1998; 105 (5A):S22–7.

45. Bianchi Porro G, Parente F, Imbesi V *et al.* Role of HP in ulcer healing and recurrence of gastric and duodenal ulcers in long term NSAID users: response to omeprazole dual therapy. Gut 1996; 39:22–6.

46. Chan FK, Sung JJ, Chung SC *et al.* Randomised trial of eradication of HP before NSAID therapy to prevent peptic ulcers. Lancet 1997; 350:975–9.

47. Podolsky I, Storms PR, Richardson CT *et al.* Gastric adenocarcinoma masquerading endsocopically as benign gastric ulcer: a five-year experience. Dig Dis Sci 1988; 33:1057–63.

48. de Boer WA. Diagnosis of *Helicobacter pylori* infection. Review of diagnostic techniques and recommendations for their use in different clinical setting. Scand J Gastroenterol 1997; 223 (Suppl):35–42.

49. Boixeda D, Gisbet JP, de Raffael L *et al.* The importance of obtaining biopsies of the gastric body in the follow-up after treatment of HP infection. Med Clin (Barc) 1995; 105:566–9.

50. Vaira D, Holton J, Menegatti M *et al.* New immunological assays for the diagnosis of HP infection. Gut 1999; 45 (Suppl 1):123–7.

51. Van Zwet AA, Thys JC, Kooistra-Smid AMD *et al.* Sensitivity of culture compared with that of PCR for detection of HP from antral biopsy samples. J Clin Microbiol 1993; 31:1918–20.

52. Savarino V, Vigneri S, Celle G. The 13C urea breath test in the diagnosis of HP infection. Gut 1999; 45 (Suppl 1):118–122.

53. Vaira D, Holton J, Menegatti M *et al.* New immunological assays for the diagnosis of HP infection. Gut 1999; 45 (Suppl 1):123–7.

54. Soll AH. Medical treatment of peptic ulcer disease – practice guidelines. JAMA 1996; 275:622–9.

55. Laine L, Martin-Sorensen M, Weinstein WM. Non-steroidal anti-inflammatory drug-associated gastric ulcers do not require *Helicobacter pylori* for their development. Am J Gastroenterol 1992; 87:1398–1402.

56. Graham DY, Lew GM, Klein PD *et al.* Effect of treatment of *Helicobacter pylori* infection on the long term recurrence of gastric or duodenal ulcer. Ann Int Med 1992; 116:705–8.

57. Forbes GM, Glaser ME, Cullen DJE *et al.* Duodenal ulcer treatment with *Helicobacter pylori* eradication: seven year follow up. Lancet 1994; 343:258–60.

58. Huang JQ, Hunt RH. Review: eradication of *Helicobacter pylori*. Problems and recommendations. J Gastroenterol Hepatol 1997; 12 (8):590–8.

59. Lind T, Velduyzen van Zanten SJO, Unge P *et al.* Eradication of *Helicobacter pylori* using one week triple therapies combining omeprazole with two antimicrobials. The MACH 1 study. *Helicobacter* 1996; 1:138–44.

 60. Malfertheiner P, Megraud F, O'Morain C *et al.* Current European concepts in the management of *Helicobacter pylori* infection – the Maastricht consensus report. Eur J Gastroenterol Hepatol 1997; 9:1–2.

61. Maton PN. Omeprazole. New Engl J Med 1991; 324:965–75.

62. Zollinger RM, Ellison EH. Primary peptic ulcerations of the jejunum associated with islet cell tumours of the pancreas. Ann Surg 1955; 142:709–23.

63. Bondeson AG, Bondeson L, Thompson NW. Stricture and perforation of the oesophagus: overlooked threats in Zollinger–Ellison syndrome. World J of Surg 1990; 14:361–3.

64. Jaffe BN. Surgery for gut hormone-producing tumours. Am J Med 1987; 82 (Suppl 5B):68–76.

65. Ellison EH, Wilson SD. The Zollinger–Ellison syndrome: re-appraisal and evaluation of 260 registered cases. Ann Surg 1964; 160:512–20.

66. Stabile BE, Passaro E. Benign and malignant gastrinoma. Am J Surg 1985; 149:144–50.

67. Zollinger RM, Ellison EC, O'Darisio TM *et al.* Thirty years of experience with gastrinoma. World J of Surg 1984; 8:427–35.

68. Norton JA, Fraker DL, Alexander HR, Venzon DJ, Doppman JL, Serrano J, Goebel SU, Peghini PL, Roy PK, Gibril F, Jensen RT. Surgery to cure the Zollinger–Ellison syndrome. New Engl J Medicine 1999; 341 (9):635–44.

69. Wu PC, Alexander HR, Bartlett DL et al. A prospective analysis of the frequency, location, and curability of ectopic (nonpancreaticoduodenal, nonnodal) gastrinoma. Surgery 1997; 122 (6):1176–82.

70. McArthur KE, Richardson CT, Barnett CC et al. Laparotomy and proximal gastric vagotomy in Zollinger–Ellison syndrome: results of a 16-year prospective study. Am J Gastroenterol 1996; 91 (6):1104–11.

71. Richardson CT, Peters MN, Feldman M et al. Treatment of Zollinger–Ellison with exploratory laparotomy, proximal gastric vagotomy and H2 receptor antagonists. A prospective study. Gastroenterology 1985; 89:357–67.

72. Jensen RT, Fraker DL. Zollinger–Ellison syndrome: advances in treatment of the gastric hypersecretion and the gastrinoma. JAMA 1994; 271:1–7.

73. Bansal R, Tierney W, Carpenter S et al. Cost effectiveness of EUS for preoperative localization of pancreatic endocrine tumors. Gastrointest Endosc 1999; 49 (1):19–25.

74. Maton PN, Miller DL, Doppman JL et al. Role of selective angiography in the management of patients with Zollinger–Ellison syndrome. Gastroenterology 1987; 92:913–18.

 75. Alexander HR, Fraker DL, Norton JA et al. Prospective study of somatostatin receptor scintigraphy and its effect on operative outcome in patients with Zollinger–Ellison syndrome. Ann Surg 1998; 228 (2):228–38.

76. Norton JA, Fraker DL, Alexander HR et al. Surgery to cure the Zollinger–Ellison syndrome. New Engl J Med 1999; 341 (9):635–44.

77. Termanini B, Gibril F, Reynolds JC et al. Value of somatostatin receptor scintigraphy: a prospective study in gastrinoma of its effect on clinical management. Gastroenterology 1997; 112 (2):335–47.

78. Norton JA, Doherty GM, Fraker DL et al. Surgical treatment of localized gastrinoma within the liver: a prospective study. Surgery 1998; 124 (6):1145–52.

79. Norton JA. Intraoperative methods to stage and localize pancreatic and duodenal tumors. Ann Oncol 1999; 10 (Suppl 4):182–4.

80. Simeone DM, Hassan A, Scheiman JM. Giant peptic ulcer: a surgical or medical disease? Surgery 1999; 126:474–8.

81. Johnston D, Wilkinson AR. Highly selective vagotomy without a drainage procedure in the treatment of duodenal ulceration. Br J Surg 1970; 57:289–95.

82. Johnston D. Operative mortality and postoperative morbidity of highly selective vagotomy. Br Med J 1975; 4:545–7.

83. Johnston D, Humphrey CS, Walker BE et al. Vagotomy without diarrhoea. Br Med J 1972; 3:788–90.

84. Jordan PH, Thornby J. Should it be parietal cell vagotomy or selective vagotomy antrectomy for treatment of duodenal ulcer? Ann Surg 1987; 205:572–87.

85. Johnston D, Axon ATR. Highly selective vagotomy for duodenal ulcer – the clinical results after 10 years. Br J Surg 1979; 66:874–8.

86. Blackett RL, Johnston D. Recurrent ulceration after highly selective vagotomy for duodenal ulcer. Br J Surg 1981; 68:705–10.

87. Donahue PE, Bombeck T, Yoshida J et al. Endoscopic congo red test during proximal gastric vagotomy. Am J Surg 1987; 153:249–55.

88. Chisholm EM, Raimes SA, Leong HT et al. Proximal gastric vagotomy and anterior seromyotomy with posterior truncal vagotomy assessed by the endoscopic congo red test. Br J Surg 1993; 80:737–9.

89. Taylor TV, Gunn AA, Macleod DAD et al. Anterior lesser curve seromyotomy with posterior truncal vagotomy for duodenal ulcer. Br J Surg 1985; 72:950–1.

90. Raimes SA, Smirniotis V, Wheldon EJ et al. Post-vagotomy diarrhoea put into perspective. Lancet 1987; 2:851–3.

91. Dorricott NJ, McNeish AR, Alexander-Williams J et al. Prospective randomised multicentre trial of proximal gastric vagotomy or truncal vagotomy and antrectomy for chronic duodenal ulcer: interim results. Br J Surg 1978; 65:152–4.

92. DeVries BC, Schattenkirk EM, Smith EEJ et al. Prospective randomised trial of proximal gastric vagotomy or truncal vagotomy and antrectomy for chronic duodenal ulcer: results after 5–7 years. Br J Surg 1983; 70:701–3.

93. Primrose JN, Axon ATR, Johnston D. Highly selective vagotomy and ulcers that fail to respond to H2 receptor antagonists. Br Med J 1988; 296:1031–5.

94. Lu Y, Hoa Y, Jia S et al. Experimental study of pylorus and pyloric vagus preserving gastrectomy. World J Surg 1993; 17:525–9.

95. Yunfu L, Oinghua Z, Yongjia W. Pylorus and pyloric vagus preserving gastrectomy treating 125 cases of peptic ulcer. Minerva Chirugia 1998; 53:889–93.

96. Bloom BS. Cross-national changes in the effects of peptic ulcer disease. Ann Int Med 1991; 114:558–62.

97. Bardhan KD, Cust G, Hinchliffe RFC *et al*. Changing patterns of admissions and operations for duodenal ulcer. Br J Surg 1989; 76:230–6.

98. Hermansson M, Sael vH, Zilling T. The surgical approach and prognostic factors after peptic ulcer perforation. Eur J Surg 1999; 165:566–72.

99. Svannes C, Lie RT, Svanes K *et al*. Adverse effects of delayed treatment for perforated peptic ulcer. Ann Surg 1994; 220:168–75.

100. Kum CK, Chong YS, Koo CC *et al*. Elderly patients with perforated peptic ulcers: factors affecting morbidity and mortality. J R Coll Surg Edin 1993; 38:344–7.

101. Taylor H. Aspiration treatment of perforated ulcers. Lancet 1951; 1:7–12.

102. Gul YA, Shine MF, Lennon F. Non-operative management of perforated duodenal ulcer. Irish J Med Sci 1999; 168 (4):254–6.

103. Crofts TJ, Park KGM, Steele RJC *et al*. A randomised trial of nonoperative treatment for perforated peptic ulcer. New Engl J Med 1989; 320 (15):970–3.

104. Donovan AJ, Berne TV, Donovan JA. Perforated duodenal ulcer: an alternative therapeutic plan. Arch Surg 1998; 133 (11):1166–71.

105. Pai D, Sharma A, Kanungo R *et al*. Role of abdominal drains in perforated duodenal ulcer patients: a prospective controlled study. Austral N Z J Surg 1999; 69 (3):210–13.

106. Abbasakoor F, Attwood SE, McGrath JP *et al*. Simple closure and follow up of H2 receptor antagonists for perforated peptic ulcer-immediate survival and symptomatic outcome. Irish Med J 1995; 88:207–9.

107. Mihmanli M, Isgor A, Kabukcuoglu F *et al*. The effect of *H. pylori* in perforation of duodenal ulcer. Hepato Gastroenterol 1998; 45 (23):1610–12.

108. Ng EKW, Lam YH, Sung JJY *et al*. Eradication of HP prevents recurrence of ulcer after simple closure of DU perforation: randomised controlled trial. Ann Surg 2000; 231:153–8.

109. Mouret P, Francois Y, Vagnal J *et al*. Laparoscopic treatment of perforated peptic ulcer. Br J Surg 1990; 77:1006.

110. Pescatore P, Halkic N, Calmes JM *et al*. Combined laparoscopic-endoscopic method using an omental plug for therapy of gastroduodenal ulcer perforation. Gastrointest Endosc 1998; 48 (4):411–14.

111. Chang YC. Abdominal wall-lifting laparoscopic simple closure for perforated peptic ulcer. Hepato Gastroenterol 1999; 46 (28):2246–8.

112. Mutter D, Evrard S, Keller P *et al*. Perforated peptic ulcer – the laparoscopic approach. Ann Chir 1994; 48:339–44.

113. Munro WS, Bajwa F, Menzies D. Laparoscopic repair of perforated duodenal ulcers with a falciform

114. ligament patch. Ann R Coll Surg Engl 1996; 78:390–1.

114. Miserez M, Eypasch E, Spangenberger W *et al*. Laparoscopic and conventional closure of perforated peptic ulcer – a comparison. Surgical Endoscopy – Ultrasound and Interventional Techniques 1996; 10:831–6.

115. Robertson GS, Wemyss-Holden SA, Maddern GJ. Laparoscopic repair of perforated peptic ulcers. The role of laparoscopy in generalised peritonitis. Ann R Coll Surg Engl 2000; 82 (1):6–10.

116. Katkhouda N, Mavor E, Mason RJ *et al*. Laparoscopic repair of perforated duodenal ulcers: outcome and efficacy in 30 consecutive patients. Arch Surg 1999; 134 (8):845–8.

117. Khoursheed M, Fuad M, Safar H *et al*. Laparoscopic closure of perforated duodenal ulcer. Surg Endosc 2000; 14 (1):56–8.

118. Naesgaard JM, Edwin B, Reiertsen O *et al*. Laparoscopic and open operation in patients with perforated peptic ulcer. Eur J Surg 1999; 165:209–14.

119. Druart ML, Van Hee R, Etienne J *et al*. Laparoscopic repair of perforated duodenal ulcer. Surg Endos 1997; 11:1017–20.

120. Johannsson B, Hallerback B, Glise H *et al*. Laparoscopic suture closure of perforated peptic ulcer; a nonrandomised comparison with open surgery. Surg Endosc 1996; 10:656–8.

121. So JBY, Kum CK, Fernandes ML *et al*. Comparison between laparoscopic and conventional omental patch repair for perforated duodenal ulcer. Surg Endos 1996; 10:1060–63.

122. Bergamaschi R, Marvik R, Johnsen G *et al*. Open vs laparoscopic repair of perforated peptic ulcer. Surg Endos 1999; 13:679–82.

123. Green FW, Kaplan M, Curtis L *et al*. Effect of acid and pepsin on blood coagulation and platelet aggregation. Gastroenterology 1978; 74:38–43.

124. Zukerman G, Welch R, Douglas A. Controlled trial of medical therapy for active upper gastrointestinal bleeding and prevention of re-bleeding. Am J Med 1984; 76:361–6.

125. Collins R, Langman M. Treatment with histamins H2 antagonists in acute upper gastrointestinal haemorrhage. New Engl J Med 1985; 314:660–66.

126. Daneshmend TK, Hawkey CJ, Langman MJ *et al*. Omeprazole versus placebo for acute upper gastrointestinal bleeding: randomised double blind controlled trial. BMJ 1992; 304 (6820):143–7.

127. Khuror MS, Yattoo GN, Javid G *et al*. Comparison of omeprazole and placebo for bleeding peptic ulcer. New Engl J Med 1997; 336:1054–8.

128. Lin HJ, Lo WC, Lee FY *et al*. A prospective randomized comparative trial showing that

omeprazole prevents rebleeding in patients with bleeding peptic ulcer after successful endoscopic therapy. Arch Int Med 1998; 158 (1):54–8.

129. Lau JYW, Sung JJY, Lee KKC *et al*. Effect of intravenous omeprazole on recurrent bleeding after endoscopic treatment of bleeding peptic ulcers. New Engl J Med 2000; 343:310–6.

130. Henry D, O'Connel D. Effects of fibrinolytic inhibitors on mortality from upper gastrointestinal haemorrhage. BMJ 1989; 298:1142–6.

131. Lamerts S, Van der Lely A, De Harder *et al*. Octreotide. N Engl J Med 1996; 334:246–54.

132. Cook DJ, Guyatt GH, Salena *et al*. Endoscopic therapy for acute non-variceal upper gastrointestinal haemorrhage: a metanalysis. Gastroenterology 1992; 102:139–48.

133. Laine L, Peterson WL. Bleeding peptic ulcer. New Engl J Med 1994; 331:717–27.

134. Lau JYW, Sung JJY, Lam YH *et al*. Endoscopic re-treatment compared with surgery in patients with recurrent bleeding after initial endoscopic control of bleeding ulcers. New Engl J Med 1999; 340:751–6.

135. Teenan RP, Murray WR. Late outcome of undersewing alone for gastric ulcer haemorrhage. Br J Surg 1990; 77:811–12.

136. Poxon VA, Keighley MR, Dykes PW *et al*. Comparison of minimal and conventional surgery in patients with bleeding peptic ulcer: a multicentre trial. Br J Surg 1991; 78 (11):1344–5.

137. Brandimarte G, Tursi A, di Cesare L *et al*. Antimicrobial treatment for peptic stenosis: a prospective study. Eur J Gastroenterol Hepatol 1999; 11 (7):731–4.

138. Griffin SM, Chung SCS, Leung JWC *et al*. Peptic pyloric stenosis treated by endoscopic balloon dilatation. Br J Surg 1989; 76:1147–8.

139. Chisholm EM, Chung SCS, Leung JWC. Peptic pyloric stenosis – after the balloon goes up! Gastrointest Endosc 1993; 37:240.

140. Wyman A, Stuart RC, Ng EKW *et al*. Laparoscopic truncal vagotomy and gastroenterostomy for pyloric stenosis. Am J Surg 1996; 171:600–03.

13 Treatment of the complications of previous upper GI surgery

John R. Anderson

INTRODUCTION

Despite better understanding of the pathophysiology of various upper gastro-intestinal disorders and improved surgical and anaesthetic techniques, there remains a group of patients in whom primary surgery fails and long-term complications develop. Failure itself is not easy to define and changing attitudes over the last 50 years have altered our perception of this concept.

In 1949 a partial gastrectomy was considered as 'probably the best treatment for peptic ulcers requiring surgery'[1] yet it carried a mortality of 10% or greater. In that era it could be argued that to leave hospital alive was considered a success. Over the next decade the justification for gastrectomy was the low ulcer-recurrence rate. In the original Visick grading system[2] recurrent ulceration was automatically and permanently a grade 4 result. At this time it must be remembered that there was no good medical treatment for peptic ulcer disease. With the discovery of the H2 receptor antagonists many patients with recurrent ulceration following surgery were satisfied with the results of their operation if the disease was ameliorated to a degree which enabled it to be controlled with medical therapy.[3,4] Non-gastrointestinal problems after surgery such as wound pain or incisional hernia were potentially disregarded when assigning the Visick grade and may be just as important to the patient as the traditional complications.[4] More recently quality of life has become the main yardstick by which results of treatment have been assessed. This in itself is not without its problems, as quality of life is peculiarly personal. While failure to some would be the inability to cope with a 'jetset' lifestyle or regular over-indulgence in alcohol, to others dissatisfaction would be the inability to carry out their daily work or to enjoy the company of their friends and family.

The reasons for failure are often obvious, but may at times be hard to find. Is the problem with the surgeon, the operation or the patient? Poor technical surgery may lead to failure, but even when the experienced surgeon carries out the same operation, there will probably still be a small group of patients in whom the operation is less successful. The multiplicity of antireflux procedures suggests that there is no operation of choice that can be used in all circumstances for all patients by all surgeons. Inappropriate choice of operation may well mean the wrong procedure for that particular patient, but equally it may also mean the wrong operation for that particular surgeon.[5] Poor choice of operation may mean carrying out *any* surgical treatment. The author has been impressed on occasions when carrying out revisional surgery for the sequelae of previous peptic ulcer surgery by the paucity of signs in the duodenum. Visick[6] was one of the first to recognise that a small percentage of patients were predestined to failure, not because of the operation, but because of poor selection and their mal-adjusted lifestyle. Johnstone *et al.*[7] introduced the term 'the albatross syndrome' to identify patients with psychological problems who are unable to accept or handle physiological problems following surgery. There is another small group of patients who need their symptoms to act as a prop or crutch to enable them to cope with life, and if this crutch is removed another will be found to take its place. Dissatisfaction with the results of surgery was at one time thought to be due to unrealistic and unrealisable expectations but in the majority of patients this has not been borne out with observation.[8]

It can be seen that a number of factors need to be taken into consideration when dealing with the failures of earlier upper gastrointestinal surgery. Continuing symptoms may not only be caused by the operation but by the patient and his lifestyle. A failure of surgery is more likely to be seen in patients with a poor preoperative quality of life – often associated with alcohol abuse, smoking or psychiatric illness – and in patients with relatively few physical complaints. Such patients respond less well to revisional surgery and may require psychosocial support, if further failure is to be avoided.

Complications of antireflux surgery

Controversy still exists as to which surgical approach is best at achieving long-term control of gastro-oesophageal reflux without inflicting new and sometimes proce-dure-specific symptoms on our patients. The common causes for failure of an antireflux procedure are technical errors in carrying out the procedure or failure to recognise or deal with oesophageal shortening due to chronic oesophagitis. Half of the symptomatic recurrences will undergo their revisional operation within 5 years of the most recent failed antireflux operation.[9] Risk factors for recurrence include elderly people, because of the poor tensile strength of their tissues, obesity, chronic obstructive airways disease and previous gastric surgery.

Preoperative evaluation

Recurrent gastro-oesophageal reflux accounts for between a third and half of the failures of anti-reflux surgery irrespective of what primary procedure is carried out. The use of absorbable sutures, insufficient mobilisation of the oesophagus, inadequate suture technique and insufficient mobilisation of the fundus are all factors involved in the partial or complete breakdown of the primary repair. Partial fundoplications may be more prone to disruption because a longer length of intra-abdominal oesophagus is required and the integrity of the procedure depends on sutures in the oesophageal wall.

Peculiar to total fundoplication is the so called 'gas-bloat' syndrome producing a sensation of post-prandial epigastric fullness occasionally associated with pain, thought to result from the inability of patients to belch or vomit. Modifications to the original Nissen total fundoplication by using a 'floppy' wrap have minimised the occurrence of the syndrome,[10,11] and its severity tends to diminish with time.[12] The other complication uniquely associated with the total wrap is the so-called 'slipped' fundoplication.[13] This results from either causal migration of the wrap down the distal oesophagus on to the upper stomach or the improper location of the initial wrap around the upper stomach itself. In the author's experience of 11 slipped fundoplications each showed little evidence of oesophageal mobilisation at reoperation, suggesting the improper location of the wrap is the commoner cause of this complication.

Gastric ulceration has also been reported following fundoplication,[14,15] probably caused by gastric stasis resulting from vagal damage. Various fistulae from stomach to adjacent viscera have been described, including the bronchial tree[16] and the left ventricle.[17] The most likely cause for these events is sutures placed too deeply in the stomach or oesophagus or tied too tightly.

Preoperative evaluation

History

A careful history is mandatory. Any new symptom developing after previous antireflux surgery requires assessment. Symptoms alone may not always determine the cause of the problem but they do give some idea of its severity. Heartburn, regurgitation and dysphagia are the commonest symptoms, but patients can present with weight loss, recurrent attacks of bronchopneumonia due to aspiration, gastrointestinal bleeding and even diarrhoea, possibly caused by inadvertent damage to the vagus nerves. The response of symptoms to general measures and specific antireflux medication will help determine which patients should be considered for revisional surgery. The patient's occupation will also have a significant bearing on the need for further surgery.

Endoscopy

Endoscopic examination of the full upper gastrointestinal tract is essential and should be carried out by the surgeon contemplating the revisional procedure. The presence of oesophagitis, despite medical management, is an important finding and the level of the gastrooesophageal junction may help guide the surgeon in determining the approach to the patient. Any previous gastric surgery needs to be endoscopically assessed and the presence of bile in the stomach or oesophagus is worthy of note. It is important to retroflex the instrument and examine the area of the gastro-oesophageal junction while carrying out the endoscopy as this may well show partial or complete disruption of a fundoplication. It can also occasionally show a partial or complete intrathoracic fundoplication as a result of failure of the crural repair or migration of the wrap secondary to oesophageal scarring and shortening. Barium contrast examination of oesophagus and stomach may occasionally be a useful adjunct in order to determine the anatomy of the area.

Details of previous surgery

It is important to review the operation summary from the original operation. The findings at revisional surgery often bear little resemblance to the description of the original operation and therefore the information contained within the original report has to be interpreted with caution. Details of specific intraoperative problems can however be useful and may assist the surgeon in selecting the approach to the revisional procedure.

Oesophageal pH and manometry

Oesophageal manometry and 24-hour pH monitoring are mandatory in the evaluation of patients with recurrent symptoms (for full details see Chapter 9). Low-amplitude recordings in the distal oesophageal high-pressure zone suggests partial or complete disruption of the previous repair. Useful information is also obtained regarding the motility characteristics of the body of the oesophagus. Occasionally an antireflux procedure will have been carried out on a patient with an unsuspected motility disorder of the oesophagus e.g. achalasia or scleroderma and this will obviously influence the surgeon's choice of reoperative procedure. 24-hour pH monitoring will quantify the degree of reflux and establish the pattern of abnormal reflux in both the supine and erect positions. Following previous gastric surgery, enterogastric reflux of bile is common and found in 80% of patients with a truncal vagotomy and drainage and 90% of patients after partial gastrectomy.[18] 24-hour pH monitoring in this situation may reveal alkaline oesophagitis, but in many patients the refluxate is neutral and may therefore be missed. Endoscopic oesophagitis in this group of patients is usually obvious. Further assessment of the degree of enterogastro-oesophageal reflux can be carried out using the HIDA test.[19] There is little difference between the symptomatic and asymptomatic groups with regard to the degree of enterogastric reflux, but in symptomatic patients a delay in clearance of the refluxate was noted.[20] When gastric retention of food and fluid is noted at endoscopy and in patients with previous gastric surgery, the surgeon should consider carrying out isotope gastric-emptying studies.

After complete evaluation of the patient, an assessment can be made as to the nature/cause of the problem and the need for further surgery can be determined. The classification described by Skinner (see **Table 13.1**) is useful in describing the causes of symptoms after antireflux surgery, but in the author's experience is less useful in determining which revisional antireflux procedure should be carried out.

Redo procedures

Few generalisations can be made about the approach and techniques for revisional antireflux surgery, as each reoperation must be tailored to individual circumstances. Frequently the final decision about which procedure can be

1.	Failure of sphincter mechanism
2.	Failure of oesophageal clearance
3.	Sphincter and clearance failure
4.	Alkaline/neutral reflux
5.	Incorrect original diagnosis

Table 13.1 *Classification of antireflux failures*

undertaken is made at the time of surgery, once the previous procedure has been taken down and the condition of the lower oesophagus and fundus has been fully appreciated. Although some authors favour a transthoracic approach[9,20] most advocate a more selective approach involving transabdominal, thoracoabdominal or a purely transthoracic approach.[21,22,23,24,25,26,27] A number of factors need to be taken into consideration when deciding the surgical approach to these patients. These include: the build of the patient and in particular the degree of obesity, the angle of the costal junction, the previous approach, the nature of the previous operation, the level of the oesophagogastric junction (as defined endoscopically and with manometry) and the degree of oesophagitis found prior to surgery. The approach to a patient presenting with recurrent reflux following a previous transabdominal fundoplication would usually be transabdominal, provided the oesophagogastric junction was below 35 cm from the incisor teeth and there were no other contraindications. Conversely a patient who had undergone a transthoracic antireflux procedure, and in whom the oesophago-gastric junction was more proximal, would almost certainly undergo a further transthoracic operation. A thoracoabdominal approach should be considered where there has been a previous complex antireflux procedure (such as a gastroplasty fundoplication) and where greater access to the abdomen may be needed (in order to carry out further gastric surgery or possibly to mobilise the jejunum or colon).

At the time of revisional surgery, the previous procedure should be taken down. The objectives of revisional surgery are to restore the gastro-oesophageal junction 3–5 cm below the diaphragm and to carry out the antireflux procedure without tension, crural approximation with adequate bites of muscle and correction of any previous gastric intervention that may compromise the result of the revisional surgery. This is especially true in patients who have undergone a previous truncal vagotomy and drainage in order to 'improve' drainage of the stomach without prior objective evidence of delayed emptying. The exact revisional procedure undertaken will be determined by the findings at laparotomy and after careful mobilisation of the proximal stomach and lower oesophagus and by the familiarity of the surgeon with the various procedures. Vagal injury is possible during reintervention and in this situation a pyloromyotomy or pyloroplasty may be advisable but should be avoided if at all possible. If a total fundoplication is the considered procedure of choice it should be performed around a large intraoesophageal bougie and should be loose and short (1–2 cm): the crural defect must be carefully repaired.

Operations with oesophageal lengthening

Shortening of the oesophagus – usually encountered in patients with longstanding reflux – is a major problem. The creation of a gastric 'neo-oesophagus' was originally reported by Collis in 1961.[28] Originally reported as an antireflux procedure for patients with oesophageal shortening and stricture formation, the long-term results of this procedure alone have been disappointing. The original modification was the addition of a Belsey procedure[29] and although this improved results, there was a high incidence of continued reflux in the long term.[30] Total fundoplication gastroplasty (the Collis–Nissen procedure) was therefore introduced to provide a more effective control of reflux.[31] In most studies the results of this procedure are superior to the Collis–Belsey procedure.[9,32]

Provided the original procedure can be taken down without significant damage to the oesophagus or devascularisation of the fundus, the gastroplasty fundoplication is probably the procedure of choice where oesophageal shortening does not allow the gastro-oesophageal junction to lie below the diaphragm without tension. It can be equally easily performed through the abdomen or chest. The use of the stapling guns within the abdomen facilitates the procedure, which should be carried out around a size Fr 55 bougie. It should be of sufficient length to enable a 3–5 cm neo-oesophagus to lie below the diaphragm, the resulting cut fundus can be totally wrapped around the gastric tube over a distance of 1–2 cm. If the gastric wall is oedematous, the sutures can be tied over pledgets to prevent them cutting out. This operation creates an artifical Barrett's oesophagus and several cases of adenocarcinoma arising within the neo-oesophagus have been reported, although the aetiological relationship between the gastroplasty and carcinoma remains unproven.[33]

An alternative approach is to reduce acid secretion and divert biliary and pancreatic secretions away from the stomach and oesophagus by carrying out a vagotomy and antrectomy with roux loop reconstruction.[34,35] This procedure is particularly useful for patients in whom it is considered hazardous to attempt further dissection of the oesophago-gastric junction, especially where the adhesions are particularly dense. It is also extremely useful in patients developing reflux oesophagitis after gastric surgery for peptic ulcer disease. Unfortunately the operation carries an incidence of post-prandial symptoms as high as 20%[36] and can occasionally be followed by the development of a stomal ulcer.

Oesophageal resection

Resection of the oesophagus should not be contemplated lightly. The indications are an undilatable stricture or a chronic oesophageal fistula following previous surgery. Resection should also be considered in a patient with poor peristaltic activity in the body of the oesophagus. Resection may also need to be considered when there is intraoperative disruption of the oesophagus or when there is evidence of devascularisation of the lower oesophagus and possibly fundus. The inability to take down a previous repair is occasionally an indication for resection but in this situation the author favours antrectomy and Roux-en-Y anastomosis if this is technically and anatomically possible. The number of previous unsuccessful antireflux operations is a poor guide to the need for oesophageal resection. The aim of resectional surgery is not the restoration of normal gastro-oesophageal physiology but its total alteration.

Following resection, the major question that remains unanswered is which is the best organ to replace the oesophagus. Transhiatal oesophagectomy with cervical oesophago-gastric anastomosis allows the patient the benefits of resection without the morbidity sometimes associated with a thoracotomy.[37] This procedure undoubtedly abolishes reflux and uses a safer cervical anastomosis; there is, however, a tendency to stenosis, although this can be minimised by constructing the anastomosis over a 46 Fr or larger intraoesophageal dilator.[38,39] The incidence of postoperative hoarseness due to recurrent laryngeal nerve damage ranges from 3.7 to 37% of patients after this procedure. This problem can be partly prevented by identifying the nerve before isolating the cervical oesophagus, and by the avoidance of metal retraction on the trachea. In the author's experience the incidence of nerve damage after transhiatal oesophagectomy is

4% and in all patients their voice was returned to virtually normal after teflon injection of the vocal cord three months postoperatively.[40] It must be noted, however, that previous attempts at antireflux surgery may preclude the use of stomach for reconstruction, especially if part of the stomach has to be removed at the time of resection.

A jejunal interposition has its advocates.[41,42] An isoperistaltic jejunal segment can be isolated on a centrally placed vascular pedicle. Often the mesentery is too short for the length of jejunum and short resections are necessary to avoid redundancy, which may cause kinking and obstruction. Many authors favour a colonic interposition.[43,44,45,46] Although the colon tends to be a passive conduit, the long-term results are excellent.[44,47,48] Functional results using colon interposition are better when the colon is anastomosed to the antrum. If colon is anastomosed to the denervated fundus, there may be problems with gastric retention.

Reflux after previous gastric surgery

Gastro-oesophageal reflux is commonly encountered after previous gastric surgery, usually for peptic ulcer disease: it may be acid, neutral or alkaline. Neutral or alkaline reflux occurs as a complication of gastrectomy and is most marked after subtotal or total gastrectomy. It is almost always accompanied by bile reflux. It can also be seen following truncal vagotomy and drainage. In contrast, acid reflux is more often seen after vagotomy; it is reported in 20–40% of patients after truncal vagotomy and drainage or proximal gastric vagotomy.[49,50] This was thought to result from damage to the phreno-oesophageal ligament and oesophago-gastric fixation, vagal denervation of the lower oesophagus and loss of the gastro-oesophageal angle. It has been shown, however, that duodenal ulcer patients have a high incidence of gastro-oesophageal reflux symptoms proven by endoscopy and 24-hour pH monitoring prior to surgery and there is no evidence that vagotomy influences these findings.[51] If the ulcer disease is cured by vagotomy, then gastro-oesophageal reflux symptoms will appear more prominent after surgery for peptic ulcer disease.

If acid reflux is diagnosed using 24-hour pH monitoring then the patient should initially be treated medically (see Chapter 10). Operative treatment is indicated after the failure of medical therapy (persistent symptoms despite good medication, unhealed oesophagitis or side effects from medical treatment) or because of the development of complications (such as stricture formation or significant ulceration). Medical therapy (bile salt binding agents, mucosal protective agents and prokinetic agents) is usually ineffective in patients with alkaline or neutral reflux; if symptoms significantly interfere with quality of life and unless contraindicated by comorbid disease, surgical treatment is usually necessary in such cases. Patients with reflux disease following previous gastric surgery need a careful appraisal of their symptoms as many will describe features of dumping, bile vomiting or diarrhoea. Although the spectrum of post-gastric surgery syndromes are well described, the majority of patients will present with a mixed clinical picture. Careful appraisal however will reveal a dominant problem and any treatment should be targeted to this after the appropriate investigations. The actual surgical treatment depends on the nature of the previous operation(s) and the type of reflux (acid, neutral or alkaline). In patients with a previous truncal vagotomy and drainage or proximal gastric vagotomy and proven acid reflux, the surgical procedure with which the surgeon is most familiar would seem to be the most appropriate procedure. The author favours a loose 1–2 cm total fundoplication in this situation. Consideration should be given to reconstruction of the pylorus in the presence of a pyloroplasty, especially where this is large or taking down a gastro–jejunostomy. Fundoplication is contraindicated in patients who have had a previous partial gastrectomy. If the left gastric pedicle was divided during the course of the original gastrectomy, then division of the short gastric vessels may render the gastric remnant ischaemic. Even with a good gastric remnant blood supply, there is usually not enough mobility of the gastric remnant to allow a loose wrap to be created without tension. In this situation a posterior gastropexy would seem the most appropriate procedure.

Alkaline or neutral reflux after vagotomy and drainage is best dealt with by taking down the drainage procedure provided the duodenum is not significantly scarred. Both these revisional procedures are potentially ulcerogenic and it is the author's practice to mobilise the oesophagus and check on the completeness of the vagotomy prior to carrying out an additional loose total fundoplication. After antrectomy or other forms of partial gastrectomy, diversion of bile and pancreatic secretion is best carried out with a 45 cm Roux loop. In patients who have undergone a previous oesophago-gastrectomy, especially where the oesophago-gastric anastomosis is within the thorax and in patients in whom reconstruction of the pylorus fails, a suprapapillary duodeno-jejunal anastomosis in conjunction with a Roux loop would seem an appropriate procedure (**Fig. 13.1**).[52] The author has now used this procedure on five occasions in patients with a previous oesophago-gastrectomy for carcinoma (more than 5 years previously) with satisfactory short-term results.

Personal experience

Between 1985 and 1995, 57 patients (35 male and 22 female) with a mean age of 46 years underwent revisional antireflux surgery. After careful preoperative evaluation, classification of the failures suggested sphincter mechanism failure in 17 patients, clearance failure in 9, combined sphincter mechanism and clearance

Figure 13.1
Pylorus preserving Roux loop – the duodenal switch operation (De Meester et al.)[52]

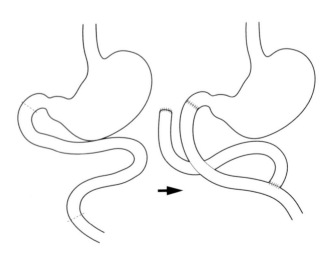

failure in 21, alkaline or neutral reflux in 9 and an incorrect original preoperative diagnosis in one patient. Four of the patients had undergone two previous anti-reflux procedures, in three a posterior gastropexy followed by a total fundoplication, and in the other a failed fundoplication had been followed by a Belsey procedure. The remaining 53 patients had undergone one previous procedure, total fundoplication in 30 (transthoracic in 6 and transabdominal in 24), a partial fundoplication in 7, an Angelchik antireflux prosthesis in 6, an Allison–type repair in 6, a posterior gastropexy in two and a transthoracic Belsey procedure in a further two. Of the 47 patients with a previous transabdominal antireflux procedure, 19 had undergone a truncal vagotomy with pyloroplasty in 13, gastro-jejunostomy in four, pyloric dilatation in one and antrectomy in the other. Three patients had also undergone a proximal gastric vagotomy. In only 5 of these 22 patients was there evidence at the time of revisional surgery of previous significant peptic ulcer disease. In the remaining 17, the vagotomy with drainage procedure if appropriate appears to have been carried out to reduce acid output and 'improve' gastric emptying.

A revisional procedure was carried out transthoracically in 15 patients, with one of these patients also undergoing a transabdominal pylorus-preserving 45 cm Roux loop (in the patient who had undergone a previous truncal vagotomy, pyloric dilatation and partial fundoplication). In this particular patient a hole was made in the posterior aspect of the oesophagus during its transthoracic mobilisation and this was managed with a Thal patch covered by a floppy total fundoplication. A transabdominal revisional procedure was carried out in the remaining 42 patients. Thirty patients underwent a floppy total fundoplication including the patient described above. In 21 patients a gastroplasty/total fundoplication was carried out and in 5 patients a posterior gastropexy was fashioned. The patient with achalasia underwent transhiatal oesophagectomy with colonic interposition. The gastro-jejunostomy was taken down in all four patients and pylorus reconstruction was undertaken in the 13 patients with a previous pyloroplasty. There were four significant operative complications, the intraoperative oesophageal rupture referred to above and three cases of splenic injury, which required splenectomy in two to control bleeding. There was no operative mortality.

After a mean follow-up of 8.3 years, 48 of the patients had a good or satisfactory outcome but in 9 the outcome was poor. Three of these patients continued to complain of intermittent dysphagia, including the patient with the oesophageal rupture. In retrospect it may have been appropriate to resect this patient's oesophagus. Six patients continued to complain of reflux-type symptoms: one following a transthoracic gastroplasty/total fundoplication and the remaining 5 following a total fundoplication – two carried out transthoracically and three carried out transabdominally. All of these 6 patients however significantly improved using proton pump inhibitors. These results compare favourably with other published studies (**Table 13.2**), but are overall not as good as the results of primary antireflux surgery.

Complications of previous ulcer surgery

The discovery of *Helicobacter pylori* as the principal causative agent in most patients with peptic ulcer disease (excluding those caused by non–steroidal anti-

Author	No of patients	Mortality	Good/satisfactory result
Skinner[20]	117	2 (1.7%)	98/115 (85%)
Rieger et al.[23]	61	2 (3%)	51/58 (87%)
Siewert et al.[22]	71	1 (1%)	60/70 (87%)
Ellis et al.[25]	101	1 (1%)	68/85 (80%)
Stirling et al.[9]	87	0	69/87 (79%)
Present series	57	0	48/57 (84%)

Table 13.2 *Published results of revisional antireflux surgery*

inflammatory drugs and aspirin) and its effective eradication has virtually eliminated the need for surgery in primary uncomplicated peptic ulcer disease.[53] However there remains a large cohort of patients operated on prior to the mid-1980s with a variety of surgical procedures, of whom a small percentage will develop further symptoms, some of which may be severely disabling. Although numerous clinical syndromes have been well described (**Table 13.3**) patients presenting with pure syndromes are uncommon. The majority present with a mixed picture, but usually have a dominant symptom complex suggesting one main problem. This needs to be elucidated by a careful and detailed history of the clinical events occurring during a bad attack.

Joint management with a gastro-enterological physician usually improves the outcome in this group of patients, in part due to better patient selection for remedial surgery. It also allows for independent assessment of the results of revisional surgery. After an accurate history, a number of detailed investigations will be required to outline the abnormal anatomy and pathophysiology in order to obtain objective evidence of the principal abnormality. The clinician involved in these patients should not become so totally focused on the previous gastric surgery but should also remember that many of the symptom complexes patients describe can also be caused by diseases of the liver, biliary tract and pancreas.

Pathophysiological problems
  Gastro-oesophageal reflux
  Recurrent ulcer
  Enterogastric reflux
  Dumping
  Reactive hypoglycaemia
  Diarrhoea
  Malabsorption

Mechanical problems
  Loop obstruction
  Small stomach syndrome
  Bezoars

Other sequelae
  Cholelithiasis
  Carcinoma

Table 13.3 *Post-peptic ulcer surgery sequelae*

Preoperative evaluation

Endoscopy

Endoscopic examination is essential and as with patients after previous antireflux surgery, it should be carried out by the surgeon considering any revisional procedure. The exact anatomy, size of the gastric remnant, size and position of any drainage procedure, the presence of enterogastric reflux of bile, recurrent ulceration, the general state of the gastric mucosa and the presence of a hiatus hernia and/or reflux oesophagitis can be assessed. All abnormalities should be biopsied. All patients should be assessed for the presence of *Helicobacter pylori*.

Radiology

Barium meal examination of the stomach is a useful adjunct where the anatomy remains unclear.

Gastrin level

The serum gastrin levels should be determined routinely in all patients with benign recurrent ulcers to exclude the Zollinger–Ellison syndrome. False-positive results can occur in patients with achlorhydria, pernicious anaemia, atrophic gastritis and after vagotomy. Hypergastrinaemia can also be seen with antral G-cell hyperplasia or gastric outlet obstruction as well as in patients with a retained antrum after a Billroth II/Polya type gastrectomy where a small cuff of antrum has been included in the duodenal 'closure' (see Chapter 12). If a retained antrum is suspected, technetium pertechnetate scan may be useful in identifying the antral mucosa.[54] There is a strong relationship between hyperparathyroidism and peptic (including recurrent) ulcer disease and consequently all patients should be screened for hypercalcaemia by multiple serum calcium measurements. The presence of hyperparathyroidism should alert the clinician to the possibility of other endocrine abnormalities associated with the multiple endocrine adenopathies.

Studies for completeness of vagotomy

Gastric acid secretory studies are not considered valuable in the assessment of patients with recurrent ulcers. Insulin-induced hypoglycaemia as a stimulant to acid production results in a large number of false-positive tests and may also be potentially dangerous. It should therefore be abandoned. Confirmation of an incomplete vagotomy and also mapping of the incomplete fibres can be carried out in a much safer and simple way by using the endoscopic congo red test. This involves giving the patient 6 µg/kg body weight of subcutaneous pentagastrin 15 minutes before carrying out the endoscopy. At endoscopy the stomach is lavaged with 200 ml of congo red (3 g/l) in 0.5% sodium bicarbonate solution. The solution must access all areas of the stomach. After aspirating excess fluid, the stomach is observed for 2 minutes. Vagally innervated parietal cells turn black and if the vagotomy is complete there should obviously be no black areas.

Gastric-emptying studies

Gastric-emptying studies may occasionally be useful. Barium meal examination may show rapid emptying of the dye from the stomach and may demonstrate gross intestinal hurry with the meal reaching the caecum within a short time of leaving the stomach. Gastric emptying is however best studied using a radioactive-labelled meal, either liquid or solid. In general, the radioactive liquid meals are easier to interpret than solid meals. The normal measured indices such as 10 minute emptying, the $T_{1/2}$ and the percentage retention after 60 minutes are often used in assessment. However after gastric surgery these indices can be misleading as the patients often show a fast initial emptying component followed by a slower component.

Dumping provocation tests

The standard dumping provocation test may be required where there is doubt about the presence of dumping. The test consists of an oral ingest of 150 ml 50% glucose solution which should precipitate symptoms and be accompanied by a fall in calculated plasma volume.[55] This test may cause severe symptoms and should be carried out in hospital under direct medical supervision.

Other tests

Oesophageal function tests (already mentioned) will be required in those patients suspected of having gastro-oesophageal reflux. Enterogastric reflux can be assessed using the HIDA scan as previously mentioned. Bacterial overgrowth following gastric resection may occasionally cause diarrhoea. Diagnosis is made by aspiration and culture of jejunal contents or by the C14 glycocholate breath test.

Various nutritional indices including weight, serum albumin, transferase, corrected serum calcium concentration should be measured in all patients. In selected patients full assessment for metabolic bone disease should be undertaken especially in post-menopausal women. A full haematological survey should be carried out including measurement of serum iron, iron binding capacity, folate and B12 levels.

Recurrent ulceration

Recurrent peptic ulceration has always been regarded as the hallmark of failure of an ulcer operation. However, while disheartening for both patient and clinician, it is in fact more easily treated that many of the other lifelong sequelae (**Table 13.3**). The frequency of ulcer recurrence varies with the operation performed and representative recurrent rates are shown in **Table 13.4**.[56,57,58,59,60,61,62] There is variability in the time interval between initial operation and the development of recurrent ulcer (**Table 13.5**).

Endoscopic confirmation of recurrence is essential as there are multiple causes for recurrent dyspeptic symptoms after ulcer surgery (**Table 13.6**). All recurrent gastric ulcers must be biopsied – early recurrence may be the result of a missed carcinoma initially where a late recurrence may represent malignancy developing in the postoperative stomach.

The various aetiological factors that can cause recurrent ulceration are shown in **Fig. 13.2**.

Medical treatment

Nowadays the first step in management of recurrent ulcers is to eradicate *Helicobacter pylori* when it is present and confirm both eradication and healing.

Operation	Recurrence rate (%)
Gastro-jejunostomy	20
Gastrectomy	3
Vagotomy and antrectomy	1
Vagotomy and drainage	10
Proximal gastric vagotomy	12

Table 13.4 *Recurrent ulcer rates after various initial operations for peptic ulcer*

Operation	Average time (years)
Gastro-jejunostomy	8
Gastrectomy	3
Vagotomy and antrectomy	1
Vagotomy and drainage	3
Proximal gastric vagotomy	3

Table 13.5 *Time interval between initial operation and recurrent ulcer*

Recurrent ulcer
Dumping
Enterogastric reflux
Biliary disease
Pancreatic disease
Gastro-oesophageal reflux
Carcinoma
Musculoskeletal pain with radiation
Non-specific pain

Table 13.6 *Causes of recurrent dyspepsia after ulcer surgery*

Ingestion of ulcerogenic drugs such as aspirin or NSAIDs must be stopped. Probably the commonest cause of recurrent ulceration in patients who are *H. pylori* negative and not ingesting noxious drugs is incomplete vagotomy. This can be confirmed using the endoscopic congo red test already described. Rarely will hyperparathyroidism, the Zollinger–Ellison syndrome or a retained antrum be the cause of recurrent ulceration, but when found treatment should obviously be directed at removing the cause.

Some patients will have life-threatening complications when the diagnosis of recurrent ulceration is first made and operation may be indicated as a life-saving

Figure 13.2
Aetiological factors in recurrent ulceration

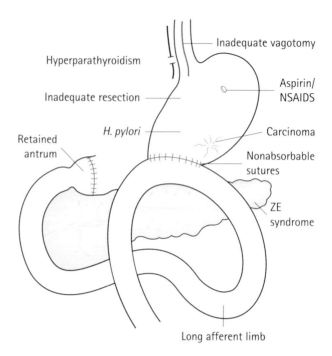

procedure. In patients presenting with dyspeptic symptoms and in whom both *Helicobacter pylori* and ulcerogenic drugs have been excluded, non-operative therapy is indicated as an ulcer that failed to respond to medical treatment pre-operatively may well now respond to such treatment.[4] Current antisecretory drugs such as the proton pump inhibitors induce virtual achlorhydria and ulcer healing is the norm. Once the ulcer has been healed and especially in *H. pylori*-negative patients, consideration should be given to long-term maintenance treatment, especially if the patient is over 60 years of age or has comorbid disease that increases anaesthetic risk.

Surgical treatment

Surgery is probably indicated in the younger patient. The patient must be fully informed about the proposed surgical procedure and its long-term implications and must be involved in the decision-making process. Mortality rates of less than 2%[63] and second recurrent ulcer rates of less than 6%[64] can be obtained by experienced gastric surgeons.

The surgical procedure for recurrent ulcer depends on the initial operation, the results of any preoperative tests and in the findings at revisional surgery. Complete examination of the duodenum, pancreas and liver is essential. If a retained antrum is found in the duodenal stump and the ulcer is less than 2 cm in diameter, excision of the antral tissue is curative.[65,66] If preoperative evaluation indicates a Zollinger–Ellison syndrome, total gastrectomy and excision of as much tumour mass as possible is indicated (see Chapter 12).

In all other patients the operation should aim to reduce acid secretion. Local ulcer excision, revision of gastro-jejunostomy or closure of perforations are attended by a high mortality rate approaching 12% and a second ulcer recurrence rate of nearly 50%.[67] It is mandatory therefore that either vagotomy and/or gastric resection be carried out. Truncal vagotomy and antrectomy is the procedure of choice where the initial operation was simple gastro-jejunostomy, truncal vagotomy and drainage or proximal gastric vagotomy. Following partial gastrectomy, the vast majority of recurrent ulcers are treated by truncal vagotomy. If the recurrent ulcer is large or complicated by bleeding, obstruction or perforation, or if the original resection is judged to be inadequate (probably less than two-thirds) then a further resection will be necessary. Vagotomy alone or with additional resection has a further ulcer recurrence rate of approximately 10%.[67] In the uncommon situation of a recurrent ulcer following truncal vagotomy and antrectomy, the ulceration is usually the result of an inadequate vagotomy. If at the time of re-exploration a large residual vagal trunk is found, revagotomy is usually adequate. If no large vagal trunks are found and the resection is thought to be inadequate, then a 70% plus gastrectomy is appropriate. If an adequate vagotomy and subtotal gastrectomy have already been carried out, total gastrectomy may be required to control the ulcer disease even in the absence of a gastrinoma.

The benign gastro-jejuno-colic fistula that occurs as a consequence of recurrent ulceration has become a rarity. This was most commonly seen after a simple gastro-jejunostomy. After demonstration of the fistula using barium studies and exclusion of carcinoma of the stomach by gastroscopy and colon by colonoscopy, most patients are best treated by truncal vagotomy and en bloc resection of the gastric antrum and fistula (including short segments of jejunum and colon) with primary anastomosis to restore gastrointestinal continuity.

Enterogastric reflux

Reflux of alkaline duodenal content into the stomach occurs following surgery which damages, bypasses or removes the pylorus. Enterogastric reflux is more common after gastrectomy, especially where reconstruction as a Billroth II gastro-jejunostomy has been carried out. Chronic exposure of the gastric mucosa to upper intestinal contents leads to typical histological changes including foveolar hyperplasia, glandular cystification, oedema of the lamina propria and vasocongestion of the mucosal capillaries, all in association with inflammatory cell infiltration.[68] These changes are worsened in the absence of the antrum because of the lack of the trophic hormone gastrin.[69] It has also been shown that when reflux is eliminated using a Roux loop, the severity of the histological gastritis is substantially reduced.[70] The vasocongestion seen histologically may have an endoscopic corollary. Gastric mucosal oedema and erythema involving more than just the peristomal area are considered to be a reasonably specific endoscopic sign of excessive enterogastric reflux. A significant correlation has been shown between the hyperaemia and the concentration of bilirubin in samples of endoscopically obtained gastric juice.[71] Less enterogastric reflux occurs following proximal gastric vagotomy.[72]

The symptoms consist of persistent epigastric discomfort, sometimes made worse by eating and frequently associated with intermittent vomiting of bile-stained fluid or food mixed with bile, usually occurring within an hour and a half of a meal. Some patients become malnourished because of inadequate food intake and anaemia develops in about a quarter of the patients as a result of chronic blood loss from the associated gastritis. Gastro-oesophageal reflux disease may also develop and this has been covered in the earlier part of this chapter.

Endoscopy shows a diffuse gastritis with an oedematous hyperaemic friable mucosa and frequently superficial erosions. Endoscopic biopsy shows typical histological features. The presence of bile in the stomach in the absence of endoscopic and histological features does not establish the diagnosis. If a technetium HIDA scan is used to obtain objective evidence, the results need to be interpreted with caution as there is little difference in the extent of enterogastric reflux between symptomatic and asymptomatic patients after gastric surgery. As previously stated, delay in emptying of the radio-active material is usually only seen in the symptomatic groups.

Medical treatment

A variety of drug therapies have been tried in symptomatic patients and apart from one exception, none have proved very effective. Cholestyramine has been shown to be an effective bile-acid binding agent *in vitro*, although the results of several therapeutic trials have been disappointing.[73,74] Antacids containing aluminium hydroxide have also been studied because of their bile-acid binding capacity but the results have been equally unimpressive. Sucralfate has been shown to protect rat gastric mucosal cells in tissue culture from the damage caused by taurocholate.[75] In clinical trials sucralfate has been shown to reduce the inflammation within the gastric mucosa but this has not been associated with any improvement in symptoms.[76] Prokinetic agents have also been used to improve clearance of the refluxate from the stomach and the occasional patient may respond. These agents may however worsen dumping and diarrhoea. Ursodeoxycholic acid has been shown in one study to almost abolish the nausea and vomiting associated with enterogastric reflux and to significantly decrease the intensity and frequency of pain.[77] It was suggested that this was due to an alteration of the bile-salt composition in the refluxate. It is interesting to note that neither the macroscopic or microscopic appearance of the gastric mucosa was affected using this drug.

Surgical treatment

Patients with severe symptoms will inevitably come to surgical revision. In patients with a previous truncal vagotomy and drainage, reversal of the drainage procedure can be undertaken provided at least one year has elapsed from the original operation. This is based on the concept that the stomach will regain some of its lost motility during this time. It should be remembered that in the early days of vagotomy, more than half of the patients with truncal vagotomy alone did well and did not require a drainage procedure. Closure of gastrojejunostomy for enterogastric reflux and bile vomiting is usually followed by improvement or complete relief in the vast majority of patients.[78] The risks of gastric stasis are minimal and conversion to a pyloroplasty should be avoided.

Reconstruction of the pylorus after pyloroplasty is a relatively straightforward operation. Having cleared the anteropyloroduodenal segment of all adhesions, the scar of the previous pyloroplasty is accurately opened. The pyloric ring is palpated and the scarred ends freshened if necessary. It is the author's practice to make a small antral gastrotomy to allow the insertion of a size 12 or 14 Hegar dilator through the area of the pyloric reconstruction into the duodenum. It is difficult to decide how narrow to make the reconstructed pyloric ring and the use of a Hegar dilator is somewhat arbitrary, but seems to work in practice. Using a double-ended monofilament suture the pyloric ring is accurately opposed around the Hegar's dilator before reapproximating the duodenum and antrum using a continuous serosubmucosal technique. Withdrawal of the Hegar's dilator allows fingertip palpation of the reconstructed pylorus prior to closure of the antral gastrotomy. The overall results of pyloric reconstruction show that 80% of patients gain a satisfactory or good result with 20% gaining no benefit.[79] In one study, only half of the patients with enterogastric reflux had a satisfactory or good response.[80] However the procedure is relatively simple and safe and should probably be the initial revisional procedure for patients with symptoms after a previous pyloroplasty.

If enterogastric reflux is not relieved, then the duodenal switch operation[52] would seem an appropriate further remedial procedure for patients whose symptoms necessitate further surgery.

In patients who have had a gastric resection or in those with a gastro-jejunostomy with pyloric stenosis, a Roux limb (approximately 45 cm in length) would seem an appropriate revisional procedure (with antrectomy in patients with pyloric stenosis). The procedure however does carry risks, as it is ulcerogenic because it diverts the buffering effect of upper gastrointestinal contents away from the gastroenteric anastomosis. It is therefore the author's practice to carry out exploration of the oesophagus at the time of Roux conversion to check on the adequacy of the vagotomy. The second problem is the development of delayed gastric emptying of solid food producing a symptom complex of satiety, epigastric pain and nonbilious vomiting that has been termed 'the Roux syndrome'. Although many patients will demonstrative objective evidence of delayed gastric emptying of solids,[81,82] this is usually of little or no clinical consequence except in a minority. The Roux syndrome is more likely to develop in patients who demonstrate delay in gastric emptying of solids prior to construction of the Roux limb and those who have a large residual gastric pouch. The syndrome may also be more likely to develop in those patients who require a completion vagotomy. Where these conditions exist, the operative procedure required is more extensive. The entire anastomosis should be resected to leave a small gastric pouch and the Roux limb should be anastomosed to the stomach as an end-to-side Polya-type gastro-jejunostomy. In those patients who develop severe symptoms from the Roux syndrome postoperatively, then the treatment is near-total resection of the gastric remnant with a Polya-type gastro-jejunostomy.

Roux diversion will control enterogastric reflux in excess of 70% of patients and recurrent jejunal ulcers can be avoided by checking and if necessary completing the truncal vagotomy as part of the operative procedure.[83,84]

Chronic afferent loop syndrome

The afferent loop syndrome obviously depends on the presence of an afferent loop and can therefore only occur after gastro-jejunostomy or a Billroth II type reconstruction after partial gastrectomy. The condition is caused by intermittent post-prandial obstruction of the afferent limb of the gastro-jejunostomy. The reason for mentioning this briefly here is that the clinical picture is very similar to that produced by enterogastric reflux (see **Table 13.7**). The problem is rarely encountered if surgeons use a short afferent jejunal loop. The cause of the obstruction may be due to anastomotic kinking, adhesions, internal herniation,

Chronic afferent loop syndrome	Enterogastric reflux
Meal-related pain – relieved by vomiting	Constant pain (worsened by eating) – not relieved by vomiting
Vomitus contains bile	Vomitus contains bile and food
Vomiting projectile	Vomiting non-projectile
Rarely associated with bleeding/anaemia	Bleeding/anaemia found in 25% of patients

Table 13.7 *Differentiation between the chronic afferent loop syndrome and enterogastric reflux*

volvulus of the afferent limb or obstruction of the gastrojejunal stoma itself. Once diagnosed the treatment is always surgical. Conversion to a Billroth I anastomosis or a Roux–en–Y reconstruction of the afferent limb have both produced good results.

Dumping

Dumping occurs to some degree after most gastric operations, but is encountered least often after proximal gastric vagotomy. The literature shows a considerable variability in the incidence of dumping after each procedure due at least partly to variations in definitions of the syndrome. A significant number of patients will develop dumping-type symptoms in the early period after their initial gastric operation but the majority have sufficient reserve to adjust to the changes without developing severe sequelae. The incidence of severe dumping after partial gastrectomy is probably around 4%, with 7% of patients developing problems after truncal vagotomy and antrectomy and about 3% after truncal vagotomy and drainage. Severe dumping has not been reported after proximal gastric vagotomy in any prospective study.

The symptoms of early dumping can be divided into vasomotor and gastrointestinal as shown in **Table 13.8**. In a severe attack, the vasomotor symptoms are usually experienced by the patient towards the end of a meal or within 15 minutes of finishing and the gastrointestinal symptoms develop a little later, but usually within 30 minutes after eating.

There is now clear evidence that dumping is associated with rapid gastric emptying leading to hyperosmolar jejunal content causing massive fluid shifts from the extracellular space into the lumen. This is associated with a significant fall in plasma volume.[55,85,86] It is also known that plasma concentrations of several gut regulatory peptides are elevated in patients with the dumping syndrome,[87,88,89,90] but it is not clear whether this is coincidental or causative.[87,88,89,90]

Taking a careful history, delineating the vasomotor and gastrointestinal components, usually makes the diagnosis of the dumping syndrome. Where there is any doubt, the patient should be encouraged to keep a diary card recording the foods eaten and the symptoms that develop thereafter. Rarely will the dumping provocation test be required and this should be carried out in hospital because of the severe and potentially life-threatening symptoms that can occur as a result of the test.

Vasomotor	**Gastrointestinal**
Palpitations	Nausea
Flushings	Vomiting
Sweating	Belching
Headache	Fullness
Weakness	Colic
Faintness	Borborygmi
Anxiety	Diarrhoea

Table 13.8 *Symptoms of early dumping*

Medical treatment

The majority of patients displaying the dumping syndrome can be managed satisfactorily by dietary manipulation. Reducing the carbohydrate content and restricting fluid intake with meals will help many of these patients. Avoiding extra salt and eating more frequent small meals may also be required. Assuming the supine posture after eating helps to slow gastric emptying and may minimise symptoms. Guar gum, a vegetable fibre, is known to reduce post-prandial hypoglycaemia in both normal[91] and diabetic[92] patients. In a small study of post-gastric surgery patients it has been shown to prevent the dumping syndrome and increase food tolerance in the majority of patients.[93] Pectin also delays gastric emptying but may precipitate attacks of diarrhoea. Somatostatin and more recently its analogue octreotide given subcutaneously prior to eating has been shown to significantly reduce or abolish the symptoms of dumping.[94,95,96] The published experience with this treatment is limited but the author has used it with success in 5 patients.

Surgical treatment

The easiest patients to manage are those with truncal vagotomy and drainage procedures. Taking down the gastro-jejunostomy[78,97] should cure or improve dumping in over 80% of patients. Reconstruction of the pylorus produces similar results.[98,99,100] After gastrectomy, a number of procedures have been advocated for dumping. The simplest and probably the best is to convert the drainage procedure to a 45 cm Roux-en-Y gastro-jejunostomy. The delay in liquid emptying after this procedure is thought to be due to myoelectrical abnormalities within the Roux limb itself causing a degree of retrograde contraction. The delay in emptying of solids is probably a result of the vagotomy leading to a degree of gastric atony and loss of the antral prepulsive force to propel solid food into the small intestine.[101,102] Reversal of the proximal 10 cm of the jejunal limb to create an antiperistaltic interposition is unnecessary and may lead to further stasis and dilatation of the interposed segment. This will worsen any symptoms of gastric retention. The author has had to undertake two operations to remove a proximal interposed jejunal segment and this is the finding of others.[103] The interposition of a segment of upper jejunum between the gastric remnant and the duodenum has been advocated. Both isoperistaltic and antiperistaltic interpositions have been used, but these procedures can be associated with serious complications and the long-term success rate is variable.[104,105] The author has had to remove one isoperistaltic jejunal interposition because of stenosis and ulceration at the duodeno-jejunal anastomosis. A 45 cm Roux-en-Y conversion was carried out.

Diarrhoea

Alteration in bowel habit occurs in the majority of patients who undergo truncal vagotomy and in most this is a change from constipation to a more regular habit with one or two motions per day. However 11% of patients following truncal vagotomy and pyloroplasty had continuous diarrhoea that significantly interfered with their lifestyle.[106] A further 20% of patients will have episodic attacks of diarrhoea more than once a week.

The aetiology of post-vagotomy diarrhoea remains poorly understood. Gastric stasis, abnormal small bowel motility, impaired biliary and pancreatic function have all been incriminated. Malabsorption, bacterial colonisation of the proximal small bowel and increased faecal excretion of bile salts and acid may all be contributing factors.[107,108] Patients who have had a cholecystectomy are more likely to develop post-vagotomy diarrhoea and have a particularly severe form.

Diarrhoea may be a component of the dumping syndrome especially in patients after gastrectomy, but in many post-vagotomy patients it is unassociated with dumping. The stool consistency varies from watery to soft and in its severe form may be explosive in onset without warning, thus leading to incontinence. Patients may be unable to distinguish between the urge to pass flatus and a bowel motion. Occasionally symptoms will be so pronounced that weight loss and malnutrition become apparent.

Investigation of these patients includes the measurement of faecal fats and vitamin B12 level. A barium enema should be carried out to rule out disorders of the colon and if bacterial overgrowth is suspected, the diagnosis may be confirmed by bacteriological examination of jejunal aspirates or by using the C14 glycocholate breath test.

Medical treatment

The treatment of post-vagotomy diarrhoea begins with dietary manipulation and in particular, the avoidance of refined carbohydrates and foods with a high fluid content. Restriction of fluid intake with meals is occasionally of benefit. Cholestyramine taken morning and evening may be of benefit especially in patients who have also had a cholecystectomy. There are however long-term complications such as megaloblastic anaemia due to folate deficiency in patients on long-term cholestyramine therapy. Codeine and diphenoxylate (Lomotil) may also be useful. Loperamide taken in small doses has proved to be successful. The treatment starts with 2 mg every morning and increases in 2 mg increments. It is uncommon for patients to require more than 4 mg a day.[109]

Surgical treatment

Closure of a gastro-jejunostomy will improve or cure diarrhoea in 80% of patients.[78] A similar improvement is seen with reconstruction of the pylorus.[80,98,100] Various intestinal interpositions to act as an intestinal brake have been advocated. The use of a 10 cm antiperistaltic jejunal segment placed 100 cm distal to the duodeno-jejunal junction has been described.[110] The reversed segment produces a delay in the passage of contents through the small bowel. A modification of this procedure using autostaples and a 20 cm segment of jejunum has been described by Poth,[111] which does not twist or rotate the mesenteric vessels. The author has treated 6 patients, three with each of the above-mentioned procedures and none has had a satisfactory result. All have undergone further surgery with removal of the reversed segment. This is also the experience of other authors.[112] The operation that has proved effective is the reverse ileal onlay graft.[112] The author has now used this procedure in 41 patients with improvement in the diarrhoea of 35. In one patient a postoperative leak from the onlay graft necessitated its removal. In the remaining 5 patients, the diarrhoea has not worsened and no other long-term complication has developed to date.

Small stomach syndrome

This usually occurs only after a high subtotal gastrectomy in which 80–90% of the stomach is removed. Non-operative treatment consists of frequent small meals, antispasmodics and mineral and vitamin replacement. Patients may also require fine-bore nasoenteric nutritional supplementation. In a small number of patients with uncontrollable symptoms, surgery may have to be considered. The reservoir jejunal interposition described by Cuschieri, a modification of the Hunt-Lawrence, is probably the procedure of choice.[113] Long-term follow-up of these patients is required as there is a tendency for the jejunal limb to elongate over several years and this can lead to stasis and ulceration.

Summary

Revisional surgery for patients with failure or complications of primary upper gastrointestinal surgery is time consuming, technically difficult and carries with it a higher morbidity and mortality rate. It is important not to rush into further surgery before developing a good rapport with the patient. The patient must be involved in the decision making process and have a realistic expectation of the outcome. When the original operation has failed, the results of remedial surgery are rarely as good as those after primary surgery. In general, the greater the number of previous procedures, the less is the likelihood of the patient becoming asymptomatic although many can be significantly improved. Careful pre-operative assessment of the patient and his/her symptoms will identify those patients in whom further surgery may be of benefit. The surgeon carrying out revisional surgery must be capable of carrying out all the remedial operations. The final decision about which procedure will be the most effective in any individual patient may well have to be made at the time of surgery when the surgeon can determine exactly what is capable of being carried out, both in terms of the abnormal anatomy and his own technical limitations. A successful outcome cannot be guaranteed but those with a significant improvement in their symptoms are frequently grateful. Converting a patient who has a gastric or oesophageal disablement into someone who can enjoy the simple pleasures of life, albeit with a few residual symptoms is also rewarding to the surgeon.

References

1. Leading article. 'Dumping' after gastrectomy. Lancet 1949; 2:613.

2. Pulvertaft CN. The results of partial gastrectomy for peptic ulcer. Lancet 1952; 1:225–31.

3. Busman DC, Munting JDK. Results of highly selective vagotomy in a non-university teaching hospital. Br J Surg 1982; 69:620–4.

4. Stanton PD, Anderson JR. Results of surgery for duodenal ulcer: assessment by patients. Br J Surg 1991; 78:815–7.

5. Adami H, Enander L, Ingvar C et al. Clinical results of 229 patients with duodenal ulcer 1–6 years after highly selective vagotomy. Br J Surg 1980; 67:29–32.

6. Visick AH. A study of the failure after gastrectomy. Ann R Coll Surg 1948; 3:266–84.

7. Johnstone FRC, Holubitsky MD, Debas HT. Postgastrectomy problems in patients with personality defects: the 'Albatross' syndrome. Can Med Ass J 1967; 96:1559–64.

8. Aagard J, Amdrup E, Aminoff D et al. A clinical and socio-medical investigation of patients 5 years after surgical treatment for duodenal ulcer. I. Behavioural consequences and psychological symptoms. Scand J Gastroenterol 1981; 16:361–8.

9. Stirling MC, Orringer MB. Surgical treatment after the failed antireflux operation. J Thorac Cardiovasc Surg 1986; 92:667–72.

10. Menguy R. A modified fundoplication which preserves the ability to belch. Surgery 1978; 84:301–7.

11. Guarner V, Martinez N, Gavino JF. Ten year evaluation of posterior fundoplasty in the treatment of gastro-esophageal reflux: long-term and comparative study of 135 patients. Am J Surg 1980; 130:200–3.

12. Bushkin FL, Nenstein CL, Parker TH et al. Nissen fundoplication for reflux peptic esophagitis. Ann Surg 1977; 185:672–7.

13. Olson RC, Lasser RB, Ansel H. The 'Slipped' Nissen. Gastroenterology 1976; 70:924.

14. Herrington JL, Meecham PW, Hunter RM. Gastric ulceration after fundic wrapping: vagal nerve entrapment, a possible causative factor. Ann Surg 1982; 195:574–81.

15. Maher JW, Cerda JJ. The role of gastric stasis in the genesis of gastric ulceration following fundoplication. World J Surg 1982; 6:794–9.

16. Hill LD, Ilves R, Stevenson JK et al. Re-operation for disruption and recurrence after Nissen fundoplication. Arch Surg 1979; 114:542–8.

17. Nakhgevany KB, Parra LA. Gastric left ventricular fistula: an unusual complication of Nissen fundoplication. Contemp Surg 1983; 23:57–60.

18. Mackie CR, Hulks G, Cuschion A. Enterogastric reflux and gastric clearance of refluxate in normal subjects and in patients with and without bile vomiting following peptic ulcer surgery. Ann Surg 1986; 204:537–42.

19. Mackie CR, Wiskey ML, Cuschien A. Milk 99mTc – EHIDA test for entero-gastric bile reflux. Br J Surg 1982; 69:101–4.

 20. Skinner DB. Surgical management after failed antireflux operations. World J Surg 1992; 16:359–63.

21. Collard JM, Verstraete L, Ott JB et al. Clinical radiological and functional results of remedial antireflux operations. Int Surg 1993; 78:2980–306.

22. Siewert JR, Stein HJ, Feussner H. Reoperations after failed antireflux procedures. Ann Chirurg Gynaecol 1995; 84:122–8.

23. Rieger NA, Jamieson GG, Britten-Jones R et al. Reoperation after failed antireflux surgery. Br J Surg 1994; 81:1159–61.

24. Stein HJ, Feussner H, Siewert JR. Failure of antireflux surgery: causes and management strategies. Am J Surg 1996; 171:36–40.

25. Ellis FH, Gibb SP, Heatley GJ. Reoperation after failed antireflux surgery. Review of 101 cases. Eur J Cardiothorac Surg 1996; 10:225–32.

26. Lim JK, Moisidis E, Munro WS et al. Re-operation for failed anti-reflux surgery. Aust NZ J Surg 1996; 66:731–3.

27. Deschamps C, Traslek VF, Allen MS et al. Long term results after reoperation for failed anti-reflux procedures. J Thorac Cardiovasc Surg 1997; 113:545–50.

28. Collis JL. Gastroplasty. Thorax 1961; 16:197–206.

29. Pearson FG, Langer B, Henderson RD. Gastroplasty and Belsey hiatus repair: an operation for the management of peptic stricture with acquired short esophagus. J Thorac Cardiovasc Surg 1971; 61:50–63.

30. Orringer MB, Sloan H. Complications and failings of the combined Collis–Belsey operation. J Thorac Cardiovasc Surg 1977; 74:726–31.

31. Pearson FG, Cooper JD, Nelms JM. Gastroplasty and fundoplication in the management of complex reflux problems. J Thorac Cardiovasc Surg 1978; 76:6650–72.

32. DeMeester TR, Johnson LF, Kent AH. Evaluation of current operations from the prevention of gastroesophageal reflux. Ann Surg 1974; 180:5511–25.

33. Pearson FG, Cooper JD, Patterson GA *et al.* Gastroplasty and fundoplication for complex reflux problems. Ann Surg 1987; 206:473–81.

34. Herrington JL, Mody B. Total duodenal diversion for the treatment of reflux esophagitis uncontrolled by repeated antireflux procedures. Ann Surg 1976; 183:636–44.

35. Royston CMS, Dowling BL, Spencer J. Antrectomy with Roux-en-Y anastomosis in the treatment of peptic oesophagitis with stricture. Br J Surg 1975; 62:605–7.

36. Perniceni T, Gaget B, Fekete R. Total duodenal diversion in the treatment of complicated peptic oesophagitis. Br J Surg 1988; 75:1108–11.

37. Orringer MB, Sloan H. Esophagectomy without thoractomy. J Thorac Cardiovasc Surg 1978; 76:643–54.

38. Orringer MB, Marshall B, Stirling MC. Transhiatal esophagectomy for benign and malignant disease. J Thorac Cardiovasc Surg 1993; 105:265–77.

39. Orringer MB, Stirling MC. Cervical esophagogastric anastomosis for benign disease: functional results. J Thorac Cardiovasc Surg 1988; 96:887–93.

40. Beik AI, Jaffray B, Anderson JR. Transhiatal oesophagectomy: a comparison of alternative techniques in 68 patients. JR Coll Surg Edinb 1996; 41:25–9.

41. Polk HC Jr. Jejunal interposition for reflux esophagitis and esophageal stricture unresponsive to valvuloplasty. World J Surg 1980; 4:731–6.

42. Wright C, Cuschien A. Jejunal interposition for benign esophageal disease. Ann Surg 1987; 205:54–60.

43. Postlethwait RW. Colonic interposition as esophageal substitution. Surg Gynaecol Obstet 1983; 145:377–83.

44. Wilkins EW Jr. Long-segment colon substitution for the esophagus. Ann Surg 1980; 192:722–5.

45. Curet Scott MJ, Ferguson MK, Little AG *et al.* Colon interposition for benign esophageal disease. Surgery 1987; 102:568–74.

46. Cerfolio RJ, Allen MS, Deschamps C *et al.* Esophageal replacement by colon interposition. Ann Thorac Surg 1995; 59:1382–4.

47. Johnson SB, MeMeester TR. Esophagectomy for benign disease: use of the colon. Adv Surg 1994; 27:317–34.

48. Peters JH, Kaner WK, Crookes PF *et al.* Esophageal resection with colon interposition for end-stage achalasia. Arch Surg 1995; 130:632–7.

49. Goligher JC, Hill GL, Kennedy TF *et al.* Proximal gastric vagotomy without drainage for duodenal ulcer: results after 5–8 years. Br J Surg 1978; 65:145–51.

50. Stoddard CJ, Vassilakis JS, Duthie HL. Highly selective vagotomy or truncal vagotomy and pyloroplasty for chronic duodenal ulceration: a randomized, prospective clinical study. Br J Surg 1978; 65:793–6.

51. Flook D, Stoddard CJ. Gastro-oesophageal reflux and oesophagitis before and after vagotomy for duodenal ulcer. Br J Surg 1985; 72:804–7.

52. DeMeester TR, Fuchs KH, Ball CS *et al.* Experimental and clinic results with proximal end-to-end duodenojejunostomy for pathological duodenogastric reflux. Ann Surg 1987; 206:414–26.

53. Warren RJ, Marshall BJ. Unidentified curved bacilli on gastric epithelium in active chronic gastritis. Lancet 1983; 1:1273–5.

54. Chaudhuri TK, Shiraqzi SS, Condon RE. Radioisotope scan: a possible aid in differentiating retained gastric antrum from Zollinger-Ellison syndrome in patients with recurrent peptic ulcer. Gastroenterology 1973; 65:697.

55. Le Quesne LP, Hobsley M, Hand BH. The dumping syndrome: factors responsible for the symptoms. Br Med J 1960; 1:141.

56. Small WP. The recurrence of ulceration after surgery for duodenal ulcer. JR Coll Surg Edinb 1964; 9:255–78.

57. Goligher JC, Pulvertaft CN, Irvin TT *et al.* Five-to-eight – year results of truncal vagotomy and pyloroplasty for duodenal ulcer. Br Med J 1972; 1:7–13.

58. Nelson PG. Surgery for duodenal ulcer: a comparison of the results of four standard operations. Med J Aust 1968; 2:522–8.

59. Price WE, Grizzle JE, Postlethwaite RW *et al.* Results of operation for duodenal ulcer. Surg Gynecol Obstet 1970; 131:233–44.

60. Anderson D, Amdrup E, Hostrup H *et al.* The Aarhus County vagotomy trial: trends in the problem of recurrent ulcer after parietal cell vagotomy and selective gastric vagotomy with drainage. World J Surg 1982; 6:86–92.

61. Blackett RL, Johnston D. Recurrent ulceration after highly selective vagotomy for duodenal ulcer. Br J Surg 1981; 68:706–10.

62. Knight CD Jr, van Heerden JA, Kelly KA. Proximal gastric vagotomy: update. Ann Surg 1983; 197:22–6.

63. Jess P, Christiansen J, Svendsen LB. Antrectomy as treatment of recurrence after vagotomy for duodenal ulcer. Am J Surg 1979; 137:338–41.

64. Kennedy T, Green WER. Stomal and recurrent ulceration: Medical or surgical management? Am J Surg 1980; 139:18–21.

65. Stuart M, Hoerr SO. Recurrent peptic ulcer following primary operations with vagotomy for

duodenal ulcer: results of surgical treatment in 42 patients. Arch Surg 1971; 103:129–32.

66. Cleator GM, Holnbitsky IB, Harrison RC. Anastomotic ulceration. Ann Surg 1974; 179:339.

67. Stabile BE, Passaro E Jr. Recurrent peptic ulceration. Gastroenterology 1976; 70:124–35.

68. Dixon MF, O'Connor HJ, Axon ATR *et al*. Reflux gastritis: distinct histopathological entity. J Clin Pathol 1986; 39:524–30.

69. Witt TR, Roseman DL, Banner BF. The role of the gastric antrum in the pathogenesis of reflux gastritis. J Surg Res 1970; 26:220–3.

70. Ritchie WP Jr. Alkaline reflux gastritis: an objective assessment of its diagnosis and treatment. Ann Surg 1980; 192:288–98.

71. Keighley MRB, Asquith P, Alexander-Williams J. Duodenogastric reflux: a cause of gastric mucosal hyperaemia and symptoms after operations for peptic ulceration. Gut 1975; 16:28–32.

72. Dewar EP, Dixon MF, Johnston D. Bile reflux and degree of gastritis after highly selective vagotomy, truncal vagotomy, and partial gastrectomy for duodenal ulcer. World J Surg 1983; 7:743–50.

73. Meshkinpour H, Elashoff J, Stewart H *et al*. Effect of cholestyramine on the symptoms of reflux gastritis. A randomized double-blind crossover study. Gastroenterology 1977; 73:441–3.

74. Nicolai JJ, Speelman P, Tytgat GN *et al*. Comparison of the combination of cholestyramine/alginate with placebo in the treatment of post-gastrectomy biliary reflux gastritis. Eur J Pharmacol 1981; 21:189–94.

75. Romano M, Razandi M, Ivey KS. Effect of sucralfate and its components on taurocholate-induced damage to rat gastric mucosal cells in tissue culture. Dig Dis Sci 1990; 35:467–76.

76. Buch KL, Weinstein WM, Hill TA *et al*. Sucralfate therapy in patient with symptoms of alkaline reflux gastritis. Am J Med 1985; 79:49–54.

77. Stefaniwsky AB, Tint GS, Speck J *et al*. Urodeoxycholic acid treatment of bile reflux gastritis. Gastroenterology 1985; 89:1000–4.

78. Green R, Spencer A, Kennedy T. Closure of gastrojejunostomy for the relief of post-vagotomy symptoms. Br J Surg 1978; 65:161–3.

79. Koruth NM, Krukowski ZH, Matheson N. Pyloric reconstruction. Br J Surg 1985; 72:808–10.

80. Martin CJ, Kennedy T. Reconstruction of the pylorus. World J Surg 1985; 6:221–5.

81. Hocking MP, Vogel SB, Falasca CA *et al*. Delayed gastric emptying of liquids and solids following Roux Y biliary diversion. Ann Surg 1981; 914:494–501.

82. Ritchie WP Jr. Alkaline reflux gastritis: late results of a controlled clinical trial. Ann Surg 1986; 203:537–44.

83. Kennedy T, Green R. Roux diversion for bile reflux following gastric surgery. Br J Surg 1978; 65:323–5.

84. Herrington JL, Sawyers JL, Whitehead WA. Surgical management of reflux gastritis. Ann Surg 1974; 180:526–37.

85. Weidner MG, Bond AG, Gobbel WG *et al*. The dumping syndrome. I. Studies in patients after gastric surgery. Gastroenterology 1959; 37:188–93.

86. Scott HW, Weidner MG, Shull J *et al*. The dumping syndrome. II. Further investigations of etiology in patients and experimental animals. Gastroenterology 1959; 37:194–9.

87. Bloom SR, Royston CMS, Thompson JPS. Enteroglucagon release in the dumping syndrome. Lancet 1972; 2:789–91.

88. Blackburn AM, Christotides ND, Ghatei MA *et al*. Elevation of plasma neurotensin in the dumping syndrome. ClinSci 1980; 59:237–43.

89. Sagor GR, Bryant MG, Ghatei MA *et al*. Release of vasoactive intestinal polypeptide in the dumping syndrome. Br Med J 1981; 282:507–10.

90. Adrian TE, Long RG, Fuessl HS *et al*. Plasma peptide YY (PYY) in dumping syndrome. Dig Dis Sci 1985; 30:1145–8.

91. Jenkins DSA, Leeds AR, Gassull MA *et al*. Decrease in postprandial insulin and glucose concentrations by guar and pectin. Ann Intern Med 1977; 86:20–23.

92. Jenkins DSA, Leeds AR, Gassull MA *et al*. Unabsorbable carbohydrates and diabetes: decrease in post-prandial hyperglycaemia. Lancet 1976; 2:172–4.

93. Harju E, Larmi TKI. Efficacy of guar gum in preventing the dumping syndrome. J Parenter Enteral Nutrition 1983; 7:470–2.

94. Long RG, Adrian TE, Bloom SR. Somatostatin and the jumping syndrome. Br Med J 1985; 290:886–9.

95. Hopman WPM, Wolberink RGJ, Lamers CBHW *et al*. Treatment of the dumping syndrome with a somatostatin analogue SMS. 201-995. Ann Surg 1988; 207:155–9.

96. Primrose JN, Johnston D. Somatostatin analogue SMS 201-995 (octreotide) as a possible solution to the dumping syndrome after gastrectomy or vagotomy. Br J Surg 1989; 76:140–4.

97. McMahon MJ, Johnston D, Hill GT *et al*. Treatment of severe side effects after vagotomy and gastroenterostomy by closure of gastroenterostomy without pyloroplasty. Br Med J 1978; 1:7–8.

98. Frederiksen HJB, Johansen TS, Christiansen PM. Post vagotomy diarrhoea and dumping treated with reconstruction of the pylorus. Scand J Gastroenterol 1980; 15:245–8.

99. Ebied FH, Ralphs DNL, Hobsley M *et al*. Dumping symptoms after vagotomy treated by reversal of pyloroplasty. Br J Surg 1982; 69:527–8.

100. Cheadle WG, Baker PR, Cuschieri A. Pyloric reconstruction for severe vasomotor dumping after vagotomy and pyloroplasty. Ann Surg 1985; 202:568–72.

101. Karlstrom L, Kelly KA. Ectopic jejunal pacemakers and gastric emptying after Roux gastrectomy: effect of intestinal pacing. Surgery 1989; 106:867–71.

102. Mattias JR, Fernandez A, Sninsky CA *et al.* Nausea, vomiting, and abdominal pain after Roux-en-Y anastomosis: motility of the jejunal limb. Gastroenterology 1985; 88:101–7.

103. Vagel SB, Hocking MP, Woodward ER. Clinical and radionuclide evaluation of Roux-Y diversion for postgastrectomy dumping. Ann J Surg 1988; 155:57–62.

104. Herrington JL Jr. Reversed jejunal segments one year after operation. Ann J Surg 1970; 119:340–2.

105. Cuschieri A. Isoperistaltic and antiperistaltic jejunal interposition for the dumping syndrome. A comparative study. J R Coll Surg Edin 1977; 22:319–42.

106. Raimes SA, Smirniotis V, Wheldon EJ *et al.* Post vagotomy diarrhoea put into perspective. Lancet 1986; 2:851–3.

107. Ballinger WF. Postvagotomy changes in the small intestine. Am J Surg 1967; 114:382–7.

108. Browning GG, Buchan KA, Mackay C. Small bowel flora and bowel habit studied at intervals following vagotomy and drainage. Br J Surg 1972; 59:908–9.

109. Wayman J, Raimes SA. Benign ulceration of the stomach and duodenum. In: Griffin SM, Raimes SA (eds). Upper gastrointestinal surgery, 1st edn. W.B. Saunders, 1997, pp. 351–2.

110. Sawyers JL, Herrington JL Jr. Treatment of postgastrectomy syndromes. Am Surg 1980; 46:201–7.

111. Herrington JL Jr, Sawyers JL. Remedial operations. In: Nyhus LM, Wastell C (eds). Surgery of the stomach and duodenum, 4th edn. Little, Brown 1986, pp. 550–5.

112. Cuschieri A. Surgical management of severe intractable postvagotomy diarrhoea. Br J Surg 1986; 73:981–4.

113. Cuschieri A. Long term evaluation of a reservoir jejunal interposition with an isoperistaltic conduit in the management of patients with a small stomach syndrome. Br J Surg 1982; 69:386–8.

14 Oesophageal emergencies

Samuel M. Dresner
S. Michael Griffin

INTRODUCTION

While the majority of oesophageal pathology has an insidious natural history, a number of conditions that affect this organ present in a dramatic manner requiring urgent medical attention. Historically, most oesophageal emergencies have resulted from spontaneous rupture, the ingestion of foreign bodies or variceal haemorrhage, although with the wider use of diagnostic and therapeutic endoscopic techniques over the last 50 years iatrogenic damage has become an increasing problem. The diverse presentations that encompass the spectrum of such oesophageal disease together with the different age groups affected have spread the management of oesophageal emergencies among a wide group of clinicians. This distribution, as well as the relative rarity of some oesophageal pathologies, has meant that in general no single clinical group or institution has amassed a large experience in their management. Critical interpretation of the literature regarding oesophageal emergencies is therefore difficult, particularly as many reports contain relatively small numbers of patients accumulated over long time periods and there are few well conducted randomised trials. This situation may improve however, as changes in the structure of service provision currently underway for upper gastrointestinal disease may afford the necessary multidisciplinary cover for all oesophageal emergencies.

This chapter will focus upon the diagnosis and management of oesophageal rupture and perforation, injuries induced as the result of ingestion of noxious agents and finally the management of food bolus and foreign body ingestion. Variceal and non-variceal oesophageal haemorrhage together with the management of specific postoperative complications related to elective oesophageal resection are discussed elsewhere.

Rupture and perforation of the oesophagus

Definitions

Perforation or rupture of the oesophagus may occur as the result of a variety of traumatic insults and it is important to clarify the different aetiological aspects of such events when discussing the management of these injuries. Historically, the literature on the subject has used a number of interchangeable terms to describe such oesophageal injuries and this has led to considerable confusion. Indeed, even the terms perforation and rupture are ambiguous as perforation is often used to describe an iatrogenic insult in an already diseased organ, whereas rupture is a term more commonly associated with a violent injury usually in an otherwise normal oesophagus. Aetiological factors described in the development of oesophageal rupture and perforation are listed in **Table 14.1**. As there are a myriad of aetiologies no classification system is ideal, although in the broadest terms there are four main categories of injury that cause oesophageal tears.

1.	*Spontaneous rupture (Boerhaave's syndrome)*	
	Post-emetic (80–90%)	Dietary indiscretion
		Ethanol excess
		Antabuse
		Hyperemesis gravidarum
	Barogenic	Parturition
		Defaecation
		Heavy weight lifting
		Heimlich manoeuvre
	Neurological disorders	Seizures
		Intracranial tumours
	Underlying disease	Infection (HSV/TB/HIV)
		Malignancy
		Ulceration (Z–E syndrome/Barrett's oesophagus)
2.	*Iatrogenic perforation*	
	Intraluminal injury	Flexible/rigid endoscopy
		Bougienage and pneumatic dilatation
		Variceal sclerotherapy/ligation
		Laser/photodynamic therapy
		Endoprosthesis insertion
		Endotracheal/nasogastric intubation
	Operative injury	Antireflux surgery
		Cardiomyotomy
		Anterior cervical spine surgery
		Thoracic aneurysm repair
		Tube thoracostomy
		Radical pneumonectomy
3.	*Traumatic perforation*	
	Penetrating	Stab injuries
		Gunshot wounds
	Blunt	Blast/compressed air injuries
		Road traffic accidents
		Cervical spine fracture/disclocation
4.	*Ingestion injuries*	
	Corrosive agents	Acid/alkali
	Foreign bodies	

Table 14.1 *Aetiology of oesophageal rupture and perforation*

1. Spontaneous oesophageal rupture, mainly encompassing the classical post-emetic 'Boerhaave's syndrome', although rupture may rarely occur spontaneously in association with oesophageal malignancy or infection.
2. Iatrogenic perforation resulting from various endoscopic or surgical interventions.
3. Traumatic perforation complicating penetrating or blunt external insults.
4. Perforation in association with the ingestion of corrosive agents or foreign bodies.

Natural history

The oesophagus lacks a serosal layer and so when a perforation or rupture involves the full thickness of the organ, retained gastric contents, saliva, digestive enzymes and microorganisms enter the mediastinum producing severe mediastinitis. The middle third of the thoracic oesophagus is adjacent to the right pleura while the lower third is in contact with the left pleura such that injuries at these specific sites will eventually lead to involvement of the respective pleural cavity. Once the parietal pleura has been breached mediastinal emphysema and fluid can contribute to the development of a hydropneumothorax, which if sufficiently large may compound cardiorespiratory insufficiency.

The site of the injury together with the degree of mediastinal contamination will determine the overall clinical features. Cervical perforations rarely produce mediastinitis unless infection tracks down the fascial planes or the retro-oesophageal space into the posterior mediastinum[1] and more commonly present with a localised perioesophageal abscess.[2] In contrast, thoracic perforations and ruptures are usually associated with widespread mediastinal dissemination of polymicrobial bacterial fluid as the result of negative intrathoracic pressure. The natural history of this continued process is fluid sequestration, sepsis, multi-organ failure and death.[3] Occasionally, if an injury remains localised, the clinical features of sepsis and shock may be absent and the presentation may be subacute (over 24 hours to 2 weeks) with chest pain and dyspnoea the predominant features. Perforation of the intra-abdominal oesophagus, as with perforation of peptic ulcer disease, usually rapidly progresses to peritonitis and death if left untreated.

The aetiology, diagnosis and management of spontaneous rupture, iatrogenic perforation and traumatic damage are presented in turn with specific reference to each type of injury. The overall management of the ingestion of corrosive agents and foreign bodies will be discussed separately.

Spontaneous rupture of the oesophagus

Historical perspective

Although there is some debate as to whether Alexander the Great died as the result of oesophageal rupture,[4] it was the Dutch physician Hermann Boerhaave who described the first recorded case of spontaneous oesophageal rupture in 1724.[5] To this day the clinical features of this condition continue to carry his name eponymously as 'Boerhaave's syndrome'. In 1946, Barrett[6] summarised Boerhaave's description of the death of Baron Jan van Wassenaer, Grand Admiral of the Dutch Fleet, a 50-year-old notorious glutton who practised the Roman habit of autoemesis by taking multiple doses of ipecacuanha to induce vomiting. Boerhaave was called to see the admiral after a particularly violent bout of vomiting during which he complained of severe chest pain and exclaimed that he had felt something burst and was sure that he would die. Over the next 18 hours the admiral became progressively more pale, tachycardic and tachypnoeic and eventually died. Postmortem examination demonstrated a rupture in an otherwise normal-looking oesophagus with roast duck and medicine within the left thoracic cavity! From 1723 onwards there were many further reports of similar cases, all uniformly fatal, until Barrett himself reported the first early diagnosis and successful surgical repair.[6]

Aetiology and pathophysiology

Although Boerhaave's syndrome classically follows prolonged or forceful vomiting, other entities that cause a sudden rise in intraoesophageal pressure such as weight lifting, defaecation or the Heimlich manoeuvre[7] may also cause oesophageal rupture, leading some authorities to describe such injuries as barogenic perforations.[8] Historical studies produced experimental ruptures similar to those encountered clinically with an average intraluminal pressure of 5 psi[9] although it is believed that the abruptness with which the rise in pressure occurs is more significant than the ultimate level of pressure attained.

Spontaneous oesophageal rupture most commonly affects the lower oesophagus as this area is entirely composed of smooth muscle fibres that spread outwards and constitute a comparatively thinner and weaker mural structure. In nearly all cases of spontaneous rupture the area of greatest susceptibility is the left posterolateral area of this region with most large series confirming this location as the commonest site of injury.[10,11,12,13,14] Most spontaneous oesophageal tears occur in the longitudinal axis (**Fig. 14.1**) although the original description by Boerhaave was of a transverse oesophageal injury.[5] The length of the rupture varies from 0.6 to 8.9 cm with the mucosal tear longer than the underlying muscular tear. The predilection for the left site is unclear although it is believed that the lack of adjacent supporting structures together with the longitudinal orientation of muscle bundles may contribute. Some authors have additionally suggested that inherent oesophageal abnormalities such as deficiencies in the muscularis mucosa[15] or motility disorders[16] may play a role, although whether they pre-exist oesophageal rupture or simply develop in response to it is unclear.

In virtually all series males are the gender predominantly affected, usually with a median age of 40–60 years, although spontaneous oesophageal rupture has been reported in children and infants.[17] There is often a strong history of previous dietary over-indulgence or excessive alcohol consumption[13] and frequently such injuries follow the ingestion of a heavy meal with alcohol. It has been suggested that the higher incidence of oesophageal rupture in alcoholics may relate to the correspondingly higher incidence of chronic oesophagitis in this group.[18]

Clinical presentation

Spontaneous oesophageal rupture usually presents with the classical Mackler's triad[9] of vomiting or retching followed by severe chest pain and the subsequent

Figure 14.1
Endoscopic appearances of the longitudinal tear seen with spontaneous oesophageal rupture.

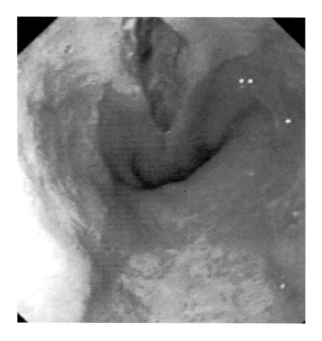

development of surgical emphysema (**Table 14.2**). These features are not always present, however, and over-reliance on Mackler's triad may lead to diagnostic delay.[8] Diagnosis based on the history alone is often difficult as 20–45% of patients have no antecedent history of vomiting[19] and the clinical features vary widely depending on the exact site of perforation.[20] A total of 80–100% of cases present with pain which, dependent on the exact site of rupture, is variable in location. Typically, the onset of rupture produces sudden, excruciating epigastric and retrosternal pain described variously as burning, crushing, knife-like tearing apart or bursting. The pain is usually located in, or radiates to, the left lower chest and is markedly exacerbated by coughing or deep inspiration, indicative of its pleuritic origin.

One of the earliest signs of spontaneous rupture is the development of mediastinal and subcutaneous emphysema. As the effects of the injury progress to a chemical and septic mediastinitis together with involvement of the pleural cavity cardiorespiratory compromise ensues. Depending on the time course, shock is not uncommon. At this stage signs may include fever, atrial fibrillation, tachypnoea, cyanosis and upper abdominal rigidity with diaphragmatic splinting. Hamman's sign (the sound of a crunch as the heart beats against air-filled tissues) has been reported.[21] Dyspnoea and respiratory distress may be further compounded by the development of unilateral or bilateral pleural effusions, pneumothoraces or hydrothorax with secondary collapse and consolidation.

1.	Vomiting or retching
2.	Chest pain
3.	Subcutaneous emphysema

Table 14.2 *Mackler's triad*

Diagnosis

Spontaneous rupture of the oesophagus is often initially mistaken for a variety of conditions the most common of which are listed in Table 14.3. A complete and accurate history is not always forthcoming, and the variety of settings in which spontaneous rupture occurs (Table 14.1) may prove misleading. The distinction between perforated peptic ulcer disease and Boerhaave's syndrome may be difficult but it is important, as the former requires a laparotomy and the latter a thoracotomy. Myocardial infarction is also frequently confused with spontaneous rupture and this can also lead to potentially disastrous therapeutic consequences; it has been noted that the coronary care unit is a dangerous place to be for the patient with non-cardiac chest pain.[22]

The presentation of Boerhaave's syndrome may also be confused with acute pancreatitis as both often occur on a background of alcohol abuse and present with vomiting, pleural effusions, and chest/abdominal pain, although a serum amylase will differentiate the majority of cases. Similarly, the respiratory symptoms associated with spontaneous oesophageal rupture may be confused with conditions such as pulmonary embolus, dissecting aortic aneurysm and spontaneous pneumothorax and pneumo-mediastinum. Above all a heightened awareness and index of suspicion as to the possibility of oesophageal rupture mimicking such conditions is required together with the systematic use of the diagnostic investigations outlined below.

Plain radiographs

The most important initial investigation for suspected oesophageal rupture is plain radiography. An urgent erect chest film will yield the most information[23] and experienced radiologists will suspect the diagnosis in over 90% of cases.[2,11,24] In rare cases of spontaneous cervical oesophageal perforation a lateral radiograph of the neck may be useful. Typical chest radiograph findings include pleural effusions, pneumo-mediastinum, subcutaneous emphysema, hydrothorax and

---

Myocardial infarction

Pancreatitis

Perforated peptic ulcer

Dissecting aortic aneurysm

Pneumonia

Spontaneous pneumothorax

Pulmonary embolism

Pericarditis

Gastric volvulus

Diaphragmatic hernia

Mesenteric thrombosis

Table 14.3 *Diseases commonly mistaken for spontaneous oesophageal rupture*

Figure 14.2
(a) and (b) Typical chest radiograph findings following spontaneous oesphageal perforation.

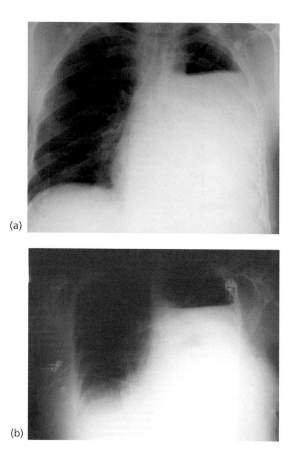

(a)

(b)

hydropneumothorax (**Fig. 14.2**).[19] Pleural effusions are found in up to 90% of chest films and an associated unilateral pneumothorax is present in the majority of these cases. Subcutaneous emphysema and mediastinal air are found less commonly and are frequently overlooked on initial films. The so-called 'V-sign of Naclerio' – mediastinal widening due to retrocardiac emphysematous dissection of fascial plains – may be an early radiographic sign.[25] The exact location of the rupture and the time interval following the insult will determine the radiographic features. Soft tissue and mediastinal emphysema can take up to 1 hour to develop and pleural effusions, particularly if sympathetic, may take several hours. In cases of intra-abdominal rupture a pneumo-peritoneum may be present.

Contrast radiography

Delays in the development of radiographic signs together with the fact that plain chest radiograph appearances will remain normal in up to 12% of patients[19] mandates further investigations if spontaneous rupture is suspected. Contrast studies are the investigation of choice and should be performed at the earliest opportunity following resuscitation and stabilisation. Swallows should be undertaken in the upright and lateral decubitus position and will demonstrate the exact site and extent of the rupture together with the size of any associated abscess cavity (**Fig. 14.3**). With the advent of water-soluble contrast media there has been a

Figure 14.3
(a) and (b) Contrast swallows demonstrating left-sided extravasation following spontaneous oesophageal perforation.

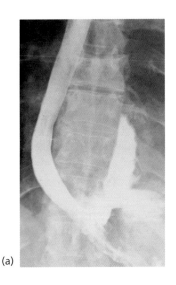

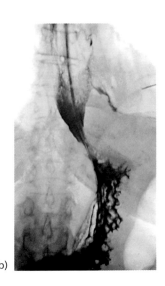

(a)   (b)

reluctance to perform barium swallows in such circumstances because of the potential risk of exacerbating mediastinal inflammation. Water-soluble agents such as gastrograffin, however, may pass through the oesophagus too quickly and many authors continue to favour the use of more viscous barium for such studies.[26] Certainly water-soluble agents may fail to detect up to 22%[27] of oesophageal ruptures and perforations and thus if an initial water-soluble study is negative it should be repeated with barium.

Despite such considerations, contrast radiography may continue to give a false-negative result in 11%[28] to 25%[29] of cases of transmural oesophageal tears. False-negative results, irrespective of the contrast medium employed, may be due to blockage of the site of rupture by oedema, clots or food particles. It is important to obtain oblique views if the anteroposterior and lateral projections are negative to ensure that a leak is not being hidden on the film by contrast material within the lumen. Additionally, extravasation may only become apparent following repetition of the contrast study after several hours if the clinical situation continues to suggest rupture but the initial contrast study failed to demonstrate it.[28]

Endoscopy

In the situation where contrast radiography is negative but the clinical suspicion of rupture remains high, flexible upper gastrointestinal videoendoscopy is particularly useful in the evaluation of the oesophagus. Not only does endoscopy accurately reveal the site and extent of oesophageal injury but it also allows full assessment of the mucosa and the extent of the laceration (**Fig. 14.1**) as well as more clearly defining any associated underlying oesophageal pathology. It has the additional advantage of allowing the safe passage of a nasogastric tube into the stomach for the subsequent drainage of secretions. Although it has been suggested that an injudicious use of endoscopy may convert small oesophageal tears into larger ones requiring surgery,[28] in experienced hands with minimal insufflation, endoscopy is a useful and safe adjunct to other diagnostic modalities.

Computerised tomography

CT may also be useful in the evaluation of oesophageal ruptures that are difficult to localise/diagnose or when contrast radiography cannot be performed. Findings that are suggestive of full thickness injury include air in the soft tissues of the mediastinum around the oesophagus, an adjacent abscess cavity, or communication of the oesophagus with adjacent mediastinal air–-fluid collections[30,31] (**Fig. 14.4**). CT of the chest may be life saving in patients with atypical presentations[32] and is probably the best radiological technique for evaluating the paraoesophageal manifestations of oesophageal rupture such as the extent of extraluminal air and fluid as well as the degree of containment of the rupture. Indeed, some authors[31] have suggested that CT may play a pivotal role in the decision to select patients for non-operative management although this remains to be more clearly defined. Instead, the current main use of CT is in the assessment of postoperative complications and the evaluation of patients who deteriorate when treated conservatively. The latter role is particularly useful as in addition to localising collections CT has the added therapeutic advantage of guiding drainage procedures.

Thoracocentesis

Analysis of any pleural fluid obtained from chest drains may prove to be the first sign that alerts the clinician to the diagnosis of Boerhaave's syndrome, particularly if the fluid contains overt food particles.[33] Additionally if the pH of such fluid is less than 6.0 or contains a high amylase count (from swallowed saliva) this will further confirm the diagnosis.

Management

General considerations

Oesophageal rupture is associated with a wide spectrum of clinical features dependent on the site, time course and degree of extraoesophageal contamination. The literature is replete with different reports on the management of such injuries and due to the relative rarity of this entity no single author has a large experience. There is thus little overall consensus on management strategies for dealing with oesophageal rupture and in most circumstances an individual management plan needs to be tailored for each patient.

Figure 14.4
(a) Left pleural collection of gas and fluid emanating from an oesophageal rupture; (b) Left basal chest drain lying within the pleural collection in the same patient.

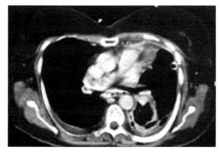

(a)

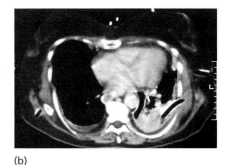

(b)

Surgical care for the injured oesophagus varies based upon the location of injury, the condition of the oesophageal tissue, any underlying disease and the overall fitness of the patient. In general, these patients should be managed by surgeons with a special interest in oesophageal disease. No single technique is suitable for all occasions so that surgeons should be versatile in all aspects of gastrointestinal and left- and right-sided thoracic surgical techniques. In addition, the decision to undertake one particular line of management must be made in the full knowledge that subsequent decisions may change according to the progress of the patient. Given the severe clinical consequences that normally accompany this type of injury all patients should be nursed in a high dependency or intensive care unit in conjunction with intensivists. Hospitals without such facilities or lacking the appropriate surgical cover should consider transfer to a regional unit at the earliest opportunity once initial resuscitation (Table 14.4) is complete.

Conservative management

Although non-operative management has been described for rare spontaneous cervical ruptures and certain contained intrathoracic injuries in patients who have demonstrated tolerance to the injury, the mainstay of treatment remains surgery. In the vast majority of true post-emetic spontaneous ruptures the degree of mediastinal contamination is so extensive that conservative management is inappropriate. Nevertheless, selected patients with spontaneous oesophageal rupture can be treated conservatively by continuing the management protocol outlined above together with tube thoracostomy and hyperalimentation using parenteral nutrition or a feeding jejunostomy. Some authors have also utilised covered self-expanding oesophageal stents to further reduce the ongoing process of mediastinal leakage[34] although the efficacy and rationale for this approach is questionable and remains to be clarified.

The exact criteria for selecting patients to be managed in this way remains controversial. Historically, most authors concluded that operative intervention was the only treatment option as there was no reliable way of predicting the

1. Central venous access and arterial line monitoring

2. Intravenous opiate analgesia

3. Urethral catheterisation

4. Intravenous fluids +/– inotropic support

5. Broad-spectrum antibiotics and antifungal agents

6. Oxygen administration

7. Nasogastric decompression (under radiological or endoscopic control)

8. Large-bore intercostal chest drainage in the appropriate thoracic cavity

9. Intravenous H2 receptor antagonists or proton pump inhibitors

10. Strictly 'nil by mouth'

Table 14.4 *Initial resuscitation for spontaneous rupture of the oesophagus*

extent of injury preoperatively[35] and the reported mortality from conservative management was 100%.[10] However, a better understanding of the pathophysiology and spectrum of disease represented by 'spontaneous rupture' together with improvements in antibiotics and intensive care facilities has resulted in an improved outlook for such patients. Larrieu and Kieffer reported a successful outcome with conservative care for a patient with spontaneous oesophageal perforation in 1975[36] and since that time numerous other reports have confirmed the validity of this approach in a select group of patients.[37,38]

It has been suggested that patients with small ruptures and contamination confined to the mediastinum[39] may be treated non-operatively although successful conservative management has been described in a patient with free left intrapleural rupture who had presented beyond 24 hours.[38] Late recognition of the rupture beyond 1–5 days has also been cited as a reason to treat conservatively[37,40] although such patients are a self-selecting group who have survived despite a failure in timely diagnosis. Many of these patients have demonstrated adequate internal drainage of a mediastinal abscess back into the oesophagus with minimal sepsis and have even recovered without a tube thoracostomy.[37,41] Similarly, drainage of the mediastinum by a nasogastric tube through the oesophageal rent[42] and other elaborate tube drainage systems have been described in isolated patients to effect conservative management. Although these data suggest that conservative management for spontaneous oesophageal rupture is a valid therapeutic option, it appears to be suitable for only a minority of patients. Surgical intervention remains the mainstay of treatment for this disease process.

Primary surgical repair

For non-cervical, non-contained oesophageal ruptures, debridement of necrotic tissue, generous irrigation and complete mediastinal and pleural drainage are fundamental parts of any operation designed for such injuries. The majority of patients with spontaneous oesophageal rupture are approached via an 8th or 9th interspace left thoracotomy and any attempt at successful primary repair should begin with the debridement of devitalised tissue and identification of the muscular and mucosal layers of the oesophagus. The mediastinal pleura should be opened to fully expose the injury and as the mucosal tear is usually longer than the muscular tear an extended myotomy and debridement may be required to allow accurate closure of the underlying mucosal defect. Most authorities recommend either a one- or two-layered anastomosis with interrupted fine absorbable sutures (**Fig. 14.5a**).[14,20]

The success of primary repair is based upon timely diagnosis, careful intraoperative assessment of tissues and meticulous surgical technique. Normal tissue that will hold sutures and has its usual tensile strength and pliability is an absolute requirement for attempted primary closure. For this reason some authorities have suggested that such techniques should only be reserved for those who are operated upon within 24 hours of the onset of symptoms.[43] However, a number of series[14,20] have challenged this concept with a recent report[14] demonstrating only one death in 9 patients treated with primary repair more than 24 hours after rupture.

Despite meticulous surgical technique, serial contrast studies in the postoperative period demonstrate continued leakage in up to 23% of patients

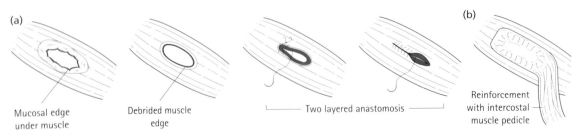

(a)

Mucosal edge
under muscle

Debrided muscle
edge

└────── Two layered anastomosis ──────┘

(b)

Reinforcement
with intercostal
muscle pedicle

Figure 14.5
(a) Primary closure and buttressing of suture line with (b) intercostal muscle flap.

following primary closure[14] with this figure rising to 50% if repair is delayed beyond 24 hours.[44] It is for this reason that many authors have suggested buttressing the primary repair in order to protect the suture line (**Fig. 14.5b**). The tissues used to reinforce the suture line have included a pleural flap, omentum, a pedicled intercostal muscle flap, the fundus of the stomach and a pericardial flap.[45] Experimental studies have documented markedly reduced rates of leakage after buttressed repair of oesophageal tears[46] and more importantly the nature of any leak using this technique may be altered from a free intrapleural leak to a contained, asymptomatic leak that will heal with observation alone. Careful surgical technique with close tissue reinforcement (as opposed to simple tacking) resulted in a clinical leak rate of only 7% and an overall mortality of only 14% in a wide spectrum of oesophageal injury treated with this technique.[45] Bufkin *et al.*[20] reported a similarly impressive 82% survival rate in a heterogeneous group of 28 patients treated with primary repair with or without reinforcement.

T-tube drainage

Although undoubtedly some cases of oesophageal rupture diagnosed at a relatively early stage can be successfully treated by primary closure, many injuries diagnosed at a late stage have tissues that are unsuitable for such repair. In such circumstances some authors prefer the approach of T-tube placement into a partially repaired rupture in order to divert all secretions via a controlled oesophago-cutaneous fistula, thus allowing healing of the surrounding tissues.[10,47] The insertion of a large lumen (6–10 mm) T-tube should be precise with the long arm directed toward the stomach and the short arm within the oesophagus, proximal to the site of injury (**Fig. 14.6**). The tube should then be brought out through a separate stab incision and secured in a lateral position and left in place for 2–3 weeks to allow development of a defined tract. Care should be taken to site the tube as far away from the aorta as possible as fatal aortic erosion from T-tube placement has been reported.[10] Gastric decompression is maintained via nasogastric tube placement or alternatively by a gastrostomy created at concomitant laparotomy at which time the formation of a feeding jejunostomy is frequently undertaken to provide enteral nutritional support.[20] This simple technique often contributes to the rapid stabilisation of a group of patients with severe sepsis. In the three detailed modern reports of T-tube drainage from the 1990s[20,47,48] 14 of 18 patients survived, a mortality rate comparable with the authors' own recently published experience employing this technique.[49]

Figure 14.6
(a) Diagramatic; (b) operative and (c) radiological views of a T-tube placement for spontaneous oesophageal rupture.

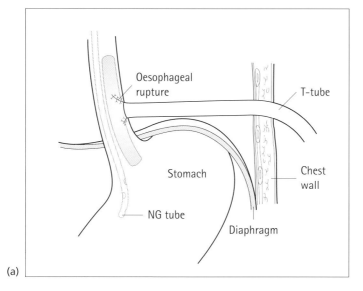

Oesophageal rupture

T-tube

Stomach

Chest wall

NG tube

Diaphragm

(a)

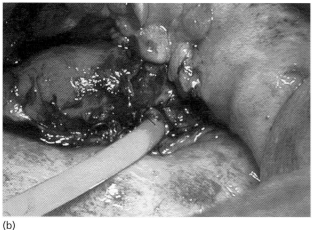

(b)

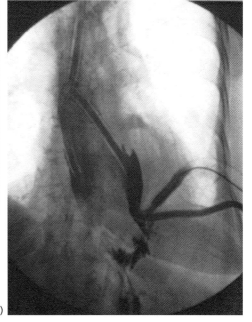

(c)

Exclusion and diversion

In addition to thoracic lavage, debridement and attempted repair some authors have advocated the technique of oesophageal exclusion and diversion[50] in order to further protect the site of oesophageal injury from oropharyngeal and gastric secretions. Distal exclusion of the oesophagus below the rupture is achieved by the use of an absorbable tie or a percutaneous 'Rumel' tourniquet brought out below the diaphragm together with a gastrostomy. At the same time a lateral side-to-side cervical oesophagostomy is performed which provides almost complete diversion because of the angulation of the proximal cervical oesophagus. The oesophageal exclusion tie usually releases at about 3 weeks; if a tourniquet is used this can be removed externally with the cervical oesophagostomy being closed under local anaesthetic at this time. The significant incidence of distal and proximal oesophageal strictures together with the need for a second operation means that this technique is rarely employed except in exceptional cases.[20]

Resection

Oesophageal resection has been successfully applied to select patients with severe mediastinal sepsis in whom oesophageal rupture has been diagnosed at a late stage.[51,52,53] Although most surgeons reserve this technique for the management of iatrogenic injuries associated with underlying oesophageal pathology, in critically ill patients with a spontaneous rupture that has caused extensive oesophageal damage it results in the rapid elimination of both the source of sepsis and the tear. In a heterogeneous series of patients containing a high percentage of spontaneous ruptures, Salo *et al.*[53] reported a mortality rate of 13% in 15 patients who underwent oesophagectomy compared to 68% for similar patients treated with primary repair. Salo performed a two-stage procedure with resection, diversion and late reconstruction using either a colonic or gastric conduit, although alimentary continuity has successfully been restored immediately in such circumstances employing either an intrathoracic[51] or cervical[52] oesophagogastric anastomosis, thus avoiding the prospect of a second operation.

Trans-oesophageal irrigation

Another technique that has been used in the context of oesophageal rupture associated with a delay in diagnosis and widespread mediastinal contamination is transoesophageal irrigation, a similar technique to that occasionally used in the management of severe necrotising pancreatitis. Santos and Frater[54] irrigated the mediastinum in 8 patients with severe oesophageal injury by passing 50–75 ml saline hourly through the oesophagus via a nasogastric tube. Irrigation served to flush bacteria, fibrin and mediastinal debris out through chest drains accurately placed near the site of the perforation. In conjunction with supportive care and broad-spectrum antibiotics 7 out of 8 patients survived with preservation of oesophageal function in 6 of the survivors.

Management algorithm

An overall management algorithm based on the available therapeutic strategies described in the literature is outlined in **Fig. 14.7**. It should be emphasised that these options are meant only as guidelines as no randomised trial has ever addressed the management of spontaneous oesophageal rupture. In most cases an individual treatment plan tailored for each patient is required and the clinician must be ready to reconsider options on a regular basis.

Rare causes of spontaneous oesophageal rupture

Primary oesophageal tumours may rarely be complicated by spontaneous rupture and perforation by invasion from contiguous primary or metastatic tumours is also well recognised. The mucosa contributes a significant amount to the strength of the oesophagus such that while intraluminal pressures of 3 to

Figure 14.7
Management algorithm for spontaneous rupture of the thoracic oesophagus.

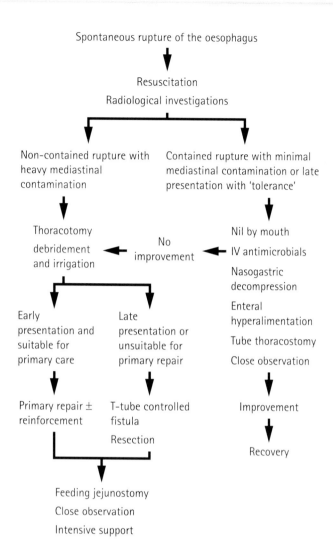

7.5 psi are required to produce rupture of an intact normal human oesophagus this falls to only 1 to 2.25 psi in the presence of oesophagitis or ulceration.[55] Thus, in the presence of severe infectious oesophagitis, usually in the immuno-compromised patient, spontaneous rupture may occur more readily. Extensive herpes simplex oesophagitis and candidal oesophagitis have been reported in association with such injuries[56,57] and a case of oesophageal erosion and rupture secondary to tuberculosis in the mediastinal lymph nodes has been reported.[58] Barrett's ulceration and Zollinger–Ellison syndrome with peptic ulcerative oesophagitis may also be causal factors in some cases of spontaneous rupture.

Other barogenic oesophageal injuries

It is likely that spontaneous oesophageal rupture represents the more severe end of a spectrum of barogenic injuries to the oesophagus. As in Boerhaave's syndrome, the pathogenesis of Mallory-Weiss tears is also believed to result from a sudden rise in intra–abdominal pressure associated with persistent vomiting and violent retching. Mallory–Weiss tears also tend to occur in similar patient groups with a strong association with alcohol abuse and the male sex.[59] Although these tears are often short (3–20 mm in length) and confined to the mucosa, their orientation and site are similar to full thickness ruptures with lacerations occurring in the longitudinal axis of the lower oesophagus, often found above a hiatal hernia.[60]

Spontaneous oesophageal intramural haematomas (also known as oesophageal apoplexy) represent another type of rare but well-recognised barogenic oesophageal injury.[61] Such haematomas form within the wall of the oesophagus as the result of trauma sustained during retching or vomiting, often after a meal.[62] Patients present with an abrupt onset of substernal or epigastric pain followed by haematemesis with dysphagia and odynophagia also being prominent symptoms. Endoscopy typically demonstrates a bluish oesophageal mucosal mass protruding into the lumen usually with an identifiable small mucosal tear, which is presumably the source of any haematemesis. Depending on the size of the lesion-contrast radiography, CT and EUS will further demonstrate the site and extent of the haematoma. A pressure-induced mechanism similar to the pathogenesis of Mallory-Weiss tears and Boerhaave's syndrome seems likely, although coagulopathy and foreign body injury may account for some cases.[61] Despite the dramatic presentation, most patients respond well to conservative management with complete resolution within 2–3 weeks in the majority of cases, although rarely surgical intervention is required.[62]

Iatrogenic perforation

Intraluminal injury

Aetiology

Medical instrumentation is the most frequent cause of oesophageal perforation, accounting for between 33% to 73% of all cases of oesophageal disruption.[2,20,43,63] Iatrogenic rupture is a well-recognised complication of rigid and flexible endoscopy and of therapeutic oesophageal dilatation.[43] Dilatation at the time of endoscopy increases the chance of perforation by as much as 10-fold with a variable risk in relation to the type of dilator used. The reported incidence for Maloney–Hurst type dilators is 0.09% but is as high as 2.2% for rigid Celestin-type dilators.[64] The use of the Savary–Gilliard dilator passed over a guide-wire under fluoroscopic control has considerably reduced this incidence with one series demonstrating no perforations in 239 dilatations of benign strictures.[65]

In the normal oesophagus, the most common location of an instrumental perforation is in the piriform fossa between the cricopharyngeus and the inferior pharyngeal constrictor muscles, where the oesophageal introitus is at its narrowest. Kyphosis of the spine, hyper-extension of the neck, cervical osteophytes and the presence of a paraoesophageal diverticulum all increase the likelihood of instrumental perforation of the cervical oesophagus.[66] More distal oesophageal perforation rarely occurs in a normal oesophagus. However, in the presence of obstructing lesions the lower thoracic oesophagus is the principal site at which perforations may occur as this is where the majority of benign and malignant strictures are found. Seventy-five to 90% of all perforations that occur during diagnostic endoscopy are found in the lower oesophagus, either in normal oesophageal tissue just above a stricture or as the result of a direct injury through the stricture itself.[67]

Pneumatic dilatation for achalasia is associated with a 1–5% incidence of perforation[68] with higher inflation pressures and previous pneumatic dilatations increasing the risk. Endoscopic variceal sclerotherapy is also associated with a perforation rate of approximately 1–6% due to delayed transmural necrosis which may occur as long as 14 days after treatment.[69] Perforation has also been reported as a complication of endoscopic variceal ligation.[70]

Palliative therapies such as endoscopic laser therapy or photodynamic therapy aimed at oesophageal tumour destruction are also associated with a perforation rate of approximately 5%[71,72] and this may also be delayed up to 1 week following treatment. The insertion of endoprostheses for the palliation of advanced or inoperable oesophageal carcinoma has been associated with a perforation rate of approximately 5%;[73] either the direct early result of dilatation and placement, or later from pressure necrosis. Newer expandable metal stents appear to have a lower perforation rate, possibly because less dilatation is required prior to their insertion.[74] Pressure necrosis leading to perforation can also rarely result from other types of non-endoscopic tube placement within the oesophageal lumen. Such events have also been reported following endotracheal intubation[75] and the use of longstanding nasogastric tubes.[76]

Clinical features and diagnosis

Although the history and mode of presentation of iatrogenic perforation is clearly different from that of spontaneous oesophageal rupture the clinical features of both conditions are similar and are entirely dependent upon the exact location and time course following injury. In most cases of instrumental perforation there will be a clear history of recent endoscopic intervention whether therapeutic or not and a high index of suspicion is required if any patient complains of suspicious symptoms in such circumstances. Intrathoracic perforations (**Fig. 14.8**) initially present with pain, fever and subcutaneous emphysema at a variable time following the endoscopic injury.[77] When cervical perforations occur, pain may localise to the neck and there may be associated dysphonia and cervical dysphagia, hoarseness and pain on cervical motion, sternocleidomastoid spasm and localised tenderness with associated cervical emphysema.[2,77] The diagnostic pathway is the same as that for spontaneous rupture of the oesophagus. A plain radiograph of the chest and/or neck followed, if any doubt exists, by a contrast swallow will delineate the injury clearly in the majority of cases.

Management

General considerations

Small instrumental cervical perforations in the hypopharynx or cervical oesophagus can usually be managed conservatively in those cases that are contained and well tolerated.[39,78] When the site of perforation cannot be found because of local inflammation, drainage only, together with intravenous antibiotics, may be adequate as cervical oesophageal fistulae will usually heal within a few days in the absence of distal luminal obstruction. However, some authorities recommend primary surgical closure through a left lateral incision anterior

Figure 14.8
Widespread extravasation of contrast material as the result of iatrogenic perforation following rigid endoscopy for a meat impaction in the lower third of the oesophagus.

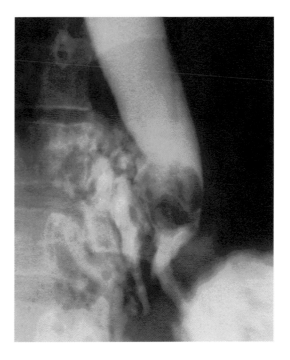

to the sternocleidomastoid exposing the oesophagus between the carotid sheath and the thyroid followed by extensive prevertebral drainage.[79] This approach is well tolerated even in the critically ill patient and may avert additional morbidity and mortality by preventing mediastinal extension of sepsis.

In general, thoracoabdominal perforations are managed along the same guidelines as those already discussed for spontaneous rupture of the oesophagus. Instrumental perforations tend to occur in patients who have been starved for upper gastrointestinal endoscopy and thus the degree of mediastinal contamination is usually considerably less than that encountered with spontaneous oesophageal rupture. In addition such injuries occur within the context of a hospital environment and, given the heightened index of suspicion following endoscopic procedures, they are more readily diagnosed at an early stage. The spectrum of disease severity is therefore often less than with spontaneous rupture making successful conservative management from iatrogenic perforations a more likely goal.

Conservative management

As with spontaneous rupture of the oesophagus the principles of non-operative management involve maintaining no food or drink to be taken. Hyperalimentation is achieved preferably via an enteral route, together with nasogastric suction and broad-spectrum intravenous antibiotics. The outcome data on the management of iatrogenic perforations using this approach is considerably more extensive than that for spontaneous oesophageal rupture. In the earliest report of conservative management instituted mostly within 24 hours of injury in 18 patients with instrumental perforations[80] only one death (5.5%) occurred, although the authors could not duplicate their results with spontaneous oesophageal rupture as the result of advanced mediastinitis in the latter group. Cameron[81] was the first to propose certain criteria to select patients for conservative management based upon his experience with a zero mortality from conservative management in 8 patients who had sustained a variety of mediastinal insults, the majority of which were postoperative disruptions diagnosed at a late stage. Cameron proposed the following criteria for selecting non-operative management: low grade fever or leucocytosis, mild pain controlled by opiate analgesia, absence of shock or systemic sepsis and a cavity confined to the mediastinum that appears to drain well into the oesophagus on contrast radiography. Many of Cameron's patients were diagnosed at a late stage (> 48 hours) and had already demonstrated tolerance to mediastinal contamination. Nevertheless, employing similar criteria Wesdorp *et al.*[67] found no deaths in 14 patients treated conservatively within a few hours of instrumental perforation and had a similar favourable outcome for a further 5 patients selected for operative management. Numerous other reports of conservative management for iatrogenic perforation have described a 0–19% mortality rate for patients with iatrogenic intrathoracic perforations selected for conservative management.[24,43,79,82,83]

Shaffer *et al.*[84] reassessed Cameron's criteria in 1992 in a comparative study between 12 patients treated conservatively and 13 patients who underwent surgery. Only one death occurred among the 25 patients and this was in the surgical cohort, although it should be noted that there were several differences in the aetiology, delay to diagnosis and clinical features at presentation between the two groups. In contrast to Cameron's observations, the authors found that pain requiring narcotic analgesia, significant fever and leucocytosis or the presence of retention or trapping of barium within the mediastinum did not preclude non-operative management. They concluded that the most relevant of Cameron's criteria was containment of the perforation within the mediastinum.

These studies support the concept that a non-operative approach may be applied to carefully selected patients with instrumental perforations in the clinical context outlined in **Table 14.5**. Even after initial selection for conservative management the decision to switch to surgical treatment should always be considered. Cameron[81] proposed that serial gastrograffin studies should be performed every

---

1. Early detection of elective instrumental perforations prior to oral alimentation

2. Absence of shock or systemic sepsis

3. Mild to moderate fever or leucocytosis

4. Pain controlled with opiate analgesia

5. Absence of crepitus, diffuse mediastinal gas, hydropneumothorax or pneumo-peritoneum

6. Mediastinal containment of perforation

7. Absence of widespread extravasation of contrast material

8. No evidence of ongoing luminal obstruction or retained foreign body

9. Patients demonstrating tolerance following diagnostic delay

10. Patients who remain clinically stable with conservative management

Table 14.5 *Guidelines for selecting non-operative management in cases of oesophageal perforation*

3–5 days to check on the progress of the patient's perforation. However, close observation of the patient's clinical condition is a more important and practical option and any deterioration should prompt either further contrast radiography or a CT scan to detect any abscess. If intrapleural collections should develop, ultrasound or CT guided drainage together with indwelling tube thoracostomy may allow the continuation of conservative management. However, in situations where the patient's condition continues to deteriorate early surgical intervention should be considered as any delay may prejudice the outcome. It should be noted that despite advances in technology and medical care a large recent series has demonstrated that iatrogenic perforation continues to carry a 19% mortality rate.[85]

Surgical management

The indications for surgical intervention for iatrogenic perforations are indicated in **Table 14.6**. In general the principles of surgical management for iatrogenic perforation of the oesophagus are similar to those described for spontaneous oesophageal rupture. Although the spectrum of surgical techniques designed to deal with the injured oesophagus apply equally in most situations, iatrogenic perforations associated with underlying oesophageal pathology such as peptic strictures, achalasia and carcinoma may require special consideration, as the mortality may be 6-fold higher.[83]

While many patients with small and well-contained perforations secondary to pneumatic dilatation for achalasia can be treated conservatively, those patients with larger injuries or with persistent distal obstruction will require surgical intervention. In such circumstances primary repair with or without reinforcement appears to have good results although there continues to be debate as to whether a further contralateral myotomy is required.[86] Similarly, perforation of a reflux-related stricture may not heal in the presence of persisting distal obstruction or appreciable continuing gastro-oesophageal reflux. Thus, if primary, reinforced or controlled repair is carried out in such circumstances adequate intraoperative stricture dilatation may need to be performed with or without a concomitant antireflux procedure if the patient's condition allows. When these goals cannot be achieved resection can be performed with reasonable results.[52]

Patients who sustain an instrumental perforation of a malignant stricture represent a unique group. Those patients with disseminated oesophageal metastatic disease or who are considered unfit for surgical resection are usually managed conservatively with the use of an endoprosthesis. This approach was successful in all but one of 35 consecutive perforations treated in this manner.[67] Similar reports of conservative management have also demonstrated the efficacy of protecting the perforation site with a covered metal stent.[74,87,88]

---

1. Clinically unstable patients with sepsis or shock

2. Heavily contaminated mediastinum and pleural space

3. Widespread intrapleural or intraperitoneal extravasation of contrast material

4. Ongoing luminal obstruction or retained foreign body

5. Failed medical therapy

Table 14.6 *Indications for surgical intervention following iatrogenic oesophageal perforation*

In the presence of localised and potentially operable perforated malignant disease the optimal management strategy is less clearly defined. Most authors have recommended resection with immediate or delayed reconstruction[20,52,89] as the only means of controlling sepsis, obtaining healing and offering long-term cure. However, this approach has consistently been associated with a high mortality rate (22–75%) and in addition such perforations may adversely affect survival, as is the case with malignant perforation elsewhere in the gastrointestinal tract including the stomach and colon. In the authors' own experience[90] resection in such circumstances can be performed with a low morbidity and mortality although in contrast to curative elective resections survival is significantly compromised suggesting that many of these patients may be better considered for non-surgical palliation.

An algorithm for the management of iatrogenic perforation in various circumstances is set out in **Fig. 14.9**.

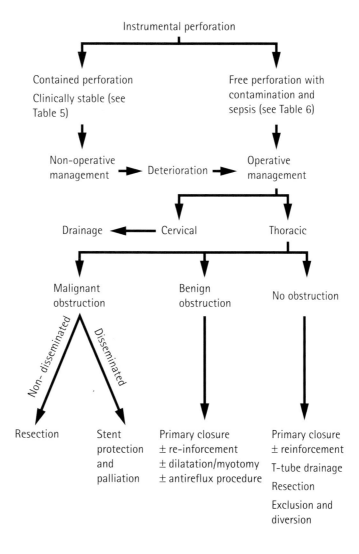

Figure 14.9
Management algorithm for iatrogenic perforation of the oesophagus.

Operative oesophageal perforation

Inadvertent damage to the oesophagus leading to perforation can result from surgery to the oesophagus itself or its contiguous structures. Oesophageal disruption due to anastomotic leaks is a specific postoperative complication and is discussed elsewhere. An incidence of leakage of 0.5% to 1.2% has been described following antireflux surgery[91] with most of these perforations complicating intrathoracic fundoplications. Previous surgery, incomplete wraps and severe active oesophagitis were associated risk factors. Although 50% of such leaks are localised and can be successfully managed conservatively, the mortality for surgery for uncontained leaks is as high as 17%.[91] Surgery for Heller's myotomy may also result in a mucosal laceration and perforation, although this is usually identified and dealt with appropriately at the time of surgery. A late complication of oesophageal surgery no longer performed includes the erosion of the Angelchik prosthesis through the oesophagus resulting in perforation.[92]

More serious complications may occur as the result of undetected intraoperative injury such as the 0.5% of cases which may complicate radical pneumonectomy[93] and the reported 0.25% incidence of oesophageal perforation following anterior spinal surgery.[94] Both emergency tracheostomy and chronic tracheostomy cuff erosion may also cause perforation or tracheo-oesophageal fistulation and segmental ischaemic oesophageal necrosis is a well-recognised complication of intrathoracic aortic aneurysm surgery. Rarely, pressure necrosis from a closed thoracostomy tube may result in perforation.[95] As with any oesophageal injury the key to successful management in such cases is early recognition and the commencement of those treatment options already discussed for the management of spontaneous rupture and instrumental perforation.

Traumatic injury to the oesophagus

Penetrating trauma

Aetiology

Traumatic perforations of the oesophagus comprise approximately 19% of all types of oesophageal injury.[29] The majority of such injuries are from penetrating wounds rather than blunt trauma, usually the result of stabbing or gunshot injuries. The oesophagus is an elusive and well-protected target, particularly within the thorax, as the depth of penetration required to sustain an injury is high. As a result, gunshot injuries prevail in the thoracic oesophagus whereas the cervical oesophagus, lacking skeletal protection, is more prone to stab injuries. This latter type of injury is by far the commonest in surviving patients as penetrating injuries that traverse the thorax may damage vital structures and determine the immediate fate of the patient.

A common presentation for knife injuries is an entrance wound in the mid-left neck with a right pneumothorax or empyema indicating a high transmediastinal injury.[96] With gunshot wounds there tends to be a high incidence of associated injuries with Pass[97] noting 39 concomitant injuries in 18 patients with gunshot-induced oesophageal perforation, the commonest being pulmonary followed by tracheobronchial. Such injuries require simultaneous attention from a multidisciplinary team including cardiothoracic surgeons.

Diagnosis

As with all other oesophageal injuries the clinical presentation will depend on the size and location of the perforation together with duration from injury and resultant contamination. In the context of trauma such perforations may be particularly difficult to diagnose as they are often overshadowed by the more dramatic and obvious features of associated visceral injuries. The importance of maintaining a high index of suspicion in such circumstances cannot be overemphasised. Subcutaneous emphysema and cervical haematomata as well as radiological evidence of mediastinal widening or retropharyngeal swelling may be overlooked or confused with associated pulmonary damage particularly with intrathoracic gunshot wounds.[97]

If oesophageal perforation is suspected then contrast radiography should be obtained initially utilising a water-soluble medium and if negative then subsequently with barium. As previously discussed there are limitations as to the efficacy of such investigations[97,98] and in many trauma situations it may be impractical to undertake contrast radiography. In such situations upper gastrointestinal videoendoscopy is particularly useful as it may identify or refute the presence of oesophageal injury such that appropriate operative management may be planned. If urgent surgery has been undertaken without the benefit of these investigations the oesophagus should be carefully inspected intraoperatively although inevitably there will be some cases that are missed and present late with mediastinal sepsis or food particles in chest drains.

Management

Virtually all transthoracic gunshot wounds will require surgical exploration and any associated cardiovascular, tracheobronchial or pulmonary injuries take precedent. With cervical stab wounds the general management philosophy is stratified thus:

1. The exploration of all wounds traversing the platysma or potentially having a transmediastinal path with the bias here being one of over-exploration rather than risking a missed injury.
2. A selective approach to exploration, relying upon the efficacy of arteriography, contrast studies, endoscopy and other modalities in order to exclude oesophageal and associated injuries.

Isolated injuries to the cervical oesophagus may be repaired via a left- or right-sided incision anterior to the sternocleidomastoid, as this will allow excellent access if unexpected vascular injuries are encountered. In general injuries to the upper or middle third of the oesophagus should be explored via a high right posterolateral thoracotomy whereas injuries to the lower third require a left-sided approach. However, this caveat may be broken if the location of clinical signs requires an ipsilateral thoracotomy or if associated injuries necessitate a median sternotomy. Once the injury has been identified the basic principles of treatment of traumatic oesophageal perforation are identical to those already described for iatrogenic and barogenic tears. Although bullet wounds are usually low velocity in civilian practice, the resultant damage may be extensive and thorough debridement and wide drainage are particularly important in this context.

Mortality

The overall mortality rate for patients with penetrating traumatic injuries of the oesophagus is 15 to 27% with a lower rate for patients with cervical oesophageal injuries (0–16%) compared with those with thoracic oesophageal injuries (30–57%).[97,99,100] Early diagnosis, location and associated vascular or tracheobronchial injuries are factors that have an impact on survival.

Blunt trauma

Blunt traumatic rupture of the oesophagus is exceedingly rare. It may result from a compressed air or blast injury that causes a rapid rise in intraoesophageal pressure against a closed or only partially relaxed lower or upper oesophageal sphincter. Blunt trauma to the upper chest or cervical area from steering wheels in road traffic accidents may result in a cervical oesophageal perforation in a similar manner[101] and perforation complicating the Heimlich manoeuvre has been reported.[7] Extreme flexion and extension of the neck as in a whiplash injury[102] or a fracture dislocation of the cervical spine[103] may also cause blunt oesophageal perforation.

The diagnosis of oesophageal rupture after blunt trauma is often hampered by the associated symptoms and signs related to severe chest or abdominal trauma. Together with the relative rarity of this condition it is not surprising that diagnostic delay occurred in up to 68% of patients in one review[104] and thus a high index of suspicion and a low threshold for contrast and endoscopic evaluation are required.

Most of the oesophageal injuries that result from blunt trauma are often similar to those resulting from barogenic or iatrogenic injuries and as such the diagnostic studies and management considerations are similar. For extensive oesophageal injury resection may be indicated with either immediate[105] or delayed reconstruction. If a cervicothoracic perforation is suspected then triple endoscopy should be performed as there may be up to a 56% incidence of associated tracheobronchial and laryngeal injury[104] requiring multidisciplinary management.

Caustic injuries

Aetiology

The ingestion of caustic substances can result in devastating injuries to the oesophagus as well as the stomach and duodenum. There is a bimodal age distribution with the majority of caustic injuries occurring in children as the result of accidental ingestion with a second, smaller peak in incidence between the ages of 20–30 years, almost always associated with suicide attempts. In Denmark the incidence of paediatric caustic ingestion has been measured at 34.6/100 000 with oesophageal burns in 15.8/100 000 and a median age of less than 3 years.[106] In the adult population the incidence is considerably lower at 1/100 000[107] with 61% representing suicide attempts and the remainder mostly accidental ingestions by alcoholics.

The severity of injury depends not only on the corrosive properties and concentration of the ingested substance but also on the quantity swallowed. In general, suicide attempts, where intent is deliberate, usually represent the more severe end of the spectrum of upper gastrointestinal injury in comparison with accidental ingestions. Serious injuries are often the result of alkali burns from cleaning agents, lye soaps or disc batteries. Strong acid is less commonly available in this country and is therefore rarely ingested. Ingestion of household bleaches in contrast is particularly common although fortunately these agents rarely cause damage to the oesophagus or stomach.[108]

Pathophysiology

In general, alkali ingestion does more harm to the oesophagus than the stomach whilst the converse is true for acid. However, if ingested in sufficient quantity either agent can inflict a potentially fatal injury to any part of the upper gastro-intestinal tract. Aspiration, which may often accompany the ingestion or subsequent expectoration of caustic substances, may additionally cause life-threatening injuries to the larynx, tracheobronchial tree or lungs.

Alkalis cause saponification of cell membrane lipids and denaturation of intracellular proteins resulting in a process of 'liquefactive necrosis' causing vascular thrombosis and local tissue damage. Deeper injury including transmural necrosis and perforation into the mediastinum or peritoneal cavity will continue until the alkali is neutralised (**Table 14.7**). The neutralising effect of gastric acid is presumably why there is a lower tendency to sustain gastric injury when ingesting alkalis. The particular properties of the ingested substance affect the site and severity of any injury with viscous caustic agents tending to produce more proximal lesions. In contrast, ingested acid usually passes rapidly through the oesophagus and although coagulation necrosis may produce a firm oesophageal eschar, pooling in the stomach produces a more severe injury.

Clinical features

The variable properties and volume of caustic agents that are ingested means that there is a different propensity to cause injury to the oropharynx, oesophagus, stomach or duodenum. Additionally, symptoms and signs will vary in relation to the time course such that early clinical features are not necessarily reliable indicators of the severity or extent of injury. Caustic burns in the oropharynx produce localised pain and oedema that may prevent oropharyngeal clearance of secretions resulting in drooling. Caustic injury to the epiglottis or larynx can present with hoarseness or stridor whereas dyspnoea is more suggestive of aspiration or

Phase	Days	Pathophysiology
Acute	1–5	Liquefactive necrosis and vascular thrombosis
Subacute	5–15	Mucosal sloughing leading to mural weakness Development of granulation tissue
Cicatrisation	15–90	Further proliferation of fibroblasts and collagen deposition potentially leading to strictures

Table 14.7 *Phases of caustic injury to the oesophagus*

tracheobronchial burns. On inspection, oropharyngeal burns may range from mild oedema and superficial erosions to extensive mucosal necrosis with pseudomembrane formation.

Oesophageal burns present with dysphagia and odynophagia and may also cause drooling due to pain or inability to swallow. Retrosternal pain radiating through to the back is a sign of a third degree burn with oesophageal perforation. Such perforations may occur within hours or up to several days after ingestion occurred. Gastric injuries are manifested by epigastric pain, retching and vomiting, often with the vomitus containing blood or necrotic tissue. Full thickness injuries to the stomach or oesophago-gastric junction may lead to perforation and peritonitis.

The acute features described above subside between 1–5 days with a further 10-day minimally symptomatic latent period. From day 15 onwards, as collagen deposition reaches its peak, dysphagia as the result of stricture formation may occur. Up to 35% of paediatric patients with a documented caustic oesophageal injury will develop a stricture[109] although in some cases it may take months or even years for strictures to develop after the initial insult. Gastric outlet obstruction may complicate fibrotic stenosis of the distal stomach following caustic injury at a similar time interval to the development of oesophageal strictures. Another late feature of caustic injury is the associated cancer incidence with an estimated 1000-fold increased risk of developing squamous carcinoma in patients with a lye stricture.[110] There appears to be a long latent period for the development of malignant change with a mean delay of 41 years such that surveillance follow-up in such patients may be impractical.

Investigations

Free mediastinal or subdiaphragmatic gas will be evident on an initial plain radiograph of the chest if oesophageal or gastric perforation has occurred and such plain films are also useful in the evaluation of potential respiratory complications. However, for the majority of patients with caustic trauma to the oesophagus endoscopy is the single most valuable assessment tool and should be undertaken within 12–24 hours of all caustic ingestions once resuscitation and respiratory optimisation are complete. Although there is a risk of iatrogenic perforation in severe oesophageal burns, especially if several days have elapsed since the injury, flexible videoendoscopy in experienced hands will identify the site and extent of mucosal injury with minimal morbidity. The endoscopic signs of caustic oesophageal injury are outlined in **Table 14.8**. The need for contrast radiography in the setting of caustic oesophageal injury has largely been circumvented by early endoscopy, although these studies still play an important role in the presence of perforation and in the later follow-up of subsequent strictures.

Management

The first priority in dealing with patients who have ingested caustic agents is to establish an adequate airway. In the presence of significant respiratory compromise endotracheal intubation or emergency tracheostomy may be required. Associated burns to the face and eyes should be treated with copious irrigation and plastic surgery or ophthalmology input sought. Patients who are asymptomatic, who

First degree	Non-ulcerative oesophagitis
	Mucosal oedema and erythema
Second degree	Severe erythema and contact haemorrhage
	Superficial, friable ulceration extending through submucosa to muscularis propria with erosions and white exudate
Third degree	Deep ulceration with possible transmural perforation
	Extensive areas of black–grey necrosis

Table 14.8 *Endoscopic findings in caustic oesophageal burns*

have no oropharyngeal burns and normal endoscopic findings, and furthermore are not suicidal may be discharged. All other patient categories require admission to hospital.

Prior to 1990 the majority of patients who were admitted to hospital having sustained a caustic oesophageal injury were routinely treated with intravenous antibiotics and steroids.

However, in a prospective randomised trial comparing a standard steroid and antibiotic regime with simple supportive care in children with caustic oesophageal injuries Anderson et al.[109] found no significant difference in outcome in terms of stricture formation.

Routine use of steroids has, therefore, now largely been abandoned and antibiotics are reserved only for selective cases of proven infection or in patients with a perforation or aspiration. Supportive care includes antisecretory medication, intravenous hydration and analgesia together with nutritional support when recovery is protracted with the enteral route used in preference to the parenteral route. In most cases the latter is achieved via a nasojejunal tube passed under endoscopic or fluoroscopic control so as to avoid inadvertent perforation. Nasojejunal tubes have the added advantage of potentially acting as a partial stent and may decrease the incidence of subsequent stricture formation.

Patients with first- and second-degree oesophageal burns are observed for laryngeal oedema or transmural progression of their injury usually over the period of 5–7 days. Diet is reintroduced gradually and once discharged, patients require a follow-up contrast swallow or repeat endoscopic evaluation looking for late strictures. For severe grade 3 burns or in those patients presenting with perforation surgical intervention is usually required as widespread necrosis leads to life-threatening mediastinitis, sepsis, tracheobronchial injury and shock. Such patients respond poorly to conservative measures and an aggressive surgical philosophy is recommended (**Fig. 14.10**).[111] An emergency oesophago-gastrectomy is performed with reconstruction using a colonic interposition graft (as the stomach is usually injured and resected) on a delayed basis 6–8 weeks later. The oesophagus may be left in situ if minimally burnt or if the trachea is involved and defunctioned with a cervical oesophagostomy and feeding jejunostomy, although a colonic bypass may still be required at a later date.

The mortality rate for such severe injuries is high, ranging from 12.9% in those treated conservatively[112] to 23% in those requiring surgery.[111] If the oesophagus is preserved in grade 3 injuries virtually all patients will go on to develop oesophageal strictures whereas this is a less common problem with milder degrees

Figure 14.10
Management algorithm for caustic oesophageal injuries.

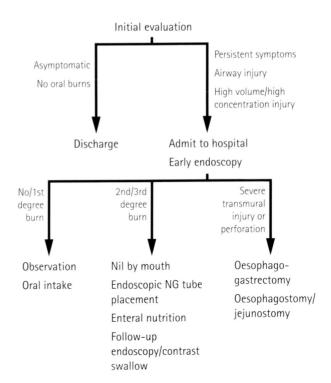

Initial evaluation

Asymptomatic
No oral burns

Persistent symptoms
Airway injury
High volume/high concentration injury

Discharge

Admit to hospital
Early endoscopy

No/1st degree burn

2nd/3rd degree burn

Severe transmural injury or perforation

Observation
Oral intake

Nil by mouth
Endoscopic NG tube placement
Enteral nutrition
Follow-up endoscopy/contrast swallow

Oesophago-gastrectomy
Oesophagostomy/jejunostomy

of caustic injury.[109] Although every effort should be made to maintain swallowing with periodic dilatation there are some patients with severe recurrent stricture formation who will inevitably require oesophageal replacement.

Foreign bodies

Epidemiology and aetiology

The oesophagus is the commonest site of foreign body impaction in the gastrointestinal tract, accounting for approximately 75% of such cases.[113] The majority of impactions occur in paediatric patients between the ages of 6 months and 3 years[113,114] with coins, toys, crayons, buttons and batteries being the most frequently ingested items. In contrast, adults usually present with meat or bone impaction with patients wearing dentures having the highest risk due to the relative tactile insensitivity of the palate that results.[113] Other adult groups at increased risk include prisoners (seeking secondary gain), alcohol and drug abusers and those with mental retardation or psychiatric disease.[113,114] Multiple foreign bodies may have been ingested and the process may be recurrent,[115] particularly in psychiatric patients and prisoners.

Typically foreign bodies lodge in areas of physiological narrowing at the level of the cricopharyngeus and cervical oesophagus, the aortic arch, the left main bronchus and the diaphragmatic hiatus. Over 80% of all impacted foreign bodies will be located in the cervical oesophagus with the remainder distributed in the middle and lower thirds.[116] Many patients with food impaction have underlying benign oesophageal pathology such as a Schatzki ring or peptic stricture,[114] whereas in contrast, malignant strictures are rarely the cause of foreign body or food impaction.[116]

Clinical presentation

Although patients who have swallowed a foreign object may present with a variety of symptoms and signs, a careful history will usually provide the diagnosis in the majority of older children and fully conscious, cooperative adults. Patients usually complain of a sticking sensation in the neck or chest and may be able to localise the level of the obstruction. Dysphagia is the commonest symptom followed by odynophagia, regurgitation, and excessive salivation and drooling.[114] In psychiatric patients and in children where a history is lacking, a high index of suspicion is required; the diagnosis should be considered in all infants and toddlers who present with refusal of feeds, gagging or chronic pulmonary aspiration. Although the majority of patients will present within hours of the ingestion, the diagnosis can be delayed for months or rarely even years in some paediatric cases.[117] Respiratory symptoms such as coughing, wheezing, stridor and dyspnoea occur in 5–15% of patients and are primarily seen in children with foreign bodies lodged in the cervical oesophagus. In adults food bolus impaction at this level may present with respiratory symptoms causing the so-called 'café-coronary' or 'steak-house syndrome' as the result of tracheal compression. Sharp, pointed objects that abrade the mucosa (e.g. fish bones) may cause a persistent foreign body sensation even after the object has been passed or extracted.

The physical examination is often unremarkable. Inability to swallow saliva and drooling indicate complete obstruction and the patient will often pinpoint pain at the suprasternal notch or xiphoid process depending on the site of impaction. Neck swelling, erythema, tenderness or crepitus are signs of oropharyngeal or proximal oesophageal perforation complicating foreign body ingestion. Clinical features of more distal perforations relate to the specific nature and site of the impacted foreign body together with the time course following its ingestion. Chronic fistulation either into the airways or major vessels causing massive haemorrhage has been reported.[118,119] Longstanding foreign bodies may induce cricoid perichondritis, perioesophagitis, oesophageal diverticula or even stenosis.[120]

Diagnosis

Plain radiographs of the neck and chest will help localise radio-opaque ingested foreign bodies (**Figs. 14.11, 14.12**) and will additionally identify signs of complications such as perforation or aspiration. Films should be obtained in both the anteroposterior and lateral projections since some objects will only be visible on the lateral view if they overlie the vertebrae. Combined views may also help distinguish whether objects are in the oesophagus or lodged within the tracheobronchial tree. In infants, more extensive plain radiographs covering the mouth to the anus may be required to identify or refute the presence of an ingested radio-opaque foreign body. Even in the absence of symptoms or physical signs a strong history should prompt the use of radiography as up to 17% of asymptomatic children with a history of coin ingestion will still be found to have a coin within the oesophagus.[121]

Figure 14.11
Ingested batteries lying in the antrum of the stomach.

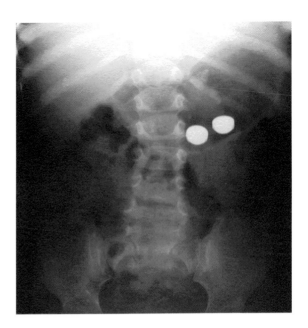

Figure 14.12
Ingested 50 pence coin.

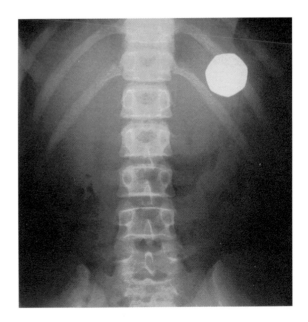

Non-radio-opaque objects such as wood, aluminium, glass and plastics may not be visible without the use of contrast agents (**Figure 14.8**). A contrast study may localise the impaction or delineate the site and extent of any associated perforation but may make subsequent endoscopy more difficult, particularly if barium is used. Hypertonic water-soluble media such as gastrograffin should be avoided if there is proximal impaction with high-grade obstruction as aspiration of this agent may provoke pulmonary oedema. Non-ionic contrast agents are preferable in such situations if a swallow is indicated. Failure to locate an object on radiography or contrast swallow mandates the use of videoendoscopy as some objects may be missed with these techniques.[121]

Management

General considerations

Although 80–90% of all ingested foreign bodies will pass through the gastro-intestinal tract uneventfully 10–20% must be removed endoscopically and 1% may need surgery.[122] Objects reaching the stomach are unlikely to pass the pylorus if they are more than 5–6 cm long or 2 cm in diameter. Similarly, elongated objects are more likely to become impacted in the duodenum making endoscopic retrieval more difficult. Foreign bodies in the oesophagus should therefore be managed expeditiously, particularly as prolonged delays have been shown to result in higher complication rates.[123]

The care of patients with foreign body ingestion is non-uniform with a variety of paediatricians, general surgeons, gastroenterologists and otolaryngologists involved depending on local policies. This fact, together with the numerous techniques described for extracting such objects dependent on their nature and site has led to considerable variation in practice. Flexible videoendoscopy is now the most commonly employed therapeutic modality and the fibreoptic endoscope has been used for foreign body extraction since the 1970s with excellent results. In comparison with rigid endoscopy, flexible endoscopy has been reported to be equally successful in the removal of foreign bodies with significantly fewer complications (5.1% versus 10% for rigid endoscopy)[124] and has therefore become the technique of choice for the majority of such objects. In addition, rigid endoscopy often requires a general anaesthetic with clear cost and risk implications. Nevertheless, many otolaryngologists and thoracic surgeons continue to employ the rigid endoscope, particularly for foreign bodies impacted in and around the cricopharyngeus as the view and therapeutic access may be superior.

Intravenous sedation or pharyngeal topical anaesthesia is employed although in younger children general anaesthesia may be indicated for flexible endoscopy. The oesophagus should be intubated under direct vision and in all patients it is critical to protect the patient's airway from obstruction or inadvertent aspiration of saliva, retained oesophageal/gastric secretions or the object itself. To this end an oesophageal overtube may be employed not only to protect the airway but also to prevent any iatrogenic damage to the oropharynx.

Specific management

Urgent endoscopic intervention is required for sharp objects and disc batteries as well as coins in the proximal oesophagus and any impaction producing complete dysphagia.[113,114] Coins in the lower third of the oesophagus will often pass spontaneously and can therefore be observed for a period of 12–24 hours. Once in the stomach the majority of coins and similarly sized objects will pass through the rest of the gastrointestinal tract without problem. Coins impacted more proximally should be extracted to relieve symptoms and prevent pressure necrosis and perforation. The 'rat-tooth' foreign body grasping forceps are required to grasp a coin securely although in their absence a standard polypectomy snare or retrieval basket may be employed. The grasped coin should be extracted under direct vision reorientating it into the frontal plane to aid safe passage through the hypopharynx.

Food impactions tend to occur in the lower oesophagus and are often associated with underlying pathology. A variety of non-endoscopic techniques have been described for the relief of such impactions including intravenous glucagon to relax oesophageal smooth muscle, topical proteolytic agents aimed at digesting the food bolus and gas-forming drinks to propel impacted food through the oesophagus. Although enthusiasts for these techniques have reported good results in select patients their wider adoption has been limited due to concerns regarding their efficacy and safety. A multicentre placebo-controlled double-blinded study of the ability of glucagon and diazepam to treat oesophageal foreign bodies found no benefit over placebo.[125] Proteolytic agents such as papain have been reported to cause fatal transmural oesophageal digestion[126] and haemorrhagic pulmonary oedema if aspirated, although in theory such enzymes only act upon non-viable tissue. Similarly, despite the apparently benign nature of effervescent agents, these too have been reported to cause oesophageal perforation.[127]

The mainstay of therapy for food impaction is endoscopy which not only allows removal of the bolus but also an immediate assessment of the underlying pathology. An impacted bolus can be removed in one piece using a polypectomy snare, retrieval basket or foreign body forceps. Occasionally, large boluses need to be broken up and removed piecemeal, using an overtube to protect the airway and facilitate repeated intubation. The temptation to push the bolus onwards should be resisted as this may lead to perforation unless the scope has already been passed distal to the bolus to assess any luminal obstruction. In the presence of a stricture either immediate or delayed endoscopic dilatation should be performed under fluoroscopic guidance depending on operator preference and the clinical situation.

Disc batteries represent a special case as electrical discharge or release of alkaline contents may cause rapid local necrosis and oesophageal perforation. If plain radiographs demonstrate a disc battery lodged in the oesophagus urgent extraction is indicated although this can be a technically difficult exercise. Batteries that are dislodged or have passed spontaneously into the stomach usually pass without complication. Objects that have sharp or pointed objects are also challenging to manage as they may cause lacerations or perforations when removed and may require intraluminal manipulation such that the pointed edge trails on removal.

Endoscopic techniques are successful in the extraction of the vast majority of foreign bodies and surgical retrieval is rarely required. Surgery is generally indicated for large objects that have failed endoscopic management, when the object has become embedded in the oesophageal wall or when there has been a perforation (Fig. 14.8).[113]

Summary

Oesophageal emergencies represent a heterogeneous group of conditions occurring as the result of a variety of different insults and aetiologies producing a wide spectrum of injury. The close proximity of the oesophagus to the vital organs, together with its relatively inaccessible position, mean that all conditions which affect this organ have a common potential for causing devastating consequences.

The complex epidemiology and presentation of oesophageal pathology has led to a large number of different subspeciality clinicians dealing with such emergencies which in turn has produced a wide array of often unproven management strategies with significant variations in outcome. In addition, oesophageal injuries are often initially misdiagnosed or mismanaged, further prejudicing a successful outcome. Only by raising the profile of these conditions through improved undergraduate and post-graduate teaching together with the concentration of expertise in multidisciplinary teams trained and equipped to deal with oesophageal emergencies can we hope to improve the outcome for what is too often a fatal event.

References

1. Burnett CM, Rosemurgy AS, Pfeiffer EA. Life-threatening acute posterior mediastinitis due to esophageal perforation. Ann Thorac Surg 1990; 49 (6):979–83.

2. Reeder LB, DeFilippi VJ, Ferguson MK. Current results of therapy for esophageal perforation. Am J Surg 1995; 169 (6):615–7.

3. Ajalat GM, Mulder DG. Esophageal perforations: The need for individual approach. Arch Surg 1984; 119 (11):1318–20.

4. Cirocco WC. Alexander the Great may have died of post-emetic esophageal perforation (Boerhaave's syndrome). J Clin Gastroenterol 1998; 26 (1):93–4.

5. Boerhaave H. Atrocis, nec descripti pruis, morbi historica: secundum medicae artis leges conscripta. Lugduni Batavorum, Boutesteniana, 1724.

6. Barrett NR. Spontaneous perforation of the oesophagus: review of the literature and report of 3 new cases. Thorax 1946; 1:48–56.

7. Haynes DE, Haynes BE, Yong YV. Esophageal rupture complicating Heimlich maneuver. Am J Emerg Med 1984; 2 (6):507–9.

8. Henderson JA, Peloquin AJ. Boerhaave revisited: spontaneous esophageal perforation as a diagnostic masquerader. Am J Med 1989; 86 (5):559–67.

9. Mackler SA. Spontaneous rupture of the esophagus: An experimental and clinical study. Surg Gynaec Obstet 1952; 95:345–50.

10. Abbott OA, Mansour KA, Logan WD Jr et al. Atraumatic so-called 'spontaneous' rupture of the esophagus. A review of 47 personal cases with comments on a new method of surgical therapy. J Thorac Cardiovasc Surg 1970; 59 (1):67–83.

11. Pate JW, Walker WA, Cole FH Jr et al. Spontaneous rupture of the esophagus: a 30-year experience. Ann Thorac Surg 1989; 47 (5):689–92.

12. Justicz AG, Symbas PN. Spontaneous rupture of the esophagus: immediate and late results. Am Surgeon 1991; 57 (1):4–7.

13. Brauer RB, Lieberman-Meffert D, Stein HJ et al. Boerhaave's syndrome analysis of the literature and report of 18 new cases. Dis Esoph 1997; 10 (1):64–8.

14. Lawrence DR, Ohri SK, Moxon RE et al. Primary oesophageal repair for Boerhaave's syndrome. Ann Thorac Surg 1999; 67 (3):818–20.

15. Kuwano H, Matsumata T, Adachi E et al. Lack of muscularis mucosa and the occurrence of Boerhaave's syndrome. Am J Surg 1989; 158 (5):420–2.

16. Salo JA, Seppala KM, Pitkaranta PP et al. Spontaneous rupture and functional state of the esophagus. Surgery 1992; 112 (5):897–900.

17. Inculet R, Clark C, Girvan D. Boerhaave's syndrome in children: a rare and unexplained combination. J Paed Surg 1996; 31 (9):1300–01.

18. Izaguirre SFS, Haggerty JT, Eckert G. Spontaneous rupture of the oesophagus. Surgery 1970; 67 (4):607–13.

19. Han SY, McElvein KB, Aldrete JS et al. Perforation of the esophagus: correlation of site and cause with plain film findings. Am J Roentgenol 1985; 145 (3):537–40.

20. Bufkin BL, Miller JI Jnr, Mansour KA. Esophageal perforation: emphasis on management. Ann Thor Surg 1996; 61:1447–51.

21. Kossick PR. Spontaneous rupture of the oesophagus. S Afr Med J 1973; 47:1807–9.

22. Hampton JR. The patient with chest pain and breathlessness. Med Int 1985; 2:661–4.

23. Appleton DS, Sandrasagra FA, Flower CDR. Perforated oesophagus: review of twenty-eight consecutive cases. Clin Radiol 1979; 30 (5):493–7.

24. Bladergroen MR, Lowe JE, Posthelwait RW. Diagnosis and recommended management of esophageal perforation and rupture. Ann Thorac Surg 1986; 42:235–9.

25. Naclerio EA. The 'V-sign' in the diagnosis of spontaneous rupture of the esophagus (an early roentgen clue). Am J Surg 1957; 93:291–8.

26. Foley MJ, Ghahremani GG, Rogers LF. Reappraisal of contrast media used to detect upper gastro-intestinal perforations: comparison of ionic water-soluble media with barium sulfate. Radiology 1982; 144 (2):231–7.

27. Buecker A, Wein BB, Neuerburg JM, Guenther RW. Esophageal perforation: comparison of use of aqueous and barium containing contrast media. Radiology 1997; 202 (3):683–6.

28. Sawyer R, Phillips C, Vakil N. Short- and long-term outcome of esophageal perforation. Gastrointest Endosc 1995; 41 (2):130–4.

29. Jones WG II, Ginsberg RJ. Oesophageal perforation: a continuing challenge. Ann Thorac Surg 1992; 53 (3):534–43.

30. Backer CL, LoCicero J III, Hartz RS et al. Computed tomography in patients with esophageal perforation. Chest 1990; 98 (5):1078–80.

31. White CS, Templeton PA, Attar S. Esophageal perforation: CT findings. Am J Roentgenol 1993; 160 (4):767–70.

32. Jaworski A, Fischer R, Lippmann M. Boerhaave's syndrome. Computed tomographic findings and diagnostic considerations. Arch Int Med 1988; 148 (1):223–4.

33. Drury M, Anderson W, Heffner JE. Diagnostic value of pleural fluid cytology in occult Boerhaave's syndrome. Chest 1992; 102 (3):976–8.

34. Yuasa N, Hattori T, Kobayashi Y et al. Treatment of spontaneous esophageal rupture with a covered self-expanding metal stent. Gastrointest Endosc 1999; 49 (6):777–80.

35. Cruci JJC, Horman MJ. Boerhaave's syndrome: The importance of early diagnosis and treatment. Ann Surg 1976; 183:401–08.

36. Larrieu AJ, Kieffer R. Boerhaave's syndrome: report of a case treated non-operatively. Ann Surg 1975; 181 (4):452–4.

37. Ivey TD, Simonwitz DA, Dillard DH et al. Boerhaave's syndrome: successful conservative management in three patients with late presentation. Am J Surg 1981; 141 (5):531–3.

38. Troum S, Lane CE, Dalton MI Jr. Surviving Boerhaave's syndrome without a thoracotomy. Chest 1994; 106 (1):297–9.

39. Tilanus HW, Bosuyt P, Schattenkerk ME et al. Treatment of oesophageal perforation: a multivariate analysis. Br J Surg 1991; 78 (5):582–5.

40. Lyons WS, Serementis MG, de Guzman VC et al. Ruptures and perforations of the esophagus: the case for conservative supportive management. Ann Thorac Surg 1978; 25 (4):346–50.

41. Anderson OS, Giustra PE. Nonoperative management of contained esophageal perforation. Arch Surg 1981; 116 (9):1214–7.

42. Hinder RA, Baskind AF, Le Grange F. A tube system for the management of ruptured oesophagus. Br J Surg 1981; 68 (3):182–4.

43. Flynn AE, Verrier ED, Way LW et al. Esophageal perforation. Arch Surg 1989; 124 (10):1211–4.

44. Nesbitt JC, Sawyers JL. Surgical management of oesophageal perforation. Ann Surg 1987; 53 (4):183–91.

45. Wright CD, Mathisen DJ, Wain JC et al. Reinforced primary repair of thoracic esophageal perforation. Ann Thorac Surg 1995; 60 (2):245–9.

46. Bryant LR, Eisman B. Experimental evaluation of intercostal pedicle grafts in esophageal repair. J Thorac Cardiovasc Surg 1965; 50 (5):626–31.

47. Mansour KA, Wenger RK. T-tube management of late esophageal perforations. Surg Gynecol Obstet 1992; 175 (6):571–2.

48. Larsson S, Pettersson G, Lepore V. Esophago-cutaneous drainage to treat late and complicated esophageal perforation. Eur J Cardiothorac Surg 1991; 5 (11):579–82.

49. Shenfine J, Dresner SM, Viswanath YKS et al. Management of spontaneous rupture of the oesophagus. Br J Surg 2000; 87:364.

50. Urschel HC Jr, Razzuk MA, Wood RE et al. Improved management of esophageal perforation: exclusion and diversion in continuity. Ann Surg 1974; 179 (5):587–91.

51. Altorjay A, Kiss J, Voros A et al. The role of esophagectomy in the management of esophageal perforations. Ann Thorac Surg 1998; 65 (5):1433–6.

52. Orringer MB, Stirling MC. Esophagectomy for esophageal disruption. Ann Thorac Surg 1990; 49 (1):35–42.

53. Salo JA, Isolauri JO, Heikkila LJ et al. Management of delayed esophageal perforation with mediastinal sepsis. Esophagectomy or primary repair? J Thorac Cardiovasc Surg 1993; 106 (6):1088–91.

54. Santos GH, Frater RW. Transesophageal irrigation for the treatment of mediastinitis produced by esophageal rupture. J Thorac Cardiovasc Surg 1986; 91 (1):57–62.

55. Derrick JR, Harrison WH, Howrad JM. Factors predisposing to spontaneous perforation of the esophagus. Surgery 1958; 43:486–90.

56. Bauer TM, Dupont V, Zimmerli W. Invasive candidiasis complicating spontaneous esophageal perforation (Boerhaave's syndrome). Am J Gastroenterol 1996; 91 (6):1248–50.

57. Cronstedt JL, Bouchama A, Hainau B et al. Spontaneous esophageal perforation in herpes simplex esophagitis. Am J Gastroenterol 1992; 87 (1):124–7.

58. Adkins MS, Raccuia JS, Acinapura AJ. Esophageal perforation in a patient with acquired immunodeficiency syndrome. Ann Thorac Surg 1990; 50 (2):299–300.

59. Sugawa C, Benishek D, Walt AJ. Mallory–Weiss syndrome: a study of 224 patients. Am J Surg 1983; 145 (1):30–3.

60. Katz PO, Salas L. Less frequent causes of upper gastro-intestinal bleeding. Gastroenterol Clin North Am 1993; 22 (4):875–89.

61. Jotte RS. Esophageal apoplexy: case report, review, and comparison with other esophageal disorders. J Emerg Med 1991; 9 (6):437–43.

62. Folan RD, Smith RE, Head JM. Esophageal haematoma and tear requiring emergency surgical intervention. A case report and literature review. Dig Dis Sci 1992; 37 (12):1918–21.

63. Ohri SK, Liakakos TA, Pathi V et al. Primary repair of iatrogenic thoracic esophageal perforation and Boerhaave's syndrome. Ann Thorac Surg 1993; 55 (3):603–6.

64. Cox JGC, Bennett JR. Benign esophageal strictures. In: Bennett JR, Hunt RH (eds) Therapeutic endoscopy and radiology of the gut, 2nd edn. Baltimore: Williams and Wilkins, 1990; p.11.

65. Monnier P, Hsieh V, Savary M. Endoscopic treatment of esophageal stenosis using Savary-Gilliard bougies: technical innovations. Acta Endosc 1985; 15:1–5.

66. Pasricha PJ, Fleischer DE, Kalloo AN. Endoscopic perforations of the upper digestive tract: a review of their pathogenesis, prevention, and management. Gastroenterol 1994; 106 (3):787–802.

67. Wesdorp IC, Bartelsman JF, Huibregtse K et al. Treatment of instrumental oesophageal perforation. Gut 1984; 25 (4):398–404.

68. Borotto E, Gaudric M, Danel B et al. Risk factors of oesophageal perforation during pneumatic dilatation for achalasia. Gut 1996; 39 (1):9–12.

69. Korula J, Pandya K, Yamada S. Perforation of esophagus after endoscopic variceal sclerotherapy. Incidence and clues to pathogenesis. Dig Dis Sci 1989; 34 (3):324–9.

70. Johnson P, Campbell D, Antonson C et al. Complications associated with endoscopic band ligation of esophageal varices. Gastrointest Endosc 1993; 39 (2):181–5.

71. Bisgaard T, Wojdemann M, Heindorff H et al. Nonsurgical treatment of esophageal perforations after endoscopic palliation in advanced esophageal cancer. Endoscopy 1997; 29 (3):155–9.

72. Lightdale CJ, Heier SK, Marcon NE et al. Photodynamic therapy with porfimer sodium versus thermal ablation therapy with Nd:YAG laser for palliation of oesophageal cancer: a multicenter randomized trial. Gastrointest Endosc 1995; 42 (6):507–12.

73. Cusumano A, Ruol A, Segalin A et al. Push-through intubation: effective palliation in 409 patients with cancer of the esophagus and cardia. Ann Thorac Surg 1992; 53 (6):1010–4.

74. Bartelsman JF, Bruno MJ, Jensema AJ et al. Palliation of patients with esophago-gastric neoplasms by insertion of a covered expandable modified Gianturco-Z endoprosthesis: experiences in 153 patients. Gastrointest Endosc 2000; 51 (2):134–8.

75. Dubost C, Kaswin D, Duranteau A et al. Esophageal perforation during attempted endotracheal intubation. J Thorac Cardiovasc Surg 1979; 78 (1):44–51.

76. Jackson RH, Payne DK, Bacon BR. Esophageal perforation due to nasogastric intubation. Am J Gastroenterol 1990; 85 (4):439–42.

77. Panzini L, Burrell MI, Traube M. Instrumental esophageal perforation: chest film findings. Am J Gastroenterol 1994; 89 (3):367–70.

78. Dolgin SR, Wykoff TW, Kumar NR et al. Conservative medical management of traumatic pharyngoesophageal perforations. Ann Oto Rhinol Laryngol 1992; 101 (3):209–15.

79. Brewer LA III, Carter R, Mulder GA et al. Options in the management of perforations of the esophagus. Am J Surg 1986; 152 (1):62–9.

80. Mengoli LR, Klassen KP. Conservative management of oesophageal perforation. Arch Surg 1965; 91:238–41.

81. Cameron JL, Kieffer RF, Hendrix TR et al. Selective nonoperative management of contained intrathoracic esophageal disruptions. Ann Thorac Surg 1979; 27 (5):404–08.

82. Sarr MG, Pemberton JH, Payne WS. Management of instrumental perforations of the esophagus. J Thorac Cardiovasc Surg 1982; 84 (2):211–8.

83. Michel L, Grillo HC, Malt RA. Operative and non-operative management of esophageal perforations. Ann Surg 1981; 194 (1):57–63.

84. Shaffer HA Jr, Valenzuela G, Mittal RK. Esophageal perforation. A reassessment of the criteria for choosing medical or surgical therapy. Arch Intern Med 1992; 152 (4):757–61.

85. Fernandez FF, Richter A, Freudenberg S, Wendl K, Manegold BC. Treatment of endoscopic esophageal perforation. Surg Endosc 1999; 13 (10):962–6.

86. Pricolo VE, Park CS, Thompson WR. Surgical repair of esophageal perforation due to pneumatic dilatation for achalasia: is myotomy really necessary? Arch Surg 1993; 128 (5):540–3.

87. Nicholson AA, Royston CM, Wedgewood K et al. Palliation of malignant oesophageal perforation and proximal oesophageal malignant dysphagia with covered metal stents. Clin Radiol 1995; 50 (1):11–4.

88. Watkinson A, Ellul J, Entwhistle K et al. Plastic-covered metallic endoprostheses in the management

of oesophageal perforation in patients with oesophageal carcinoma. Clin Radiol 1995; 50 (5):304–9.

89. Adam DJ, Thompson AM, Walker WS et al. Oesophago-gastrectomy for iatrogenic perforation of oesophageal and cardia carcinoma. Br J Surg 1996; 83 (10):1429–32.

90. Dresner SM, Lamb PJ, Vishwanath YKS et al. Oesophagectomy following iatrogenic perforation of operable oesophageal carcinoma. Br J Surg 2000; 87 (S1):29.

91. Urschel JD. Gastroesophageal leaks after antireflux operations. Ann Thorac Surg 1994; 57 (5):1229–32.

92. Albin J, Noel T, Allan K, Khalil KG. Intra-thoracic esophageal perforation with the Angelchick antireflux prosthesis: report of a new complication. Gastrointest Radiol 1985; 10 (4):330–2.

93. Sethi GK, Takaro T. Esophago-pleural fistula following pulmonary resection. Ann Thorac Surg 1978; 25 (1):74–81.

94. Newhouse KE, Lindsey RW, Clark CR et al. Esophageal perforation following anterior cervical spine surgery. Spine 1989; 14 (10):1051–3.

95. Shapira OM, Aldea GS, Kupferscmid J et al. Delayed perforation of the esophagus by a closed thoracostomy tube. Chest 1993; 104 (6):1897–8.

96. Shama DM, Odell J. Penetrating neck trauma with tracheal and oesophageal injuries. Br J Surg 1984; 71 (7):534–6.

97. Pass LJ, LeNarz LA, Schreiber JT et al. Management of esophageal gunshot wounds. Ann Thorac Surg 1987; 44 (3):243–6.

98. Glatterer MS Jr, Toon RS, Ellestad C et al. Management of blunt and penetrating external esophageal trauma. J Trauma-Inj Infec Crit Care 1985; 25 (8):784–92.

99. Defore WW Jr, Mattox KL, Hansen HA et al. Surgical management of penetrating injuries of the esophagus. Am J Surg 1977; 134 (6):734–8.

100. Symbas PN, Tyras DH, Hatcher CR Jr et al. Penetrating wounds of the esophagus. Ann Thorac Surg 1972; 13 (6):552–8.

101. Hagan WE. Pharyngoesophageal perforations after blunt trauma to the neck. Otolaryngol Head Neck Surg 1983; 91 (6):620–6.

102. Rotstein OD, Rhame FS, Molina E et al. Mediastinitis after whiplash injury. Can J Surg 1986; 29 (1):54–6.

103. Reddin A, Mirvis SE, Diaconis JN. Rupture of the cervical esophagus and trachea associated with cervical spine fracture. J Trauma-Inj Infec Crit Care 1987; 27 (5):564–6.

104. Beal SL, Pottmeyer EW, Spisso JM. Esophageal perforation following external blunt trauma. J Trauma-Inj Infec Crit Care 1988; 28 (10):1425–32.

105. Sabanathan S, Eng J, Richardson J. Surgical management of intrathoracic oesophageal rupture. Br J Surg 1994; 81 (6):863–5.

106. Christesen HB. Epidemiology and prevention of caustic ingestion in children. Acta Paediatr 1994; 83 (2):212–5.

107. Christesen HB. Caustic ingestion in adults – epidemiology and prevention. J Toxicol Clin Toxicol 1994; 32 (5):557–68.

108. Wasserman RL, Ginsburg CM. Caustic substance injuries. J Paed 1985; 107 (2):169–74.

109. Anderson KD, Rouse TM, Randolph JG. A controlled trial of corticosteroids in children with corrosive injury of the esophagus. New Engl J Med 1990; 323 (10):637–40.

110. Appelqvist P, Salmo M. Lye corrosion carcinoma of the esophagus: a review of 63 cases. Cancer 1980; 45 (10):2655–8.

111. Andreoni B, Farina ML, Biffi R, Crosta C. Esophageal perforation and caustic injury: emergency management of caustic ingestion. Dis Esoph 1997; 10 (2):95–100.

112. Zargar SA, Kochhar R, Nagi B et al. Ingestion of strong corrosive alkalis: spectrum of injury to upper gastrointestinal tract and natural history. Am J Gastroenterol 1992; 87 (3):337–41.

113. Webb WA. Management of foreign bodies in the upper gastrointestinal tract; update. Gastrointest Endosc 1995; 41 (1):39–51.

114. Ginsberg GG. Management of ingested foreign objects and food bolus impaction. Gastrointest Endosc 1995; 41 (1):33–8.

115. Webb WA. Management of foreign bodies of the upper gastrointestinal tract. Gastroenterol 1988; 94 (1):204–6.

116. Nandi P, Ong GB. Foreign body in the oesophagus: review of 2394 cases. Br J Surg 1978; 65 (1):5–9.

117. Fernandes ET, Hollabaugh RS, Boulden T. Mediastinal mass and radiolucent esophageal foreign body. J Pediatr Surg 1989; 24 (11):1135–6.

118. Wu MH, Lai WW. Aortoesophageal fistula induced by foreign bodies. Ann Thorac Surg 1992; 54:155–6.

119. Rajesh PB, Goiti JJ. Late onset tracheo-oesophageal fistula following a swallowed dental plate. Eur J Cardiothorac Surg 1993; 7 (12):661–2.

120. Doolin EJ. Esophageal stricture: an uncommon complication of foreign bodies. Ann Oto Rhinol Laryngol 1993; 102 (11):863–6.

121. Hodge D III, Tecklenburg F, Fleisher G. Coin ingestion. Does every child need a radiograph? Ann Emerg Med 1985; 14 (5):443–6.

122. Anonymous. Guideline for the management of ingested foreign bodies. American Society for Gastrointestinal Endoscopy. Gastrointest Endosc 1995; 42 (6):622–5.

123. Chaikhouni A, Kratz JM, Crawford PA. Foreign bodies of the esophagus. Am Surg 1985; 51 (4):173–9.

124. Berggreen PJ, Harrison E, Sanowski RA *et al.* Techniques and complications of esophageal foreign body extraction in children and adults. Gastrointest Endosc 1993; 39 (5):626–30.

125. Tibbling L, Bjorkhoel A, Jansson E *et al.* Effect of spasmolytic drugs on esophageal foreign bodies. Dysphagia 1995; 10 (2):126–7.

126. Holsinger JW, Fuson RL, Sealy WC. Esophageal perforation following meat impaction and papain ingestion. JAMA 1968; 204:734–5.

127. Smith JC, Janower ML, Geiger AH. Use of glucagon and gas-forming agents in acute esophageal food impaction. Radiology 1986; 159 (2):567–8.

15 The surgical management of morbid obesity

John N. Baxter

INTRODUCTION

Obesity surgery – often termed bariatric surgery – dates from the 1950s when the term referred to various forms of small bowel bypass; since then, it has evolved considerably. Like many surgical procedures it has been influenced by the laparoscopic revolution, with many of the available procedures being under-taken laparoscopically by various proponents. While enthusiasm for bariatric surgery has waxed and waned over the years it is making a vigorous comeback with the realisation that it is the only effective long-term treatment for patients with morbid obesity who have a much reduced life expectancy compared to age-gender-matched controls of a normal weight.[1] It is only relatively recently that society has realised that obesity is a major cause of early death with the economic costs of its complications running into billions of dollars annually.[2]

Conservative treatment fails in >95% of morbidly obese patients. Unfortunately most health-care systems are slow to realise (or more likely do not want to) the value of weight reduction by surgical methods and the whole area has been driven into the private sector as a result – an enormous mistake for the public health-care system. It is the challenge for the next decade to convince funders of health care that in a strictly economic sense bariatric surgery repre-sents value for money and should be part of the core surgical services. A recent prospective cost-effectiveness analysis of vertical banded gastroplasty (VBG) from The Netherlands concluded that VBG resulted in a gain of quality-adjusted life years and lower health service costs hence it should be continued from a societal point of view.[3]

 The forthcoming publication of the results of the Swedish Obese Subjects (SOS) study will provide the most robust data for furthering the case for bariatric surgery.[4]

While there have been at least 30 surgical procedures described for weight reduction this chapter will focus on operative techniques and results of some of the currently used operations being mindful that there are many other procedures: space precludes discussion but they have been well reviewed elsewhere.[5]

General considerations

This type of surgery should not be undertaken lightly since it is demanding, difficult and expensive. Patients need to be properly selected and counselled. In order to do all of this effectively, it is mandatory for this surgery to be carried out under the auspices of or within a multidisciplinary team (**Table 15.1**). Clearly the surgeon needs to be properly trained and should preferably be an upper gastrointestinal surgeon. Accreditation of these procedures, which helps to maintain standards, is mandatory in many countries. As with most forms of surgery the bariatric surgeon must perform the procedures reasonably frequently to stay competent and maintain the skills of the team. One of the most difficult issues with this form of surgery is overcoming the prejudice which still exists about morbidly obese patients and even the surgeons who perform bariatric procedures.[6] There is still a feeling in many circles that these patients do not have a 'real' problem other than a lack of eating discipline. This reveals a gross lack of knowledge about the pathophysiology of morbid obesity, the complex genetic aspects of which have recently become obvious with the recognition of genetic defects on all 22 pairs of autosomes, 10 of which are dominant.

 There is now voluminous literature attesting to the fact that morbid obesity is an inborn error of metabolism manifested by an impaired satiety mechanism and an increased conversion of calories to fat rather than dissipation as body heat.[7,8,9,10]

The chances of an effective medical treatment being discovered in the near future are bleak, although we live in hope. A further problem, especially in the United Kingdom, is finding enough operating time to perform these procedures in a health service that struggles to cope with its present workload. As a consequence many procedures are being driven into the private sector depriving patients who cannot afford them of their benefit.

The multidisciplinary team that manages these patients must audit their results and be prepared to discuss with patients their personal results and complication rates. There are many anecdotal reports of the value of self-help patient counselling groups in helping patients deal with any post-surgical problems and in maintaining their diets. The use of a psychologist or psychiatrist is advantageous to help weed out frankly psychotic patients or patients who may not be suited to long-term follow-up.

- Bariatric surgeon

- Dietician

- Physician with a special interest in obesity

- Anaesthetist with a special interest in anaesthesia of the morbidly obese

- Psychologist or counsellor

- Nursing staff with special training

Table 15.1 *A bariatric surgery team*

Selection of patients for surgery

Morbid obesity (sometimes called clinically severe obesity or class III obesity) is defined as a patient who has a body mass index (BMI) > 40 kg/m². The comorbidity that morbidly obese patients suffer from is well known (**Table 15.2**) and it is important to understand those comorbid conditions that can be improved by bariatric surgery (**Table 15.2**). Data from the Framingham study shows that even as little as a 10% weight reduction results in a 20% reduction in the risk of heart disease.[11] The most striking effect of weight-reducing surgery is the report by Pories demonstrating that 83% of type II diabetics achieve cure after gastric bypass.[12] In his series he achieved a remarkable 96% follow-up at 14 years. Another study revealed a three-times greater mortality in type II diabetics after medical treatment compared with a surgically treated group.[13] There is also ample evidence from the literature of improvement – and in many cases cure of – sleep apnoea syndrome,[14] high blood pressure, dyslipidaemias,[15] joint problems

Diabetes mellitus (Type II)*

High blood pressure*

Dyslipidaemia*

Obstructive sleep apnoea*

Venous and lymphatic stasis*

Osteoarthritis*

Decreased mobility*

Increased cancer risk (endometrium, prostate, breast, colorectal, cervix, ovary)

Increased risk of cardiac and cerebral vascular events*

Chronic respiratory hypoventilation (Pickwickian syndrome)*

Hypertrophic cardiomyopathy*

Pseudotumour cerebri (idiopathic intracranial hypertension)*

Poor quality of life*

Increased neuroses*

Chronic cholecystitis

Thromboembolic disease

Urinary stress incontinence*

Gastro-oesophageal reflux disease*

Obesity-related pulmonary hypertension

Hernia

Table 15.2 *Comorbidity of morbid obesity (those conditions with * have been shown to be improved by bariatric surgery)*

and hypertrophic cardiomyopathy.[16] Of critical importance is the fact that mortality rate is directly related to weight with obesity *per se* being a risk factor in addition to the associated comorbidity. Furthermore, there is evidence that the increased risk of death with morbid obesity reverts to a normal risk following successful weight reduction surgery.[17]

The International Federation for Surgery of Obesity (IFSO) has devised strict criteria of eligibility for bariatric surgery (**Table 15.3**). The counselling process prior to surgery must be thorough and be supported by literature. There are also many useful Internet Websites which provide valuable information but any physician or surgeon should approve these personally before advising patients to view them. The patient must understand that the operation alone does not cure them but requires a concurrent diet. The patient must also agree to postoperative follow-up for life and satisfy the dietician in the team that he or she fully understands the associated dietary aspects of the treatment. There is controversy about the value of formal psychiatric evaluation of all surgical patients. It is the author's practice only to seek specialised psychological evaluation where the team thinks that the patient may have a significant premorbid psychological problem such as a frank psychosis.

One of the most difficult areas is the anaesthetic evaluation and risk assessment of morbidly obese patients with serious comorbidity. In general terms it is difficult in the really high-risk patient to weigh up the true risk of perioperative death with therapeutic gain — the decision usually being made in an *ad hoc* manner. Hopefully further studies will allow evaluation of this difficult area.

Another problematic area is the ability to quantify the added value to the patient of having surgery. Although most patients come seeking surgical treatment after years of failed conservative management they must have realistic expectations of what surgery has to offer. They must understand that it is not a cosmetic procedure but rather aimed at prolonging life by reducing the chance of premature death to which they are exposed. It is assumed that reduction of their excess weight always extrapolates to improved survival, an assumption which is likely to be true, but we need further evidence for it. It can be justified when operating on a patient with a BMI 35–39 who is not technically morbidly obese providing they have a comorbid condition which is clearly improved by weight loss (**Table 15.2**). Whether it is justifiable to operate on patients with a BMI <35 with serious comorbid disease treatable by weight reduction needs evaluation.

- BMI > 40
- BMI 35–40 with comorbid condition improved by weight loss
- Age 18–55
- Fit for surgery
- Minimum 5 years morbid obesity
- Failed conservative treatment
- No alcoholism or psychosis
- Agrees to lifelong follow-up

Table 15.3 *Criteria for considering bariatric surgery*

Since around 80% of patients seeking surgery are female they should be counselled not to become pregnant within 2 years of bariatric surgery because of the suspicion that rapid weight loss may be detrimental to a foetus. Should a patient become pregnant following successful bariatric surgery the surgeon should have a close liaison with the obstetrician since the latter is often unaware of the nutritional problems that may supervene.[18]

Outline of surgical gastric procedures

The surgical options are broadly divided into gastric restrictive procedures with or without a malabsorption component. Pure gastric restrictive procedures usually consist of a gastroplasty (usually vertical banded) or gastric banding. Gastric bypass procedures usually involve the creation of gastric pouch with a Roux-en-Y gastro-jejunal anastomosis with varying lengths of limbs. Some proponents of bypass procedures reinforce the gastric outlet stoma with an additional band to prevent dilatation. Biliopancreatic diversion with or without a duodenal switch are favoured by some surgeons for their very good outcome although they are big operations and should probably be reserved for patients who have failed conventional surgery. Occasionally a jejuno-ileal bypass may be considered, especially where it may be technically impossible to do any other procedure – providing it is of the Cleator type (*vide infra*) good results can be expected. During most bariatric procedures a cholecystectomy should be performed because of the high incidence of gallstones at the time of surgery or during the follow-up period.

The importance of counselling patients about the nutritional requirements following surgery cannot be overestimated. All patients need to take an adequate diet in protein, calories and micronutrients. Pure gastric restrictive procedures such as vertical banded gastroplasty (VBG) or gastric banding all cause weight loss by restricting intake; the patient has to chew the food well and eat slowly to avoid vomiting – a form of aversion therapy. Where the patient has persistent vomiting a protein-calorie malnutrition and/or vitamin deficiency state can occur, hence it is usual to prescribe added vitamins for all patients. Gastric bypass procedures, while having some gastric restriction, also have a variable element of malabsorption depending on the length of the bypass. As a result these patients are at risk of developing iron and vitamin B12 deficiency as well as reduced vitamin D and calcium absorption. Hence, it is particularly important for these patients to have lifelong vitamin and mineral supplements.

The general complications of bariatric surgery are similar to abdominal surgery in a high-risk patient. Peritonitis due to anastomotic leakage is the most dangerous complication and is often difficult to diagnose, needing a high degree of suspicion when the patient is not recovering as expected. There should be a very low threshold for repeating contrast studies when leakage is suspected or even reoperation if there is any remaining uncertainty. Abdominal wall hernias are common after open procedures, occurring in 10–20% of patients. They should be repaired, preferably using a mesh technique, when the weight loss has stabilised.

When the excess weight loss has stabilised at around 24 months many patients complain of problems with redundant skin flaps especially around the anterior abdominal wall. It will often be necessary to refer these patients to a plastic surgeon for 'body sculpturing' if it is thought desirable.

Preoperative considerations

When bariatric surgery is contemplated it is necessary to assess fitness for surgery. All patients should have a complete cardiorespiratory examination and investigations including electrocardiogram, chest radiography, respiratory function tests, arterial blood gases, echocardiogram if indicated and routine baseline blood tests. An epidural anaesthetic is preferable where open surgery is contemplated, although it may be difficult to carry out in some patients. Some surgeons do not like epidural anaesthesia where the small intestine is being used as in a bypass because of the spasm that often occurs. All patients must receive thromboprophylaxis as they are hypercoagulable and more prone to pulmonary embolism, which is the most common cause of death following this form of surgery. When deciding to perform any particular procedure it is advisable to seek permission to perform an alternative procedure should circumstances dictate at surgery that the intended procedure is contraindicated or not possible to perform. Antibiotic prophylaxis is advisable for all procedures.

Most surgical wards dealing with these patients have special beds and frames that can cope with the increased weight of these patients. In the operating theatre, tables must be able to withstand the increased weight. For open surgery special deep-bladed retractors such as the Omnitract®-type are essential for safe surgery. For laparoscopic surgery some special instrumentation is usually necessary although most procedures can be done without it.

Some patients may need to have an intensive care unit bed booked if it is thought that postoperative ventilation is a possibility. Most patients, however, will not need this facility and can be managed in a high dependency unit with monitoring including pulse oximetry.

Procedures

Pure gastric restriction

Vertical banded gastroplasty (VBG)

Although a VBG can be performed laparoscopically most surgeons prefer to do this as an open procedure since the former is technically difficult. The principle of the operation is to create a pouch about 15–20 ml in volume with an outlet stoma of 4.75–5.0 cm (**Fig. 15.1**). In order to do this the author recommends the following technique:

- Place patient on operating table supine with about 20° head-up tilt (reverse Trendelberg).
- Make a midline skin incision and then use a fat-splitting technique to expose the anterior sheath of the rectus muscle.
- Divide the right triangular ligament and fold back left lobe of liver.
- Insert Omnitract® or similar retractor to display gastro-oesophageal junction (GOJ).

Figure 15.1
*Vertical banded
gastroplasty*

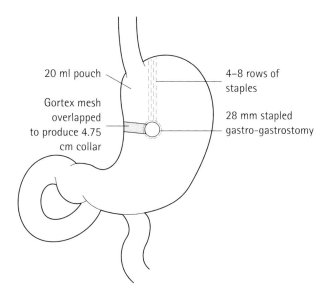

20 ml pouch

Gortex mesh
overlapped
to produce 4.75
cm collar

4–8 rows of
staples

28 mm stapled
gastro-gastrostomy

- Divide gastrophrenic ligament and open up angle of His.
- Divide gastrocolic ligament to allow access to lesser sac.
- Divide adhesions from stomach to posterior wall of lesser sac and use finger to break out at angle of His.
- Insert 32 Fr bougie and measure 5 cm down from GOJ and 3 cm in from lesser curve – mark with a diathermy burn.
- Take anvil from 28 mm stapler and insert it from lesser sac posteriorly through stomach at site of diathermy burn or closer to lesser curve keeping the anvil snug up against the bougie, emerging anteriorly – attach rest of the stapler then fire creating a gastro-gastrostomy.
- Oversew gastro-gastrostomy to prevent bleeding.
- Insert a linear 90 mm stapler (four staple rows) without a blade into gastro-gastrostomy up to angle of His to create vertical staple line – ensure the whole length of stomach is stapled. A second firing for security should be used – 8 rows of staples in all.
- Insert with bougie *in situ* a Gortex® band 6.75 × 1.0 cm long through gastro-gastrostomy around lesser curve (being careful to separate fat from lesser curve) – leaving the ends to overlap by 1 cm (**Fig. 15.2**). Suture in two layers as shown in **Fig. 15.2** to allow for postoperative dilatation if necessary without complete rupture of the band.
- Cover gastric band with a tongue of greater omentum.
- Insert a nasogastric tube for 24 hours.
- Check for bleeding then close abdomen with a running non-absorbable suture.
- Allow free fluids postoperatively.

While there are many minor variations on the technique above it has been stan-dardised more than any other bariatric operation. Some surgeons prefer to use more staple lines while others prefer to divide the stomach instead (gastric partitioning). A double application of a 4-row linear stapler giving 8 rows of staples, appears to have reduced staple-line disruption to a minimum. Some

Figure 15.2
*The technique of
band fixation for a
vertical banded
gastroplasty*

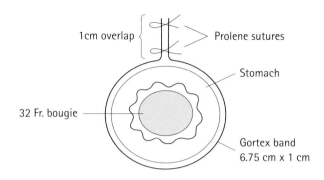

1cm overlap — Prolene sutures

Stomach

32 Fr. bougie —

Gortex band
6.75 cm x 1 cm

surgeons prefer a 5 cm circumference stoma rather than the 4.75 cm used above by the author. Measuring the pouch volume and pressure has been recommended by some authors but others find it does not add to the procedure. Similarly leak testing with methylene blue has been recommended by some surgeons although it is probably not necessary if the procedure has been straightforward.

Patients should immediately start on their fluid diet gradually increasing the viscosity of the food over the next 3 months. Close dietary follow-up is necessary with monitoring of weight loss. Added vitamins are essential. Food intolerance or persistent vomiting usually settles although occasionally a dilatation is necessary. The most common early postoperative complication is wound infection despite the use of antibiotic prophylaxis.

Adjustable gastric banding

There are currently two major choices of adjustable gastric band:

- The American Lap-Band® (BioEnterics, Carpenteria, California, USA) formerly known as Adjustable Silicone Gastric Band (ASGB). This changed its name when the method of insertion evolved to a laparoscopic technique.
- The Swedish Adjustable Gastric Band (SAGB) (Obtech Medical AG, St-Antons-Gasse, Switzerland).

Both bands can be inserted by an open or laparoscopic technique, the latter becoming the method of choice. There have been > 23 000 Lap-Bands inserted worldwide with many published reports attesting to its efficacy. Either band is essentially a collar of silicone containing a bladder, which can be inflated with saline, that is placed around the upper stomach just below the GOJ (**Fig. 15.3**) The saline inflation of the band is carried out by inserting a special needle into a reservoir implanted under the skin on the rectus sheath. The choice of gastric band is a matter of personal preference but there is some evidence that the Lap-Band® may have fewer complications than the SAGB[19,20] although this has not been proven by a randomised comparison. The obvious attractions of the gastric band technique are:

1. Possible insertion by a laparoscopic technique with the advantages of less pain, fewer wound complications, shorter hospital stay and earlier return to normal activity;
2. Reversibility if a non-surgical cure is ever found for morbid obesity.
3. The ability to calibrate the stoma;

Figure 15.3
Adjustable gastric band with reservoir

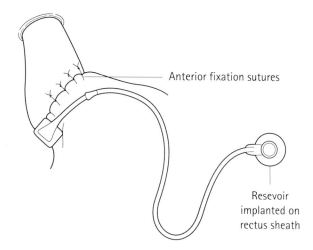

Anterior fixation sutures

Resevoir implanted on rectus sheath

4. It is less destructive to the stomach.

While the first of these advantages is obvious the latter three are less clear e.g. some patients do not trust themselves with a procedure that is potentially reversible. The main disadvantages are the steep learning curve for laparoscopic insertion and the cost of the prosthesis.

There is an urgent need for a good health-services economic evaluation of gastric bands preferably compared with other bariatric procedures and conservative treatment.

Most emerging data suggest that the gastric band is as efficient as a VBG although more long-term data are still needed. The longest a band has remained in a patient is around 8 years. There have been occasional reports in the literature of non-adjustable bands which can be placed laparoscopically but more experience is needed with them before they can be properly assessed.[21]

The principles of patient selection for this procedure are the same as for any bariatric procedure. During the learning curve it is mandatory to have attended a course on how to insert the band which includes watching bands being inserted. When starting out it is a good idea to insert the first few with an open technique as this may become necessary during the learning curve of laparoscopic insertion. It is not wise to embark on laparoscopic band insertion unless the surgeon is accomplished at laparoscopic hiatal surgery.

Open technique (Lap-Band®)

The essential steps for the open technique using the Lap-Band® are listed below. There are several differences in the technique for the SAGB.

- Perform laparotomy as for VBG above including insertion of retractor.
- Anaesthetist inserts calibration tube into stomach and inflates balloon to 15 ml then impacts tube into the GOJ.
- Make a diathermy mark on the lesser curve adjacent to the equator of the gastric balloon – then deflate balloon and pull calibration tube into oesophagus.

- Divide gastro-phrenic ligament then start dissecting at angle of His backwards towards the lesser curve in the bare area of the stomach *above* the lesser sac.
- Commence dissection of a retrogastric tunnel from the lesser curve at the previously marked site – use of a long blunt slightly curved instrument is valuable here. It is important not to enter the lesser sac.
- When the tunnel is complete pass a long curved forcep through the tunnel and grasp the previously prepared band and position it in the tunnel.
- Reinsert the gastric calibration tube and inflate the balloon as before, then close the band around the pressure sensor on the distal end of the calibration tube. The gastrostenometer should not light up beyond the second light – if it does then too much tissue has been included in the band and it will need to be repositioned.
- Apply 3–4 fixation sutures to stabilise the band anteriorly (and a few posteriorly if the lesser sac has accidentally been entered).
- Make a separate transverse incision on the rectus sheath at the site chosen to place the reservoir then leaving a reasonable amount of tubing in the abdomen bring the tubing through and attach to the previously prepared reservoir. It is wise to reinforce the connection with non-absorbable ties.
- The reservoir must be sutured flat on the rectus sheath being careful that it does not rotate.
- Close the abdomen in the usual manner (as for a VBG).

The need to use the gastrostenometer is often debated by surgeons since with experience it is highly unusual to incorporate too much tissue. The author suspects that in time this refinement will be dropped from the technique.

It is usual to leave the band deflated for 6–8 weeks before commencing inflating which is best done by a radiologist using imaging and the special needle provided. The titration of inflation with dysphagia is an iterative process with most patients' needing two or three inflations to get the optimal degree of dysphagia for solids.

Like a VBG the procedure must be accompanied by a parallel 700 calorie-diet with the patient eating slowly and chewing the food well.

The SAGB has a slightly different point of insertion being usually placed through a window in the lesser omentum under the fold of the left gastric artery aiming to come out the angle of His as for the Lap-Band®. The SAGB thus incorporates more tissue and is not closed around a pressure measuring device. Because the band does not have a locking device like the Lap-Band it is necessary to suture it to prevent it unlocking.

Laparoscopic technique (Lap-Band®)

As with any laparoscopic technique it is necessary to have the correct equipment before embarking on this procedure. No special long instruments are necessary although the Lap-Band® closing instrument for locking the band makes the operation easier. The most difficult part of the operation is making the retrogastric tunnel with confidence because of the potential for perforating the stomach. There have been several instruments developed for the retrogastric dissection from which the surgeon needs to decide which one they prefer. The technique is essentially the same as for the open technique apart from the need for an abdominal laparotomy incision.

- The patient should be positioned as for an antireflux procedure with the surgeon standing between the legs and the patient given a 30° head-up tilt.
- The pneumo-peritoneum is made with a Veress needle remembering that the baseline pressure in these patients is often high, at around 8–10 mmHg. The Veress needle is more safely inserted in the left upper quadrant just below the rib cage where the peritoneum is more firmly attached to the posterior surface of the abdominal wall.
- Trocars are inserted as shown in **Fig. 15.4**.
- The left lobe of the liver is best retracted with a Nathanson® liver retractor system (large size) which gives excellent access to the GOJ although any fan-type retractor can be used.
- The calibration tube is inserted as for the open procedure and the diathermy mark made.
- The dissection of the angle of His is best carried out after the gastrophrenic ligament has been divided.
- The retrogastric tunnel is then made very cautiously using a blunt instrument – the author preferring a closed Endo-Roticular®.
- When the tunnel is made the previously prepared band is inserted into the abdomen through the 15 mm (or 18 mm) port – being careful not to damage it.
- When the band is positioned around the calibration tube pressure device it is closed using the special closing tool.
- Using an intracorporeal suturing technique the band is fixed anteriorly as for the open technique.
- The tubing is then delivered through one of the dissection port sites which has been enlarged. The tubing is then attached to the reservoir which is then sutured to the rectus sheath.
- All wounds are closed after deflation of the pneumo-peritoneum.

Figure 15.4
The sites for laparoscopic port insertion for gastric banding

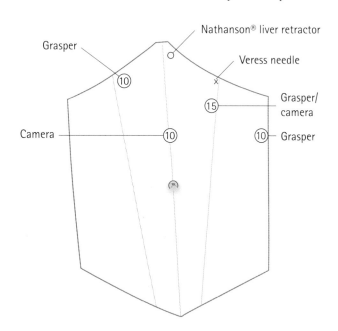

In the super-obese patient (BMI > 50) there is often a lot of fat in the left upper quadrant which frustrates visualisation of the dissection area. This can be made easier by inserting a suture into the fat and exteriorising the suture in the lower left abdomen to hold the fat away from the dissection area. The positioning of posterior sutures to stabilise the band if the lesser sac is entered is possible but they are often difficult to place. Some surgeons use other techniques for posterior fixation such as placement of a roll of mesh Marlex.[22]

Complications of gastric bands

With evolution of the techniques for insertion, complications rates have decreased significantly. With the Lap-Band® the pouch has been made increasingly smaller and emphasis placed on making a small retrogastric tunnel through the bare area of the stomach above the lesser sac which facilitates posterior fixation. Several anterior sutures also help prevent prolapse of the stomach with band rotation and subsequent obstruction. There have been rare reports of band erosion into the stomach with the Lap-Band®, a complication which appears more common with the SAGB.[19] A recent very honest report on complications following SAGB insertion indicated that, similar to the Lap-Band® experience, complication rates are falling with evolution of the insertion technique and attention to detail.[19] Infection of the reservoir site and band failure have also been reported but they are very rare.

Gastric restriction plus malabsorption

Gastric bypass

Surgeons who prefer gastric bypass usually base their arguments on the better long-term outcome after this technique compared to pure gastric restrictive techniques. The gastric bypass technique is especially popular in the USA where there are many excellent reports attesting to its efficacy. Unfortunately there is very little standardisation of the technique and very little agreement on the best type of bypass which makes it difficult to make any recommendation to the reader – every surgeon claiming that their modification is the best.[23] Anyone contemplating performing this type of surgery is well advised to learn from observing an experienced gastric bypass surgeon and adopting their technique. The present author prefers the technique favoured by the Mayo clinic,[24] although there are many other excellent techniques.

One objection that many surgeons have to gastric bypass is the fact that the majority of the stomach is not available for direct visualisation should the patient later develop dyspeptic symptoms. Worry concerning delayed diagnosis of gastric cancer is a theoretical problem about which there has been more ink spilt than blood. Some surgeons advise a preoperative gastroscopy as a baseline which appears sensible. Gastric bypass is usually performed as an open procedure because of the technical difficulty in performing it laparoscopically although there are many excellent exponents of the latter, especially Lonroth from Sweden.[25]

Selection of patients for this form of surgery is controversial. Some surgeons perform it as their sole bariatric procedure while others reserve it for the super-obese or those patients who are predominantly sweet-eaters – the bypass causing

Figure 15.5
*Nomenclature for
gastric bypass limbs*

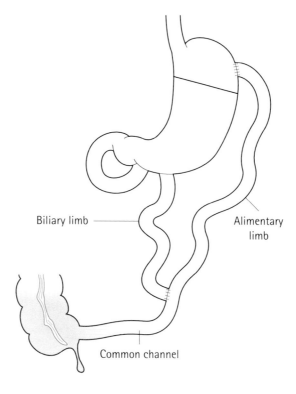

Biliary limb

Alimentary
limb

Common channel

them to dump and hence adding an increased aversion element to the procedure. There is also considerable variation in the length of the alimentary limb (**Fig. 15.5**), with some surgeons tailoring the lengths according to the preoperative BMI. There is a gradually emerging consensus that the optimal length of the alimentary limb should be about 200 cm for the morbidly obese with longer limbs for the super-obese (distal Roux-en-Y gastric bypass). Another area of controversy appears to be whether to reinforce the gastric stoma with a band to prevent dilatation. This appears to be carried out more commonly in short limb gastric bypasses than in long limb bypasses.[26]

Gastric bypass (Mayo technique)

The following account is the author's technique (**Fig. 15.6**) based on the method of Sarr.[24]

- Open abdomen as described above for a VBG.
- Make an opening in the gastrocolic ligament then divide adhesions from the stomach to the posterior wall of the lesser sac.
- The gastrophrenic ligament is divided then the angle of His dissected backwards towards the lesser curve.
- A calibration tube is then passed as for the gastric band above and inflated with 15 ml fluid – a mark is then made on the lesser curve at the inferior margin of the balloon.
- A 1 cm hole is made in the lesser omentum adjacent to the lesser curve at the marked site then a retrogastric tunnel made to the angle of His similar to that described for gastric banding.

Figure 15.6
Gastric bypass –
Mayo technique
(after Sarr)[24]

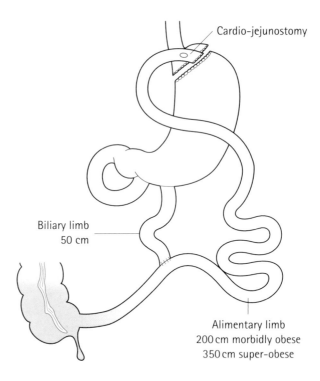

Cardio-jejunostomy

Biliary limb
50 cm

Alimentary limb
200 cm morbidly obese
350 cm super-obese

- A Roux limb is then constructed starting 40–50 cm distal to the DJ flexure. The Roux limb is brought retrocolic and tested for length making sure that there is no tension.
- Gastric division is then made using a linear 90 mm stapler with a blade, being careful to completely transect the stomach. Both suture lines are oversewn in a continuous non-inverting manner.
- The anvil of a 21 mm circular stapler is inserted into the anterior wall of the gastric pouch keeping at least 1.5 cm away from the staple line – 2–0 prolene is used to close the gastrotomy around the shaft of the anvil.
- The rest of stapler in then inserted into the Roux limb and at the anti-mesenteric border in a suitable place the shaft is brought through the wall then attached to the anvil.
- The stapler is fired and the doughnuts inspected. The anastomosis (cardio-jejunostomy) should be reinforced with an absorbable suture regardless of completeness of the doughnuts – the end of the Roux limb is closed with a linear stapler and the end oversewn.
- The enteroenterostomy is made at 300–350 cm distal to the gastro-jejunal anastomosis in the super-obese and at 200 cm for the morbidly obese.
- A gastrostomy in the blind stomach remnant is then performed and the abdomen closed with looped nylon after placement of a tube drain to the left subhepatic space. The gastrostomy tube is removed at 6 weeks.

When undertaking this procedure for the first few times it is tempting to make the gastric pouch larger because this is easier to do. This should, however, be resisted as the smaller the size of the pouch the less the acid secretion and hence the incidence of stomal ulceration. Leak from the gastro-jejunal anastomosis should never be more than 2% and is usually less in most series.[27] Obstruction of the excluded segment is very rare in the largest reported series.[27] Subphrenic abscess and accidental splenectomy should be less than 2% while mortality rates should be less than 1%.[27]

Biliopancreatic diversion

This procedure – probably the most efficient of all bariatric procedures – was developed in Italy by Scopinario[28] who has now performed more than 2000 procedures over a 20-year period (**Fig. 15.7**). However, it is also the most destructive bariatric procedure if a gastric resection is included (and this is usually advised). Nevertheless, it is much favoured by some exponents of the technique because of the excellent results. Protein–calorie malnutrition (PCM) is a real long-term complication if these patients are lost to follow-up and it should not be contemplated in an unreliable patient.

The procedure was developed because of the dissatisfaction with jejunoileal bypass procedures, in particular, the creation of a bypassed limb with its attendant complications. Scopinario currently adapts the size of gastric pouch and lengths of various limbs in an *ad hoc* manner dictated by personal experience.[28]

The essential features of the technique are:

- The stomach is displayed as described for a VBG.
- The gastric pouch is made around 150 ml by marking 15 cm from the GOJ on the greater curve side and 3 cm from the GOJ on the lesser curve side then using a stapler to perform a 75% distal gastrectomy – the duodenal staple line is oversewn.

Figure 15.7
Biliopancreatic bypass

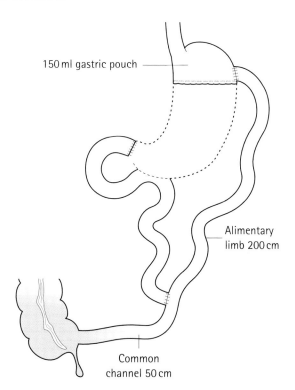

150 ml gastric pouch

Alimentary limb 200 cm

Common channel 50 cm

- The caecum is mobilised to allow for increased mobility – the ileum is marked 50 cm and 250 cm proximal to ileocaecal valve and then divided at the latter point.
- The pancreatico-biliary limb (see **Fig. 15.7**) is anastomosed at the 50 cm mark and the proximal ileum brought retrocolic and a gastroileostomy performed to the gastric pouch.
- The abdomen is closed with looped nylon after insertion of a drain to the duodenal stump.

During the early postoperative period patients often experience some minor dumping features (not vasomotor symptoms) but this usually settles within a year probably because of intestinal adaptation. Patients undergoing a BPD have to understand that they can absorb only minimal fat, little starch, sufficient protein but nearly all mono- and disaccharides, short-chain trigylcerides and alcohol. Most patients have loose foul-smelling stools. The late complication of anaemia requires iron and multivitamin preparations to be taken. Stomal ulceration requires prophylaxis with acid inhibitors, especially if the gastric pouch is large. Thiamine must also be taken routinely to prevent neurological complications. Protein-calorie malnutrition is the most serious complication of this procedure which is usually characterised by hypoalbuminaemia, anaemia, oedema, asthenia and alopecia which requires 2–3 weeks of careful parenteral therapy.[28]

Despite this procedure being complex it has much to recommend it in selected patients and should be studied more in order to find its place in the management of morbid obesity. If it is not the primary operation for morbid obesity then it may have a place in revisional surgery when other procedures have failed. If the stomach is not resected it becomes in effect a gastric bypass with a long alimentary limb (distal Roux-en-Y bypass).

Biliopancreatic diversion with a duodenal switch

The idea of this operation is to decrease the side effects of the BPD while still maintaining the good weight-reducing effects.[29] Essentially a sleeve gastrectomy is performed which maintains the antropyloric motor activity while reducing the parietal cell mass (**Fig. 15.8**). Maintaining a small segment of duodenum also protects against marginal ulceration. The essential principles of the operation are:

- The stomach is displayed as for a VBG above.
- All short gastric vessels are transected from the pylorus to the oesophagus freeing up the greater curve.
- The duodenum is mobilised very carefully for about 5 cm distal to the pylorus.
- A 40 Fr dilator is passed orally into the stomach then the duodenum. Using several firings of a linear stapler, the stomach is vertically resected about one fingerbreadth from the dilator. The staple line is then oversewn.
- The duodenum is then transected with a linear stapler as far distally as possible and the distal end oversewn.
- The ileum is then marked at 100 cm and 250 cm proximal to the ileocaecal valve – the ileum is then divided at the 250 cm mark with a linear stapler.
- The distal ileum is then brought retrocolic up to the divided duodenum then anastomosed very carefully end-to-end to the proximal duodenum. This is a

Figure 15.8
*Biliopancreatic
bypass with a
duodenal switch*

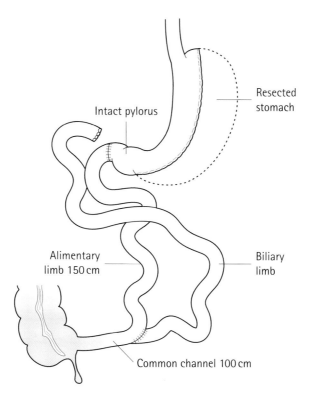

Resected stomach

Intact pylorus

Alimentary
limb 150 cm

Biliary
limb

Common channel 100 cm

difficult anastomosis to perform and can be simplified by suturing the posterior layer first of both closed stapled ends with a running seromuscular suture
then removing the staples and finishing the anastomosis anteriorly.

● The proximal ileum is then anastomosed end-to-side to the ileum at the
  50 cm mark.

Most patients eat normally following this procedure without any vomiting.
Indeed, there is evidence that the digestive side effects are less with the duodenal
switch than with a straight BPD and that there is more patient satisfaction.[29]
Nevertheless, similar follow-up and supplements must be prescribed as for a
straight BPD.

Miscellaneous procedures

Jejuno-ileal bypass (JIB)

Although JIBs of various forms were the favoured operation of the 1950s and
60s they have now fallen from grace as about one-third needed to be reversed
because of side effects, in some cases progressive and leading to death. Although
weight loss was excellent, on balance the risks of the procedure were generally
considered too great. Most of the serious complications were attributed to the
bypass segment jejuno–ileum in a way that has yet defied complete understanding. Despite several ingenious modifications of the technique to avert bypass
problems there still remains dissatisfaction with the technique. However, Cleator's
group from Vancouver have continued to use JIB using their own modification

Figure 15.9
Jejunoileal bypass (after Cleator)[30]

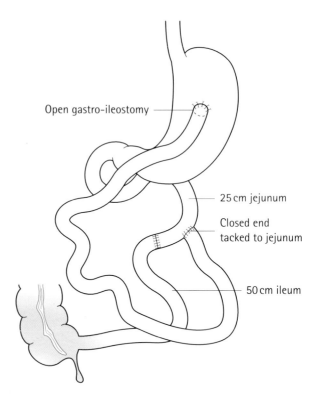

Open gastro-ileostomy

25 cm jejunum

Closed end tacked to jejunum

50 cm ileum

of the technique (**Fig. 15.9**) and have published results which are excellent.[30] In their hands the insertion of the blind limb into stomach would appear to have solved the problem of bypass complications. There may still be a place for this modification of the procedure which needs to be confirmed by other workers. The author has occasionally used it where access is very difficult for a gastric bypass or other procedure especially in the extremely obese (BMI > 60). Indeed, there is another recent report in the literature supporting JIB on the basis of excellent long-term results providing follow-up can be guaranteed to detect complications early.[31]

Essential features of this operation are:

- Access is gained with an upper abdominal midline incision.
- A point is chosen 25 cm distal to the duodenal-jejunal flexure and the bowel divided with a linear stapler.
- The ileum is then measured 50 cm from the ileocaecal valve and divided with a linear stapler. The distal end is then anastomosed end-to-end with the proximal jejunum. Some mobilisation of the small bowel mesentery may be necessary.
- The proximal stapled end of the defunctioned bowel is then lightly sutured to the proximal jejunum about 5 cm proximal to the jejuno-ileal anasto-mosis (**Fig. 15.9**).
- The distal end of the defunctioned bowel is then brought antecolic (through a window in the greater omentum) and anastomosed as high as possible on the anterior gastric wall using a single layer technique.
- The abdomen is closed without any drainage.

Gastric balloons

A gastric balloon essentially acts as an artificial bezoar by partially filling the stomach and causing an increase in satiety and hence reduction of food intake. The balloon allows the patient to eat normal food rather than a liquid or semi-solid diet. Weight loss of 25–30 kg can be expected although there are several patients who cannot tolerate the balloon and request its removal. In general terms gastric balloons have little place in the permanent management of morbid obesity since they are only a stop-gap procedure which ceases to have an effect when the balloon eventually deflates, usually after about 6 months. However, as part of a diet programme it may help patients adhere to the diet and increase chances of long-term success although there are little data to this effect.

There is evidence that modest weight loss preoperatively (10–20%) reduces the incidence of post-operative complications.[32] The bariatric surgeon may find a role in using a balloon as a temporary procedure to reduce weight enough to allow a more conventional procedure to take place, especially laparoscopic gastric banding. During laparoscopic dissection in the super-obese there is more difficulty in determining the level of dissection since the calibration tube is difficult to visualise. Indeed, there is some evidence from one study that a gastric balloon used preoperatively in these patients may be useful although much more convincing data are needed.[33] In this study there were no conversions to open banding procedures after prior use of gastric balloons in super- and super-super obese patients.[33] If the waiting list is long a gastric balloon may prevent further weight increase until surgery is carried out. Furthermore, it has been argued that use of a gastric balloon may tease out those patients who do not conform to a diet since they will lose little if any weight with a balloon and hence be bad surgical candidates. This notion of using the results of gastric balloon insertion as a predictor of good long-term results from bariatric surgery needs evaluation.

Although gastric balloons have been around for a long time they have been recently rediscovered with claims of improved performance. They are inserted under sedation using a gastroscope and inflated with saline to around 500–700 ml volume. Many patients cannot tolerate them despite post-procedure cocktails of antiemetics and thus require removal which is often not easy. However, when they are deployed satisfactorily they can result in quite impressive weight loss and when they deflate a further balloon can be inserted, although it is not clear how many and how often this can be repeated.

Results of bariatric surgery

The crucial element in assessing the efficacy of any bariatric procedure is usually defined as the percentage of initial excess weight (IEW) that the patient has lost. Theoretically a patient can lose 100% of their IEW and return to a normal BMI. Invariably, however, this never occurs except for a BPD where this is not uncommon. Most other procedures result in a variable IEW loss usually being a function of how well the patient adheres to the associated diet and degree of physical activity. By general consensus the definition of success is defined as reduction of IEW by 50% – an arbitrary definition. Recently it has been questioned as to whether absolute weight loss is the right variable with which to define success since many patients are more interested in reduction of risk factors for comorbidity rather than absolute weight loss. For example, reduction in the need for antidiabetic treatment, normalisation of blood pressure, reduction in serum lipids, improvement in mobility and quality of life and so on may be more valuable determinants of success. Notwithstanding the above most reported results for ease of description relate to absolute reduction in IEW which obviously disadvantages an operation performed in a super-obese patient. Weight loss usually reaches a maximum at 18–24 months after surgery.

Table 15.4 shows the average excess IEW loss from selected reports in the literature of the various bariatric procedures described above. It is generally accepted that gastric bypass procedures result in around an extra 10% loss of IEW when compared with pure gastric restrictive procedures. The critical question often posed by doubters of the surgical approach regards the durability of the bariatric procedure, given that the patients are never cured of their problem. Reports from surgeons invariably have good follow-up for the first 2 years then increasingly poor follow-up at 5 years. The International Bariatric Surgery Register, which has over 75 surgeons who have contributed over 14 600 bariatric surgery procedures, has only a 15% follow-up at 5 years! It is usual for sceptics to assume that patients who do not return for follow-up are probably failures although there is no evidence that this is so. Equally they may not return for follow-up because they have a stable lower weight and are happy with their result. The best follow-up in the literature is that of Poires from the USA who has a remarkable 96% follow-up at 14 years and reported that surgery (gastric bypass) is still as effective as when initially carried out.[12] A critical analysis of most published follow-up data following a VBG or gastric bypass reveals a slight drift upwards of weight with increasing follow-up but weight still remains well below the definition of successful surgery. Sceptics have to compare this with the effectiveness of conservative treatment.

It is commonly assumed that good weight reduction will be matched by improvements in risk factors for comorbidity. Although there are good data to support this notion, it still requires confirmation as to whether this translates to improved longevity. However, it is reasonable to extrapolate data from medical studies in non-morbidly obese patients where it has been shown unequivocally that weight reduction increases length of life. One relatively recent study in morbidly obese patients treated surgically revealed improvement in quality of life.[34]

 Much-needed data will become available when the SOS study reports and this data may change the attitude to bariatric surgery forever.

Vertical banded gastroplasty[41]	58% at 5 years
Gastric banding[42]	55% at 6 years
Gastric bypass[41]	68% at 5 years
Biliopancreatic diversion[43]	77% at 8 years
Biliopancreatic diversion with duodenal switch[44]	70% at 8 years
Jejuno-ileal bypass (Cleator)[30]	57% at 2 years

Table 15.4 *Results of bariatric procedures (mean percentage initial excess weight lost)*

The SOS study is a cohort study comparing conservative with surgical treatment in 2000 patients in each arm of the study.[4] Around 1800 patients have been recruited so far into each arm and the follow-up will be for 10 years. At 2 years the surgically treated patients lost an average of 35 kg compared with no weight loss in the conservative arm. Several reports of emerging data from their recent meetings suggest overwhelming evidence of the efficacy of bariatric surgery compared with conservative treatment – with the benefits outweighing the risks of surgery, providing the surgery maintains > 15% of weight reduction at 8 years. The SOS research group have reported the usual improvement in diabetes, high blood pressure and lipid abnormalities and also reduction in left ventricular mass, improvement in cardiac function and reduction in atherosclerosis rates in the surgical patients compared with those treated medically. In addition they also found a lower incidence of sick leave and disability payouts in surgical patients.

An area of controversy is whether the age at surgery should be limited to those under 55 when there are data that suggest that patients over 55 at the time of surgery have a sustained improvement in morbidity when followed for 6 years.[35] In highly selected and well-motivated patients over 55 there can be compelling reasons for operating but each patient much be assessed individually by the team.

Revisional bariatric surgery

Despite properly carried out surgery there is always a failure rate for a variety of reasons – technical failures, the patient 'out-eating' the operation, unacceptable side effects, lack of desired effect and so on. When counselling the patient about the possibility of repeat-surgery then they must be warned of the increased morbidity and mortality attendant on such surgery. There have been several publications, largely from the USA, dealing with this difficult area.[36,37,38] The options are varied and have to be tailored according to the primary operation, the desired outcome and the reason for failure.

Laparoscopically placed gastric bands can be repositioned laparoscopically in skilled hands. Minor problems with port-site infection usually require disconnection and reservoir replacement after an interval. Although technical failures are now relatively uncommon following VBG performed according to the above technique there is still a steady small incidence of band problems (usually they are too tight) and staple-line disruptions. A tight band can be replaced if it does not respond to endoscopic dilatation, which appears to be successful in around 50% of cases. A ruptured staple line can be restapled or preferably the stomach can be divided when this is carried out to prevent further rupture. There is a low threshold among some surgeons to convert the VBG to some form of gastric bypass when there has been a staple line rupture.[38] This is especially the case where there has been band erosion into the stomach. Failure to lose sufficient weight or alternatively the onset of PCM after a gastric bypass usually requires a revision of the common channel to a larger or smaller length as required.

Whatever surgical strategy is decided upon when further surgery is undertaken it is vital to allow plenty of operative time, plan the approach well and have various options available. This surgery will test the surgeon's ability to the maximum and hence should not be undertaken lightly if he or she is not experienced and confident.

Summary

Morbid obesity is a disease, and it is just as valid to use surgery in its cure as is it with any other disease. Overcoming the prejudice that exists against the obese is an ongoing challenge for the bariatric surgeon. There is a real need to mainstream bariatric surgery into training programmes. Only when it becomes a recognised element of training will it become more accepted by the surgical community.[39]

Based on the foregoing it is difficult to advise a surgeon about the best procedure for any given patient. There is probably no one operation which is uniquely suitable for every patient although laparoscopic banding because of its simplicity and relative 'non-invasiveness' is becoming the first choice for many surgeons. If this operation is not successful then a more aggressive procedure can be chosen. The author's personal algorithm expresses this view (**Fig. 15.10**) although other bariatric surgeons may prefer to stick to the operation of which they have had most experience and know to produce good results. Whatever operation is chosen it is important that the surgeon is properly trained as exemplified by the recent International Federation for the Surgery of Obesity Cancun statement which lays down strict criteria for training and accreditation.[40] The need for a team approach with lifelong follow-up to assist in the maintenance of weight loss and the detection of long-term nutritional problems cannot be overestimated.

Figure 15.10
Suggested algorithm for managing morbid obesity

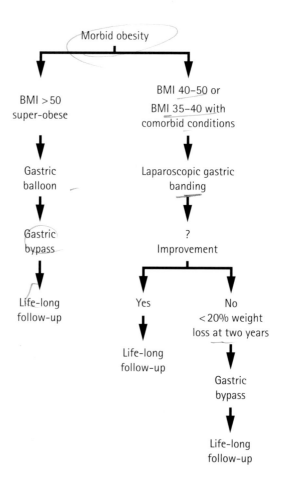

References

1. Lew EA, Garfinkel L. Variations in mortality by weight among 750 000 men and women. J Chronic Dis 1979; 32:563–76.

2. Colditz GA. Economic costs of obesity. Am J Clin Nutr 1992; 55:S503–7.

3. Gemert WG, Adang EMM, Kop M *et al*. A prospective cost-effectiveness analysis of vertical banded gastroplasty for the treatment of morbid obesity. Obesity Surg 1999; 9:484–91.

 4. Sjostrum L, Larsson B, Backaman L *et al*. Swedish Obese Subjects (SOS). Recruitment for an intervention study and a selected description of the obese state. Int J Obes 1992; 16:465–79.

5. Dietel M (ed). Surgery for the morbidly obese patient. 1st edn. London: Lea and Febiger, 1989.

6. Cowan GSM. What do patients, families and society expect from the bariatric surgeon? Obesity Surg 1998; 8:77–85.

7. Zhang Y, Proenca R, Maffei M *et al*. Positional cloning of the mouse obese gene and its human homologue. Nature 1994; 372:425–8.

8. Stephens TW, Basinsky M, Bristow PK *et al*. The role of neuropeptide Y in the antiobesity action of the obese gene product. Nature 1995; 377:530–2.

9. Arch JRS, Kaumann AJ. β3 and atypical α-adrenoceptors. Med Res Rev 1993; 13:663–729.

10. Ravussin E, Lillioja S, Knowler WC *et al*. Reduced rate of energy expenditure as a risk factor for body-weight gain. N Eng J Med 1988; 318:467–72.

11. Kannel WB, Gordon T. Obesity and cardiovascular disease. London: Churchill Davidson, 1974.

 12. Pories WJ, Swanson MS, MacDonald KG *et al*. Who would have thought it? An operation proves to be the most effective therapy for adult-onset diabetes mellitus. Ann Surg 1995; 222:339–52.

13. MacDonald KG, Long DS, Swanson MS *et al*. The gastric bypass operation reduces the progression and mortality of non-insulin dependent diabetes mellitus. J Gastrointest Surg 1997; 1:213–20.

14. Kyzer S, Charuzi I. Obstructive sleep apnoea in the obese. World J Surg 1998; 22:998–1001.

15. Cowan GSM, Buffington CK. Significant changes in blood pressure, glucose and lipids with gastric bypass surgery. World J Surg 1998; 22:987–92.

16. Karason K, Wallentin I, Larsson B *et al*. Effect of obesity and weight loss on cardiac function and valvular performance. Obesity Research 1998; 6:422–9.

17. Benotti PN, Hollingshead J, Mascioli EA *et al*. Gastric restrictive operations for morbid obesity. Am J Surg 1989; 157:150–5.

18. Deitel M. Pregnancy after bariatric surgery. Obesity Surg 1998; 8:465–6.

19. Forsell P, Hallerback B, Glise H *et al*. Complications following Swedish Adjustable Gastric Banding: A long-term follow-up. Obesity Surg 1999; 9:11–16.

20. Westling A, Bjurling K, Ohrvall M *et al*. Silicone-adjustable gastric banding: disappointing results. Obesity Surg 1998; 8:467–74.

21. Kasalicky M, Fried M, Peskova M. Some complications after laparoscopic nonadjustable gastric banding. Obesity Surg 1999; 9:443–5.

22. O'Brien PE, Brown WA, Smith PJ *et al*. Prospective study of a laparoscopically placed, adjustable gastric band in the treatment of morbid obesity. Br J Surg 1999; 85:113–8.

23. Talieh J, Kirgan D, Fisher BL. Gastric bypass for morbid obesity: a standard surgical technique by consensus. Obesity Surg 1997; 7:198–202.

24. Sarr MG. Vertical disconnected Roux-en-Y gastric bypass. Dig Surg 1996; 13:45–9.

25. Lonroth H, Dalenbeck J. Other laparoscopic bariatric procedures. World J Surg 1998; 22:964–8.

26. Fobi MAL. Rediscovering the wheel in obesity surgery. Obesity Surg 1997; 7:370–2.

27. Capella RF, Capella JF. Reducing early technical complications in gastric bypass surgery. Obesity Surg 1997; 7:149–57.

 28. Scopinaro N, Adami GF, Marinari GM *et al*. Biliopancreatic diversion. World J Surg 1998; 22:936–46.

29. Marceau P, Hould FS, Lebel S *et al*. Biliopancreatic diversion with duodenal switch. World J Surg 1998; 22:947–54.

 30. Cleator IGM, Gourlay RH. Ileogastrostomy for morbid obesity. Can J Surg 1988; 31:114–6.

31. Slyvan A, Sjolund B, Janunger KG. Favourable long-term results with the end-to-side jejunoileal bypass. Obesity Surg 1995; 5:357–63.

32. Pasulka PS, Bistrian BR, Benotti PN *et al*. The risks of surgery in obese patients. Ann Intern Med 1986; 104:540–6.

33. Weiner R, Gutberlet H, Bockhorn H. Preparation of extremely obese patients for laparoscopic gastric banding by gastric-balloon therapy. Obesity Surg 1999; 9:261–4.

34. Isacsson A, Frederiksen SG, Nilsson P *et al*. Quality of life after gastroplasty is normal: A controlled study. Eur J Surg 1997; 163:181–6.

35. MacGregor AM, Rand CS. Gastric surgery in morbidly obesity. Outcome in patients aged 55 years and older. Arch Surg 1993; 128:1153–7.

36. Capella RF, Capella JF. Converting vertical banded gastroplasty to a lesser curvature gastric bypass: technical considerations. Obesity Surg 1998; 8:218–24.

37. van Gemert WG, van Wersch MM, Greve JWM *et al.* Revisional surgery after failed vertical banded gastroplasty: Restoration of vertical banded gastroplasty or conversion to gastric bypass. Obesity Surg 1998; 8:21–8.

38. Sugerman HJ, Kellum JM, DeMaria EJ *et al.* Conversion of failed or complicated vertical banded gastroplasty to gastric bypass in morbid obesity. Am J Surg 1996; 171:263–9.

39. Buchwald H. Mainstreaming bariatric surgery. Obesity Surg 1999; 9:462–70.

40. Cowan GSM. The Cancun IFSO statement on bariatric surgeon qualifications. Obesity Surg 1998; 8:86.

41. Dietel M. Overview of operations for morbid obesity. World J Surg 1998; 22:913–8.

42. Belachew M. Legrand M, Vincenti V *et al.* Laparoscopic adjustable gastric banding. World J Surg 1998; 22:955–63.

43. Scopinaro N, Gianetti D, Adami G *et al.* Biliopancreatic diversion for obesity at eighteen years. Surgery 1996; 119:261–8.

44. Hess DS, Hess DW. Biliopancreatic diversion with a duodenal switch. Obesity Surg 1998; 8:267–82.

INDEX

Page numbers in *italic* refer to figures and tables: those in **bold** indicate main discussion.
This index is in letter-by-letter order whereby spaces and hyphens between words are ignored in the alphabetization.
vs denotes differential diagnosis, or comparisons.